Memmler's The Human Body in Health and Disease

Tenth Edition

Barbara Janson Cohen

Jason James Taylor
contributor

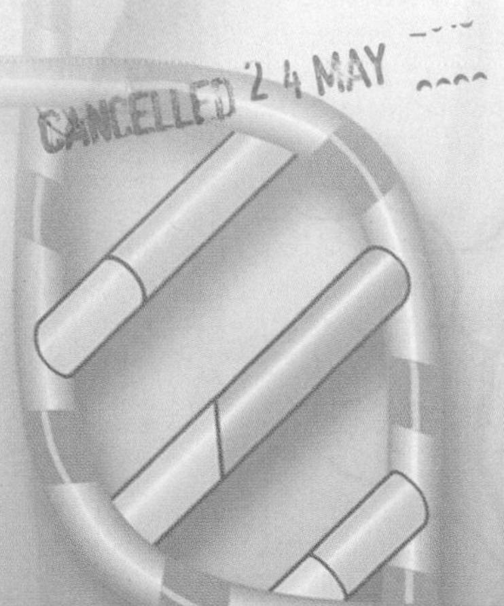

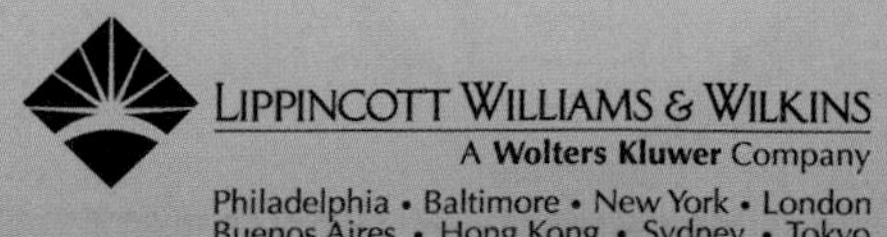

Senior Acquisitions Editor: *John Goucher*
Senior Development Editor: *Dana Knighten*
Associate Production Manager: *Kevin Johnson*
Associate Marketing Manager: *Hilary Henderson*
Cover and Interior Designer: *Armen Kojoyian*
Compositor: *Maryland Composition, Inc.*
Printer: *R.R. Donnelley & Sons-Willard*

351 West Camden Street
Baltimore, MD 21201

530 Walnut Street
Philadelphia, PA 19106

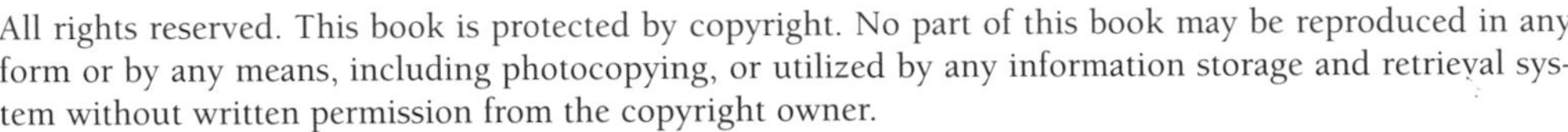

The publisher is not responsible (as a matter of product liability, negligence, or otherwise) for any injury resulting from any material contained herein. This publication contains information relating to general principles of medical care that should not be construed as specific instructions for individual patients. Manufacturers' product information and package inserts should be reviewed for current information, including contraindications, dosages, and precautions.

Printed in the United States of America

Library of Congress Cataloging-in-Publication Data

Cohen, Barbara J.
Memmler's The human body in health and disease.-- 10th ed. / Barbara Janson Cohen ; Jason J. Taylor, contributor.
p. ; cm.
Summary: "A low-level introductory text on basic human anatomy and physiology with disease coverage for HP students in programs including medical assisting, surg tech, massage, certified nursing assistant, respiratory tech, and the like. Organized by body system; includes BOB CD with Stedman's pronunciations, selected figures (from text) in DHA engine, and student review questions" – Provided by publisher.
Includes bibliographical references and index.
ISBN 0-7817-4232-3 (softcover) – ISBN 0-7817-5171-3 (hardcover)
1. Human physiology. 2. Physiology, Pathological. 3. Human anatomy. I. Title: Human body in health and disease. II. Taylor, Jason J. III. Title.
[DNLM: 1. Physiology. 2. Anatomy. 3. Pathology. QT 104 C678m 2005]
QP34.5.M48 2005
612–dc22

2004027634

The publishers have made every effort to trace the copyright holders for borrowed material. If they have inadvertently overlooked any, they will be pleased to make the necessary arrangements at the first opportunity.

To purchase additional copies of this book, call our customer service department at (800) 638-3030 or fax orders to (301) 824-7390. International customers should call (301) 714-2324.

Visit Lippincott Williams & Wilkins on the Internet: http://www.LWW.com. Lippincott Williams & Wilkins customer service representatives are available from 8:30 am to 6:00 pm, EST.

10 9 8 7 6 5 4 3 2 1

Reviewers

We gratefully acknowledge the generous contributions of the reviewers whose names appear in the list that follows. These instructors were kind enough to read the text thoroughly and make suggestions for improvement. Their comments determined many of the changes in content and direction for this revision, such as the increased number and types of learning aids, addition of new art and revisions to existing art, a stronger focus on teaching and learning anatomic and medical terminology, and an increased emphasis on physiology and the interrelatedness of structure and function. We hope they will be pleased with the results of their hard work in this 10th edition of *Memmler's The Human Body in Health and Disease.*

LaVon Barrett, RN, BSN
Amarillo College
Amarillo, TX

Nina Beaman, MS, CMA, RNC
Allied Health Program Area Coordinator
Bryant and Stratton College
Richmond, VA

Mark Andrew Bloom, BS, MS
Instructor of Biology
Texas Christian University
Fort Worth, TX

Kathleen Bode, RN, MS
Chair, Division of Health
Flint Hills Technical College
Emporia, KS

William J. Burke, BA
Madison Area Technical College
Madison, WI
Blackhawk Area Technical College
Monroe, WI

Patti Calk, MEd, LOTR
University of Louisiana at Monroe
Monroe, LA

Kathy Carson, RPH
The Cleveland Institute of Dental-Medical Assistants, Inc.
Mentor, OH

Michelle Cleary, PhD
Florida International University
Miami, FL

Stephen M. Colarusso, BS, NCTMB, ACST
Director of Education
Charles of Italy School of Massage Therapy
Lake Havasu City, AZ

Zoe Hanson Cujak, BSN, MEd
Associate Dean, Service Occupations
Fox Valley Technical College
Appleton, WI

Katherine Fukuyama, BSN, MEd
Vancouver Community College
Vancouver, British Columbia, Canada

Glenn Grady, MEd, BSMT (ASCP), CMA
Allied Health Department Chair
Miller-Motte Technical College
Wilmington, NC

Kerry Hull, PhD
Associate Professor
Department of Biology
Bishop's University
Lennoxville, Quebec, Canada

Tammee Neuhaus, MLT
Minnesota School of Health Sciences
Apple Valley, MN

Debra J. Paul, BAM, CMA
Medical Assisting Program Instructor
IVY Tech State College
South Bend, IN

Lisa S. Reed, RN, MS, CNOR
Department Chairperson for Surgical Technology
New England Institute of Technology
Warwick, RI

Dyal N. P. Singh, BSc (Honors), MSc, PhD
Professor of Anatomy
Director of Neuroscience
Ross University School of Medicine
Dominica, West Indies

Rox Ann Sparks, RN, BSN, MICN
Vocational Nursing Instructor
Merced College
Merced, CA

Alan H. Stephenson, BS, MS, PhD
Chair, Science Department
Edgecombe Community College
Tarboro, NC

Jean A. Zorko, MS, BSMT (ASCP)
Assistant Professor, Science
Stark State College of Technology
Canton, OH

Preface

Memmler's The Human Body in Health and Disease is a textbook for introductory-level health professions and nursing students who need a basic understanding of anatomy and physiology, the interrelationships between structure and function, and the effects of disease on body systems.

Like preceding editions, the 10th edition remains true to Ruth Memmler's original vision. Designed for health professions and nursing students, the features and content specifically meet the needs of those who may be starting their health career preparation with little or no science background. This book's primary goals are:

- To provide the essential knowledge of human anatomy, physiology, and the effects of disease, at an ideal level of detail, and in language that is clear and understandable.
- To illustrate the concepts discussed with anatomic art that depicts the appropriate level of detail with accuracy, simplicity, and elegance, and that is integrated seamlessly with the narrative.
- To incorporate the most recent scientific findings into the fundamental material on which Ruth Memmler's classic text is based.
- To include pedagogy designed to enhance interest in and understanding of the concepts presented.
- To teach the basic anatomic and medical terminology used in healthcare settings, preparing students to function efficiently in their chosen health career.
- To present an integrated teaching-learning package that includes all of the elements necessary for a successful learning experience.

This revision is the direct result of in-depth market feedback solicited to tell us what instructors and students at this level most need. We listened carefully to the feedback, and the results we obtained are integrated into every feature of this book. The text itself has been thoroughly revised and updated to reflect the latest accepted scientific thought in each area of the book. Because visual learning devices are so important to students at this level, this edition also features a completely revamped and expanded art program that includes revised versions of many of the figures from previous editions as well as numerous all-new, full-color anatomic line drawings and photographs. Last but not least, these features appear in an all-new design that makes the content more user-friendly and accessible than ever.

Organization and Structure

Like previous editions, the 10th edition uses a body systems approach to the study of the normal human body and how disease affects it. The book is divided into seven units, grouping related information and body systems together as follows:

- Unit I, The Body as a Whole (Chapters 1–4), focuses on the body's organization; basic chemistry needed to understand body functions; cells and their functions; and tissues, glands, and membranes.
- Unit II, Disease and the First Line of Defense (Chapters 5 and 6), presents information on disease, organisms that produce disease, and the integumentary system, which is the body's first line of defense against injury and disease.
- Unit III, Movement and Support (Chapters 7 and 8), includes the skeletal and muscular systems.
- Unit IV, Coordination and Control (Chapters 9–12), focuses on the nervous system, the sensory system, and the endocrine system.
- Unit V, Circulation and Body Defense (Chapters 13–17), includes the blood, the heart and heart disease, blood vessels and circulation, the lymphatic system, and the immune system.
- Unit VI, Energy: Supply and Use (Chapters 18–22), includes the respiratory system, the digestive system, metabolism, nutrition, temperature control, body fluids, and the urinary system.
- Unit VII, Perpetuation of Life (Chapters 23–25), covers the male and female reproductive systems, development and birth, and heredity and hereditary diseases.

The main Glossary defines the chapters' boldfaced terms, and a Glossary of Word Parts is a reference tool that not only teaches basic medical and anatomic terminology but also helps students learn to recognize unfamiliar terms. Appendixes include a variety of supplementary information that students will find useful as they work with the text, including answers to the Chapter Checkpoint questions and Zooming In illustration questions (Appendix 6) that are found in every chapter.

Pedagogic Features

Every chapter contains pedagogy that has been designed with the health professions and nursing student in mind (the User's Guide that follows the Preface provides a "guided tour" of these features and their pedagogic benefits).

- **Learning Outcomes:** Chapter objectives on the first page of every chapter help the student organize and prioritize learning.

- **Selected Key Terms:** List that accompanies the Learning Outcomes presents the most important terms covered in the chapter.
- **Chapter Checkpoints:** Brief questions at the end of main sections test and reinforce the student's recall of key information in that section.
- **"Zooming In" questions** (*NEW* to this edition): Questions with the figure legends test and reinforce the student's understanding of concepts depicted in the illustration. They are set in red to increase their visibility.
- **Phonetic pronunciations:** Easy-to-learn phonetic pronunciations are spelled out in the narrative, appearing in parentheses directly following many terms—no need for students to understand dictionary-style diacritical marks. (See the "Guide to Pronunciation" below.)
- **Special interest boxes:** Each chapter contains three special interest boxes focusing on topics that augment chapter content. The book includes five kinds of boxes altogether:
  - *A Closer Look:* Provide additional in-depth scientific detail on topics in or related to the chapter.
  - *Clinical Perspective:* Focus on diseases and disorders relevant to the chapter, exploring what happens to the body when the normal structure-function relationship breaks down.
  - *Health Professions* (*NEW* to this edition): Describe various careers in the health professions, highlighting the reasons why students need a thorough grounding in anatomy and physiology.
  - *Hot Topic* (*NEW* to this edition): Focus on current trends and research, reinforcing the link between anatomy and physiology and related news coverage that students may have seen.
  - *Health Maintenance:* Offer supplementary information on health and wellness issues.
- **Figures:** The greatly expanded and revised art program includes full-color anatomic line art, both new and revised, with a level of detail that matches that of the narrative. Also *NEW* to this edition are additional photomicrographs, radiographs, and other scans, included to give students a "preview" of what they might see in real-world healthcare settings.
- **Tables:** The numerous *NEW* and revised tables in this edition summarize key concepts and information in an easy-to-review form.
- **Color figure and table numbers** (*NEW* to this edition): Figure and table numbers appear in color in the narrative, helping students quickly find their place after stopping to look at an illustration or table. Figure callouts appear in blue type, and table callouts, in red.
- **Word Anatomy** (*NEW* to this edition): Organized by chapter headings, this chart groups various word parts used in terms found in the chapter. This learning tool helps students build vocabulary and promotes recognition of even unfamiliar terms based on a knowledge of common word parts.
- **Summary:** Outline-format summary provides a concise overview of chapter content, aiding in study and test preparation.
- **Questions for Study and Review:** Study questions have been thoroughly revised and organized hierarchically into three *NEW* levels in this edition (answers appear on the Instructor's Resource CD in the Instructor's Manual):
  - *Building Understanding:* Includes fill-in-the-blank, matching, and multiple choice questions that test factual recall.
  - *Understanding Concepts:* Includes short-answer questions (define, describe, compare/contrast) that test and reinforce understanding of concepts.
  - *Conceptual Thinking:* Includes short-essay questions that promote critical thinking skills.

Guide to Pronunciation

The stressed syllable in each word is shown with capital letters. The vowel pronunciations are as follows:

Any vowel at the end of a syllable is given a long sound, as follows:

a as in say
e as in be
i as in nice
o as in go
u as in true

A vowel followed by a consonant and the letter e (as in rate) also is given a long pronunciation.

Any vowel followed by a consonant receives a short pronunciation, as follows:

a as in absent
e as in end
i as in bin
o as in not
u as in up

Summary

In short, the 10th edition of *Memmler's The Human Body in Health and Disease* builds on the successes of the previous nine editions by offering clear, concise narrative into which accurate, aesthetically pleasing anatomic art has been woven. We have made every effort to respond thoughtfully and thoroughly to reviewers' and instructors' comments, offering the ideal level of detail for students preparing for a career in the health professions and nursing, and the pedagogic features that best support it. We hope you will agree that the 10th edition of *Memmler's* is the best ever.

User's Guide

In today's health careers, a thorough understanding of human anatomy and physiology is more important than ever. *Memmler's The Human Body in Health and Disease* not only provides the conceptual knowledge you'll need but also teaches you how to apply it. This User's Guide introduces you to the features and tools that will enhance your learning experience.

A unifying theme of this text is the relationship between structure and function, and how they differ in health and disease. We've woven that theme into the book's design and approach. Take a few minutes to look through the text and get acquainted with its organization. The two tables of contents provide a framework for your learning: the Brief Contents gives a wide-angle view of the book's "skeleton"—the units and chapters—while the detailed Contents focuses in on the individual "bones," the topics themselves. As with the different body systems, specific topics build on each other from chapter to chapter, with each supporting the ones that follow.

Next, take a look at the chapters themselves. We've included some important tools to help you learn about anatomy and physiology and apply your new knowledge:

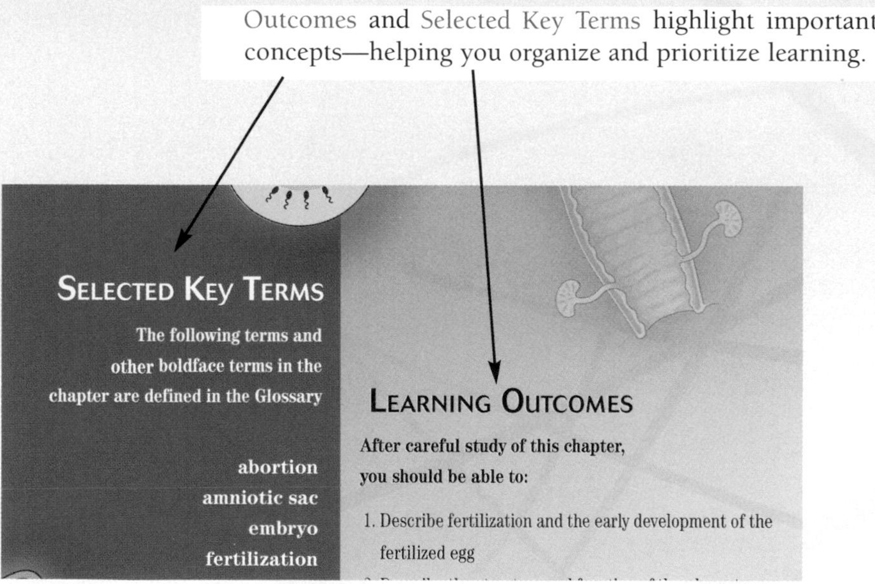

Outcomes and Selected Key Terms highlight important concepts—helping you organize and prioritize learning.

Health Professions boxes focus on a variety of health careers—showing how the knowledge of anatomy and physiology is applied in real-world jobs.

Box 1-3 · Health Professions

Health Information Technicians

Every time a patient receives medical treatment, information is added to the patient's medical record, which includes data about symptoms, medical history, test results, diagnoses, and treatment. **Health information technicians** organize and manage these records, working closely with physicians, nurses, and other health professionals to ensure that medical records provide a complete, accurate basis for quality patient care.

Accurate medical records are also essential for administrative purposes. Health information technicians assign a **code** to each diagnosis and procedure a patient receives, and this information is used for accurate patient billing. In addition, health information technicians analyze medical records to discover trends in health and disease. This research can be used to improve patient care, manage costs, and help establish new medical treatments.

Health information technicians need a strong clinical knowledge base. A thorough background in medical terminology is essential when reading and interpreting medical records. Anatomy and physiology are definitely required!

Most health information technologists work in hospitals and long-term care facilities. Others work in medical clinics, government agencies, insurance companies, and consulting firms. Job prospects are promising because of the growing need for healthcare. In fact, health information technology is projected to be one of the fastest growing careers in the United States. For more information about this profession, contact the American Health Information Management Association.

Hot Topic boxes provide cutting-edge content on trends and research—giving a view to what is happening in the larger scientific community.

Box 8-2 Hot Topics

Anabolic Steroids: Winning at All Costs?

Anabolic steroids mimic the effects of the male sex hormone testosterone by promoting metabolism and stimulating growth. These drugs are legally prescribed to promote muscle regeneration and prevent atrophy from disuse after surgery. However, athletes also purchase them illegally, using them to increase muscle size and strength and improve endurance.

When steroids are used illegally to enhance athletic performance, the doses needed are large enough to cause serious side effects. They increase blood cholesterol levels, which may lead to atherosclerosis, heart disease, kidney failure, and stroke. Steroids damage the liver, making it more susceptible to disease and cancer, and suppress the immune system, increasing the risk of infection and cancer. In men, steroids cause impotence, testicular atrophy, low sperm count, infertility, and the development of female sex characteristics such as breasts (gynecomastia). In women, steroids disrupt ovulation and menstruation and produce male sex characteristics such as breast atrophy, enlargement of the clitoris, increased body hair, and deepening of the voice. In both sexes steroids increase the risk for baldness and, especially in men, cause mood swings, depression and violence.

Clinical Perspective boxes focus on physical disorders and related body processes as well as techniques used in clinical settings—providing additional content on diseases and their treatments.

Box 7-1 Clinical Perspectives

Landmarking: Seeing With Your Fingers

Most body structures lie beneath the skin, hidden from view except in dissection. A technique called **landmarking** allows health care providers to visualize hidden structures without cutting into the patient. Bony prominences, or landmarks, can be palpated (felt) beneath the skin to serve as reference points for locating other structures. Landmarking is used during physical examinations and surgeries, when giving injections, and for many other clinical procedures. The lower tip of the sternum, the xiphoid process, is a reference point in the administration of cardiopulmonary resuscitation (CPR).

Practice landmarking by feeling for some of the other bony prominences. You can feel the joint between the mandible and the temporal bone of the skull (the temporomandibular joint, or TMJ) anterior to the ear canal as you move your lower jaw up and down. Feel for the notch in the sternum (breast bone) between the clavicles (collar bones). Approximately 4 cm below this notch you will feel a bump called the sternal angle. This prominence is an important landmark because its location marks where the trachea splits to deliver air to both lungs. Move your fingers lateral to the sternal angle to palpate the second ribs, important landmarks for locating the heart and lungs. Feel for the most lateral bony prominence of the shoulder, the acromion process of the scapula (shoulder blade). Two to three fingerbreadths down from this point is the correct injection site into the deltoid muscle of the shoulder. Place your hands on your hips and palpate the iliac crest of the hip bone. Move your hands forward until you reach the anterior end of the crest, the anterior superior iliac spine (ASIS). Feel for the part of the bony pelvis that you sit on. This is the ischial tuberosity. It and the ASIS are important landmarks for locating safe injection sites in the gluteal region.

A Closer Look boxes provide additional detail on selected topics from the text—focusing in on the details of structure and function.

Box 13-1 A Closer Look

Hemoglobin: Door to Door Oxygen Delivery

The hemoglobin molecule is a protein made of four chains of amino acids (the globin part of the molecule), each of which holds an iron-containing heme group. Each of the four hemes can bind one molecule of oxygen.

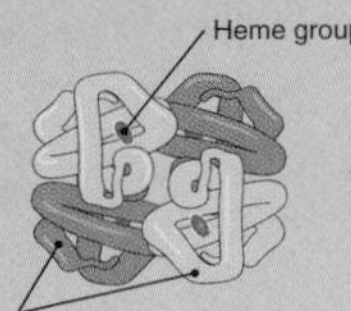

Hemoglobin. This protein in red blood cells consists of four amino acid chains (globins), each with an oxygen-binding heme group.

Hemoglobin allows the blood to carry much more oxygen than it could were the oxygen simply dissolved in the plasma. A red blood cell contains about 250 million hemoglobins, each capable of binding four molecules of oxygen. So, a single red blood cell can carry about one billion oxygen molecules! Hemoglobin reversibly binds oxygen, picking it up in the lungs and releasing it in the body tissues. Active cells need more oxygen and also generate heat and acidity. These changing conditions promote the release of oxygen from hemoglobin into metabolically active tissues.

Immature red blood cells (erythroblasts) produce hemoglobin as they mature into erythrocytes in the red bone marrow. When the liver and spleen destroy old erythrocytes they break down the released hemoglobin. Some of its components are recycled, and the remainder leaves the body as a brown fecal pigment called stercobilin. In spite of some conservation, dietary protein and iron are still essential to maintain supplies.

Health Maintenance boxes cover common health issues—offering useful information about how to keep the body healthy.

Box 5-2 · Health Maintenance

The Cold Facts about the Common Cold

Every year, an estimated one billion Americans suffer from the symptoms of the common cold—runny nose, sneezing, coughing, and headache. Although most cases are mild and usually last about a week, colds are the leading cause of doctor visits and missed days at work and school.

Colds are caused by a viral infection of the mucous membranes of the upper respiratory tract. More than 200 different viruses are known to cause cold symptoms. While most colds occur in winter, scientists have found that cold weather does not increase the risk of "catching" a cold; the incidence is probably higher in winter because people spend more time indoors, increasing the chances that the virus will spread from person to person.

Colds spread primarily from contact with a contaminated surface. When an infected person coughs or sneezes, small droplets of water filled with viral particles are propelled through the air. One unshielded sneeze may spread hundreds of thousands of viral particles several feet. Depending upon temperature and humidity, these particles may live as long as 3 to 6 hours, and others who touch the contaminated surface may pick up the particles on their hands.

To help prevent the transmission of cold viruses:

- Avoid close contact with someone who is sneezing or coughing.
- Wash hands frequently to remove any viral particles you may have picked up.
- Avoid touching or rubbing your eyes, nose, or mouth with contaminated hands.
- Clean contaminated surfaces with disinfectant.

There are currently no medically proven cures for the common cold, and treatments only ease the symptoms. Because viruses cause the common cold, antibiotics are of no benefit. Getting plenty of rest and drinking lots of fluids are the best ways to speed recovery.

The second type of bone tissue, called **spongy**, or **cancellous, bone** has more spaces than compact bone. It is made of a meshwork of small, bony plates filled with red marrow. Spongy bone is found at the epiphyses (ends) of the long bones and at the center of other bones. Figure 7-4 shows a photograph of both compact and spongy tissue in a bone section.

Checkpoint questions test your understanding of the chapter's key points—helping you review as you proceed through the chapter.

Checkpoint 7-1 A long bone has a long, narrow shaft and two irregular ends. What are the scientific names for the shaft and the ends of a long bone?

Checkpoint 7-2 What are the two types of osseous (bone) tissue and where is each type found

7

Thumbtabs make it fast and easy to find a chapter—and they're color-coded by unit!

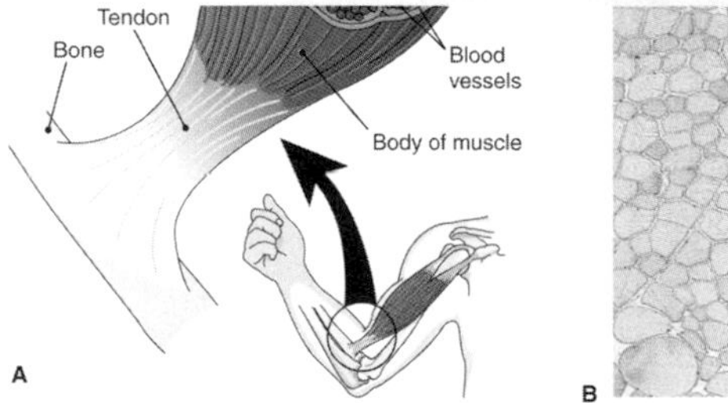

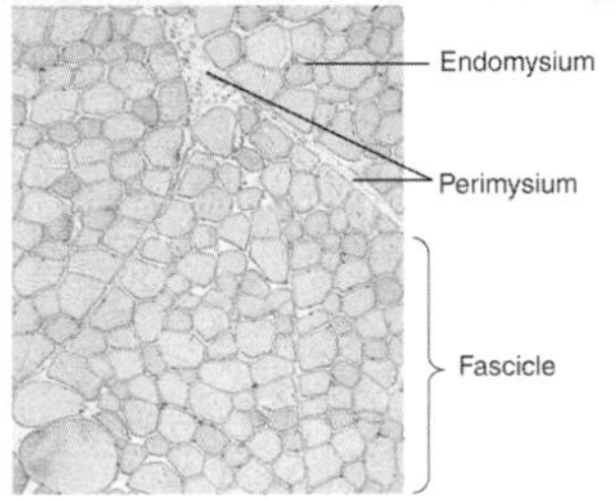

Figure 8-1 **Structure of a skeletal muscle.** Connective tissue coverings are shown. (B, Reprinted with permission from Gartner LP, Hiatt JL. Color Atlas of Histology. 3rd ed. Philadelphia: Lippincott Williams & Wilkins, 2000.) *ZOOMING IN ✦ What is the innermost layer of connective tissue in a muscle? What layer of connective tissue surrounds a fascicle of muscle fibers?*

Zooming In questions ask you to focus in on the illustration's details and answer questions based on what you see—reviewing important concepts and honing your conceptual thinking.

Phonetic pronunciations follow selected terms—helping you say the term correctly without having to stop and look up complicated pronunciation symbols.

head of the femur is the **greater trochanter** (tro-KAN-ter), used as a surface landmark. The **lesser trochanter**, a smaller elevation, is located on the medial side. On the posterior surface there is a long central ridge, the **linea aspera**, which is a point for attachment of hip muscles.

- The **patella** (pah-TEL-lah), or kneecap (see Fig. 7-1), is embedded in the tendon of the large anterior thigh muscle, the quadriceps femoris, where it crosses the

Figure numbers in blue make it easy to find your place after stopping to look at the figure.

The Word Anatomy chart helps you learn to recognize new terms based on your knowledge of word parts—building vocabulary.

Word Anatomy

Medical terms are built from standardized word parts (prefixes, roots and suffixes). Learning the meanings of these parts can help you remember words and interpret unfamiliar terms.

WORD PART	MEANING	EXAMPLE
Bones		
dia-	through, between	The *diaphysis*, or shaft, of a long bone is between the two ends, or epiphyses.
oss, osse/o	bone, bone tissue	*Osseous* tissue is another name for bone tissue.
oste/o	bone, bone tissue	The *periosteum* is the fibrous membrane around a bone.
-clast	break	An *osteoclast* breaks down bone in the process of resorption.
Divisions of the Skeleton		
para-	near	The *paranasal* sinuses are near the nose.
pariet/o	wall	The *parietal* bones form the side walls of the skull.
cost/o	rib	*Intercostal* spaces are located between the ribs.
supra-	above, superior	The *supraspinous* fossa is a depression superior to the spine of the scapula
infra-	below, inferior	The *infraspinous* fossa is a depression inferior to the spine of the scapula.
meta-	near, beyond	The *metacarpal*

Summary

I. Types of muscle
- A. Smooth muscle
  - **1.** In walls of hollow organs, vessels, and respiratory passageways
  - **2.** Cells tapered, single nucleus, nonstriated
  - **3.** Involuntary; produces peristalsis; contracts and relaxes slowly
- B. Cardiac muscle
  - **1.** Muscle of heart wall
  - **2.** Cells branch; single nucleus; lightly striated
  - **3.** Involuntary; self-excitatory
- C. Skeletal muscle
  - **1.** Most attached to bones and move skeleton
  - **2.** Cells long, cylindrical; multiple nuclei; heavily striated
  - **3.** Voluntary; contracts and relaxes rapidly

II. Muscular system
- **1.** Functions
  - a. Movement of skeleton
  - b. Maintenance of posture
  - c. Generation of heat
- **3.** Isometric contractions—tension increases, but muscle does not shorten

III. Mechanics of muscle movement
- **1.** Attachments of skeletal muscles
  - a. Tendon—cord of connective tissue that attaches muscle to bone
    - (1) Origin—attached to more fixed part
    - (2) Insertion—attached to moving part
  - b. Aponeurosis—broad band of connective tissue that attaches muscle to bone or other muscle
- A. Muscles work together
  - **1.** Prime mover—performs movement
  - **2.** Antagonist—produces opposite movement
  - **3.** Synergists—steady body parts and assist prime mover
- B. Levers and body mechanics—muscles function with skeleton as lever systems
  - **1.** Components
    - a. Lever—bone
    - b. Fulcrum—joint
    - c. Force—muscle contraction

The Summary provides a quick review of key points in outline form—helping you prepare for exams.

Questions for Study and Review cover chapter content thoroughly—testing your recall of facts, reinforcing understanding of concepts, and teaching critical thinking.

Questions for Study and Review

Building Understanding

Fill in the blanks

1. The shaft of a long bone is called the ______.
2. The structural unit of compact bone is the ______.
3. Red bone marrow manufactures ______.
4. Bones are covered by a connective tissue membrane called ______.
5. Bone matrix is produced by ______.

Matching

Match each numbered item with the most closely related lettered item.

___ 6. A rounded bony projection
___ 7. A sharp bony prominence
___ 8. A hole through bone
___ 9. A bony depression
___ 10. An air-filled bony cavity

a. condyle
b. foramen
c. fossa
d. sinus
e. spine

Multiple choice

___ 11. On which of the following bones would the mastoid process be found?
a. occipital bone
b. femur

___ 15. Which of the following synovial joints describes the hip?
a. gliding
b. hinge
c. pivot

The bonus CD contains a Human Body Review Atlas of electronic images and an Audio Pronunciations Glossary. The Altas, which contains the most important illustrations from the text, is a convenient study tool that lets you review and test your understanding of key body structures. The Glossary lets you hear the correct pronunciation of key terms from the text and practice saying them yourself, preparing you to communicate effectively in the healthcare setting.

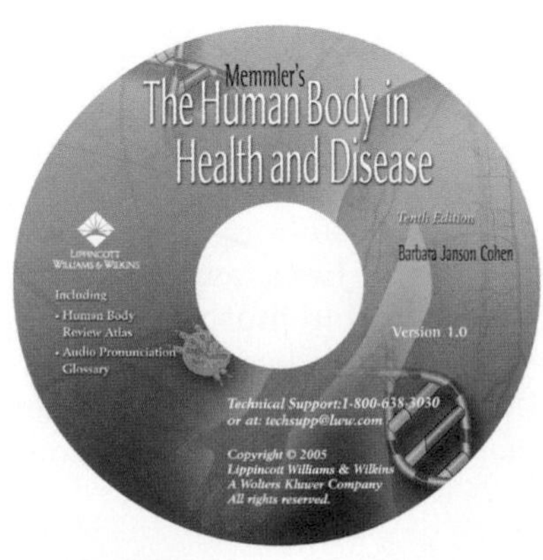

Ancillaries

A complete teaching and learning package is available for both faculty and students. For more information, please visit the text's companion website at http://connection.LWW.com/memmler, or contact your local LWW representative.

- Free Instructor's Manual packaged with Instructor's Resource CD, which includes a Brownstone test generator, image collection, PowerPoint™ slides, and the Instructor's Manual files (0-7817-5392-9).
- Free transparency set (0-7817-6167-0).
- Free course preparation assistance for instructors and tutoring for students, powered by Smarthinking™, an online support service featuring access to live e-structors. To demo this service, please visit the web site listed above.
- Online course materials and management powered by WebCT and Blackboard. To demo the online course, please visit the web site listed above.
- Student Study Guide available for purchase either alone (0-7817-5172-1) or packaged with the text (0-7817-6207-3).

Acknowledgments

To prepare a textbook, an author needs the assistance of many skilled people. This is my opportunity to thank those who have helped with revisions for the 10th edition of *Memmler's The Human Body in Health and Disease*. My editor, John Goucher, has guided this project through from start to finish and showed great skills in putting out fires. Senior Development Editor Dana Knighten kept her eye on the big picture as well as the tiniest details—and everything in between. Jason Taylor gave advice on the entire manuscript and also wrote the special interest boxes and chapter summary questions. Kerry Hull's contribution as a reviewer landed her the job of writing all of the ancillary materials, assisted by Ancillary Editor Molly Ward. Elizabeth Connolly and Jennifer Clements kept the art program on track, managing all of the electronic art files.

My thanks to all the many reviewers, listed separately, who made such valuable and detailed comments on the text. Their insights and advice truly guided every aspect of this new edition.

Enormous thanks to Craig Durant and Dragonfly Media Group for their brilliant work on the art program. They understood our needs, often better than we did, and rendered art astonishing in its clarity, instructional value, and beauty of design.

And as always, thanks to my husband Matthew, currently an instructor in anatomy and physiology, for his advice on, and contributions to the text.

Barbara Janson Cohen

Brief Contents

Contents

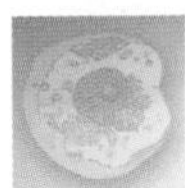

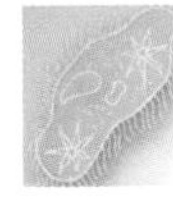

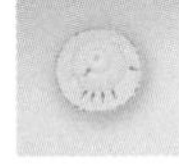

Unit VII

PERPETUATION OF LIFE

unit I

The Body as a Whole

This unit presents the basic levels of organization within the human body. Included is a description of the smallest units of life, called cells. Similar cells are grouped together as tissues, which are combined to form organs. Organs, in turn, work together in the various body systems, which together satisfy the needs of the entire organism. A short survey of chemistry, which deals with the composition of all matter and is important for the understanding of human physiology, is incorporated into this unit. These chapters prepare the student for the more detailed study of individual body systems in the units that follow.

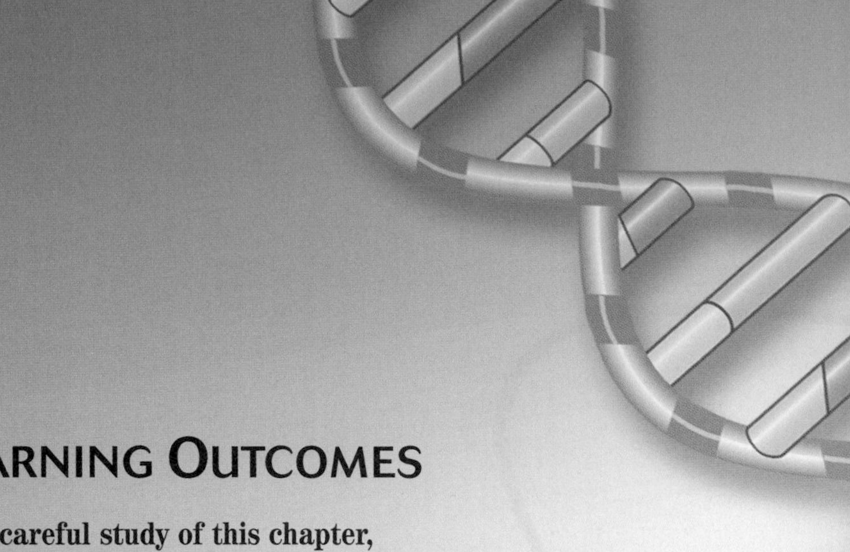

Selected Key Terms

The following terms and other boldface terms in the chapter are defined in the Glossary

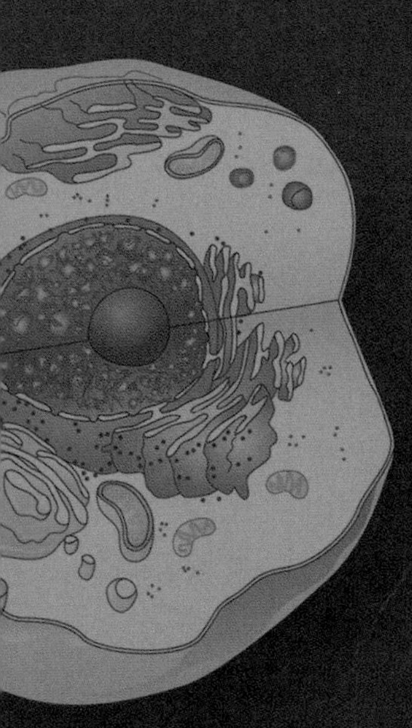

anabolism
anatomy
ATP
catabolism
cell
disease
dissect
feedback
gram
homeostasis
liter
metabolism
meter
organ
pathology
physiology
system
tissue

Learning Outcomes

After careful study of this chapter, you should be able to:

1. Define the terms *anatomy*, *physiology*, and *pathology*
2. Describe the organization of the body from chemicals to the whole organism
3. List 11 body systems and give the general function of each
4. Define *metabolism* and name the two phases of metabolism
5. Briefly explain the role of ATP in the body
6. Differentiate between extracellular and intracellular fluids
7. Define and give examples of homeostasis
8. Compare negative feedback and positive feedback
9. List and define the main directional terms for the body
10. List and define the three planes of division of the body
11. Name the subdivisions of the dorsal and ventral cavities
12. Name and locate subdivisions of the abdomen
13. Name the basic units of length, weight, and volume in the metric system
14. Define the metric prefixes kilo-, *centi-*, *milli-*, and *micro-*
15. Show how word parts are used to build words related to the body's organization (see Word Anatomy at the end of the chapter)

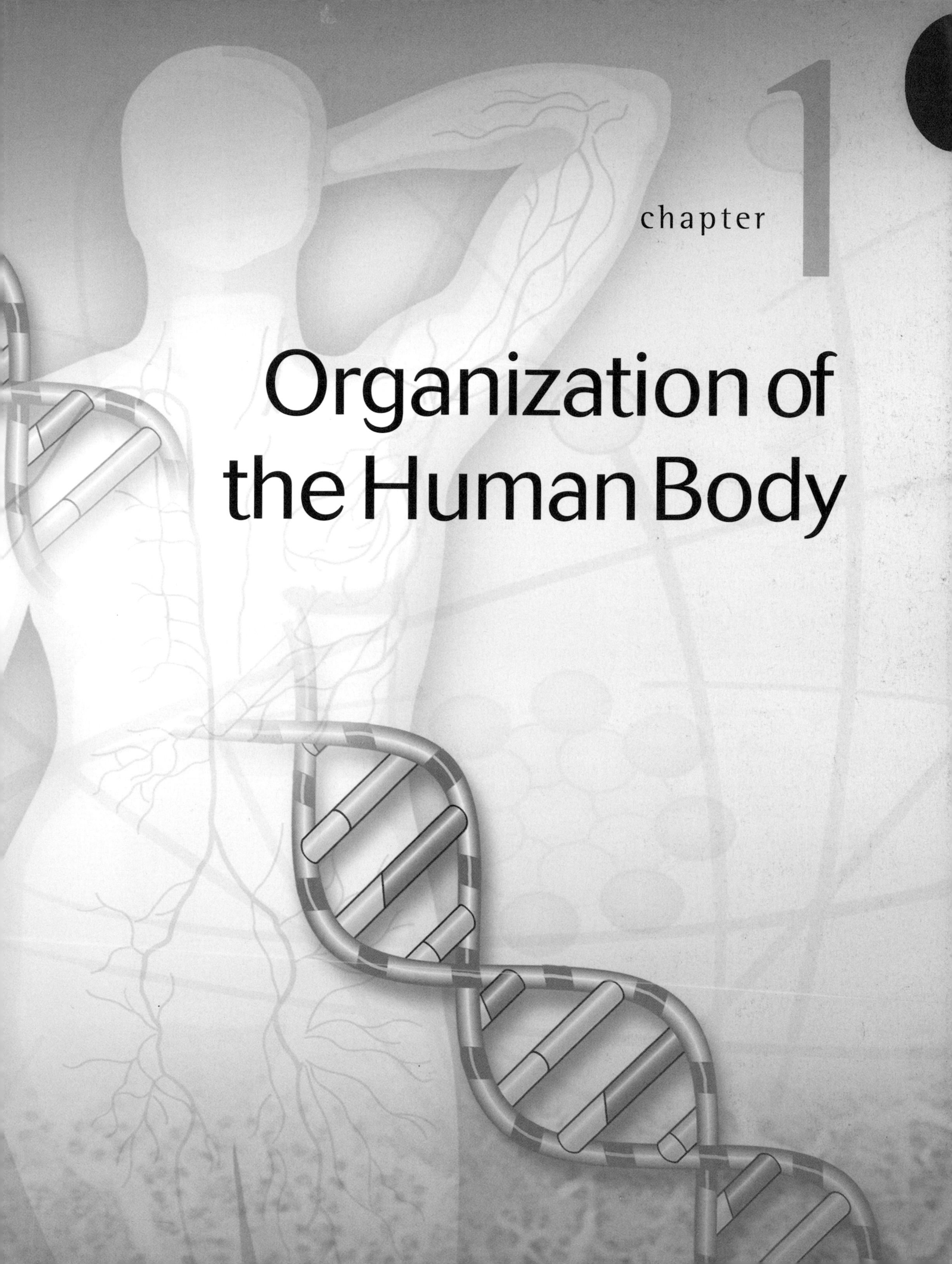

chapter 1

Organization of the Human Body

Studies of the normal structure and functions of the body are the basis for all medical sciences. It is only from understanding the normal that one can analyze what is going wrong in cases of disease. These studies give one an appreciation for the design and balance of the human body and for living organisms in general.

Studies of the Human Body

The scientific term for the study of body structure is **anatomy** (ah-NAT-o-me). The *–tomy* part of this word in Latin means "cutting," because a fundamental way to learn about the human body is to cut it apart, or **dissect** (dis-sekt) it. **Physiology** (fiz-e-OL-o-je) is the term for the study of how the body functions, and is based on a Latin term meaning "nature." Anatomy and physiology are closely related—that is, form and function are intertwined. The stomach, for example, has a pouch-like shape because it stores food during digestion. The cells in the lining of the stomach are tightly packed to prevent strong digestive juices from harming underlying tissue. Anything that upsets the normal structure or working of the body is considered a **disease** and is studied as the science of **pathology** (pah-THOL-o-je).

Levels of Organization

All living things are organized from very simple levels to more complex levels (Fig. 1-1). Living matter is derived from simple chemicals. These chemicals are formed into the complex substances that make living **cells**—the basic units of all life. Specialized groups of cells form **tissues,** and tissues may function together as **organs.** Organs working together for the same general purpose make up the body **systems.** All of the systems work together to maintain the body as a whole organism.

Checkpoint 1-1 In studying the human body, one may concentrate on its structure or its function. What are these two studies called?

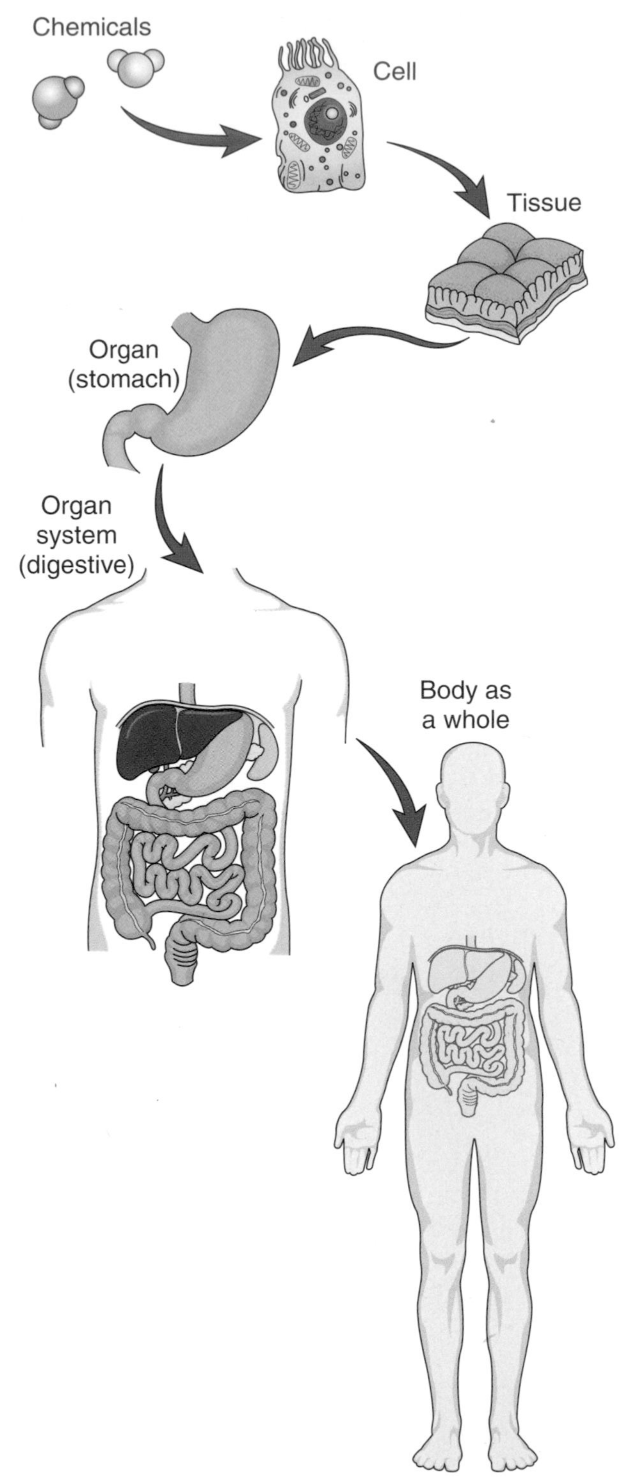

Figure 1-1 **Levels of organization.** The organ shown is the stomach, which is part of the digestive system.

Body Systems

Most studies of the human body are organized according to the individual systems, as listed below, grouped according to their general functions.

- Protection, support, and movement
  - The **integumentary** (in-teg-u-MEN-tar-e) **system.** The word ***integument*** (in-TEG-u-ment) means skin. The skin with its associated structures is considered a separate body system. The structures associated with the skin include the hair, the nails, and the sweat and oil glands.
  - The **skeletal system.** The basic framework of the body is a system of 206 bones and the joints between them, collectively known as the **skeleton.**
  - The **muscular system.** The muscles in this system are attached to the bones and produce movement of the skeleton. These skeletal muscles also give the body structure, protect organs, and maintain posture. The two other types of muscles are smooth muscle, present in the walls of body or-

gans, such as the stomach and intestine, and cardiac muscle, which makes up the wall of the heart.

- Coordination and control
  - The **nervous system.** The brain, the spinal cord, and the nerves make up this complex system by which the body is controlled and coordinated. The organs of special sense (the eyes, ears, taste buds, and organs of smell), together with the receptors for pain, touch, and other generalized senses, receive stimuli from the outside world. These stimuli are converted into impulses that are transmitted to the brain. The brain directs the body's responses to these outside stimuli and also to stimuli coming from within the body. Such higher functions as memory and reasoning also occur in the brain.
  - The **endocrine** (EN-do-krin) **system.** The scattered organs known as endocrine glands are grouped together because they share a similar function. All produce special substances called hormones, which regulate such body activities as growth, food utilization within the cells, and reproduction. Examples of endocrine glands are the thyroid, pituitary, and adrenal glands.
- Circulation
  - The **cardiovascular system.** The heart and blood vessels make up the system that pumps blood to all the body tissues, bringing with it nutrients, oxygen, and other needed substances. This system then carries waste materials away from the tissues to points where they can be eliminated.
  - The **lymphatic system.** Lymphatic vessels assist in circulation by bringing fluids from the tissues back to the blood. Organs of the lymphatic system, such as the tonsils, thymus gland, and the spleen, play a role in immunity, protecting against disease. The lymphatic system also aids in the absorption of digested fats through special vessels in the intestine. The fluid that circulates in the lymphatic system is called lymph. The lymphatic and cardiovascular systems together make up the circulatory system.
- Nutrition and fluid balance
  - The **respiratory system.** This system includes the lungs and the passages leading to and from the lungs. The purpose of this system is to take in air and conduct it to the areas designed for gas exchange. Oxygen passes from the air into the blood and is carried to all tissues by the cardiovascular system. In like manner, carbon dioxide, a gaseous waste product, is taken by the circulation from the tissues back to the lungs to be expelled.
  - The **digestive system.** This system comprises all the organs that are involved with taking in nutrients (foods), converting them into a form that body cells can use, and absorbing these nutrients into the circulation. Organs of the digestive system include the mouth, esophagus, stomach, intestine, liver, and pancreas.
  - The **urinary system.** The chief purpose of the urinary system is to rid the body of waste products and excess water. The main components of this system are the kidneys, the ureters, the bladder, and the urethra. (Note that some waste products are also eliminated by the digestive and respiratory systems and by the skin.)
- Production of offspring
  - The **reproductive system.** This system includes the external sex organs and all related internal structures that are concerned with the production of offspring.

The number of systems may vary in different lists. Some, for example, show the sensory system as separate from the nervous system. Others have a separate entry for the immune system, which protects the body from foreign matter and invading organisms. The immune system is identified by its function rather than its structure and includes elements of both the cardiovascular and lymphatic systems. Bear in mind that even though the systems are studied as separate units, they are interrelated and must cooperate to maintain health.

Metabolism and Its Regulation

All the life-sustaining reactions that go on within the body systems together make up **metabolism** (meh-TAB-o-lizm). Metabolism can be divided into two types of activities:

- In **catabolism** (kah-TAB-o-lizm), complex substances are broken down into simpler compounds (Fig. 1-2). The breakdown of the nutrients in food yields simple chemical building blocks and energy to power cell activities.
- In **anabolism** (ah-NAB-o-lizm), simple compounds are used to manufacture materials needed for growth, function, and repair of tissues. Anabolism is the building phase of metabolism.

The energy obtained from the breakdown of nutrients is used to form a compound often described as the "energy currency" of the cell. It has the long name of **adenosine triphosphate** (ah-DEN-o-sene tri-FOS-fate), but is

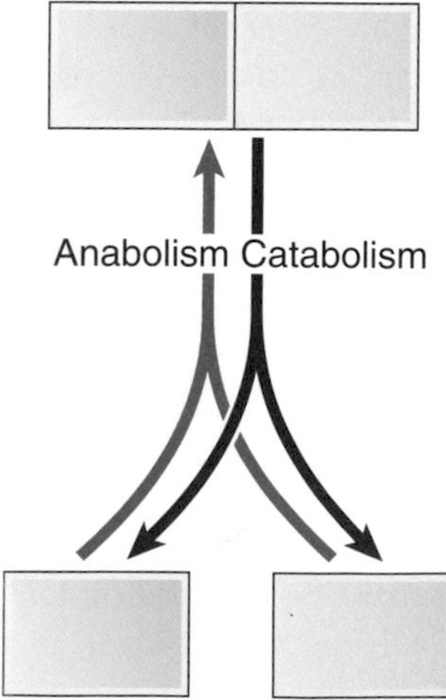

Figure 1-2 **Metabolism.** In catabolism substances are broken down into their building blocks. In anabolism simple components are built into more complex substances.

Box 1-1 **Clinical Perspectives**

Homeostatic Imbalance: When Feedback Fails

Each body structure contributes in some way to homeostasis, often through feedback mechanisms. The nervous and endocrine systems are particularly important in feedback. The nervous system's electrical signals react quickly to changes in homeostasis, while the endocrine system's chemical signals (hormones) react more slowly but over a longer time. Often both systems work together to maintain homeostasis.

As long as feedback keeps conditions within normal limits, the body remains healthy, but if feedback cannot maintain these conditions, the body enters a state of *homeostatic imbalance*. Moderate imbalance causes illness and disease, while severe imbalance causes death. At some level, all illnesses and diseases can be linked to homeostatic imbalance.

For example, feedback mechanisms closely monitor and maintain normal blood pressure. When blood pressure rises, negative feedback mechanisms lower it to normal limits. If these mechanisms fail, *hypertension* (high blood pressure) develops. Hypertension further damages the cardiovascular system and, if untreated, may lead to death. With mild hypertension, lifestyle changes in diet, exercise, and stress management may lower blood pressure sufficiently, whereas severe hypertension often requires drug therapy. The various types of antihypertensive medication all help negative feedback mechanisms lower blood pressure.

Feedback mechanisms also regulate body temperature. When body temperature falls, negative feedback mechanisms raise it back to normal limits, but if these mechanisms fail and body temperature continues to drop, *hypothermia* develops. Its main effects are uncontrolled shivering, lack of coordination, decreased heart and respiratory rates, and, if left untreated, death. Cardiac surgeons use hypothermia to their advantage during open-heart surgery by cooling the body. This stops the heart and decreases its blood flow, creating a motionless and bloodless surgical field.

commonly abbreviated **ATP.** Chapter 20 has more information on metabolism and ATP.

Homeostasis

Normal body function maintains a state of internal balance, an important characteristic of all living things. Such conditions as body temperature, the composition of body fluids, heart rate, respiration rate, and blood pressure must be kept within set limits to maintain health. (See Box 1-1, Homeostatic Imbalance: When Feedback Fails.) This steady state within the organism is called **homeostasis** (ho-me-o-STA-sis), which literally means "staying (stasis) the same (homeo)."

Fluid Balance Our bodies are composed of large amounts of fluids. The amount and composition of these fluids must be regulated at all times. One type of fluid bathes the cells, carries nutrient substances to and from the cells, and transports the nutrients into and out of the cells. This type is called **extracellular fluid** because it includes all body fluids outside the cells. Examples of extracellular fluids are blood, lymph, and the fluid between the cells in tissues. A second type of fluid, **intracellular fluid**, is contained within the cells. Extracellular and intracellular fluids account for about 60% of an adult's weight. Body fluids are discussed in more detail in Chapter 21.

Feedback The main method for maintaining homeostasis is **feedback**, a control system based on information returning to a source. We are all accustomed to getting feedback about the results of our actions and using that information to regulate our behavior. Grades on tests and assignments, for example, may inspire us to work harder if they're not so great or "keep up the good work" if they are good.

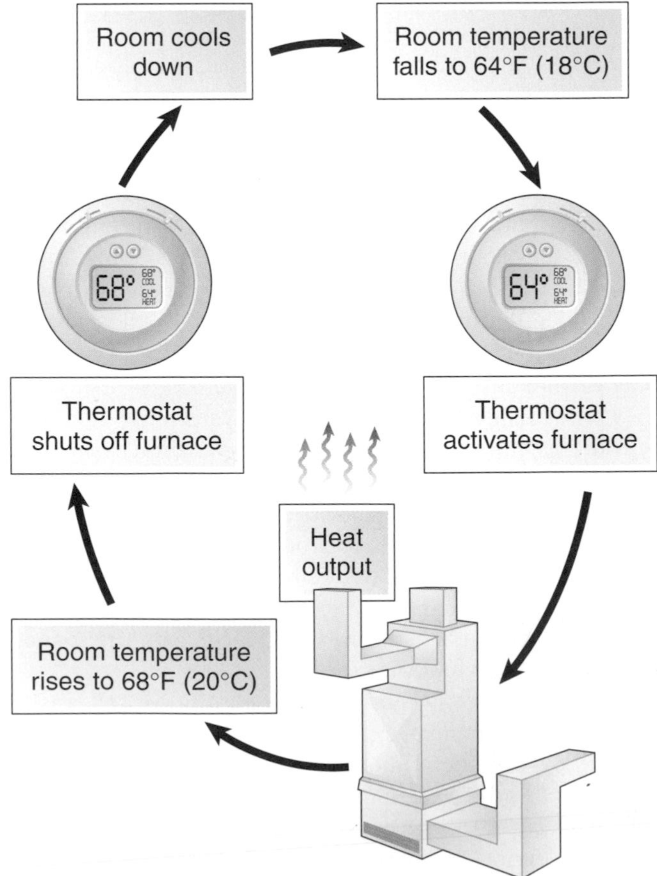

Figure 1-3 **Negative feedback.** A home thermostat illustrates how this type of feedback keeps temperature within a set range.

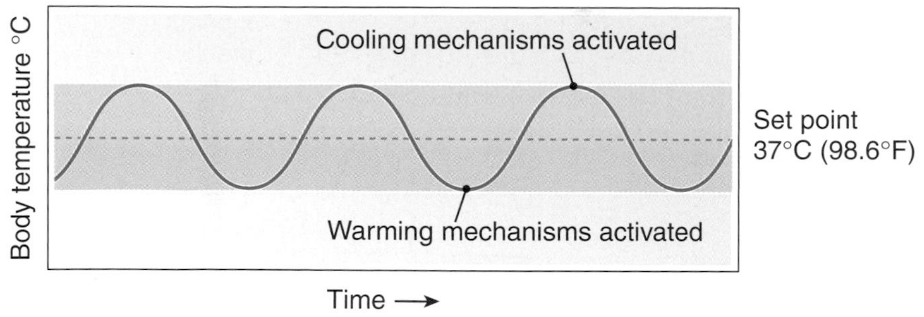

Figure 1-4 Negative feedback and body temperature. Body temperature is kept at a set point of 37° C by negative feedback acting on a center in the brain.

Most feedback systems keep body conditions within a set normal range by reversing any upward or downward shift. This form of feedback is called **negative feedback**, because actions are reversed. A familiar example of negative feedback is the thermostat in a house (Fig. 1-3). When the house temperature falls, the thermostat triggers the furnace to turn on and increase the temperature; when the house temperature reaches an upper limit, the furnace is shut off. In the body, a center in the brain detects changes in temperature and starts mechanisms for cooling or warming if the temperature is above or below the average set point of 37° C (98.6° F) (Fig. 1-4).

As another example, when glucose (a sugar) increases in the blood, the pancreas secretes insulin, which causes body cells to use more glucose. Increased uptake of glucose and the subsequent drop in blood sugar level serves as a signal to the pancreas to reduce insulin secretion (Fig. 1-5). As a result of insulin's action, the secretion of insulin is reversed. This type of self-regulating feedback loop is used in the endocrine system to maintain proper levels of hormones, as described in Chapter 12.

A few activities involve **positive feedback**, in which a given action promotes more of the same. The process of childbirth illustrates positive feedback. As the contractions of labor begin, the muscles of the uterus are stretched. The stretching sends nervous signals to the pituitary gland to release the hormone oxytocin into the blood. This hormone stimulates further contractions of the uterus. As contractions increase in force, the uterine muscles are stretched even more, causing further release of oxytocin. The escalating contractions and hormone release continue until the baby is born. In positive feedback, activity continues until the stimulus is removed or some outside force interrupts the

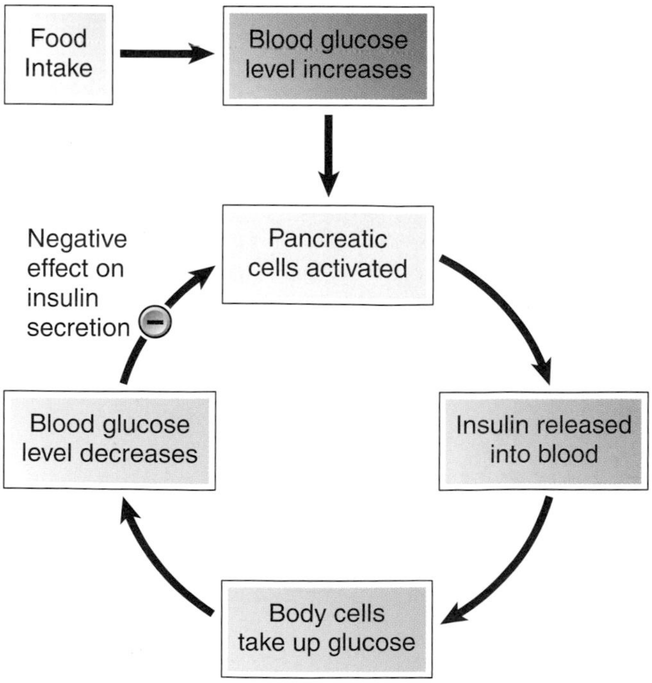

Figure 1-5 Negative feedback in the endocrine system. Glucose utilization regulates insulin production by means of negative feedback.

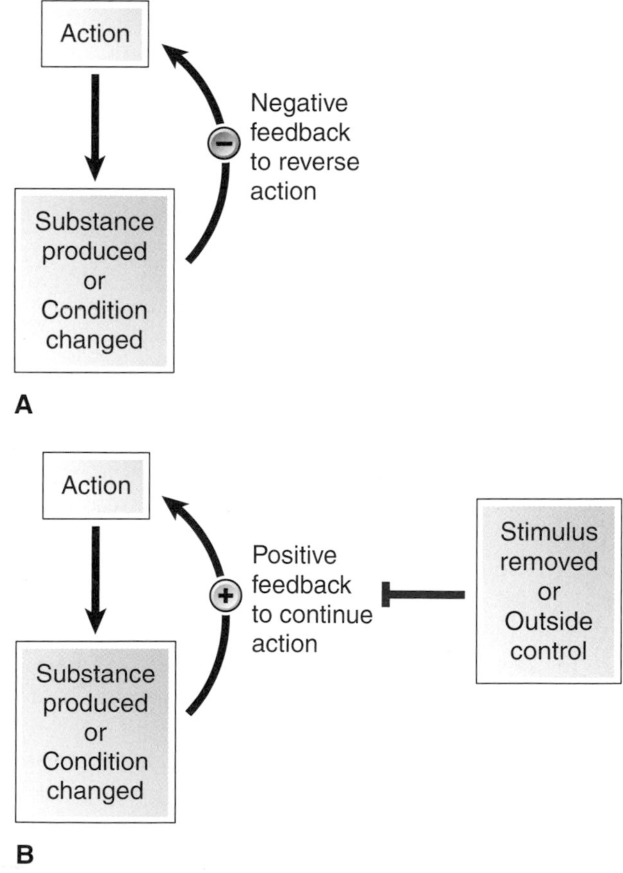

Figure 1-6 Comparison of positive and negative feedback. **(A)** In negative feedback, the result of an action reverses the action. **(B)** In positive feedback, the result of an action stimulates further action. Positive feedback continues until the stimulus is removed or an outside force stops the cycle.

activity. Positive and negative feedback are compared in Figure 1-6.

The Effects of Aging

With age, changes occur gradually in all body systems. Some of these changes, such as wrinkles and gray hair, are obvious. Others, such as decreased kidney function, loss of bone mass, and formation of deposits within blood vessels, are not visible. However, they may make a person more subject to injury and disease. Changes due to aging will be described in chapters on the body systems.

Checkpoint 1-2 Metabolism is divided into a breakdown phase and a building phase. What are these two phases called?

Checkpoint 1-3 What type of system is used primarily to maintain homeostasis?

Directions in the Body

Because it would be awkward and inaccurate to speak of bandaging the "southwest part" of the chest, a number of terms are used universally to designate position and directions in the body. For consistency, all descriptions assume that the body is in the **anatomical position.** In this posture, the subject is standing upright with face front, arms at the sides with palms forward, and feet parallel, as shown by the smaller illustration in Figure 1-7.

Directional Terms

The main terms for describing directions in the body are as follows (see Fig. 1-7):

- **Superior** is a term meaning above, or in a higher position. Its opposite, **inferior,** means below, or lower. The heart, for example, is superior to the intestine.
- **Ventral** and **anterior** have the same meaning in humans: located toward the belly surface or front of the body. Their corresponding opposites, **dorsal** and **posterior,** refer to locations nearer the back.
- **Cranial** means nearer to the head. **Caudal** means nearer to the sacral region of the spinal column (*i.e.*, where the tail is located in lower animals), or, in humans, in an inferior direction.
- **Medial** means nearer to an imaginary plane that passes through the midline of the body, dividing it into left and right portions. **Lateral,** its opposite, means farther away from the midline, toward the side.
- **Proximal** means nearer the origin of a structure; **distal,** farther from that point. For example, the part of your thumb where it joins your hand is its proximal region; the tip of the thumb is its distal region.

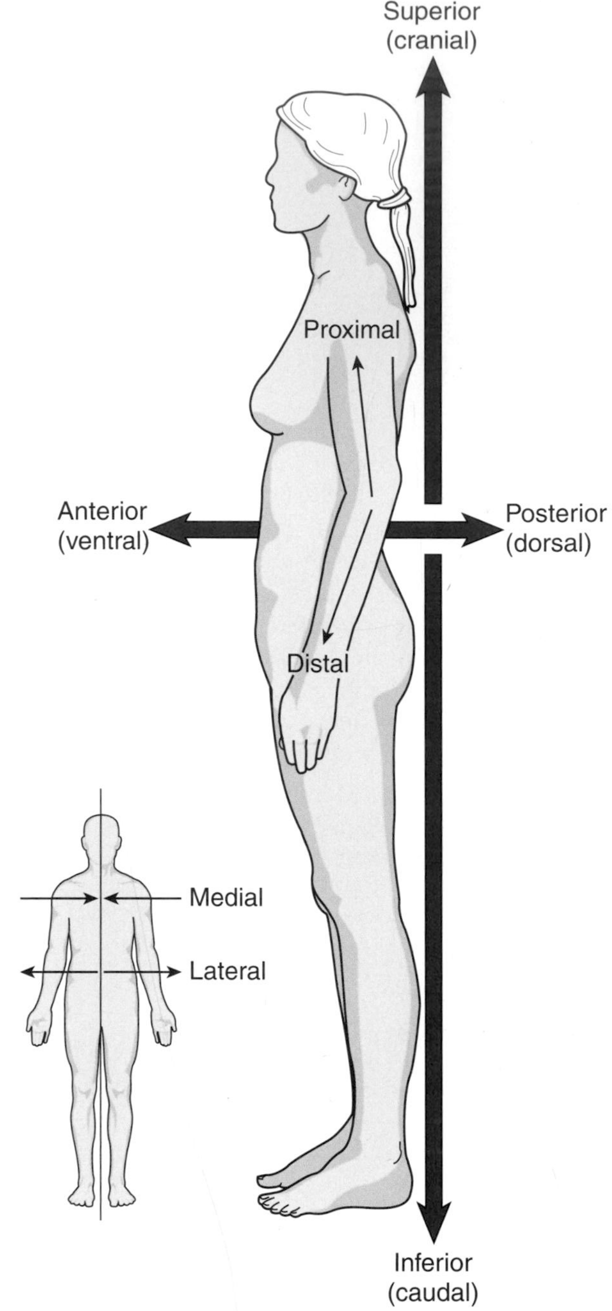

Figure 1-7 Directional terms. *ZOOMING IN ✦ What is the scientific name for the position in which the small figure is standing?*

Planes of Division

To visualize the various internal structures in relation to each other, anatomists can divide the body along three planes, each of which is a cut through the body in a different direction (Fig. 1-8).

- The **frontal plane.** If the cut were made in line with the ears and then down the middle of the body, you would see an anterior, or ventral (front), section and a poste-

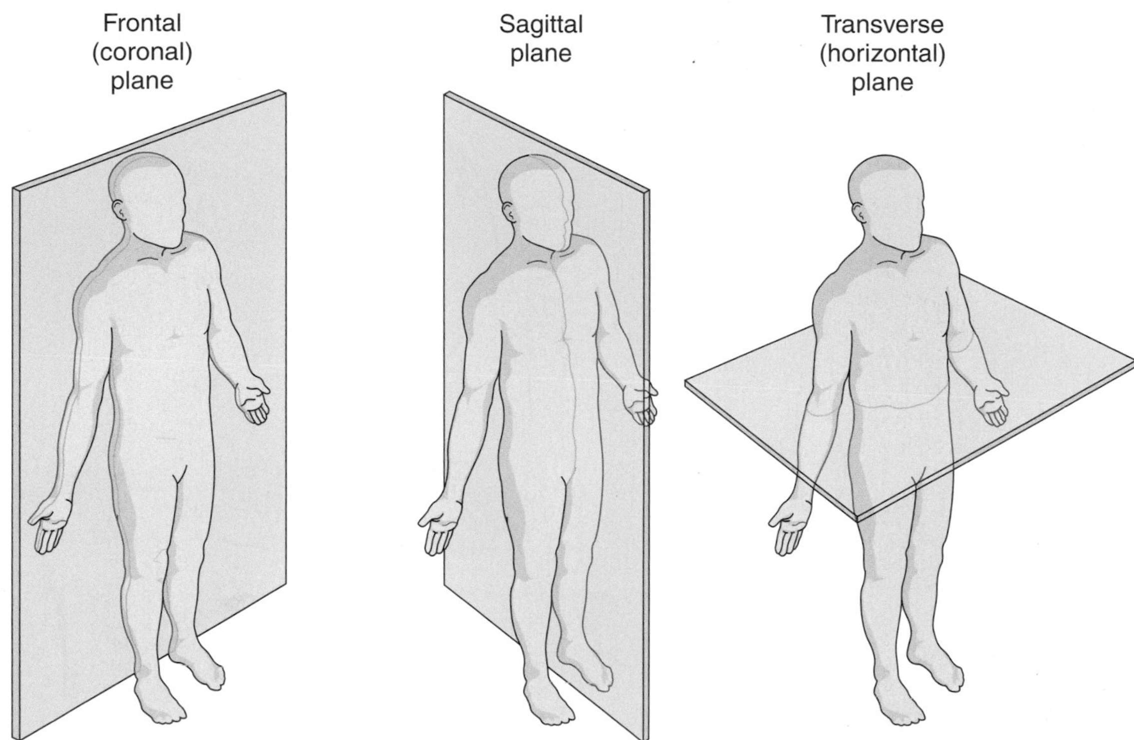

Figure 1-8 Planes of division. *ZOOMING IN ✦ Which plane divides the body into superior and inferior parts? Which plane divides the body into anterior and posterior parts?*

rior, or dorsal (back), section. Another name for this plane is *coronal plane.*

- The **sagittal** (SAJ-ih-tal) **plane.** If you were to cut the body in two from front to back, separating it into right and left portions, the sections you would see would be sagittal sections. A cut exactly down the midline of the body, separating it into equal right and left halves, is a **midsagittal** section.
- The **transverse plane.** If the cut were made horizontally, across the other two planes, it would divide the body into a superior (upper) part and an inferior (lower) part. There could be many such cross-sections, each of which would be on a transverse plane, also called a *horizontal plane.*

Tissue Sections Some additional terms are used to describe sections (cuts) of tissues, as used to prepare them for study under the microscope (Fig. 1-9). A cross section (see figure) is a cut made perpendicular to the long axis of an organ, such as a cut made across a banana to give a small round slice. A longitudinal section is made parallel to the long axis, as in cutting a banana from tip to tip to make a slice for a banana split. An oblique section

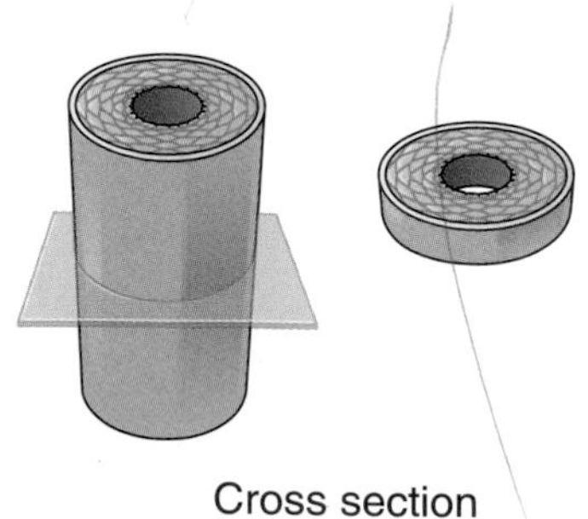

Cross section

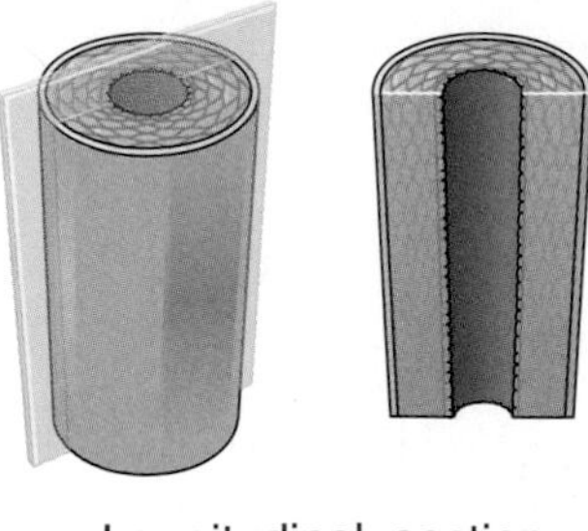

Longitudinal section

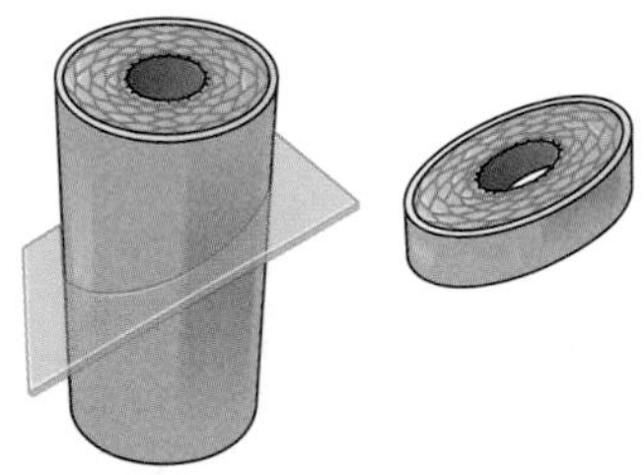

Oblique section

Figure 1-9 Tissue sections.

Box 1-2 **Hot Topics**

Medical Imaging: Seeing Without Making a Cut

Three imaging techniques that have revolutionized medicine are radiography, computed tomography, and magnetic resonance imaging. With them, physicians today can "see" inside the body without making a single cut. Each technique is so important that its inventor received a Nobel Prize.

The oldest is radiography (ra-de-OG-rah-fe), in which a machine beams x-rays (a form of radiation) through the body onto a piece of film. Like other forms of radiation, x-rays damage body tissues, but modern equipment uses extremely low doses. The resulting picture is called a radiograph. Dark areas indicate where the beam passed through the body and exposed the film, whereas light areas show where the beam did not pass through. Dense tissues (bone, teeth) absorb most of the x-rays, preventing them from exposing the film. For this reason, radiography is commonly used to visualize bone fractures and tooth decay as well as abnormally dense tissues like tumors. Radiography does not provide clear pictures of soft tissues because most of the beam passes through and exposes the film, but contrast media can help make structures like blood vessels and hollow organs more visible. For example, barium sulfate (which absorbs x-rays) coats the digestive tract when ingested.

Computed tomography (CT) is based on radiography and also uses very low doses of radiation. During a CT scan, a machine revolves around the patient, beaming x-rays through the body onto a detector. The detector takes numerous pictures of the beam and a computer assembles them into transverse sections, or "slices." Unlike conventional radiography, CT produces clear images of soft structures such as the brain, liver, and lungs. It is commonly used to visualize brain injuries and tumors, and even blood vessels when used with contrast media.

Magnetic resonance imaging uses a strong magnetic field and radiowaves. So far, there is no evidence to suggest that MRI causes tissue damage. The MRI patient lies inside a chamber within a very powerful magnet. The molecules in the patient's soft tissues align with the magnetic field inside the chamber. When radiowaves beamed at the region to be imaged hit the soft tissue, the aligned molecules emit energy that the MRI machine detects, and a computer converts these signals into a picture. MRI produces even clearer images of soft tissue than does computed tomography and can create detailed pictures of blood vessels without contrast media. MRI can visualize brain injuries and tumors that might be missed using CT.

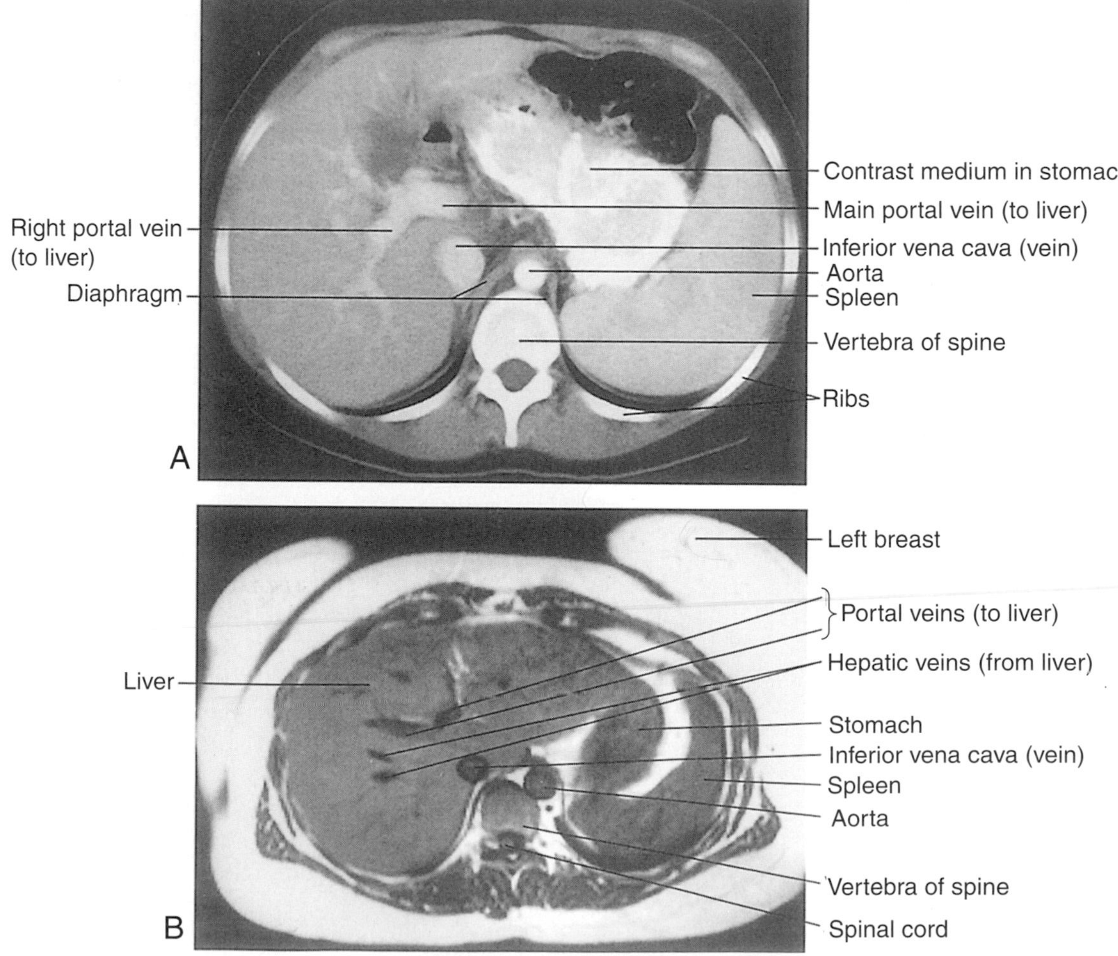

Figure 1-10 **Cross-sections in imaging.** Images taken across the body through the liver and spleen by **(A)** computed tomography (CT) and **(B)** magnetic resonance imaging (MRI). (Reprinted with permission from Erkonen WE. Radiology 101: Basics and Fundamentals of Imaging. Philadelphia: Lippincott Williams & Wilkins, 1998.)

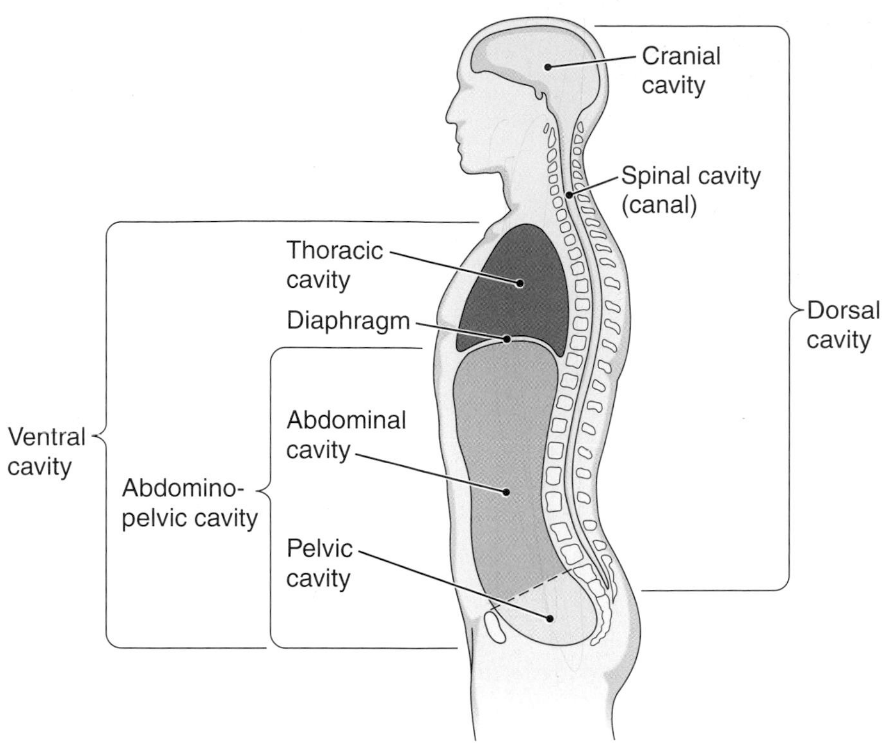

Figure 1-11 **Body cavities, lateral view.** Shown are the dorsal and ventral cavities with their subdivisions. *ZOOMING IN ✦ What cavity contains the diaphragm?*

Checkpoint 1-4 What are the three planes in which the body can be cut? What kind of a plane divides the body into two equal halves?

is made at an angle. The type of section used will determine what is seen under the microscope, as shown with a blood vessel in Figure 1-9.

These same terms are used for images taken by techniques such as computed tomography (CT) or magnetic resonance imaging (MRI). (See Box 1-2, Medical Imaging: Seeing Without Making a Cut). In imaging studies, the term cross section is used more generally to mean any two-dimensional view of an internal structure obtained by imaging, as shown in Figure 1-10.

Body Cavities

Internally, the body is divided into a few large spaces, or **cavities,** which contain the organs. The two main cavities are the **dorsal cavity** and **ventral cavity** (Fig. 1-11).

Dorsal Cavity

The dorsal body cavity has two subdivisions: the **cranial cavity,** containing the brain, and the **spinal cavity (canal),** enclosing the spinal cord. These two areas form one continuous space.

Ventral Cavity

The ventral cavity is much larger than the dorsal cavity. It has two main subdivisions, which are separated by the **diaphragm** (DI-ah-fram), a muscle used in breathing. The **thoracic** (tho-RAS-ik) **cavity** is located superior to (above) the diaphragm. Its contents include the heart, the lungs, and the large blood vessels that join the heart. The heart is contained in the pericardial cavity, formed by the pericardial sac; the lungs are in the pleural cavity, formed by the pleurae, the membranes that enclose the lungs (Fig. 1-12). The **mediastinum** (me-de-as-TI-num) is the space between the lungs, including the organs and vessels contained in that space.

The **abdominopelvic** (ab-dom-ih-no-PEL-vik) **cavity** (see Fig. 1-11) is located inferior to (below) the diaphragm. This space is further subdivided into two regions. The superior portion, the **abdominal cavity**, contains the stomach, most of the intestine, the liver, the gallbladder, the pancreas, and the spleen. The inferior portion, set off by an imaginary line across the top of the hip bones, is the **pelvic cavity.** This cavity contains the urinary bladder, the rectum, and the internal parts of the reproductive system.

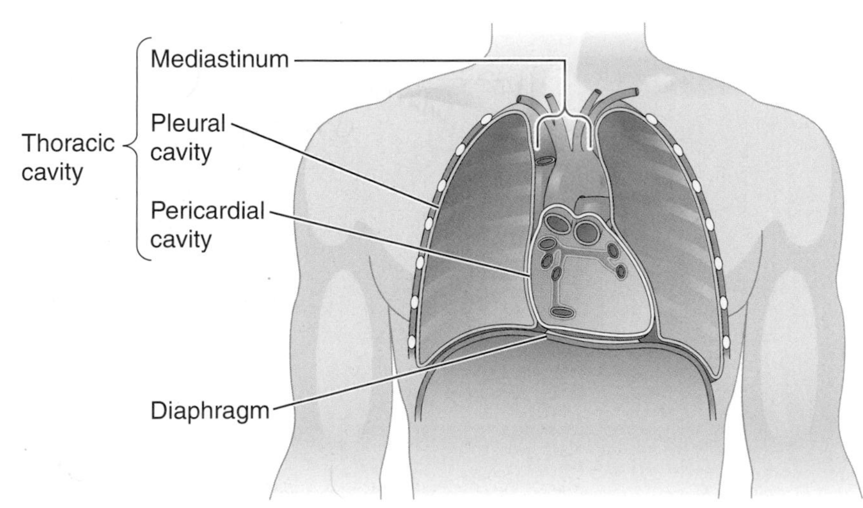

Figure 1-12 **The thoracic cavity.** Shown are the pericardial cavity, which contains the heart, and the pleural cavity, which contains the lungs.

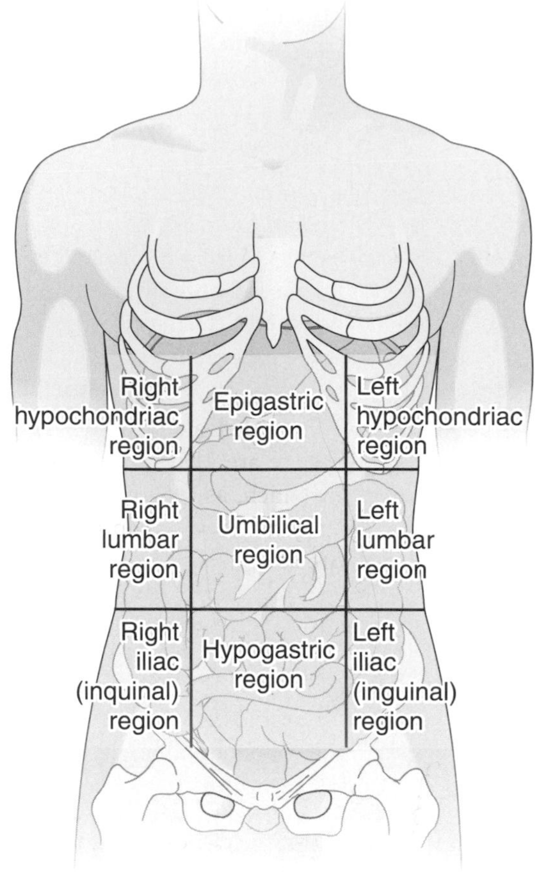

Figure 1-13 **The nine regions of the abdomen.**

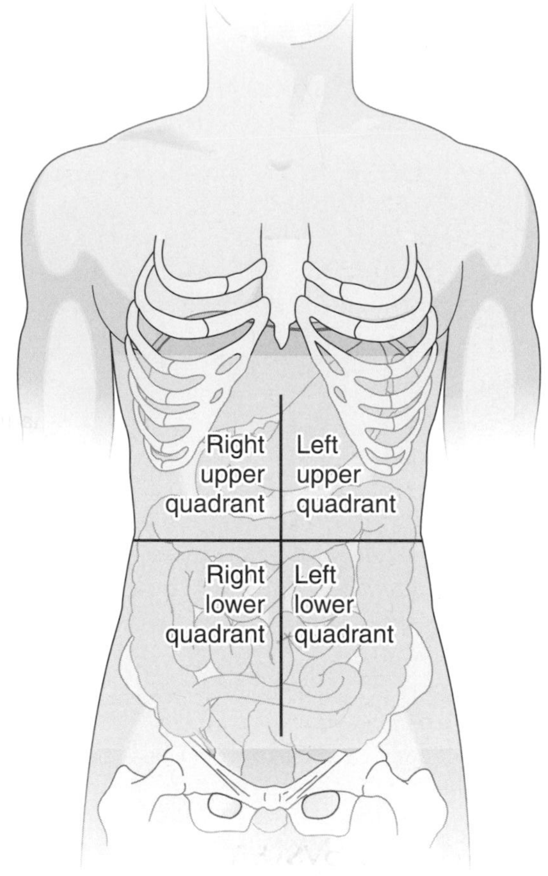

Figure 1-14 **Quadrants of the abdomen.** The organs within each quadrant are shown.

Checkpoint 1-5 There are two main body cavities, one posterior and one anterior. Name these two cavities.

Regions of the Abdomen It is helpful to divide the abdomen for examination and reference into nine regions (Fig. 1-13).

The three central regions, from superior to inferior are:

- the **epigastric** (ep-ih-GAS-trik) **region**, located just inferior to the breastbone
- the **umbilical** (um-BIL-ih-kal) **region** around the umbilicus (um-BIL-ih-kus), commonly called the *navel*

Box 1-3 · Health Professions

Health Information Technicians

Every time a patient receives medical treatment, information is added to the patient's medical record, which includes data about symptoms, medical history, test results, diagnoses, and treatment. **Health information technicians** organize and manage these records, working closely with physicians, nurses, and other health professionals to ensure that medical records provide a complete, accurate basis for quality patient care.

Accurate medical records are also essential for administrative purposes. Health information technicians assign a **code** to each diagnosis and procedure a patient receives, and this information is used for accurate patient billing. In addition, health information technicians analyze medical records to discover trends in health and disease. This research can be used to improve patient care, manage costs, and help establish new medical treatments.

Health information technicians need a strong clinical knowledge base. A thorough background in medical terminology is essential when reading and interpreting medical records. Anatomy and physiology are definitely required!

Most health information technologists work in hospitals and long-term care facilities. Others work in medical clinics, government agencies, insurance companies, and consulting firms. Job prospects are promising because of the growing need for healthcare. In fact, health information technology is projected to be one of the fastest growing careers in the United States. For more information about this profession, contact the American Health Information Management Association.

- the **hypogastric** (hi-po-GAS-trik) **region**, the most inferior of all the midline regions

The regions on the right and left, from superior to inferior, are:

- the **hypochondriac** (hi-po-KON-dre-ak) **regions**, just inferior to the ribs
- the **lumbar regions**, which are on a level with the lumbar regions of the spine
- the iliac, or **inguinal** (IN-gwih-nal), **regions**, named for the upper crest of the hipbone and the groin region, respectively

A simpler but less precise division into four quadrants is sometimes used. These regions are the right upper quadrant (RUQ), left upper quadrant (LUQ), right lower quadrant (RLQ), and left lower quadrant (LLQ) (Fig. 1-14). (See Box 1-3, Health Information Technicians, for description of a profession that uses anatomical, physiological, and medical terms.)

Checkpoint 1-6 Name the three central regions and the three left and right lateral regions of the abdomen.

The Metric System

Now that we have set the stage for further study of the body's structure and function, we should take a look at the metric system, because this system is used for all scientific measurements. The drug industry and the healthcare industry already have converted to the metric system, so anyone who plans a career in healthcare should be acquainted with metrics.

The metric system is like the monetary system in the United States. Both are decimal systems based on multiples of the number 10. One hundred cents equal one dollar; one hundred centimeters equal one meter. Each multiple in the decimal system is indicated by a prefix:

kilo = 1000

centi = 1/100

milli = 1/1000

micro = 1/1,000,000

Units of Length

The basic unit of length in the metric system is the **meter** (m). Using the prefixes above, 1 kilometer is equal to 1000 meters. A centimeter is 1/100 of a meter; stated another way, there are 100 centimeters in 1 meter. The United States has not changed over to the metric system, as was once expected. Often, measurements on packages, bottles, and yard goods are now given according to both scales. In this text, equivalents in the more familiar units of inches and feet are included along with the metric units for comparison. There are 2.5 centimeters (cm) or 25 millimeters (mm) in 1 inch, as shown in Figure 1-15. Some equivalents that may help you to appreciate the size of various body parts are as follows:

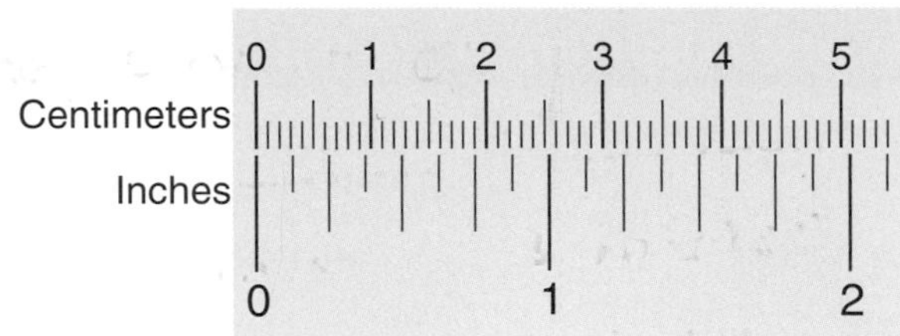

Figure 1-15 **Comparison of centimeters and inches.**

1 mm = 0.04 inch, or 1 inch = 25 mm

1 cm =0.4 inch, or 1 inch = 2.5 cm

1 m = 3.3 feet, or 1 foot = 30 cm

Units of Weight

The same prefixes used for linear measurements are used for weights and volumes. The **gram** (g) is the basic unit of weight. Thirty grams are about equal to 1 ounce, and 1 kilogram to 2.2 pounds. Drug dosages are usually stated in grams or milligrams. One thousand milligrams equal 1 gram; a 500-milligram (mg) dose would be the equivalent of 0.5 gram (g), and 250 mg is equal to 0.25 g.

Units of Volume

The dosages of liquid medications are given in units of volume. The basic metric measurement for volume is the **liter** (L) (LE-ter). There are 1000 milliliters (mL) in a liter. A liter is slightly greater than a quart, a liter being equal to 1.06 quarts. For smaller quantities, the milliliter is used most of the time. There are 5 ml in a teaspoon and 15 mL in a tablespoon. A fluid ounce contains 30 mL.

Temperature

The Celsius (centigrade) temperature scale, now in use by most countries and by scientists in this country, is discussed in Chapter 20.

A chart of all the common metric measurements and their equivalents is shown in Appendix 1. A Celsius-Fahrenheit temperature conversion scale appears in Appendix 2.

Checkpoint 1-7 Name the basic units of length, weight, and volume in the metric system.

Word Anatomy

Medical terms are built from standardized word parts (prefixes, roots, and suffixes). Learning the meanings of these parts can help you remember words and interpret unfamiliar terms.

WORD PART	MEANING	EXAMPLE
Studies of the Human Body		
-tomy	cutting, incision of	*Anatomy* can be revealed by making incisions in the body.
dis-	apart, away from	To *dissect* is to cut apart.
physi/o	nature, physical	*Physiology* is the study of how the body functions.
path/o	disease	*Pathology* is the study of disease.
Body Processes		
cata-	down	*Catabolism* is the breakdown of complex substances into simpler ones.
ana-	upward, again, back	*Anabolism* is the building up of simple compounds into more complex substances.
home/o-	same	*Homeostasis* is the steady state (sameness) within an organism.
stat	stand, stoppage, constancy	In *homeostasis*, "-stasis" refers to constancy.

Summary

I. Studies of the human body

1. Anatomy—study of structure
2. Physiology—study of function
3. Pathology—study of disease

A. Levels of organization—chemicals, cell, tissue, organ, organ system, whole organism

II. Body systems

1. Integumentary system—skin and associated structures
2. Skeletal system—support
3. Muscular system—movement
4. Nervous system—reception of stimuli and control of responses
5. Endocrine system—production of hormones for regulation of growth, metabolism, reproduction
6. Cardiovascular system—movement of blood for transport
7. Lymphatic system—aids in circulation, immunity, and absorption of digested fats
8. Respiratory system—intake of oxygen and release of carbon dioxide
9. Digestive system—intake, breakdown, and absorption of nutrients
10. Urinary system—elimination of waste and water
11. Reproductive system—production of offspring

III. Metabolism and its regulation

1. Metabolism—all the chemical reactions needed to sustain life
2. Catabolism—breakdown of complex substances into simpler substances; release of energy from nutrients
   a. ATP (adenosine triphosphate)—energy compound of cells
3. Anabolism—building of body materials

A. Homeostasis—steady state of body conditions
   1. Fluid balance
      a. Extracellular fluid—outside the cells
      b. Intracellular fluid—inside the cells
   2. Feedback—regulation by return of information within a system
      a. Negative feedback—reverses an action
      b. Positive feedback—promotes continued activity

B. Effects of aging—changes in all systems

IV. Directions in the body

1. Anatomical position—upright, palms forward, face front, feet parallel

A. Directional terms
   1. Superior—above or higher; inferior—below or lower
   2. Ventral (anterior)—toward belly or front surface; dorsal (posterior)—nearer to back surface
   3. Cranial—nearer to head; caudal—nearer to sacrum
   4. Medial—toward midline; lateral—toward side
   5. Proximal—nearer to point of origin; distal—farther from point of origin

B. Planes of division
   1. Body divisions
      a. Sagittal—from front to back, dividing the body into left and right parts
         (1) Midsagittal—exactly down the midline
      b. Frontal (coronal)—from left to right, dividing the body into anterior and posterior parts
      c. Transverse—horizontally, dividing the body into superior and inferior parts
   2. Tissue sections
      a. Cross section—perpendicular to long axis
      b. Transverse section—parallel to long axis
      c. Oblique section—at an angle

V. Body cavities

A. Dorsal cavity—contains cranial and spinal cavities for brain and spinal cord
B. Ventral cavity
   1. Thoracic—chest cavity
      a. Divided from abdominal cavity by diaphragm
      b. Contains heart and lungs
      c. Mediastinum—space between lungs and the organs contained in that space
   2. Abdominopelvic
      a. Abdominal—upper region containing stomach, most of intestine, pancreas, liver, spleen, and others
      b. Pelvic—lower region containing reproductive organs, urinary bladder, rectum
      c. Nine regions of the abdomen
         (1) Central—epigastric, umbilical, hypogastric
         (2) Lateral (right and left)—hypochondriac, lumbar, iliac (inguinal)
      d. Quadrants—abdomen divided into four regions

VI. The metric system—based on multiples of 10

1. Basic units
   a. Meter—length
   b. Gram—weight
   c. Liter—volume
2. Prefixes—indicate multiples of 10
   a. Kilo—1000 times
   b. Centi—1/100th (0.01)
   c. Milli—1/1000th (0.001)
   d. Micro—1/1,000,000 (0.000001)

A. Units of length
B. Units of weight
C. Units of volume
D. Temperature—measured in Celsius (centigrade) scale

Questions for Study and Review

Building Understanding

Fill in the blanks

1. Tissues may function together as ______.
2. Glands that produce hormones belong to the ______ system.
3. The eyes are located ______ to the nose.
4. Normal body function maintains a state of internal balance called ______.
5. The basic unit of volume in the metric system is the ______.

Matching

Match each numbered item with the most closely related lettered item.

___ 6. One of two systems that control and coordinate other systems
___ 7. The system that brings needed substances to the body tissues
___ 8. The system that converts foods into a form that body cells can use
___ 9. The cavity that contains the liver
___ 10. The cavity that contains the urinary bladder

a. nervous system
b. abdominal cavity
c. cardiovascular system
d. pelvic cavity
e. digestive system

Multiple choice

___ 11. The study of normal body structure is
   a. homeostasis
   b. anatomy
   c. physiology
   d. pathology

___ 12. Fluids contained within cells are described as
   a. intracellular
   b. ventral
   c. extracellular
   d. dorsal

___ 13. A type of feedback in which a given action promotes more of the same is called
   a. homeostasis
   b. biofeedback
   c. positive feedback
   d. negative feedback

___ 14. The cavity that contains the mediastinum is the
   a. dorsal
   b. ventral
   c. abdominal
   d. pelvic

___ 15. The foot is located ______ to the knee.
   a. superior
   b. inferior
   c. proximal
   d. distal

Understanding Concepts

16. Compare and contrast the studies of anatomy and physiology. Would it be wise to study one without the other?
17. List in sequence the levels of organization in the body from simplest to most complex. Give an example for each level.

18. Compare and contrast the anatomy and physiology of the nervous system with that of the endocrine system.
19. What is ATP? What type of metabolic activity releases the energy used to make ATP?
20. Compare and contrast intracellular and extracellular fluids.
21. Explain how an internal state of balance is maintained in the body.
22. List the subdivisions of the dorsal and ventral cavities. Name some organs found in each subdivision.

Conceptual Thinking

23. The human body is organized from very simple levels to more complex levels. With this in mind describe why a disease at the chemical level can have an effect on organ system function.
24. When glucose levels in the blood drop below normal the pancreas releases a hormone called glucagon. Using your understanding of negative feedback, discuss the possible role of glucagon in blood glucose homeostasis.
25. Your patient's chart reads: "Patient reports pain in right lower quadrant of abdomen. X-ray reveals mass in right iliac region." Locate this region on yourself and explain why it is important for health professionals to use anatomical terminology when describing the human body.

Selected Key Terms

The following terms and other boldface terms in the chapter are defined in the Glossary

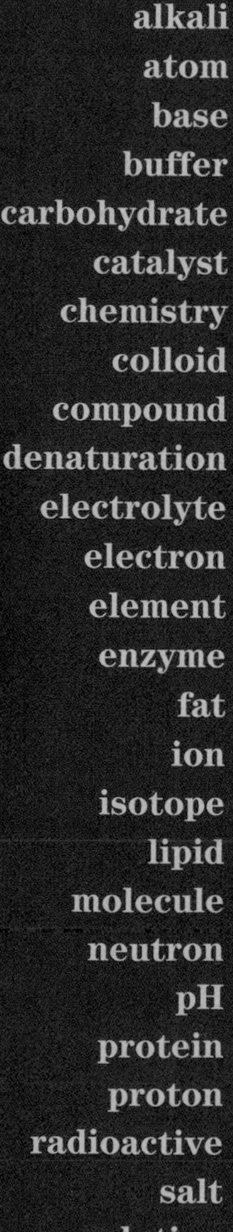

acid
alkali
atom
base
buffer
carbohydrate
catalyst
chemistry
colloid
compound
denaturation
electrolyte
electron
element
enzyme
fat
ion
isotope
lipid
molecule
neutron
pH
protein
proton
radioactive
salt
solution
suspension
valence

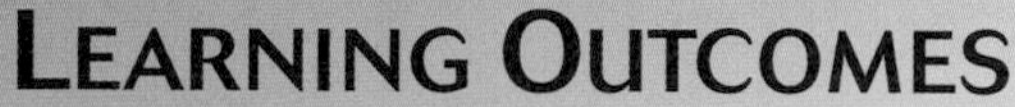

Learning Outcomes

After careful study of this chapter, you should be able to:

1. Define an element
2. Describe the structure of an atom
3. Differentiate between molecules and compounds
4. Explain why water is so important to the body
5. Define *mixture*; list the three types of mixtures and give two examples of each
6. Differentiate between ionic and covalent bonds
7. Define an electrolyte
8. Define the terms acid, *base*, and *salt*
9. Explain how the numbers on the pH scale relate to acidity and basicity (alkalinity)
10. Define *buffer* and explain why buffers are important in the body
11. Define *radioactivity* and cite several examples of how radioactive substances are used in medicine

12 List three characteristics of organic compounds

13. Name the three main types of organic compounds and the building blocks of each
14. Define *enzyme*; describe how enzymes work
15. Show how word parts are used to build words related to chemistry, matter, and life (see Word Anatomy at the end of the chapter)

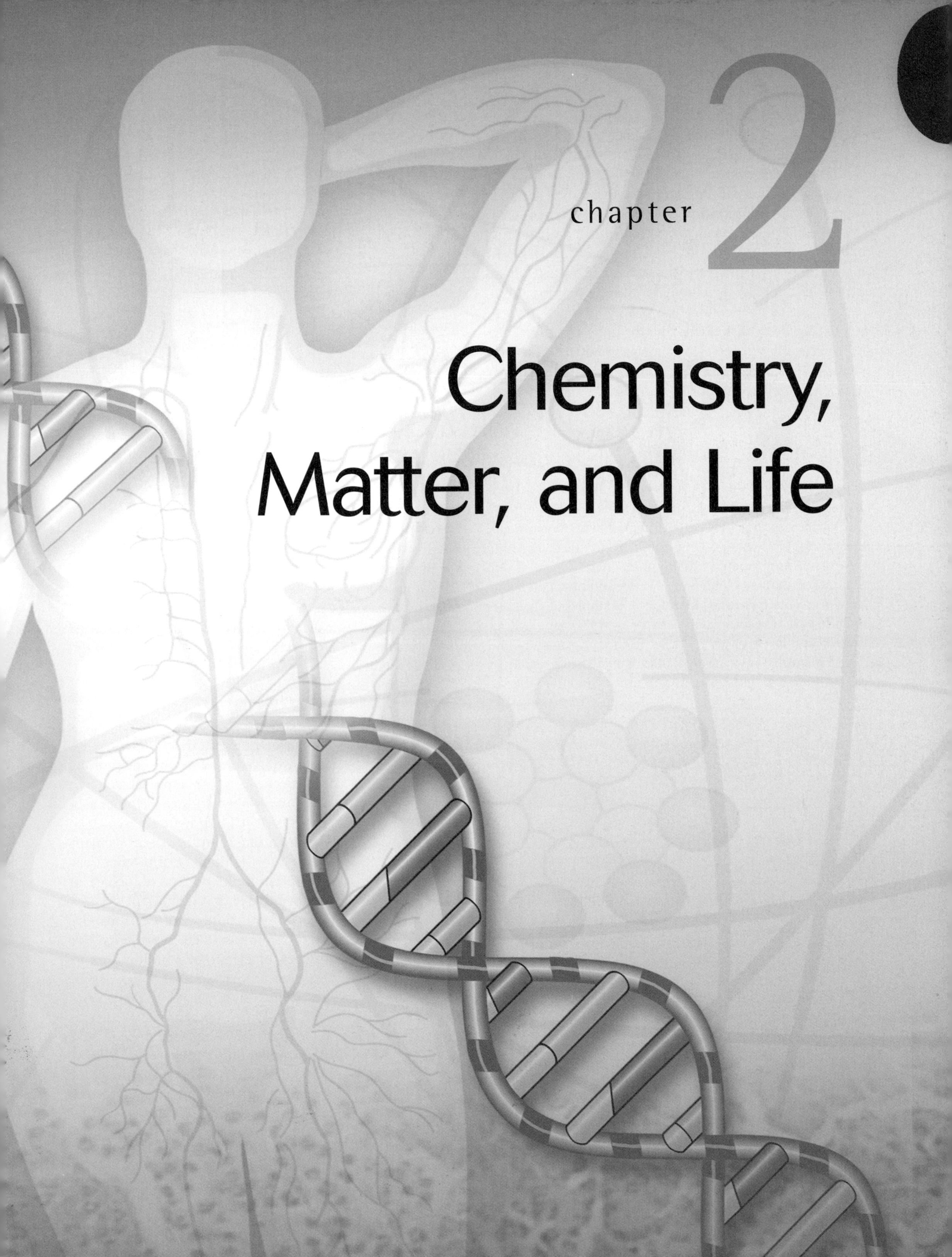

chapter 2

Chemistry, Matter, and Life

Greater understanding of living organisms has come to us through **chemistry**, the science that deals with the composition and properties of matter. Knowledge of chemistry and chemical changes helps us understand the normal and abnormal functioning of the body. The digestion of food in the intestinal tract, the production of urine by the kidneys, the regulation of breathing, and all other body activities involve the principles of chemistry. The many drugs used to treat diseases are chemicals. Chemistry is used for the development of drugs and for an understanding of their actions in the body.

To provide some insights into the importance of chemistry in the life sciences, this chapter briefly describes elements, atoms and molecules, compounds, and mixtures, which are fundamental forms of matter.

Elements

Matter is anything that takes up space, that is, the materials from which all of the universe is made. Elements are the substances that make up all matter. The food we eat, the atmosphere, water—everything around us, everything we can see and touch, is made of elements. There are 92 naturally occurring elements. (Twenty additional elements have been created in the laboratory.) Examples of elements include various gases, such as hydrogen, oxygen, and nitrogen; liquids, such as mercury used in barometers and other scientific instruments; and many solids, such as iron, aluminum, gold, silver, and zinc. Graphite (the so-called "lead" in a pencil), coal, charcoal, and diamonds are different forms of the element carbon.

Elements can be identified by their names or their chemical symbols, which are abbreviations of the modern or Latin names of the elements. Each element is also identified by its own number, which is based on the structure of its subunits, or atoms. The periodic table is a chart used by chemists to organize and describe the elements. Appendix 3 shows the periodic table and gives some information about how it is used. Table 2-1 lists some elements found in the human body along with their functions.

Table 2•1 Some Common Chemical Elements*

NAME	SYMBOL	FUNCTION
Oxygen	O	Part of water; needed to metabolize nutrients for energy
Carbon	C	Basis of all organic compounds; in carbon dioxide, the waste gas of metabolism
Hydrogen	H	Part of water; participates in energy metabolism, acid–base balance
Nitrogen	N	Present in all proteins, ATP (the energy compound), and nucleic acids (DNA and RNA)
Calcium	Ca	Builds bones and teeth; needed for muscle contraction, nerve impulse conduction, and blood clotting
Phosphorus	P	Active ingredient in the energy-storing compound ATP; builds bones and teeth; in cell membranes and nucleic acids
Potassium	K	Nerve impulse conduction; muscle contraction; water balance and acid–base balance
Sulfur	S	Part of many proteins
Sodium	Na	Active in water balance, nerve impulse conduction, and muscle contraction
Chlorine	Cl	Active in water balance and acid–base balance; found in stomach acid
Iron	Fe	Part of hemoglobin, the compound that carries oxygen in red blood cells

**The elements are listed in decreasing order by weight in the body.*

Atoms

The subunits of elements are **atoms**. These are the smallest complete units of matter. They cannot be broken down or changed into another form by ordinary chemical and physical means. These subunits are so small that millions of them could fit on the sharpened end of a pencil.

Atomic Structure Despite the fact that the atom is such a tiny particle, it has been carefully studied and has been found to have a definite structure. At the center of the atom is a nucleus, which contains positively charged electrical particles called **protons** (PRO-tonz) and noncharged particles called **neutrons** (NU-tronz). Together, the protons and neutrons contribute nearly all of the atom's weight.

In orbit outside the nucleus are **electrons** (e-LEK-tronz) (Fig. 2-1). These nearly weightless particles are negatively charged. It is the electrons that determine how the atom will react chemically. The protons and electrons of an atom always are equal in number, so that the atom as a whole is electrically neutral.

The **atomic number** of an element is equal to the number of protons that are present in the nucleus of each of its atoms. Because the number of protons is equal to the number of electrons, the atomic number also represents the number of electrons whirling around the nucleus. Each element has a specific atomic number. No two elements share the same number. In the Periodic Table of the Elements (see Appendix 3) the atomic number is located at the top of the box for each element.

The positively charged protons keep the negatively charged electrons in orbit around the nucleus by means of the opposite charges on the particles. Positively (+) charged protons attract negatively (−) charged electrons.

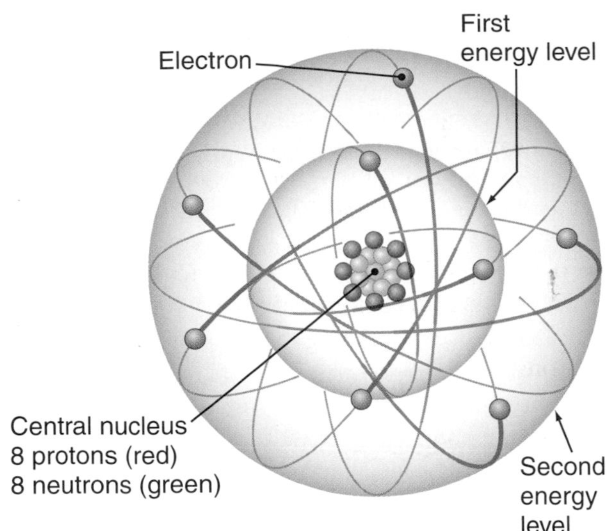

Figure 2-1 Representation of the oxygen atom. Eight protons and eight neutrons are tightly bound in the central nucleus. The eight electrons are in orbit around the nucleus, two at the first energy level and six at the second. *ZOOMING IN ✦ How does the number of protons in this atom compare with the number of electrons?*

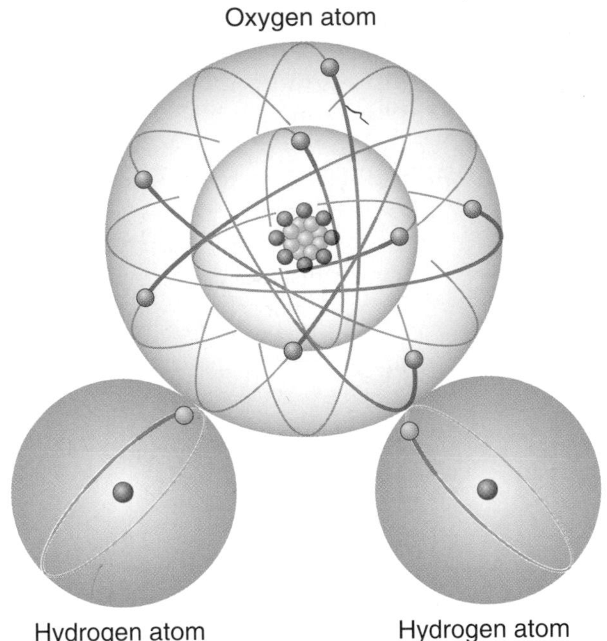

Figure 2-2 Formation of water. When oxygen reacts, two electrons are needed to complete the outermost energy level, as shown in this reaction with hydrogen to form water. *ZOOMING IN ✦ How many hydrogen atoms bond with an oxygen atom to form water?*

Checkpoint 2-1 What are atoms?

Checkpoint 2-2 What are three types of particles found in atoms?

Energy Levels The electrons of an atom orbit at specific distances from the nucleus in regions called energy levels. The first energy level, the one closest to the nucleus, can hold only two electrons. The second energy level, the next in distance away from the nucleus, can hold eight electrons.

More distant energy levels can hold more than eight electrons, but they are stable (nonreactive) when they have eight.

The electrons in the energy level farthest away from the nucleus give the atom its chemical characteristics. If the outermost energy level has more than four electrons but less than its capacity of eight, the atom normally completes this level by gaining electrons. In the process, it becomes negatively charged, because it has more electrons than protons. The oxygen atom illustrated in Figure 2-1 has six electrons in its second, or outermost, level. When oxygen enters into chemical reactions, it gains two electrons, as when it reacts with hydrogen to form water (Fig. 2-2). The oxygen atom then has two more electrons than protons.

If the outermost energy level has fewer than four electrons, the atom normally loses those electrons. In so doing, it becomes positively charged, because it now has more protons than electrons.

The number of electrons lost or gained by atoms of an element in chemical reactions is known as the **valence** of that element (from a Latin word that means "strength"). The outermost energy level, which determines the combining properties of the element, is the valence level. Valence is reported as a number with a + or – to indicate whether electrons are lost or gained in chemical reactions. Remember that electrons carry a negative charge, so when an atom gains electrons it becomes negatively charged and when an atom loses electrons it becomes positively charged. For example, the valence of oxygen, which gains two electrons in chemical reactions, is shown as O^{2-}.

Molecules and Compounds

A **molecule** (MOL-eh-kule) is formed when two or more atoms unite on the basis of their electron structures. A molecule can be made of like atoms—the oxygen molecule is made of two identical atoms—but more often a molecule is made of atoms of two or more different elements. For example, a molecule of water (H_2O) contains one atom of oxygen (O) and two atoms of hydrogen (H) (see Fig. 2-2).

Substances composed of two or more different elements are called **compounds.** Molecules are the smallest subunits of a compound. Each molecule of a compound contains the elements that make up that compound in the proper ratio. Some compounds are made of a few elements in a simple combination. For example, the gas carbon monoxide (CO) contains 1 atom of carbon (C) and 1 atom of oxygen (O). Other compounds are very large and complex. Such complexity characterizes many of the compounds found in living organisms. Some proteins, for example, have thousands of atoms.

It is interesting to observe how different a compound is from any of its constituents. For example, a molecule of liquid water is formed from oxygen and hydrogen, both of which are gases. Another example is a crystal sugar, glucose ($C_6H_{12}O_6$). Its constituents include 12 atoms of the gas hydrogen, 6 atoms of the gas oxygen, and 6 atoms of the solid element carbon. The component gases and the solid carbon do not in any way resemble the glucose.

Checkpoint 2-3 What are molecules?

The Importance of Water

Water is the most abundant compound in the body. No plant or animal, including the human, can live very long without it. Water is of critical importance in all physiological processes in body tissues. A deficiency of water, or dehydration (de-hi-DRA-shun), can be a serious threat to health. Water carries substances to and from the cells and makes possible the essential processes of absorption, exchange, secretion, and excretion. What are some of the properties of water that make it such an ideal medium for living cells?

- Water can dissolve many different substances in large amounts. For this reason, it is called the **universal solvent.** Many of the materials needed by the body, such as gases, minerals, and nutrients, dissolve in water to be carried from place to place. Substances, such as salts, that mix with or dissolve in water are described as *hydrophilic* ("water-loving"); those, such as fats, that repel and do not dissolve in water are described as *hydrophobic* ("water-fearing").
- Water is stable as a liquid at ordinary temperatures. Water does not freeze until the temperature drops to 0° C (32° F) and does not boil until the temperature reaches 100° C (212° F). This stability provides a constant environment for body cells. Water can also be used to distribute heat throughout the body and to cool the body by evaporation of sweat from the body surface.
- Water participates in chemical reactions in the body. It is needed directly in the process of digestion and in many of the metabolic reactions that occur in the cells.

Checkpoint 2-4 What is the most abundant compound in the body?

Mixtures: Solutions and Suspensions

Not all elements or compounds combine chemically when brought together. The air we breathe every day is a mixture of gases, largely nitrogen, oxygen, and carbon dioxide, along with smaller percentages of other substances. The constituents in the air maintain their identity, although the proportions of each may vary. Blood plasma is also a mixture in which the various components maintain their identity. The many valuable compounds in the plasma remain separate entities with their own properties. Such combinations are called **mixtures**—blends of two or more substances (Table 2-2).

A mixture formed when one substance dissolves in another is called a **solution.** One example is salt water. In a solution, the component substances cannot be distinguished from each other and they remain evenly distributed throughout; that is, the mixture is homogeneous (ho-mo-JE-ne-us). The dissolving substance, which in the body is water, is the **solvent.** The substance dissolved, salt in the case of salt water, is the **solute.** An **aqueous** (A-kwe-us) **solution** is one in which water is the solvent. Aqueous solutions of glucose, salts, or both of these together are used for intravenous fluid treatments.

In some mixtures, the substance distributed in the background material is not dissolved and will settle out unless the mixture is constantly shaken. This type of non-uniform, or heterogeneous (het-er-o-JE-ne-us), mixture is called a **suspension.** The particles in a suspension are separate from the material in which they are dispersed, and they settle out because they are large and heavy. Examples of suspensions are milk of magnesia, finger paints, and, in the body, red blood cells suspended in blood plasma.

Table 2•2 Mixtures

TYPE	DEFINITION	EXAMPLE
Solution	Homogeneous mixture formed when one substance (solute) dissolves in another (solvent)	Table salt (NaCl) dissolved in water; table sugar (sucrose) dissolved in water
Suspension	Heterogeneous mixture in which one substance is dispersed in another, but will settle out unless constantly mixed	Red blood cells in blood plasma; milk of magnesia
Colloid	Heterogeneous mixture in which the suspended material remains evenly distributed based on the small size and opposing charges of the particles	Blood plasma; cytosol

One other type of mixture is of importance in the body. Some organic compounds form **colloids,** in which the molecules do not dissolve yet remain evenly distributed in the suspending material. The particles have electrical charges that repel each other, and the molecules are small enough to stay in suspension. The fluid that fills the cells (cytosol) is a colloidal suspension, as is blood plasma.

Many mixtures are complex, with properties of solutions, suspensions, and colloidal suspensions. Blood plasma has dissolved compounds, making it a solution. The red blood cells and other formed elements give blood the property of a suspension. The proteins in the plasma give it the property of a colloidal suspension. Chocolate milk also has all three properties.

Checkpoint 2-5 Both solutions and suspensions are types of mixtures. What is the difference between them?

Chemical Bonds

When discussing the structure of the atom, we mentioned the positively charged (+) protons that are located in the nucleus and the equal number of orbiting negatively charged (−) electrons that neutralize the protons (Fig. 2-3 A). Atoms interact, however, to reach a stable number of electrons in the outermost energy level. These chemical interactions alter the neutrality of the atoms and also form a bond between them. In chemical reactions, electrons may be transferred from one atom to another or may be shared between atoms.

Ionic Bonds

When electrons are transferred from one atom to another, the type of bond formed is called an **ionic** (i-ON-ik) **bond.** The sodium atom, for example, tends to lose the single electron in its outermost shell (Fig. 2-3 B), leaving an outermost shell with a stable number of electrons (8). Removal of a single electron from the sodium atom leaves one more proton than electrons, and the atom then has a single net positive charge. The sodium atom in this form is symbolized as Na^+. An atom or group of atoms with a positive or negative charge is called an **ion** (I-on). Any ion that is positively charged is a **cation** (CAT-i-on).

Alternately, atoms can gain electrons so that there are more electrons than protons. Chlorine, which has seven electrons in its outermost energy level, tends to gain one electron to fill the level to its capacity. Such an atom of chlorine is negatively charged (Cl^-) (see Fig. 2-3 B). (Chemists refer to this charged form of chlorine as *chloride.)* Any negatively charged ion is an **anion** (AN-i-on).

Let us imagine a sodium atom coming in contact with a chlorine atom. The chlorine atom gains an electron from the sodium atom, forming an ionic bond. The two newly formed ions (Na^+ and Cl^-), because of their opposite charges, attract each other to produce the compound sodium chloride, ordinary table salt (Fig. 2-3 C).

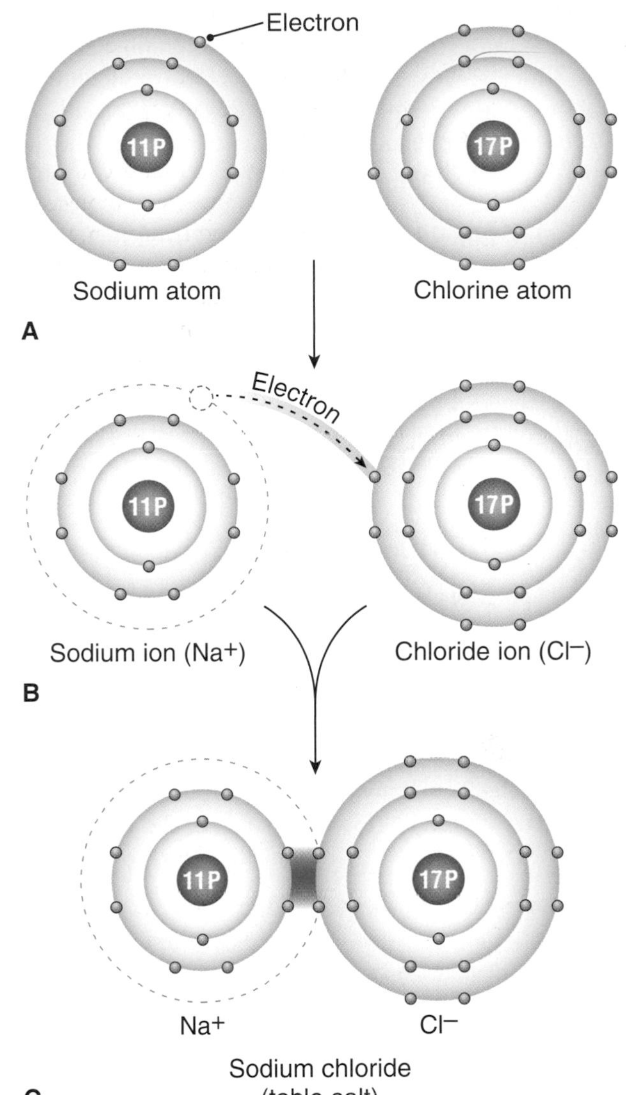

Figure 2-3 Ionic bonding. (A) A sodium atom has 11 protons and 11 electrons. A chlorine atom has 17 protons and 17 electrons. **(B)** A sodium atom gives up one electron to a chlorine atom in forming an ionic bond. The sodium atom now has 11 protons and 10 electrons, resulting in a positive charge of one. The chlorine becomes negatively charged by one, with 17 protons and 18 electrons. **(C)** The sodium ion (Na+) is attracted to the chloride ion (Cl-) in forming the compound sodium chloride (table salt).

Electrolytes Ionically bonded substances, when they go into solution, separate into charged particles. Compounds formed by ionic bonds that release ions when they are in solution are called **electrolytes** (e-LEK-tro-lites). Note that in practice, the term *electrolytes* is also used to refer to the ions themselves in body fluids. Electrolytes include a variety of salts, such as sodium chloride and potassium chloride. They also include acids and bases, which are responsible for the acidity or alkalinity of body fluids, as described later in this chapter. Electrolytes must be present in exactly the right quantities in the fluid within the cell (intracellular fluid) and the fluid outside the cell (extracellular fluid), or very damaging effects will result, preventing the cells in the body from functioning properly.

Ions in the Body Many different ions are found in body fluids. Calcium ions (Ca^{2+}) are necessary for the clotting of blood, the contraction of muscle, and the health of bone tissue. Bicarbonate ions (HCO_3^-) are required for the regulation of acidity and alkalinity of body fluids. The stable condition of the normal organism, homeostasis, is influenced by ions.

Because ions are charged particles, electrolyte solutions can conduct an electric current. Records of electric currents in tissues are valuable indications of the functioning or malfunctioning of tissues and organs. The **electrocardiogram** (e-lek-tro-KAR-de-o-gram) and the **electroencephalogram** (e-lek-tro-en-SEF-ah-lo-gram) are graphic tracings of the electric currents generated by the heart muscle and the brain, respectively (see Chapters 10 and 14).

Checkpoint 2-6 What happens when an electrolyte goes into solution?

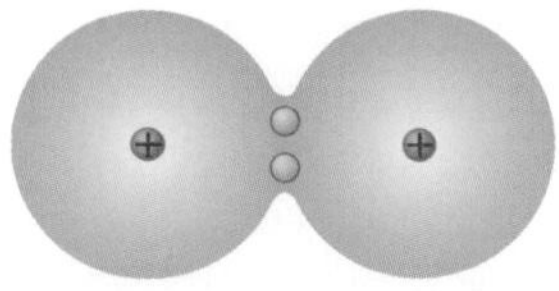

Figure 2-4 A nonpolar covalent bond. The electrons involved in the bonding of a hydrogen molecule are equally shared between the two atoms of hydrogen. The electrons orbit evenly around the two. *ZOOMING IN ✦ How many electrons are needed to complete the energy level of each hydrogen atom?*

Covalent Bonds

Although ionic bonds form many chemical compounds, a much larger number of compounds are formed by another type of chemical bond. This bond involves not the exchange of electrons but a sharing of electrons between the atoms in the molecule and is called a **covalent bond.** This name comes from the prefix *co-*, meaning "together," and *valence*, referring to the electrons involved in chemical reactions between atoms. In a covalently bonded molecule, the valence electrons orbit around both of the atoms, making both of them stable. Covalent bonds may involve the sharing of one, two, or three pairs of electrons between atoms.

In some covalently bonded molecules, the electrons are equally shared, as in the case of a hydrogen molecule (H_2) and other molecules composed of atoms of the same element (Fig. 2-4). Electrons may also be shared equally in some

Box 2-1 A Closer Look

Hydrogen Bonds: Strength in Numbers

In contrast to ionic and covalent bonds, which hold atoms together, hydrogen bonds hold molecules together. Hydrogen bonds are much weaker than ionic or covalent bonds—in fact, they are more like "attractions" between molecules. While ionic and covalent bonds rely on electron transfer or sharing, hydrogen bonds form bridges between two molecules. A hydrogen bond forms when a slightly positive hydrogen atom in one molecule is attracted to a slightly negative atom in another molecule. Even though a single hydrogen bond is weak, many hydrogen bonds between two molecules can be strong.

Hydrogen bonds hold water molecules together, with the slightly positive hydrogen atom in one molecule attracted to a slightly negative oxygen atom in another. Many of water's unique properties come from its ability to form hydrogen bonds. For example, hydrogen bonds keep water liquid over a wide range of temperatures, which provides a constant environment for body cells.

Hydrogen bonds form not only between molecules but also within large molecules. Hydrogen bonds between regions of the same molecule cause it to fold and coil into a specific shape, as in the process that creates the precise three-dimensional structure of proteins. Because a protein's structure determines its function in the body, hydrogen bonds are essential to protein activity.

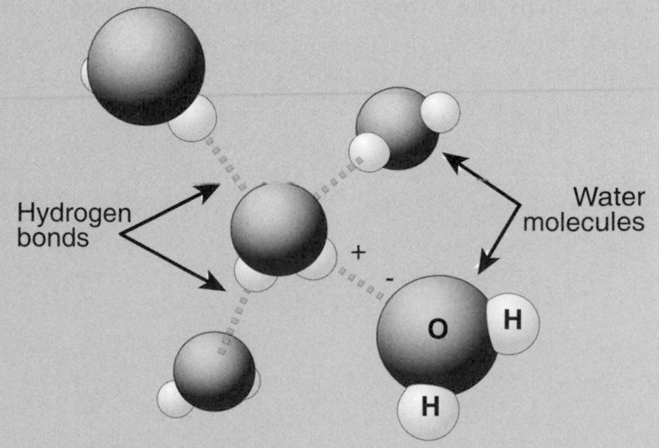

Hydrogen bonds. The bonds shown here are holding water molecules together.

molecules composed of different atoms, methane (CH_4), for example. If electrons are equally shared in forming a molecule, the electrical charges are evenly distributed around the atoms and the bond is described as a *nonpolar covalent bond*. That is, no part of the molecule is more negative or positive than any other part of the molecule. More commonly, the electrons are held closer to one atom than the other, as in the case of water (H_2O), shown in Figure 2-2. In a water molecule, the shared electrons are actually closer to the oxygen at any one time making that region of the molecule more negative. Such bonds are called *polar covalent bonds*, because one part of the molecule is more negative and one part is more positive at any one time. Anyone studying biological chemistry (biochemistry) is interested in covalent bonding because carbon, the element that is the basis of organic chemistry, forms covalent bonds with a wide variety of different elements. Thus, the compounds that are characteristic of living things are covalently bonded compounds. For a description of another type of bond, see Box 2-1, Hydrogen Bonds: Strength in Numbers.

Checkpoint 2-7 How is a covalent bond formed?

Compounds: Acids, Bases, and Salts

An **acid** is a chemical substance capable of donating a hydrogen ion (H^+) to another substance. A common example is hydrochloric acid, the acid found in stomach juices:

HCl	→	H^+	+	Cl^-
(hydrochloric acid)		(hydrogen ion)		(chloride ion)

A **base** is a chemical substance, usually containing a hydroxide ion (OH^-), that can accept a hydrogen ion. A base is also called an **alkali** (AL-kah-li). Sodium hydroxide, which releases hydroxide ion in solution, is an example of a base:

NaOH	→	Na^+	+	OH^-
(sodium hydroxide)		(sodium ion)		(hydroxide ion)

A reaction between an acid and a base produces a **salt**, such as sodium chloride:

$$HCl + NaOH \rightarrow NaCl + H_2O$$

The pH Scale

The greater the concentration of hydrogen ions in a solution, the greater is the acidity of that solution. The greater the concentration of hydroxide ion (OH^-), the greater the basicity (alkalinity) of the solution. Based on changes in the balance of ions in solution, as the concentration of hydrogen ions increases, the concentration of hydroxide ions decreases. Conversely, as the concentration of hydroxide ions increases, the concentration of hydrogen ions decreases. Acidity and alkalinity are indicated by **pH** units, which represent the relative concentrations of hydrogen and hydroxide ions in a solution. The pH units are listed on a scale from 0 to 14, with 0 being the most acidic and 14 being the most basic (Fig. 2-5). A pH of 7.0 is neutral. At pH 7.0 the solution has an equal number of hydrogen and hydroxide ions. Pure water has a pH of 7.0. Solutions that measure less than 7.0 are acidic; those that measure above 7.0 are alkaline (basic).

Because the pH scale is based on multiples of 10, each pH unit on the scale represents a 10-fold change in the number of hydrogen and hydroxide ions present. A solution registering 5.0 on the scale has 10 times the number of hydrogen ions as a solution that registers 6.0. The pH 5.0 solution also has one tenth the number of hydroxide ions as the solution of pH 6.0. A solution registering 9.0 has one tenth the number of hydrogen ions and 10 times the number of hydroxide ions as one registering 8.0. Thus, the lower the pH reading, the greater is the acidity, and the higher the pH, the greater is the alkalinity.

Blood and other body fluids are close to neutral but are slightly on the alkaline side, with a pH range of

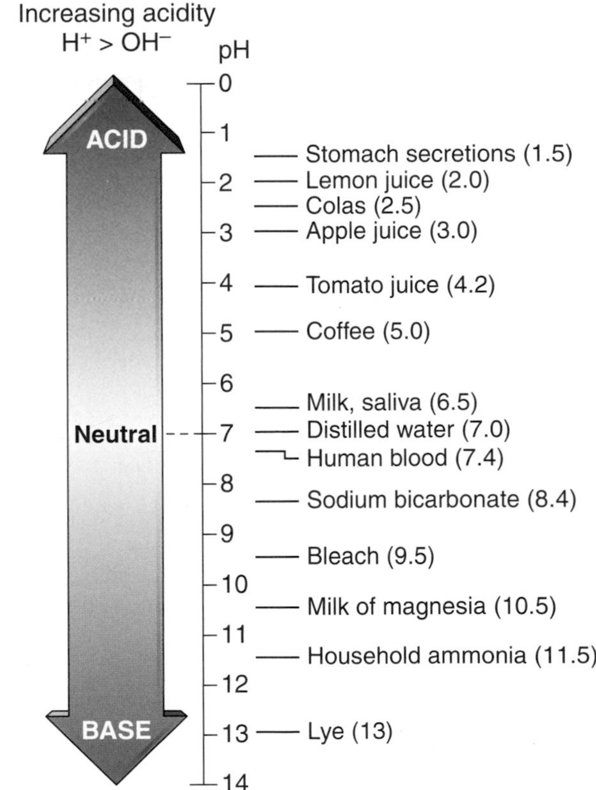

Figure 2-5 The pH scale. Degree of acidity or alkalinity is shown in pH units. This scale also shows the pH of some common substances. *ZOOMING IN ✦ What happens to the amount of hydroxide ion (OH^-) present in a solution when the amount of hydrogen ion (H^+) increases?*

7.35 to 7.45. Urine averages pH 6.0 but may range from 4.6 to 8.0 depending on body conditions and diet. Figure 2-5 shows the pH of some other common substances.

Because body fluids are on the alkaline side of neutral, the body may be considered to be in an acidic state even if the pH does not drop below 7.0. For example, if the pH falls below 7.35 but is still greater than 7.0, one is described as being in an acidic state known as *acidosis*. Thus, within a narrow range of the pH scale, physiologic acidity may differ from acidity from a chemical standpoint.

An increase in pH to readings greater than 7.45 is termed *alkalosis*. Any shifts in pH to readings above or below the normal range can be dangerous, even fatal.

Buffers

If a person is to remain healthy, a delicate balance must exist within the narrow limits of acidity and alkalinity of body fluids. This balanced chemical state is maintained in large part by **buffers.** Chemicals that serve as buffers form a system that prevents sharp changes in hydrogen ion concentration and thus maintains a relatively constant pH. Buffers are important in maintaining stability in the pH of body fluids. More information about body fluids, pH, and buffers can be found in Chapter 21.

Checkpoint 2-8 The pH scale is used to measure acidity and alkalinity of fluids. What number is neutral on the pH scale? What kind of compound measures lower than this number? Higher?

Checkpoint 2-9 What is a buffer?

Isotopes and Radioactivity

Elements may exist in several forms, each of which is called an **isotope** (I-so-tope). These forms are alike in their numbers of protons and electrons, but differ in their atomic weights because of differing numbers of neutrons in the nucleus. The most common form of oxygen, for example, has eight protons and eight neutrons in the nucleus, giving the atom an atomic weight of 16 atomic mass units (amu). But there are some isotopes of oxygen with only six or seven neutrons in the nucleus and others with 9-11 neutrons. The isotopes of oxygen thus range in weight from 14 to 19 amu.

Some isotopes are stable and maintain constant characteristics. Others disintegrate (fall apart) and give off rays of atomic particles. Such isotopes are said to be **radioactive.** Radioactive elements may occur naturally, as is the case with isotopes of the very heavy elements radium and uranium. Others may be produced artificially by placing the atoms of lighter, non-radioactive elements in accelerators that smash their nuclei together.

Use of Radioactive Isotopes

The rays given off by some radioactive elements, also called *radioisotopes*, are used in the treatment of cancer because they have the ability to penetrate and destroy tissues. Radiation therapy is often given by means of machines that are able to release tumor-destroying particles. The sensitivity of the younger, dividing cells in a growing cancer allows selective destruction of these abnormal cells with minimal damage to normal tissues. Modern radiation instruments produce tremendous amounts of energy (in the multimillion electron-volt range) and yet can destroy

Box 2-2 **Hot Topics**

Radioactive Tracers: Medicine Goes Nuclear

Like radiography, computed tomography, and MRI, **nuclear medicine imaging** (NMI) offers a noninvasive way to look inside the body. An excellent diagnostic tool, NMI shows not only structural details but also provides information about body function. NMI can diagnose cancer, stroke, and heart disease earlier than techniques that provide only structural information.

NMI uses **radiotracers**, radioactive substances that specific organs absorb. For example, radioactive iodine is used to image the thyroid gland, which absorbs more iodine than any other organ. After a patient ingests, inhales, or is injected with a radiotracer, a device called a gamma camera detects the radiotracer in the organ under study and produces a picture, which is used in making a diagnosis. Radiotracers are broken down and eliminated through urine or feces, so they leave the body quickly. A patient's exposure to radiation in NMI is usually considerably lower than with x-ray or CT scan.

Three NMI techniques are **positron emission tomography** (PET), **bone scanning**, and the **thallium stress test**. PET is often used to evaluate brain activity by measuring the brain's use of radioactive glucose. PET scans can reveal brain tumors because tumor cells are often more metabolically active than normal cells and thus absorb more radiotracer. Bone scanning detects radiation from a radiotracer absorbed by bone tissue with an abnormally high metabolic rate, such as a bone tumor. The thallium stress test is used to diagnose heart disease. A nuclear medicine technologist injects the patient with radioactive thallium, and a gamma camera images the heart during exercise and then rest. When compared, the two sets of images help to evaluate blood flow to the working, or "stressed," heart.

deep-seated cancers without causing serious skin reactions.

In radiation treatment, a radioactive isotope, such as cobalt 60, is sealed in a stainless steel cylinder and mounted on an arm or crane. Beams of radioactivity are then directed through a porthole to the area to be treated. Implants containing radioactive isotopes in the form of needles, seeds, or tubes also are widely used in the treatment of different types of cancer.

In addition to its therapeutic values, irradiation is extensively used in diagnosis. X-rays penetrate tissues and produce an image of their interior on a photographic plate. Radioactive iodine and other "tracers" taken orally or injected into the bloodstream are used to diagnose abnormalities of certain body organs, such as the thyroid gland (see Box 2-2, Radioactive Tracers: Medicine Goes Nuclear). Rigid precautions must be followed by healthcare personnel to protect themselves and the patient when using radiation in diagnosis or therapy because the rays can destroy both healthy and diseased tissues.

Checkpoint 2-10 Some isotopes are stable; others break down to give off atomic particles. What word is used to describe isotopes that give off radiation?

Chemistry of Living Matter

Of the 92 elements that exist in nature, only 26 have been found in living organisms. Most of these are elements that are light in weight. Not all are present in large quantity. Hydrogen, oxygen, carbon, and nitrogen are the elements that make up about 96% of the body by weight (Fig. 2-6). Nine additional elements, calcium, sodium, potassium, phosphorus, sulfur, chlorine, magnesium, iron, and iodine make up most of the remaining 4% of the elements in the body. The remaining 13, including zinc, selenium, copper, cobalt, chromium, and others, are present in extremely small (trace) amounts totaling about 0.1% of body weight.

Organic Compounds

The chemical compounds that characterize living things are called **organic compounds.** All of these contain the element **carbon.** Because carbon can combine with a variety of different elements and can even bond to other carbon atoms to form long chains, most organic compounds consist of large, complex molecules. The starch found in potatoes, the fat in the tissue under the skin, hormones, and many drugs are examples of organic compounds. These large molecules are often formed from simpler molecules called *building blocks,* which bond together in long chains.

The main types of organic compounds are carbohydrates, lipids, and proteins. (Another category, the nucleic acids, which are important in cellular functions, are discussed in Chapter 3.) All of these organic compounds contain carbon, hydrogen, and oxygen as their main ingredients.

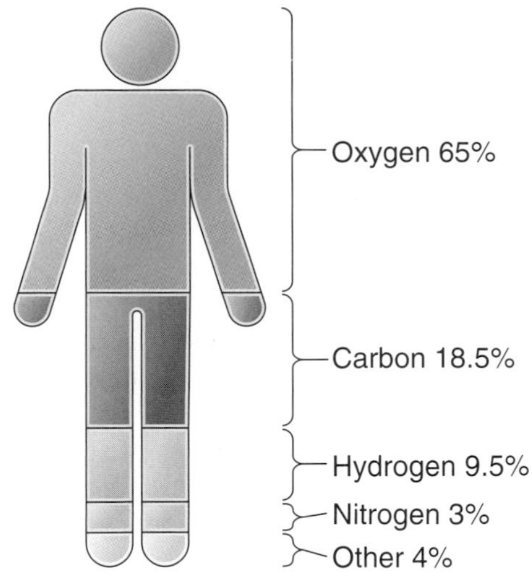

Figure 2-6 **Chemical composition of the body by weight.**

Carbohydrates, lipids, and proteins, in addition to minerals and vitamins, must be taken in as part of a normal diet. These compounds are discussed further in Chapters 19 and 20.

Checkpoint 2-11 Where are organic compounds found?

Checkpoint 2-12 What element is the basis of organic chemistry?

Carbohydrates The basic units of carbohydrates are simple sugars, or **monosaccharides** (mon-o-SAK-ah-rides) (Fig. 2-7 A). **Glucose** (GLU-kose), a simple sugar that circulates in the blood as a nutrient for cells, is an example of a monosaccharide. Two simple sugars may be linked together to form a **disaccharide** (Fig. 2-7 B), as represented by sucrose, table sugar. More complex carbohydrates, or **polysaccharides** (Fig. 2-7 C), consist of many simple sugars linked together with multiple side chains. Examples of polysaccharides are starch, which is manufactured in plant cells, and **glycogen** (GLI-ko-jen), a storage form of glucose found in liver cells and skeletal muscle cells. Carbohydrates in the form of sugars and starches are important sources of energy in the diet.

Lipids Lipids are a class of organic compounds mainly found in the body as **fat.** Fats provide insulation for the body and protection for organs. In addition, fats are the main form in which energy is stored.

Simple fats are made from a substance called **glycerol** (GLIS-er-ol), commonly known as glycerin, in combination with fatty acids (Fig. 2-8 A). One fatty acid is attached

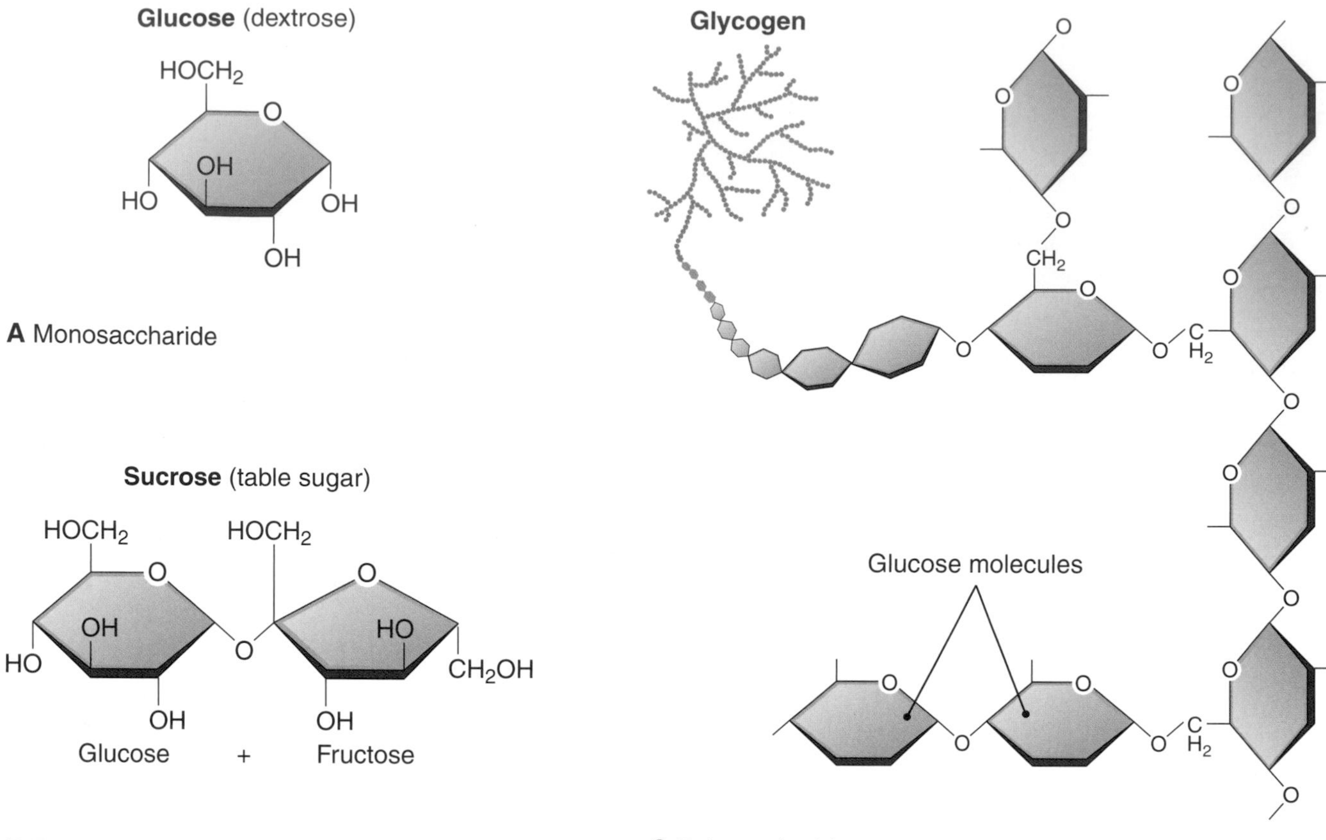

Figure 2-7 Examples of carbohydrates. A monosaccharide **(A)** is a simple sugar. A disaccharide **(B)** consists of two simple sugars linked together, whereas a polysaccharide **(C)** consists of many simple sugars linked together in chains. *ZOOMING IN ✦ What are the building blocks of disaccharides and polysaccharides?*

to each of the three carbon atoms in glycerol, so simple fats are described as **triglycerides** (tri-GLIS-er-ides). **Phospholipids** (fos-fo-LIP-ids) are complex lipids containing the element phosphorus. Among other functions, phospholipids make up a major part of the membrane around living cells. **Steroids** are lipids that contain rings of carbon atoms. They include **cholesterol** (ko-LES-ter-ol), another component of cell membranes (Fig. 2-8 B); the steroid hormones, such as cortisol, produced by the adrenal gland; the sex hormones, such as testosterone, produced by the testes; and estrogen and progesterone, produced by the ovaries.

Proteins All **proteins** (PRO-tenes) contain, in addition to carbon, hydrogen, and oxygen, the element **nitrogen** (NI-tro-jen). They may also contain sulfur or phosphorus. Proteins are the structural materials of the body, found in muscle, bone, and connective tissue. They also make up the pigments that give hair, eyes, and skin their color. It is protein that makes each individual physically distinct from others.

Proteins are composed of building blocks called **amino** (ah-ME-no) **acids** (Fig. 2-9 A). Although there are only about 20 different amino acids found in the body, a vast number of proteins can be made by linking them together in different sized molecules and in different combinations.

Each amino acid contains an acid group (COOH) and an amino group (NH_2), the part of the molecule that has the nitrogen. Many amino acids link together to form a polypeptide, which is then arranged into a particular shape. The polypeptide chain is coiled into a helix and may then be pleated or folded back on itself. Several chains also may be folded together (see Fig. 2-9 B). The overall shape of a protein is important to its function, as can be seen in the activity of enzymes.

> **Checkpoint 2-13** What are the three main categories of organic compounds?

Enzymes **Enzymes** (EN-zimes) are proteins that are essential for metabolism. They serve as **catalysts** in the hun-

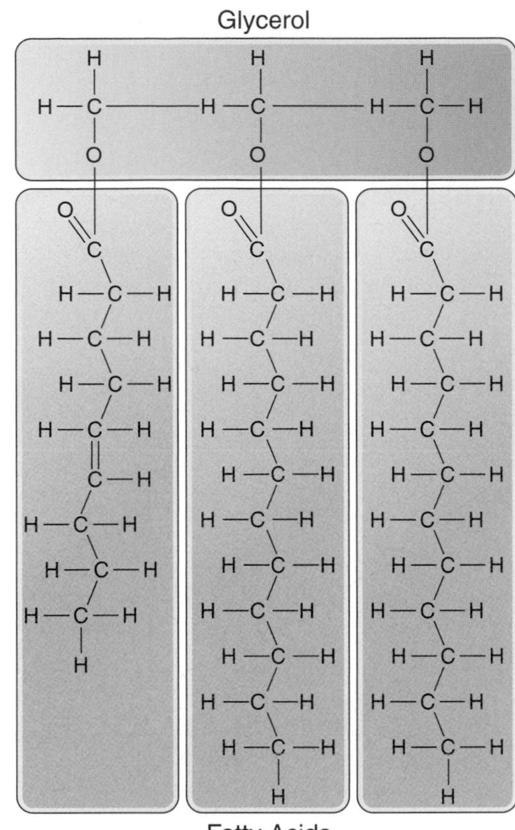

A Triglyceride (a simple fat)

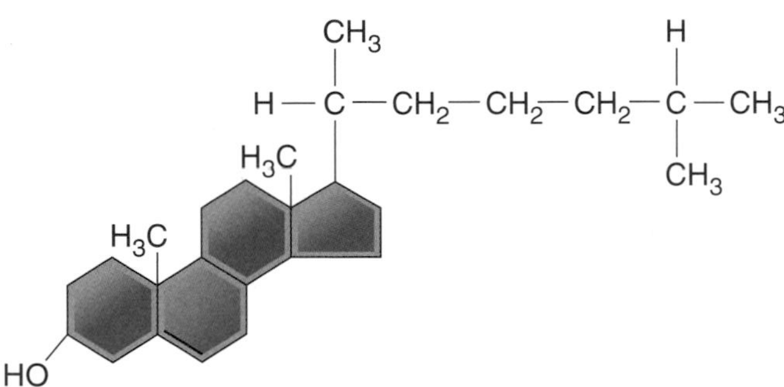

B Cholesterol (a steroid)

Figure 2-8 **Lipids. (A)** A triglyceride, a simple fat, contains glycerol combined with three fatty acids. **(B)** Cholesterol is a type of steroid, a lipid that contains rings of carbon atoms. *ZOOMING IN ✦ How many carbon atoms are in glycerol?*

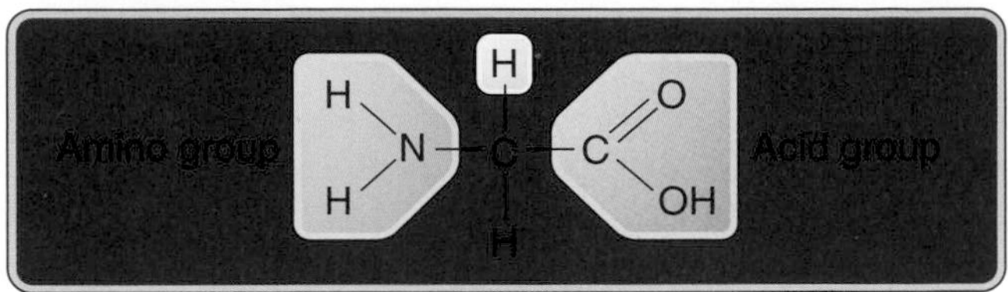

Simple amino acid

A

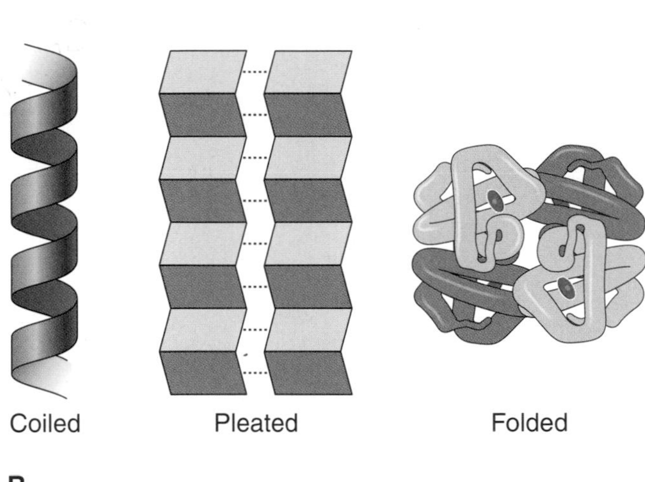

B

Figure 2-9 **Proteins. (A)** Amino acids are the building blocks of proteins. **(B)** Some shapes of proteins. *ZOOMING IN ✦ What part of an amino acid contains nitrogen?*

dreds of reactions that take place within cells. Without these catalysts, which speed the rate of chemical reactions, metabolism would not occur at a fast enough rate to sustain life. Because each enzyme works only on a specific substance, or **substrate**, and does only one specific chemical job, many different enzymes are needed. Like all catalysts, enzymes take part in reactions only temporarily; they are not used up or changed by the reaction. Therefore, they are needed in very small amounts. Many of the vitamins and minerals required in the diet are parts of enzymes.

The shape of the enzyme is important in its action. The enzyme's form must match the shape of the substrate or substrates the enzyme combines with in much the same way as a key fits a lock. This so-called "lock-and-key" mechanism is illustrated in Figure 2-10. Harsh conditions, such as extremes of temperature or pH, can alter the shape of an enzyme and stop its action. The alteration of any protein so that it can no longer function is termed **denaturation.** Such an event is always harmful to the cells.

You can usually recognize the names of enzymes because, with few exceptions, they end with the suffix *-ase*. Examples are lipase, protease, and oxidase. The first part of the name usually refers to the substance acted on or the type of reaction in which the enzyme is involved.

> **Checkpoint 2-14** Enzymes are proteins that act as catalysts. What is a catalyst?

For a description of professions that require knowledge of chemistry, see Box 2-3, Pharmacists and Pharmacy Technicians.

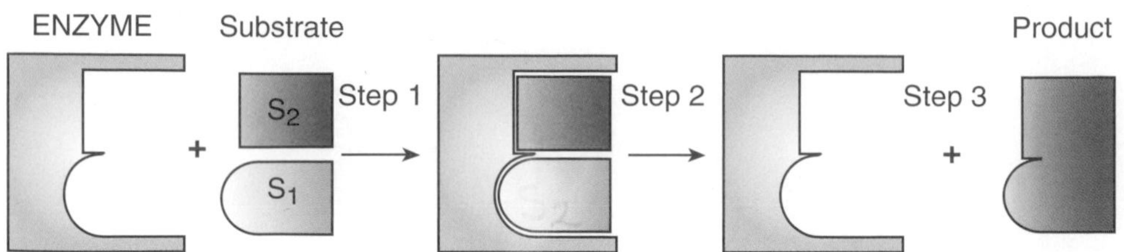

Figure 2-10 Diagram of enzyme action. The enzyme combines with substrate 1 (S_1) and substrate 2 (S_2). Once a new product is formed from the substrates, the enzyme is released unchanged. ***ZOOMING IN ✦ How does the shape of the enzyme before the reaction compare with its shape after the reaction.***

Box 2-3 · Health Professions

Pharmacists and Pharmacy Technicians

Medications are chemicals designed to treat illness and improve quality of life. The role of pharmacists and pharmacy technicians is to ensure that patients receive the correct medication and the education they need to use it effectively and derive the intended health benefits.

As key members of the healthcare team, pharmacists need a strong clinical background with a thorough understanding of chemistry, anatomy, and physiology. Pharmacists not only dispense prescription medications and monitor patients' responses to them, they also educate patients about their appropriate use. They share their expertise with other health professionals and also participate in clinical research on drugs and their effects.

Pharmacy technicians also require a thorough understanding of chemistry, anatomy, and physiology to assist pharmacists with their duties. State rules and regulations vary, but pharmacy technicians may perform many of the tasks related to dispensing medications, such as preparing them and packaging them with appropriate labels and instructions for use.

Most pharmacists and pharmacy technicians work in retail pharmacies, whereas others work in hospitals and long-term care facilities. Job prospects are promising because of the growing need for healthcare. In fact, pharmacy is projected to be one of the fastest growing careers in the United States. For more information about careers in pharmacy, contact the American Association of Colleges of Pharmacy.

Word Anatomy

Medical terms are built from standardized word parts (prefixes, roots, and suffixes). Learning the meanings of these parts can help you to remember words and interpret unfamiliar terms.

WORD PART	MEANING	EXAMPLE
Molecules and Compounds		
hydr/o	water	*Dehydration* is a deficiency of water.
phil	to like	*Hydrophilic* substances "like" water—they mix with or dissolve in it.
-phobia	fear	*Hydrophobic* substances "fear" water—they repel and do *not* dissolve in it.
hom/o	same	*Homogeneous* mixtures are the same throughout.
heter/o-	different	*Heterogeneous* solutions are different (not uniform) throughout.
aqu/e	water	In an *aqueous* solution, water is the solvent.
Chemical Bonds		
co-	together	*Covalent* bonds form when atoms share electrons.
Chemistry of Living Matter		
sacchar/o	sugar	A *monosaccharide* consists of one simple sugar.
mon/o-	one	In *monosaccharide*, "mono-" refers to one.
di-	twice, double	A *disaccharide* consists of two simple sugars.
poly-	many	A *polysaccharide* consists of many simple sugars.
glyc/o	sugar, glucose, sweet	*Glycogen* is a storage form of glucose. It breaks down to release (generate) glucose.
tri-	three	*Triglycerides* have one fatty acid attached to each of three carbon atoms.

WORD PART	MEANING	EXAMPLE
Chemistry of Living Matter		
de-	remove	*Denaturation* of a protein removes its ability to function (changes its nature).
-ase	suffix used in naming enzymes	A *lipase* is an enzyme that acts on lipids.

Summary

I. Elements—substances from which all matter is made
A. Atoms—subunits of elements
  1. Atomic structure
    a. Protons—positively charged particles in the nucleus
    b. Neutrons—noncharged particles in the nucleus
    c. Electrons—negatively charged particles in energy levels around the nucleus
  2. Energy levels—orbits that hold electrons at specific distances from the nucleus
    a. Valence—number of electrons lost or gained in chemical reactions

II. Molecules and compounds
  1. Molecules—combinations of two or more atoms
  2. Compounds—substances composed of different elements
A. The importance of water—solvent; stable; essential for metabolism
B. Mixtures: solutions and suspensions
  1. Mixtures: blend of two or more substances
  2. Solution: substance (solute) remains evenly distributed in solvent (*e.g.*, salt in water); homogeneous
  3. Suspension—material settles out of mixture on standing (*e.g.*, red cells in blood plasma); heterogeneous
  4. Colloid—particles do not dissolve but remain suspended (*e.g.*, cytosol)

III. Chemical bonds
A. Ionic bonds—formed by transfer of electrons from one atom to another
  1. Electrolytes
    a. Ionically bonded substances
    b. Separate in solution into charged particles (ions); cation positive and anion negative
    c. Conduct electric current
  2. Ions in body fluids important for proper function
B. Covalent bonds—formed by sharing of electrons between atoms
  1. Nonpolar—equal sharing of electrons (*e.g.*, hydrogen gas, H_2)
  2. Polar—unequal sharing of electrons (*e.g.*, water, H_2O)

IV. Compounds: acids, bases and salts
  1. Acids—donate hydrogen ions
  2. Bases—accept hydrogen ions
  3. Salts—formed by reaction between acid and base
A. The pH scale
  1. Measure of acidity or alkalinity of a solution
  2. Scale goes from 0 to 14
    a. 7 is neutral; below 7 is acidic; above 7 is alkaline (basic)
B. Buffer—maintains constant pH of a solution

V. Isotopes and radioactivity
  1. Isotopes—forms of an element that differ in atomic weights (number of neutrons)
    a. Radioactive isotope gives off rays of atomic particles
A. Use of radioactive isotopes
  1. Cancer therapy
  2. Diagnosis—tracers, x-rays

VI. Chemistry of living matter
A. Organic compounds—all contain carbon
  1. Carbohydrates (*e.g.*, sugars, starches); made of simple sugars (monosaccharides)
  2. Lipids (*e.g.*, fats, steroids); fats made of glycerol and fatty acids
  3. Proteins (*e.g.*, structural materials, enzymes); made of amino acids
    a. Enzymes—organic catalysts

Questions for Study and Review

Building Understanding

Fill in the blanks

1. The basic units of matter are ______.
2. The atomic number is the number of______ in an atom's nucleus.
3. A mixture of solute dissolved in solvent is called a(n) ______.
4. Blood has a pH of 7.35 to 7.45. Gastric juice has a pH of about 2.0. The more alkaline fluid is ______.
5. Proteins that catalyze metabolic reactions are called ______.

Matching

Match each numbered item with the most closely related lettered item.

___6. A simple carbohydrate such as glucose
___7. A complex carbohydrate such as glycogen
___8. An important component of cell membranes
___9. A hormone such as estrogen
___10. The basic building block of protein

a. polysaccharide
b. phospholipid
c. steroid
d. amino acid
e. monosaccharide

Multiple choice

___11. Red blood cells "floating" in plasma are an example of a mixture called a
   a. compound
   b. suspension
   c. colloid
   d. solution

___12. The most abundant compound in the body is
   a. carbohydrate
   b. protein
   c. lipid
   d. water

___13. A compound that releases ions when it is in solution is called a(n)
   a. solvent
   b. electrolyte
   c. anion
   d. colloid

___14. A chemical capable of donating hydrogen ions to other substances is called a(n)
   a. acid
   b. base
   c. salt
   d. catalyst

___15. Organic compounds always contain the element
   a. oxygen
   b. carbon
   c. nitrogen
   d. phosphorus

Understanding Concepts

16. Compare and contrast the following terms:
   a. element and atom
   b. molecule and compound
   c. proton, neutron, and electron
   d. anion and cation
   e. ionic bond and covalent bond
   f. acid and base

17. What are some of the properties of water that make it an ideal medium for living cells?

18. Explain the importance of ions in the structure and function of the human body.

19. What is pH? Discuss the role of buffers in maintaining pH homeostasis in the body.

20. Compare and contrast carbohydrates and proteins.

21. Describe three different types of lipid.

22. Define the term *enzyme* and discuss the relationship between enzyme structure and enzyme function.

Conceptual Thinking

23. Based on your understanding of strong acids and bases, why does the body have to be kept at a close-to-neutral pH?

24. Mrs. Alvarez has thyroid cancer and is undergoing radiation therapy. During one of her treatments she tells you that she had hoped her initial "thyroid scan" would have killed all of the cancer. Explain the difference between radiation therapy and nuclear medicine imaging.

25. Why do we need enzymes, when usually heat is used to speed up chemical reactions?

Selected Key Terms

The following terms and other boldface terms in the chapter are defined in the Glossary

active transport
cancer
chromosome
cytology
cytoplasm
diffusion
DNA
endocytosis
gene
interphase
isotonic
micrometer
microscope
mitochondria
mitosis
mutation
nucleotide
nucleus
organelle
osmosis
phagocytosis
plasma membrane
ribosome
RNA

Learning Outcomes

After careful study of this chapter, you should be able to:

1. List three types of microscopes used to study cells
2. Describe the function and composition of the plasma membrane
3. Describe the cytoplasm of the cell, including the name and function of the main organelles
4. Describe the composition, location, and function of the DNA in the cell
5. Compare the function of three types of RNA in the cells
6. Explain briefly how cells make proteins
7. Name and briefly describe the stages in mitosis
8. Define eight methods by which substances enter and leave cells
9. Explain what will happen if cells are placed in solutions with concentrations the same as or different from those of the cell fluids
10. Define *cancer*
11. List several risk factors for cancer
12. Show how word parts are used to build words related to cells and their functions (see Word Anatomy at the end of the chapter)

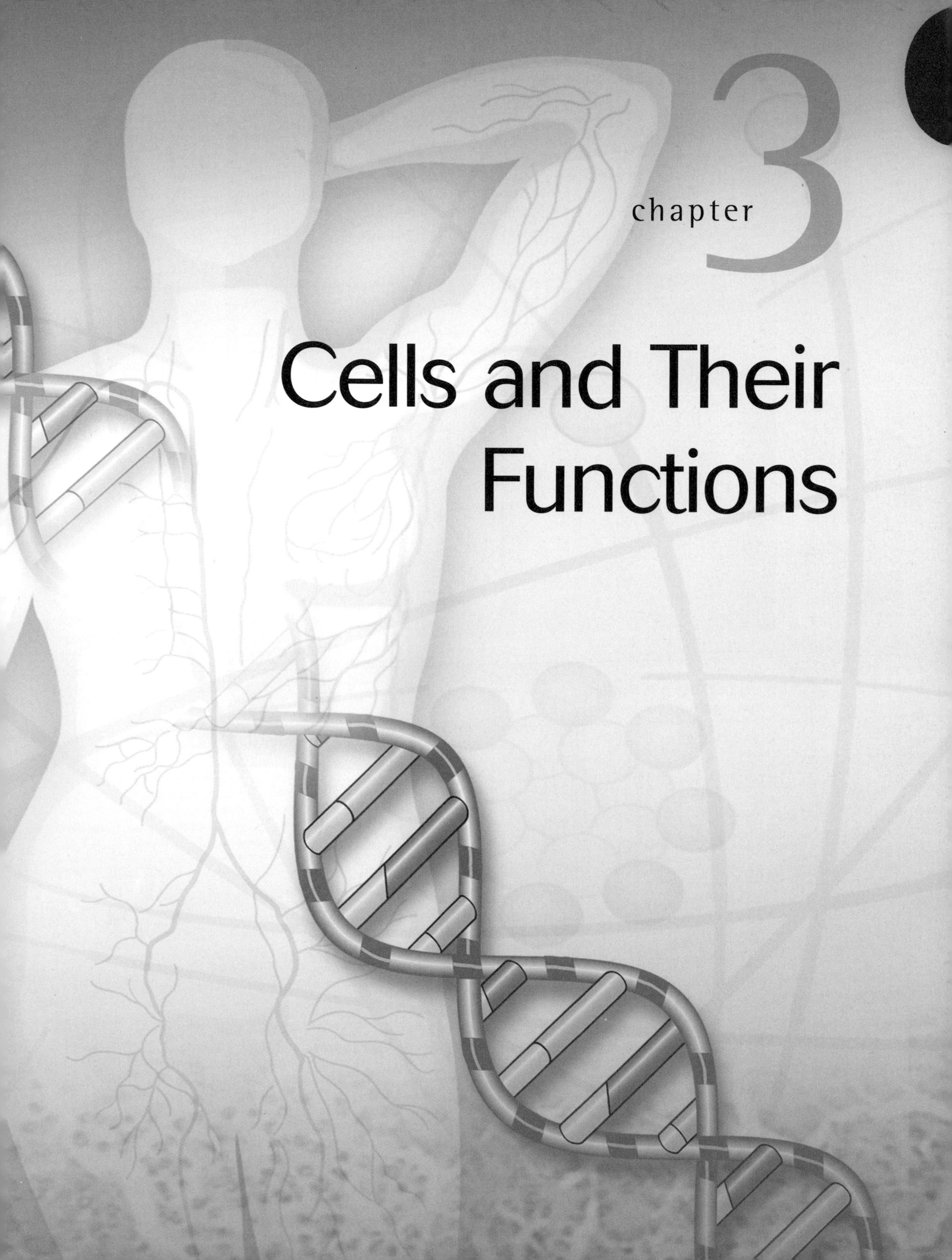

chapter 3

Cells and Their Functions

The Role of Cells

The **cell** (sel) is the basic unit of all life. It is the simplest structure that shows all the characteristics of life, including organization, metabolism, responsiveness, homeostasis, growth, and reproduction. In fact, it is possible for a single cell to live independently of other cells. Examples of some free-living cells are microscopic organisms such as protozoa and bacteria, some of which produce disease. In a multicellular organism, cells make up all tissues. All the activities of the human body, which is composed of trillions of cells, result from the activities of individual cells. Cells produce all the materials manufactured within the body. The study of cells is **cytology** (si-TOL-o-je).

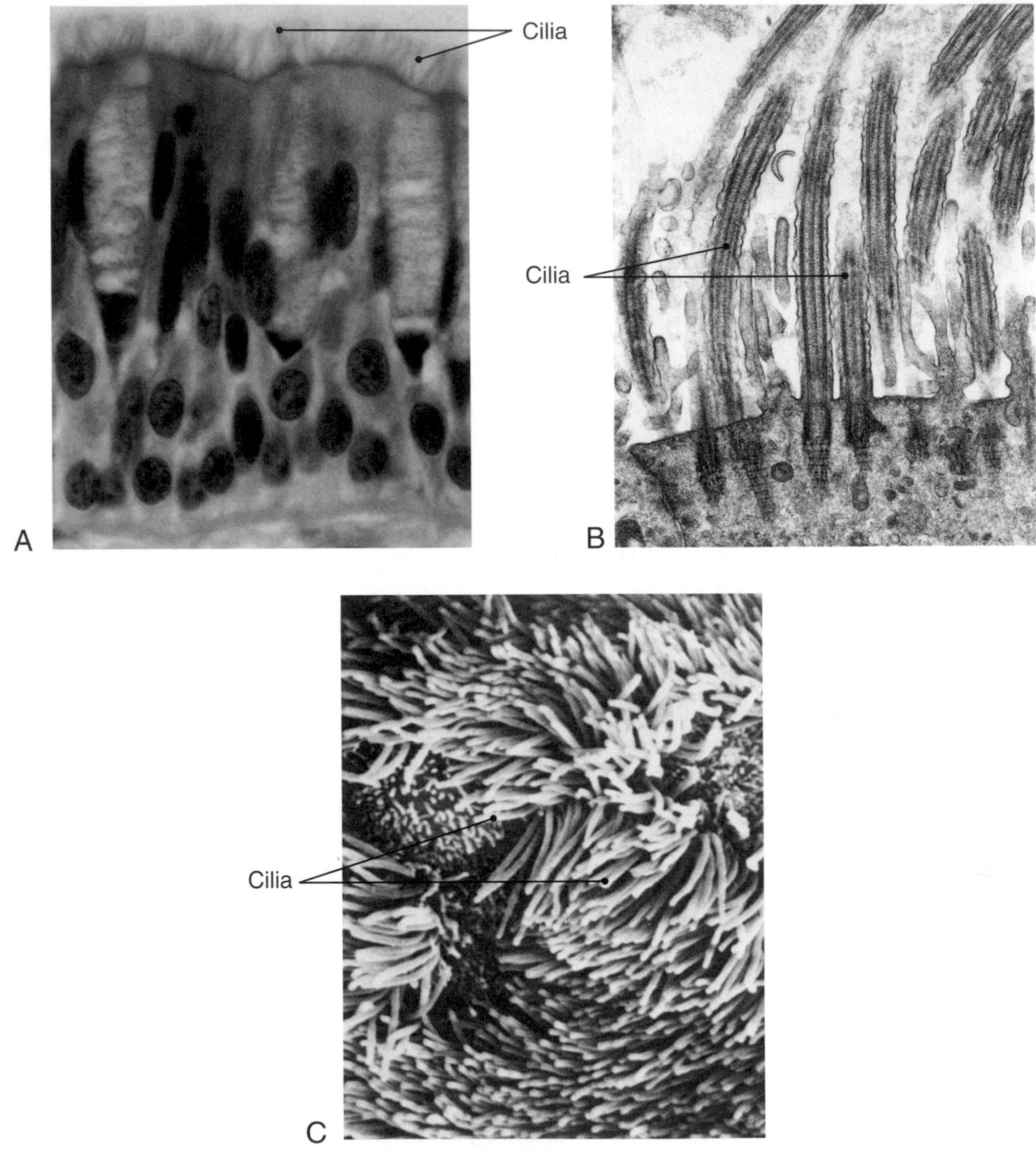

Figure 3-1 Cilia photographed under three different microscopes. (A) Cilia (hairlike projections) in cells lining the trachea under the highest magnification of a compound light microscope (1000×) **(B)** Cilia in the bronchial lining viewed with a transmission electron microscope (TEM). Internal components are visible at this much higher magnification. **(C)** Cilia on cells lining an oviduct as seen with a scanning electron microscope (SEM) (7000×). A three dimensional view can be seen. (A, Reprinted with permission from Cormack DH. Essential histology. 2nd ed. Philadelphia: Lippincott Williams & Wilkins, 2001. B, Reprinted with permission from Quinton P, Martinez R, eds. Fluid and electrolyte transport in exocrine glands in cystic fibrosis. San Francisco: San Francisco Press, 1982. C, Reprinted with permission from Hafez ESE, ed. Scanning electron microscopic atlas of mammalian reproduction. Tokyo: Igaku Shoin, 1975.) ***ZOOMING IN ✦ Which microscope shows the most internal structure of the cilia? Which shows the cilia in three dimensions?***

Microscopes

The outlines of cells were first seen in dried plant tissue almost 350 years ago. Study of their internal structure, however, depended on improvements in the design of the **microscope**, a magnifying instrument needed to examine structures not visible with the naked eye. The single-lens microscope used in the late 17th century was later replaced by the **compound light microscope** most commonly used in laboratories today. This instrument, which can magnify an object up to 1000 times, has two lenses and uses visible light for illumination. A much more powerful microscope, the **transmission electron microscope** (TEM), uses an electron beam in place of visible light and can magnify an image up to 1 million times. Another type of microscope, the **scanning electron microscope** (SEM), does not magnify as much (100,000×) and shows only surface features, but gives a three-dimensional view of an object. Figure 3-1 shows some cell structures viewed with each of these types of microscopes. The structures are cilia, short, hairlike projections from the cell that move nearby fluids. The metric unit used for microscopic measurements is the **micrometer** (MI-kro-me-ter), formerly called a micron. This unit is 1/1000 of a millimeter and is symbolized with the Greek letter mu (μ), as μm.

Before a scientist can examine cells and tissues under a microscope, he or she must usually color them with special dyes called **stains** to aid in viewing. These stains produce the variety of colors seen in pictures of cells and tissues taken under a microscope.

Checkpoint 3-1 The cell is the basic unit of life. What characteristics of life does it show?

Checkpoint 3-2 Name three types of microscopes.

Cell Structure

Just as people may look different but still have certain features in common—two eyes, a nose, and a mouth, for example—all cells share certain characteristics. Refer to Figure 3-2 as we describe some of the parts that are common to most animal cells. Table 3-1 summarizes information about the main cell parts.

Plasma Membrane

The outer limit of the cell is the **plasma membrane**, formerly called the *cell membrane* (Fig. 3-3). The plasma membrane not only encloses the cell contents but also participates in many cellular activities, such as growth, reproduction, and interactions between cells, and is especially important in regulating what can enter and leave the cell. The main substance of this membrane is a double layer of lipid molecules, described as a bilayer. Because these lipids contain the element phosphorus, they are called **phospholipids**. Some molecules of cholesterol, another type of lipid, are located between the phospholipids. Cholesterol strengthens the membrane.

A variety of different proteins float within the lipid bilayer. Some of these proteins extend all the way through the membrane, and some are located near the inner or outer surfaces of the membrane. The importance of these proteins will be revealed in later chapters, but they are listed here along with their functions (Table 3-2):

- Channels—pores in the membrane that allow specific substances to enter or leave. Certain ions travel through channels in the membrane.

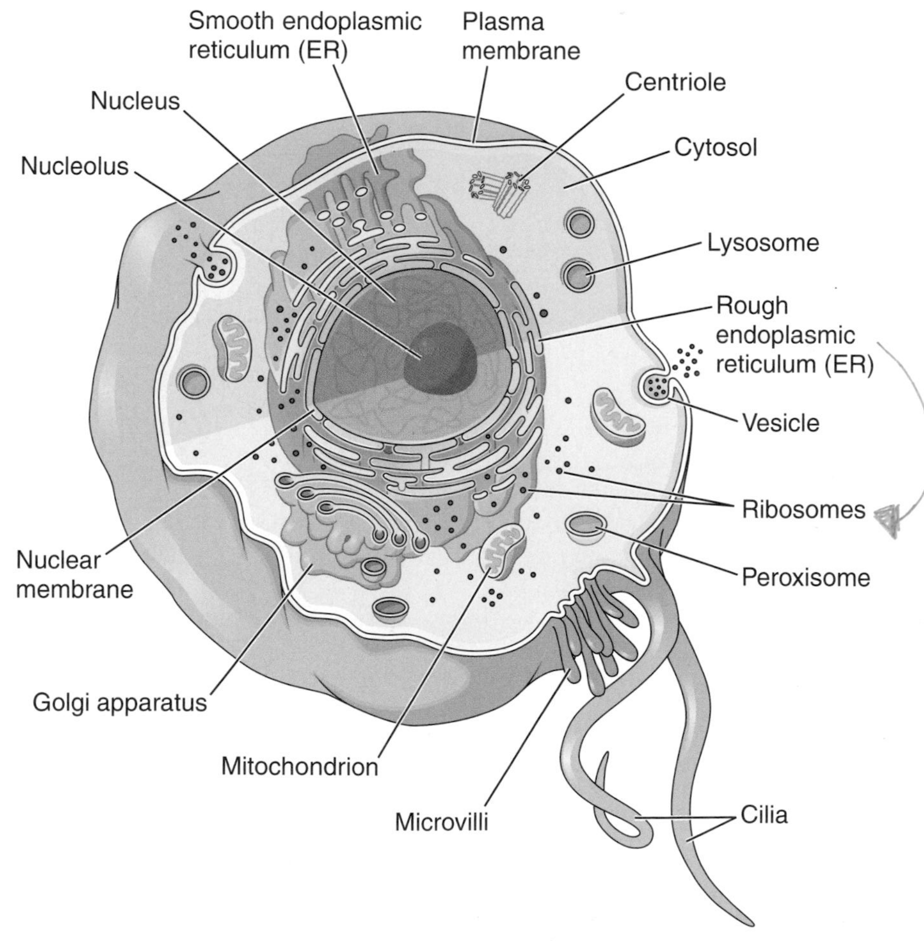

Figure 3-2 A generalized animal cell, sectional view. *ZOOMING IN ✦ What is attached to the ER to make it look rough? What is the liquid part of the cytoplasm called?*

Table 3•1 Cell Parts

NAME	DESCRIPTION	FUNCTION
Plasma membrane	Outer layer of the cell; composed mainly of lipids and proteins	Encloses the cell contents; regulates what enters and leaves the cell; participates in many activities, such as growth, reproduction, and interactions between cells
Microvilli	Short extensions of the cell membrane	Absorb materials into the cell
Nucleus	Large, dark-staining organelle near the center of the cell, composed of DNA and proteins	Contains the chromosomes, the hereditary units that direct all cellular activities
Nucleolus	Small body in the nucleus; composed of RNA, DNA, and protein	Makes ribosomes
Cytoplasm	Colloidal suspension that fills the cell from the nuclear membrane to the plasma membrane	Site of many cellular activities, consists of cytosol and organelles
Cytosol	The fluid portion of the cytoplasm	Surrounds the organelles
Endoplasmic reticulum (ER)	Network of membranes within the cytoplasm. Rough ER has ribosomes attached to it; smooth ER does not.	Rough ER sorts proteins and forms them into more complex compounds; smooth ER is involved with lipid synthesis
Ribosomes	Small bodies free in the cytoplasm or attached to the ER; composed of RNA and protein	Manufacture proteins
Mitochondria	Large organelles with folded membranes inside	Convert energy from nutrients into ATP
Golgi apparatus	Layers of membranes	Makes compounds containing proteins; sorts and prepares these compounds for transport to other parts of the cell or out of the cell
Saclike bodies	Small, membrane-enclosed bodies	Store materials, transport materials through the plasma membrane, or destroy waste material
Lysosomes	Small sacs of digestive enzymes	Digest substances within the cell
Peroxisomes	Membrane-enclosed organelles containing enzymes	Break down harmful substances
Vesicles	Small membrane-bound bubbles in the cytoplasm	Store materials and move materials into or out of the cell in bulk
Centrioles	Rod-shaped bodies (usually two) near the nucleus	Help separate the chromosomes during cell division
Surface projections	Structures that extend from the cell	Move the cell or the fluids around the cell
Cilia	Short, hairlike projections from the cell	Move the fluids around the cell
Flagellum	Long, whiplike extension from the cell	Moves the cell

- Transporters—shuttle substances from one side of the membrane to the other. Glucose, for example, is carried into cells using transporters.
- Receptors—points of attachment for materials coming to the cell in the blood or tissue fluid. Some hormones, for example, must attach to receptors on the cell surface before they can act upon the cell, as described in Chapter 12 on the endocrine system.
- Enzymes—participate in reactions occurring at the plasma membrane.
- Linkers—give structure to the membrane and help attach cells to other cells.
- Cell identity markers—proteins unique to an individual's cells. These are important in the immune system and are also a factor in transplantation of tissue from one person to another.

Carbohydrates are present in small amounts in the plasma membrane, combined either with proteins (glycoproteins) or with lipids (glycolipids). These carbohydrates help cells to recognize each other and to stick together.

In some cells, the plasma membrane is folded out into multiple small projections called **microvilli** (mi-kro-VIL-li). Microvilli increase the surface area of the membrane, allowing for greater absorption of materials from the cell's environment, just as a sponge absorbs water. Microvilli are found on cells that line the small intestine, where they promote absorption of digested foods into the circulation. They are also found on kidney cells, where they reabsorb materials that have been filtered out of the blood.

> **Checkpoint 3-3** The outer limit of the cell is a complex membrane. What is the main substance of this membrane and what are three types of materials found within the membrane?

The Nucleus

Just as the body has different organs to carry out special functions, the cell contains specialized structures that perform different tasks. These structures are called **or-**

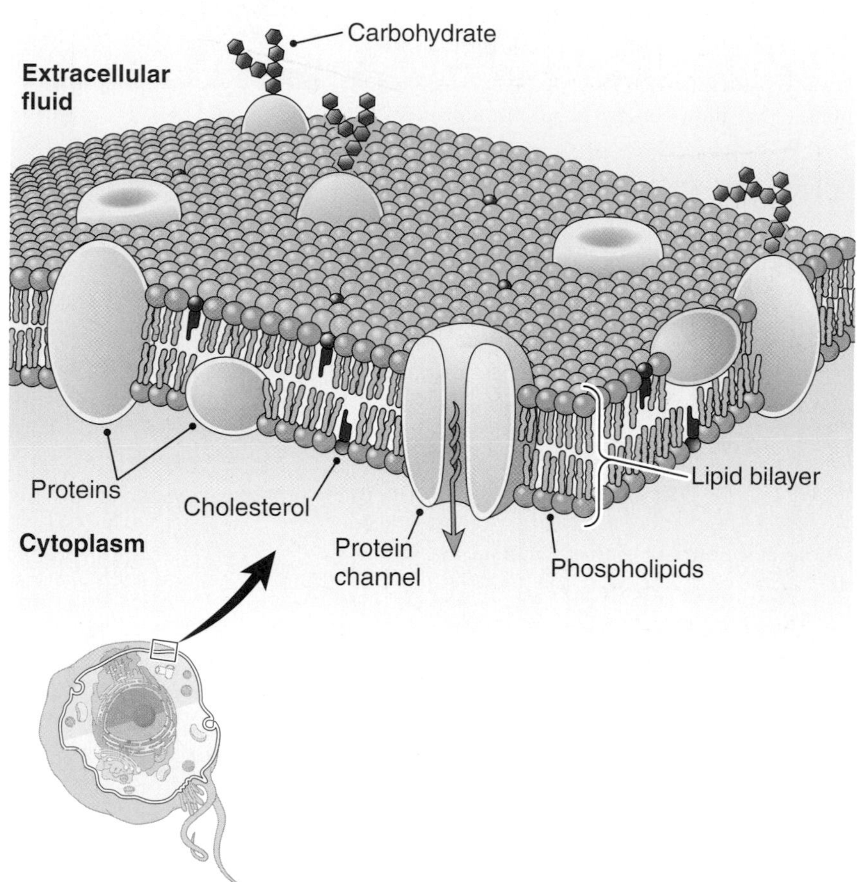

Figure 3-3 **The plasma membrane.** This drawing shows the current concept of its structure. *ZOOMING IN ✦ How many layers make up the main substance of the plasma membrane?*

ganelles, which means "little organs." The largest of the organelles is the **nucleus** (NU-kle-us).

The nucleus is often called the *control center* of the cell because it contains the chromosomes, the threadlike units of heredity that are passed on from parents to their offspring. It is information contained in the **chromosomes** (KRO-mo-somes) that governs all cellular activities, as described later in this chapter. Most of the time, the chromosomes are loosely distributed throughout the nucleus, giving that organelle a uniform, dark appearance when stained and examined under a microscope (see Fig. 3-2). When the cell is dividing, however, the chromosomes tighten into their visible threadlike forms.

Within the nucleus is a smaller globule called the **nucleolus** (nu-KLE-o-lus), which means "little nucleus." The job of the nucleolus is to assemble ribosomes, small bodies outside the nucleus that are involved in the manufacture of proteins.

Checkpoint 3-4 What are cell organelles?

Checkpoint 3-5 Why is the nucleus called the control center of the cell?

The Cytoplasm

The remaining organelles are part of the **cytoplasm** (SI-to-plazm), the material that fills the cell from the nuclear membrane to the plasma membrane. The liquid part of the cytoplasm is the **cytosol**, a suspension of nutrients, minerals, enzymes, and other specialized materials in water. The main organelles are described here (see Table 3-1).

The **endoplasmic reticulum** (en-do-PLAS-mik re-TIK-u-lum) is a network of membranes located between the nuclear membrane and the plasma membrane. Its name literally means "network" (reticulum) "within the cytoplasm" (endoplasmic), but for ease, it is almost always called simply the **ER**. In some areas, the ER appears to have an even surface, and is described as *smooth ER*. This type of ER is involved with the synthesis of lipids. In other areas, the ER has a gritty, uneven surface, causing it to be described as *rough ER*. The texture of rough ER comes from small bodies, called **ribosomes** (RI-bo-somz), attached to its surface. Ribosomes are necessary for the manufacture of proteins, as described later. They may be attached to the ER or be free in the cytoplasm.

The **mitochondria** (mi-to-KON-dre-ah) are large organelles that are round or bean-shaped with folded membranes on the inside. Within the mitochondria, the energy from nutrients is converted to energy for the cell in the form of ATP. Mitochondria are the "power plants" of the cell. Active cells, such as muscle cells or sperm cells, need lots of energy and thus have large numbers of mitochondria.

Another organelle in a typical cell is the **Golgi** (GOL-je) **apparatus** (also called Golgi complex), a stack of membranous sacs involved in sorting and modifying proteins and then packaging them for export from the cell.

Several types of organelles appear as small sacs in the cytoplasm. These include **lysosomes** (LI-so-somz), which contain digestive enzymes. Lysosomes remove waste and foreign materials from the cell. They are also involved in destroying old and damaged cells as needed for repair and remodeling of tissue. **Peroxisomes** (per-OK-sih-somz) have enzymes that destroy harmful substances produced in metabolism (see Box 3-1, Lysosomes and Peroxisomes: Cellular Recycling). **Vesicles** (VES-ih-klz) are small, membrane-bound bubbles used for storage. They can be used to move materials into or out of the cell, as described later.

Table 3•2 Proteins in the Plasma Membrane and Their Functions

TYPE OF PROTEIN	FUNCTION	ILLUSTRATION
Channels	Pores in the membrane that allow passage of specific substances, such as ions	
Transporters	Shuttle substances, such as glucose, across the membrane	
Receptors	Allow for attachment of substances, such as hormones, to the membrane	
Enzymes	Participate in reactions at the surface of the membrane	
Linkers	Give structure to the membrane and attach cells to other cells	
Cell identity markers	Proteins unique to a person's cells; important in the immune system and in transplantation of tissue from one person to another	

Box 3-1 Clinical Perspectives

Lysosomes and Peroxisomes: Cellular Recycling

Two organelles that play a vital role in cellular disposal and recycling are lysosomes and peroxisomes. **Lysosomes** contain enzymes that break down carbohydrates, lipids, proteins, and nucleic acids. These powerful enzymes must be kept within the lysosome because they would digest the cell if they escaped. In a process called **autophagy** (aw-TOF-ah-je), the cell uses lysosomes to safely recycle cellular structures, fusing with and digesting worn out organelles. The digested components then return to the cytoplasm for reuse. Lysosomes also break down foreign material, as when cells known as **phagocytes** *(FAG-o-sites)* engulf bacteria and then use lysosomes to destroy them. The cell may also use lysosomes to digest itself during **autolysis** (aw-TOL-ih-sis), a normal part of development. Cells that are no longer needed "self-destruct" by releasing lysosomal enzymes into their own cytoplasm.

Peroxisomes are small membranous sacs that resemble lysosomes but contain different kinds of enzymes. They break down toxic substances that may enter the cell, such as drugs and alcohol, but their most important function is to break down free radicals. These substances are byproducts of normal metabolic reactions but can kill the cell if not neutralized by peroxisomes.

Disease may result if either lysosomes or peroxisomes are unable to function. In Tay-Sachs disease, nerve cells' lysosomes lack an enzyme that breaks down certain kinds of lipids. These lipids build up inside the cells, causing malfunction that leads to brain injury, blindness, and death. Disease may also result if lysosomes or peroxisomes function when they should not. Some investigators believe this is the case in autoimmune diseases, in which the body develops an immune response to its own cells. Phagocytes engulf the cells and lysosomes destroy them. In addition, body cells themselves may self-destruct through autolysis. The joint disease rheumatoid arthritis is one such example.

Centrioles (SEN-tre-olz) are rod-shaped bodies near the nucleus that function in cell division. They help to organize the cell and divide the cell contents during this process.

Surface Organelles

Some cells have structures projecting from their surface that are used for motion. **Cilia** (SIL-e-ah) are small, hairlike projections that wave, creating movement of the fluids around the cell. For example, cells that line the passageways of the respiratory tract have cilia that move impurities out of the system. Ciliated cells in the female reproductive tract move the egg cell along the oviduct toward the uterus.

A long, whiplike extension from the cell is a **flagellum** (flah-JEL-lum). The only type of cell in the human body that has a flagellum is the sperm cell of the male. Each human sperm cell has a flagellum that is used to propel the sperm cell toward the egg in the female reproductive tract.

Cellular Diversity

Although all body cells have some fundamental similarities, individual cells may vary widely in size, shape, and composition according to the function of each. The average cell size is 10 to 15 μm, but cells may range in size from the 7 μm of a red blood cell to the 200 μm or more in the length of a muscle cell.

Cell shape is related to cell function (Fig. 3-4). A neuron (nerve cell) has long fibers that transmit electrical energy from place to place in the nervous system. Cells in surface layers have a modified shape that covers and protects the tissue beneath. Red blood cells are small and round, which lets them slide through tiny blood vessels. They also have a thin outer membrane to allow for passage of gases into and out of the cell. As red blood cells mature, they lose the nucleus and most of the other organelles, making the greatest possible amount of space available to carry oxygen.

Aside from cilia and flagella, most human cells have all the organelles described above. These may vary in number, however. For example, cells producing lipids have lots of smooth ER. Cells that secrete proteins have lots of ribosomes and a prominent Golgi apparatus. All active cells have lots of mitochondria to manufacture the ATP needed for energy.

Checkpoint 3-6 What are the two types of organelles used for movement, and what do they look like?

Protein Synthesis

Because protein molecules play an indispensable part in the structure and function of the body, we need to identify the cellular substances that direct the production of proteins. As noted, the hereditary units that govern the cell are the chromosomes in the nucleus. Each chromosome in turn is divided into multiple subunits, called **genes** (Fig. 3-5). It is the genes that carry the messages for the development of particular inherited characteristics, such as brown eyes, curly hair, or blood type, and they do so by directing the manufacture of proteins in the cell.

Nucleic Acids: DNA and RNA

The genes are distinct segments of the complex organic chemical that makes up the chromosomes, a substance called **deoxyribonucleic** (de-ok-se-RI-bo-nu-kle-ik) **acid**, or **DNA**. DNA is composed of subunits called **nucleotides** (NU-kle-o-tides) (see Fig. 3-5). A related compound, **ribonucleic** (RI-bo-nu-kle-ik) **acid**, or **RNA**, which also

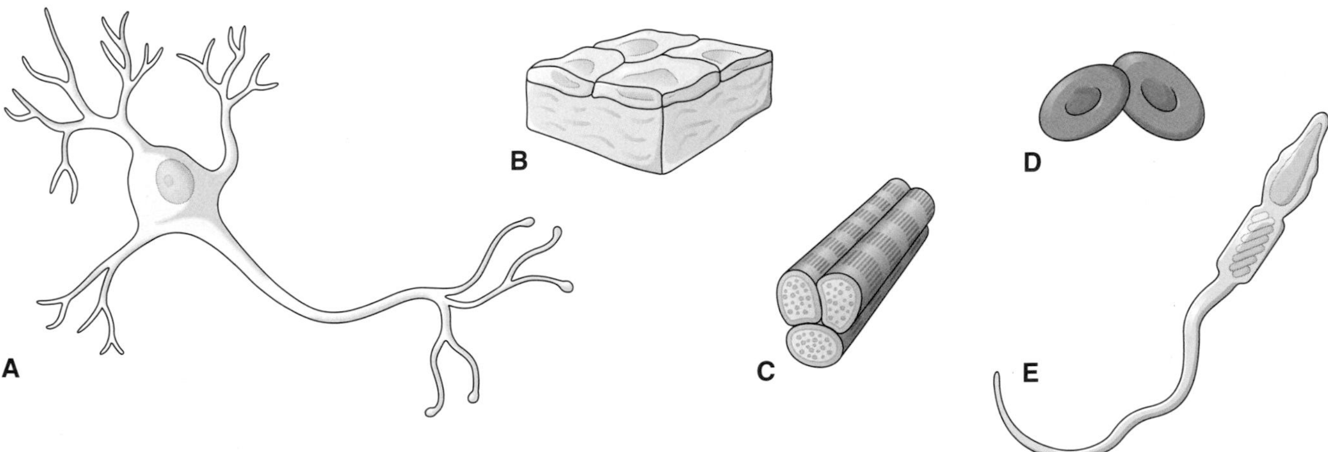

Figure 3-4 **Cellular diversity.** Cells vary in structure according to their functions. **(A)** A neuron has long extensions that pick up and transmit electrical impulses. **(B)** Epithelial cells cover and protect underlying tissue. **(C)** Muscle cells have fibers that produce contraction. **(D)** Red blood cells lose most organelles, which maximizes their oxygen-carrying capacity, and have a small, round shape that lets them slide through blood vessels. **(E)** A sperm cell is small and light and swims with a flagellum. ***ZOOMING IN ✦ Which of the cells shown would best cover a large surface area?***

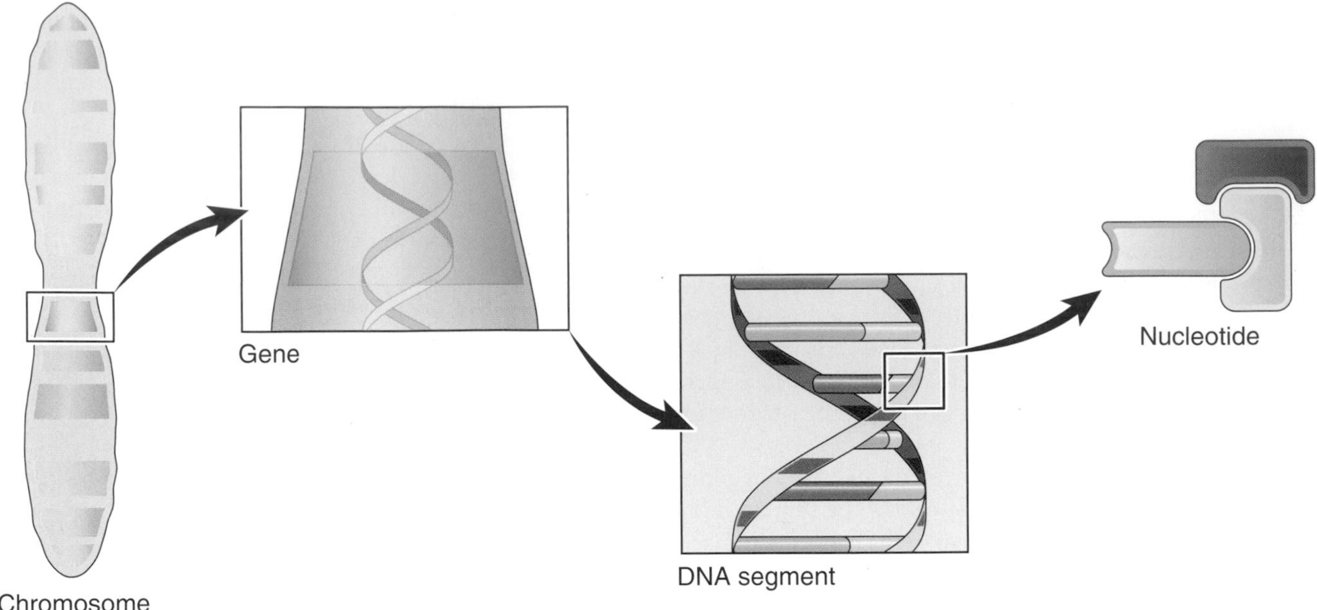

Figure 3-5 **Subdivisions of a chromosome.** A gene is a distinct region of a chromosome. The entire chromosome is made of DNA. Nucleotides are the building blocks of DNA.

participates in protein synthesis but is not part of the chromosomes, is also composed of nucleotides. There are four different nucleotides in DNA and four in RNA, but only three of these are common to both. Both DNA and RNA have the nucleotides adenine (A), guanine (G), and cytosine (C), but DNA has thymine (T), whereas RNA has uracil (U). Table 3-3 compares the structure and function of DNA and RNA.

Moving one step deeper into the structure of the nucleic acids, each nucleotide is composed of four units:

- A sugar, which in RNA is ribose and in DNA is a ribose that is missing one oxygen atom (that is, deoxyribose)
- A phosphorus-containing portion, or phosphate
- A nitrogen-containing portion known as a nitrogen base

The sugar and phosphate alternate to form a long chain to which the nitrogen bases are attached. It is variation in the nitrogen bases that accounts for the differences in the five different nucleotides.

DNA Most of the DNA in the cell is organized into chromosomes within the nucleus (a small amount of DNA is in the mitochondria located in the cytoplasm). Looking at Figure 3-6, which shows a section of a chromosome, you can see that the DNA exists as a double strand. Visualizing the complete molecule as a ladder, the sugar and phosphate units of the nucleotides make up the "side rails" of the ladder, and the nitrogen bases project from the side rails to make up the "steps" of the ladder. The two DNA strands are paired very specifically according to the identity of the nitrogen bases in the nucleotides. The adenine (A) nucleotide always pairs with the thymine (T) nucleotide; the guanine (G) nucleotide always pairs with the cytosine (C) nucleotide. The two strands of DNA are held together by weak bonds (hydrogen binds; see Box

Table 3•3 Comparison of DNA and RNA

	DNA	RNA
Location	Almost entirely in the nucleus	Almost entirely in the cytoplasm
Composition	Nucleotides: adenine (A), guanine (G), cytosine (C), thymine (T) Sugar: deoxyribose	Nucleotides: adenine (A), guanine (G), cytosine (C), uracil (U) Sugar: ribose
Structure	Double-stranded helix formed by nucleotide pairing A-T; G-C	Single strand
Function	Makes up the chromosomes, hereditary units that control all cell activities; divided into genes that carry the nucleotide codes for the manufacture of proteins	Manufacture proteins according to the nucleotide codes carried in the DNA; three types: messenger RNA (mRNA), ribosomal RNA (rRNA), and transfer RNA (tRNA)

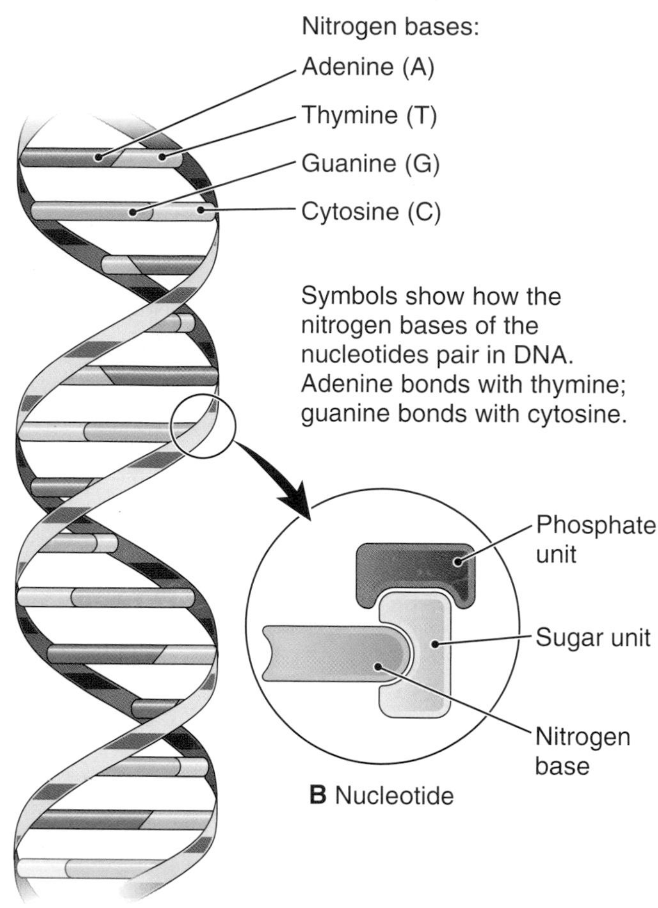

Figure 3-6 Structure of DNA. (A) This schematic representation of a chromosome segment shows the paired nucleic acid strands twisted into a double helix. **(B)** Each structural unit, or nucleotide, consists of a phosphate unit and a sugar unit attached to a nitrogen base. The sugar unit in DNA is deoxyribose. There are four different nucleotides in DNA. Their arrangement "spells out" the genetic instructions that control all activities of the cell. *ZOOMING IN ✦ Two of the DNA nucleotides (A and G) are larger in size than the other two (T and C). How do the nucleotides pair up with regard to size?*

2-1). The doubled strands then coil into a spiral, giving DNA the descriptive name *double helix.*

The message of the DNA that makes up the individual genes is actually contained in the varying pattern of the four nucleotides along the strand. The nucleotides are like four letters in an alphabet that can be combined in different ways to make a variety of words. The words represent the amino acids used to make proteins, and a long string of words makes up a gene. Each gene thus codes for the building of amino acids into a specific cellular protein. Remember that all enzymes are proteins, and enzymes are essential for all cellular reactions. DNA is thus the master blueprint for the cell.

In light of observations on cellular diversity, you may wonder how different cells in the body can vary in appearance and function if they all have the same amount and same kind of DNA. The answer to this question is that only portions of the DNA in a given cell are active at any one time. In some cells, regions of the DNA can be switched on and off, under the influence of hormones, for example. However, as cells differentiate during development and become more specialized, regions of the DNA are permanently shut down, leading to the variations in the different cell types. Scientists now realize that the control of DNA action throughout the life of the cell is a very complex matter involving not only the DNA itself but proteins as well.

Checkpoint 3-7 What are the building blocks of nucleic acids?

Checkpoint 3-8 What category of compounds does DNA code for in the cell?

The Role of RNA A blueprint is only a guide. The information it contains must be interpreted by appropriate actions, and RNA is the substance needed for these steps. RNA is much like DNA except that it exists as a single strand of nucleotides and has the nucleotide uracil (U) instead of thymine (T). Thus, when RNA pairs up with another molecule of nucleic acid to manufacture proteins, as explained below, adenine (A) bonds with uracil (U) in the RNA instead of thymine (T).

A detailed account of protein synthesis is beyond the scope of this book, but a highly simplified description and illustrations of the process are presented. The process begins with the transfer of information from DNA to RNA in the nucleus, a process known as *transcription* (Fig. 3-7). Before transcription begins, the DNA breaks its weak bonds and uncoils into single strands. Then a matching strand of RNA forms along one of the DNA strands by the process of nucleotide pairing. (For example, if the DNA strand reads CGAT, the corresponding mRNA will read GCUA. Recall that RNA uses the nucleotide U instead of A.) When complete, this messenger RNA (mRNA) leaves the nucleus and travels to a ribosome in the cytoplasm (Fig. 3-8). Recall that ribosomes are the site of protein synthesis in the cell.

Ribosomes are composed of a type of RNA called ribosomal RNA (rRNA) and also protein. At the ribosomes, the genetic message now contained within mRNA is decoded to build amino acids into the long chains that form proteins, a process termed *translation.* This final step requires a third type of RNA, transfer RNA (tRNA), small molecules present in the cytoplasm (see Fig. 3-8). Each transfer RNA carries a specific amino acid that can be added to a protein chain. A nucleotide code on each tRNA determines whether or not its amino acid will be added. After the amino acid chain is formed, it must be coiled and folded into the proper shape for that protein, as noted in Chapter 2. Table 3-4 summarizes information on the

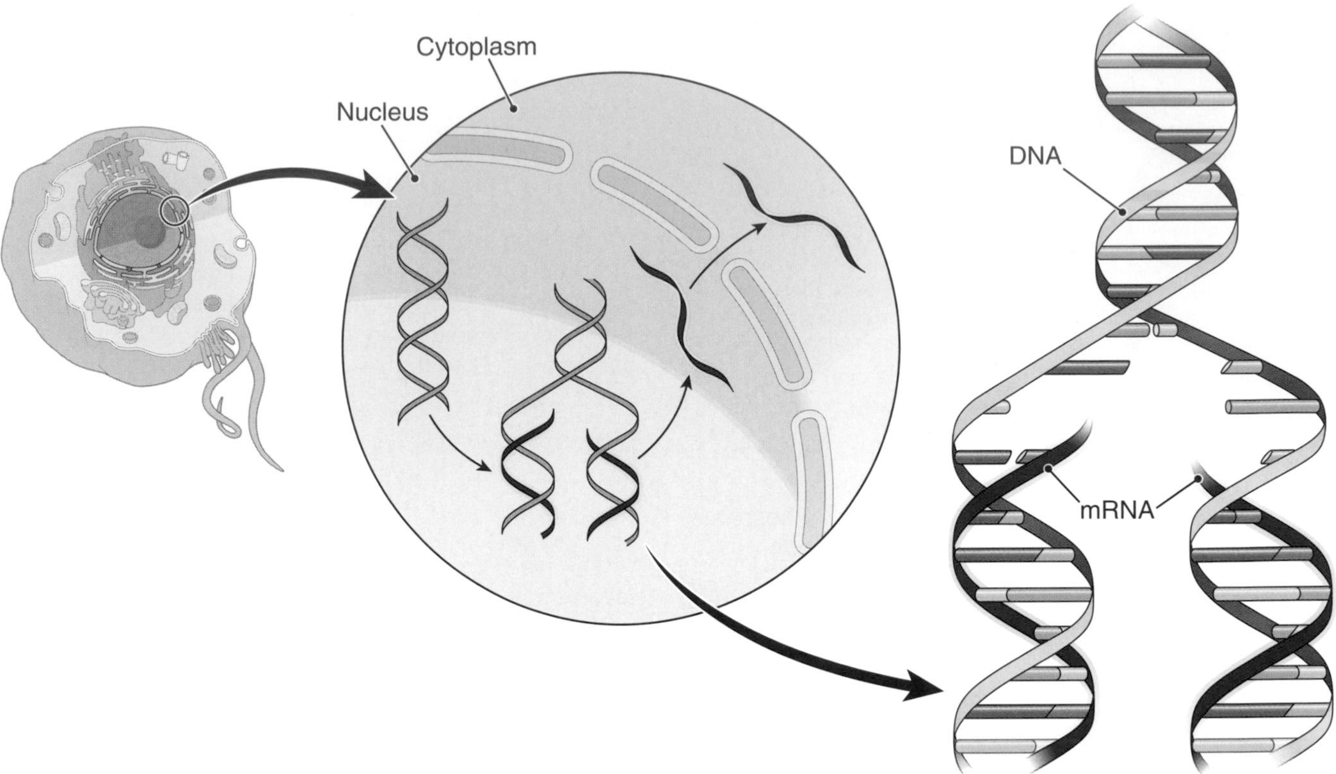

Figure 3-7 **Transcription.** In the first step of protein synthesis the DNA code is transcribed into messenger RNA (mRNA) by nucleotide base pairing. An enlarged view of the nucleic acids during transcription shows how mRNA forms according to the nucleotide pattern of the DNA. Note that adenine (A, red) in DNA bonds with uracil (U, brown) in RNA.

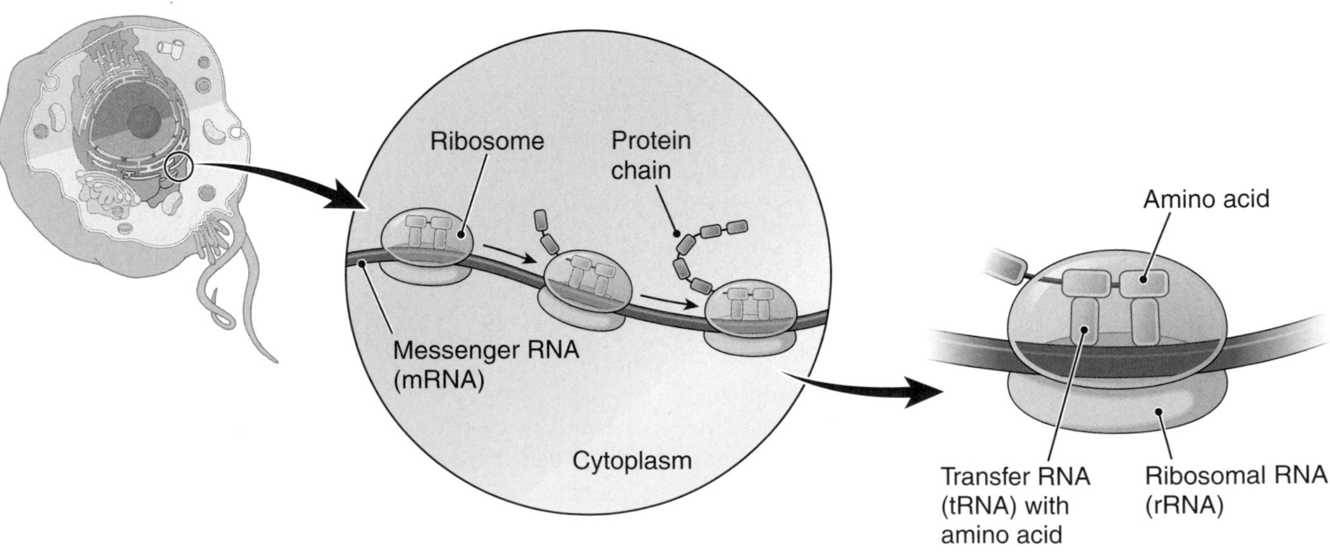

Figure 3-8 **Translation.** In protein synthesis, messenger RNA (mRNA) travels to the ribosomes in the cytoplasm. The information in the mRNA codes for the building of proteins from amino acids. Transfer RNA (tRNA) molecules bring amino acids to the ribosomes to build each protein.

Table 3•4 RNA

TYPES	FUNCTION
Messenger RNA (mRNA)	Is built on a strand of DNA in the nucleus and transcribes the nucleotide code; moves to cytoplasm and attaches to a ribosome
Ribosomal RNA (rRNA)	With protein makes up the ribosomes, the sites of protein synthesis in the cytoplasm; involved in the process of translating the genetic message into a protein
Transfer RNA (tRNA)	Works with other forms of RNA to translate the genetic code into protein; each molecule of tRNA carries an amino acid that can be used to build a protein at the ribosome

different types of RNA. Also see Box 3-2, Proteomics: So Many Proteins, So Few Genes.

Checkpoint 3-9 What three types of RNA are active in protein synthesis?

Cell Division

For growth, repair, and reproduction, cells must multiply to increase their numbers. The cells that form the sex cells (egg and sperm) divide by the process of *meiosis* (mi-O-sis), which cuts the chromosome number in half to prepare for union of the egg and sperm in fertilization. If not for this preliminary reduction, the number of chromosomes in the offspring would constantly double. The process of meiosis is discussed in Chapter 23. All other body cells, known as *somatic cells*, divide by the process of **mitosis** (mi-TO-sis). In this process, described below, each original parent cell becomes two identical daughter cells.

Before mitosis can occur, the genetic information (DNA) in the parent cell must be doubled, so that each of the two new daughter cells will receive a complete set of chromosomes. For example, a cell that divides by mitosis in the human body must produce two cells with 46 chromosomes each, the same number of chromosomes that was present in the original parent cell. DNA duplicates during **interphase**, the stage in the life of a cell between one mitosis and the next. During this phase, DNA uncoils from its double-stranded form, and each strand takes on a matching strand of nucleotides according to the pattern of A-T, G-C pairing. There are now two strands, each identical to the original double helix. The strands are held together at a region called the *centromere* (SEN-tro-mere) until they separate during mitosis. A typical cell lives in interphase for most of its cycle and spends only a relatively short period in mitosis. For example, a cell reproducing every 20 hours spends only about 1 hour in mitosis and the rest of the time in interphase.

Checkpoint 3-10 What must happen to the DNA in a cell before mitosis can occur? During what stage in the life of a cell does this occur?

Stages of Mitosis

Although mitosis is a continuous process, distinct changes can be seen in the dividing cell at four stages (Fig. 3-9).

- In **prophase** (PRO-faze), the doubled strands of DNA return to their tightly wound spiral organization and

Box 3-2 Hot Topics

Proteomics: So Many Proteins, So Few Genes

To build the many different proteins that make up the body, cells rely on instructions encoded in genes on chromosomes. Collectively, all the different genes on all the chromosomes make up the **genome**. Genes contain the instructions for making proteins, while the proteins themselves perform the body's functions.

Scientists are now studying the human **proteome**—all the proteins that can be expressed in a cell—to help them understand the proteins' structure and function. Unlike the genome, the proteome changes as the cell's activities and needs change. In 2003, after a decade of intense scientific activity, investigators mapped the entire human genome and realized that it contained only 35,000 genes, far fewer than initially expected. How could this relatively small number of genes code for several million proteins? They concluded that genes were not the whole story.

Gene transcription is only the beginning of protein synthesis. In response to cell conditions, enzymes can snip newly transcribed mRNA into several pieces, each of which a ribosome can use to build a different protein. After each protein is built, enzymes can further modify the amino acid strands to produce several more different proteins. Other molecules help the newly formed proteins to fold into precise shapes and interact with each other, resulting in even more variations. Thus, while a gene may code for a specific protein, modifications after gene transcription can produce many more unique proteins. There is much left to discover about the proteome, but scientists hope that future research will lead to new techniques for detecting and treating disease.

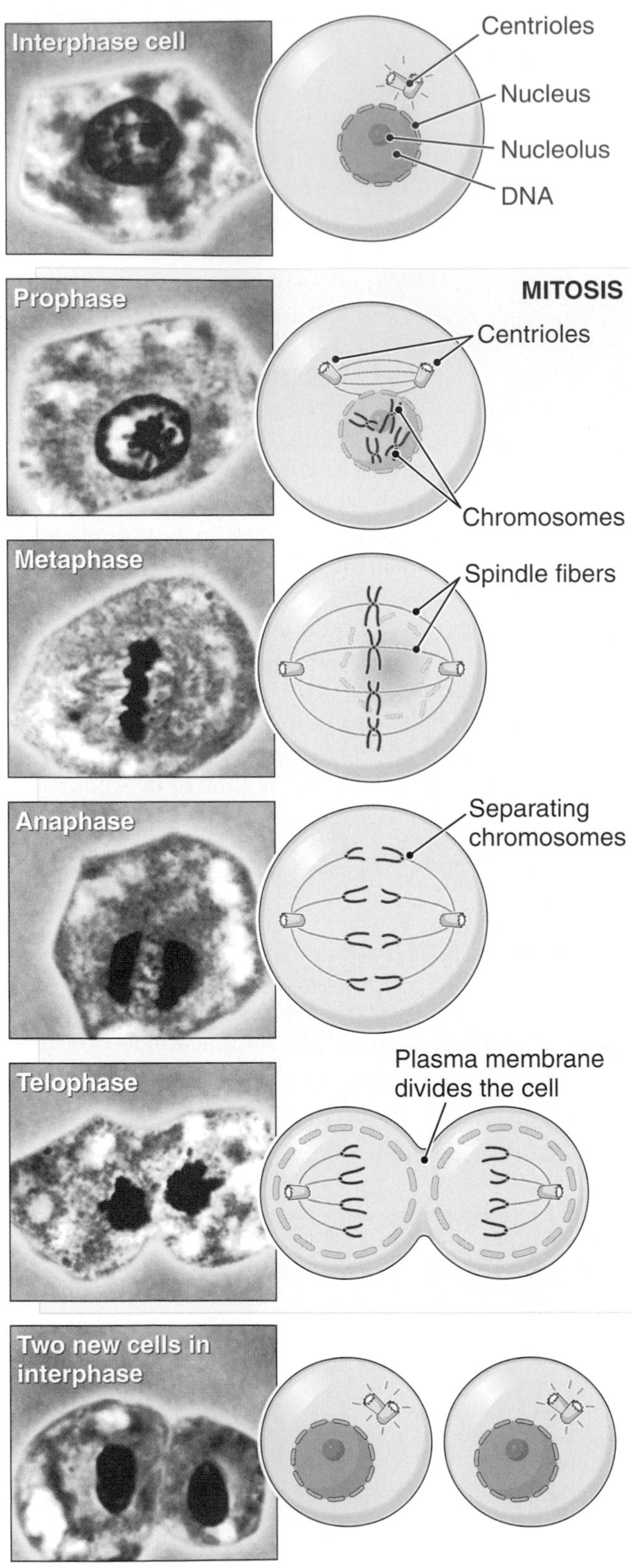

Figure 3-9 **The stages of mitosis.** When it is not dividing, the cell is in interphase. The cell shown is for illustration only. It is not a human cell, which has 46 chromosomes. (Photomicrographs reprinted with permission from Cormack DH. Essential Histology. 2nd ed. Philadelphia: Lippincott Williams & Wilkins, 2001.) *ZOOMING IN ✦ **If the original cell shown has 46 chromosomes, how many chromosomes will each new daughter cell have?***

become visible under the microscope as dark, thread-like chromosomes. The nucleolus and the nuclear membrane begin to disappear. In the cytoplasm, the two centrioles move toward opposite ends of the cell and a spindle-shaped structure made of thin fibers begins to form between them.

- In **metaphase** (MET-ah-faze), the chromosomes line up across the center (equator) of the cell attached to the spindle fibers.
- In **anaphase** (AN-ah-faze), the centromere splits and the duplicated chromosomes separate and begin to move toward opposite ends of the cell.
- As mitosis continues into **telophase** (TEL-o-faze), a membrane appears around each group of separated chromosomes, forming two new nuclei.

Also during telophase, the plasma membrane pinches off to divide the cell. The midsection between the two areas becomes progressively smaller until, finally, the cell splits in two. There are now two new cells, or daughter cells, each with exactly the same kind and amount of DNA as was present in the parent cell. In just a few types of cells, skeletal muscle cells for example, the cell itself does not divide following nuclear division. The result, after multiple mitoses, is a giant single cell with multiple nuclei. This pattern is extremely rare in the human body.

During mitosis, all the organelles, except those needed for the division process, temporarily disappear. After the cell splits, these organelles reappear in each daughter cell. Also at this time, the centrioles usually duplicate in preparation for the next cell division.

Body cells differ in the rate at which they reproduce. Some, such as nerve cells and muscle cells, stop dividing at some point in development and are not replaced if they die. They remain in interphase. Others, such as blood cells, sperm cells, and skin cells, multiply rapidly to replace cells destroyed by injury, disease, or natural wear-and-tear. Cells that multiply slowly may be triggered to divide when tissue is injured, as in repair of a bone fracture.

Immature cells that retain the ability to divide and mature when necessary are known as **stem cells** (see Box 4-1 in Chapter 4). All blood cells, for example, are produced from stem cells in the red bone marrow. Research has been done on stimulating stem cells to divide into various cell types in the laboratory, but these studies have been controversial. Although it may be possible some day to use such cells to replace cells injured by disease, some people consider these studies to be unethical.

Checkpoint 3-11 What are the four stages of mitosis?

Movement of Substances Across the Plasma Membrane

The plasma membrane serves as a barrier between the cell and its environment. Nevertheless, nutrients, oxygen, and many other substances needed by the cell must be

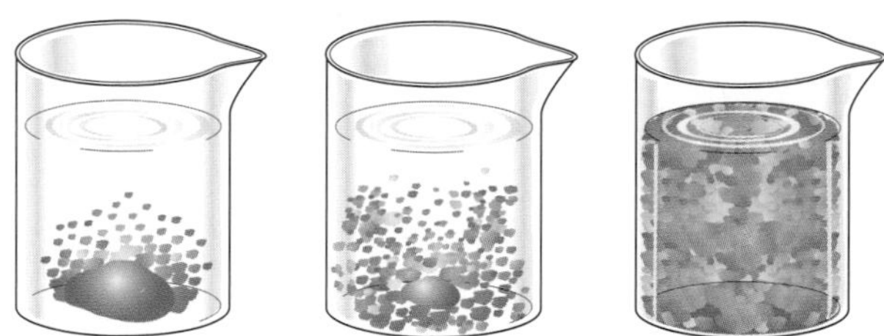

Figure 3-10 **Diffusion of a solid in a liquid.** The molecules of the solid tend to spread evenly throughout the liquid as they dissolve.

taken in and waste products must be eliminated. Clearly, some substances can be exchanged between the cell and its environment through the plasma membrane. For this reason, the plasma membrane is described at a simple level as **semipermeable** (sem-e-PER-me-ah-bl). It is permeable, or passable, to some molecules but impassable to others. Some particles, proteins for example, are too large to travel through the membrane unaided.

The ability of a substance to travel through the membrane is based on several factors. Molecular size is the main factor that determines passage through the membrane, but solubility and electrical charge are also considerations. Water, a tiny molecule, is usually able to penetrate the membrane with ease. Nutrients, however, must be split into small molecules by the process of digestion so that they can travel through the plasma membrane. Sucrose (table sugar), for example, is converted to glucose and fructose, smaller molecules that enter the cell and serve as sources of energy.

Various physical processes are involved in exchanges through the plasma membrane. One way of grouping these processes is according to whether they do or do not require cellular energy.

Movement That Does Not Require Cellular Energy

The adjective *passive* describes movement through the plasma membrane that does not require energy output by the cell. Passive mechanisms depend on the internal energy of the moving particles or the application of some outside source of energy. The methods include:

- **Diffusion** is the constant movement of particles from a region of relatively higher concentration to one of lower concentration. Just as couples on a crowded dance floor spread out into all the available space to avoid hitting other dancers, diffusing substances spread throughout their available space until their concentration everywhere is the same—that is, they reach equilibrium (Fig. 3-10). This movement from higher to lower concentrations uses the internal energy of the particles and does not require cellular energy, just as a sled will move from the top to the bottom of a snowy hill. The particles are said to follow their *concentration gradient* from higher concentration to lower concentration.

  When substances diffuse through a membrane, such as the intact plasma membrane, passage is limited to those particles small enough to pass through spaces between molecules in the membrane, as shown with a large-scale example in Figure 3-11. In the body, soluble materials, such as nutrients, electrolytes, gases, and waste materials, are constantly moving into or out of the cells by diffusion.
- **Osmosis** (os-MO-sis) is a special type of diffusion. The term applies specifically to the diffusion of water through a semipermeable membrane. The water molecules move, as expected, from an area where there are more of them to an area where there are fewer of them.

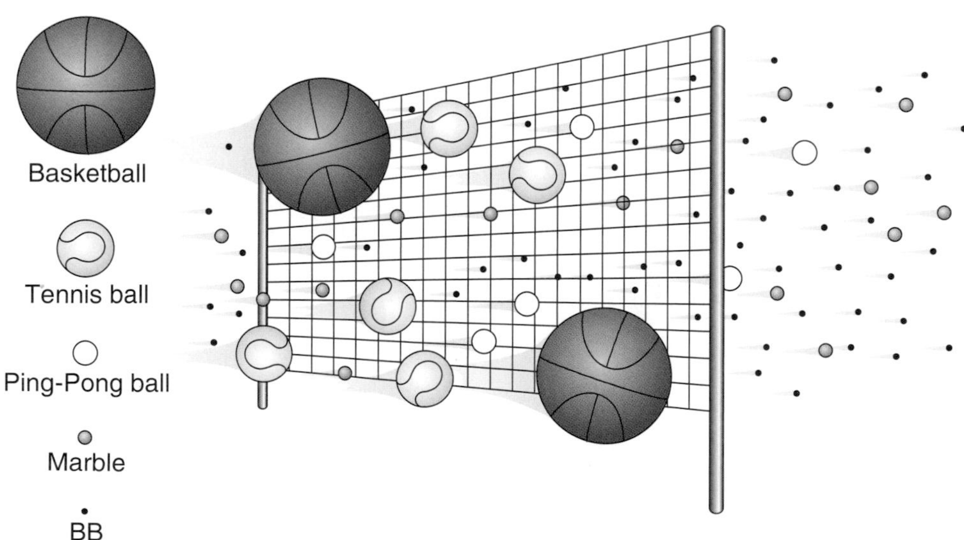

Figure 3-11 **Diffusion through a semipermeable membrane.** In this example, large objects (basketballs, tennis balls) cannot pass through the net, whereas the smaller ones (ping-pong balls, marbles, BBs) can. In the human body, large particles in the blood, such as proteins and blood cells, cannot pass through the walls of the capillaries, whereas small particles, such as nutrients, electrolytes, and gases can. *ZOOMING IN* ✦ ***If this picture represented diffusion in the body, what would the net be?***

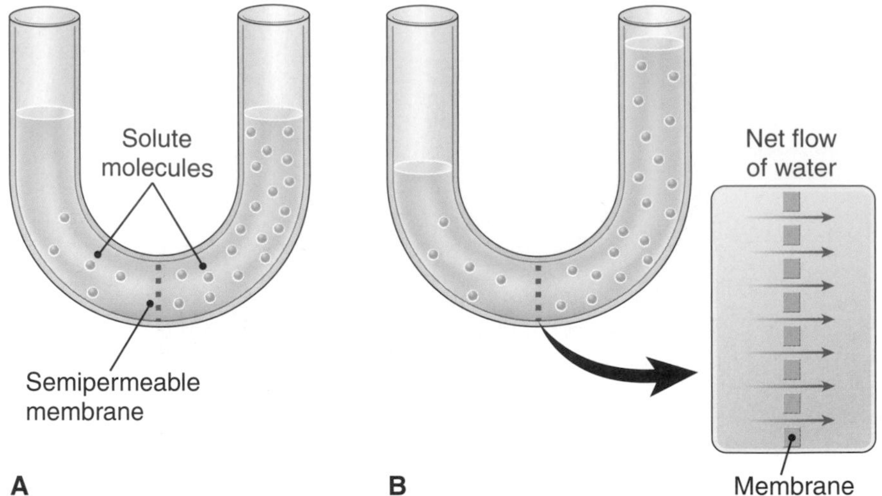

Figure 3-12 **A simple demonstration of osmosis.** Solute molecules are shown in yellow. All of the solvent (blue) is composed of water molecules. **(A)** Two solutions with different concentrations of solute are separated by a semipermeable membrane. Water can flow through the membrane, but the solute cannot. **(B)** Water flows into the more concentrated solution, raising the level of the liquid in that side. *ZOOMING IN ✦ What would happen in this system if the solute could pass through the membrane?*

That is, the solvent (the water molecules) moves from an area of lower *solute* concentration to an area of higher *solute* concentration (Fig. 3-12).

For a physiologist studying the flow of water across membranes, as in exchange of fluids through capillaries in the circulation, it is helpful to know the direction in which water will flow and at what rate it will move. A measure of the force driving osmosis is called the *osmotic pressure*. This force can be measured, as illustrated in Figure 3-13, by applying enough pressure to the surface of a liquid to stop the inward flow of water by osmosis. The pressure needed to counteract osmosis is the osmotic pressure. In practice, the term osmotic pressure is used to describe the tendency of a solution to draw water into it. This force is directly related to concentration: the higher the concentration of a solution, the greater is its tendency to draw water in.

- **Filtration** is the passage of water containing dissolved materials through a membrane as a result of a mechanical ("pushing") force on one side (Fig. 3-14). One example of filtration in the body is the movement of materials out of the capillaries and into the tissues under the force of blood pressure (see Chapter 15). Another example occurs in the kidneys as materials are filtered out of the blood in the first step of urine formation (see Chapter 22).
- **Facilitated diffusion** is the movement of materials across the plasma membrane in the direction of the concentration gradient (from higher to lower concentration) but using transporters to move the material at a faster rate (Fig. 3-15). Glucose, the sugar that is the main energy source for cells, moves through the plasma membrane by means of facilitated diffusion.

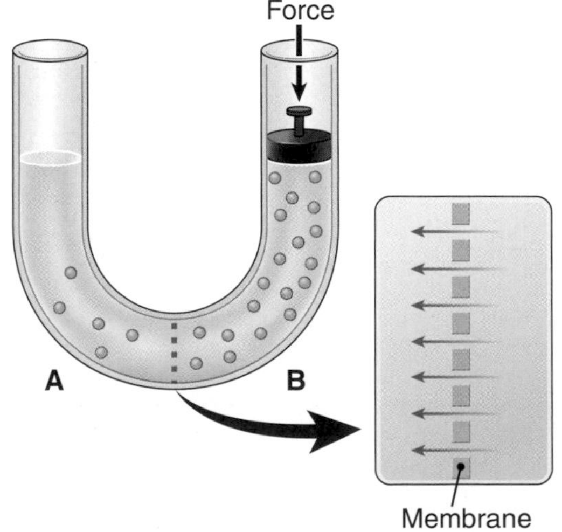

Figure 3-13 **Osmotic pressure.** Osmotic pressure is the force needed to stop the flow of water by osmosis. Pressure on the surface of the fluid in side B counteracts the osmotic flow of water from side A to side B. *ZOOMING IN ✦ What would happen to osmotic pressure if the concentration of solute were increased on side B of this system?*

Movement That Requires Cellular Energy

Movement across the membrane that requires energy is describes as *active*. These methods include:

- **Active transport.** The plasma membrane has the ability to move small solute particles into or out of the cell opposite to the direction in which they would normally flow by diffusion. That is, the membrane moves them against the concentration gradient from an area where they are in relatively lower concentration to an area where they are in higher concentration. Because this

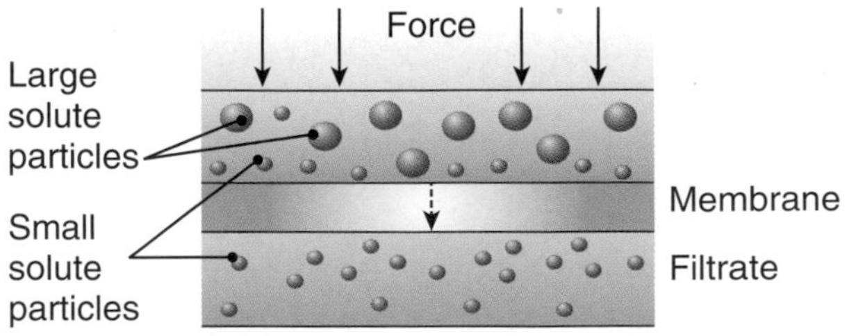

Figure 3-14 **Filtration.** A mechanical force pushes a substance through a membrane, although the membrane limits which particles can pass through based on size. The small particles go through the membrane and appear in the filtered solution (filtrate).

movement goes against the natural flow of particles, it requires energy, just as getting a sled to the top of a hill requires energy. It also requires proteins in the cell membrane that act as **transporters** for the particles.

This process of active transport is one important function of the living cell membrane. The nervous system and muscular system, for example, depend on the active transport of sodium, potassium, and calcium ions for proper function. The kidneys also carry out active transport in regulating the composition of urine. By means of active transport, the cell can take in what it needs from the surrounding fluids and remove materials from the cell. Because the cell membrane can carry on active transport, the membrane is most accurately described, not as simply semipermeable, but as **selectively permeable.** It regulates what can enter and leave based on the needs of the cell.

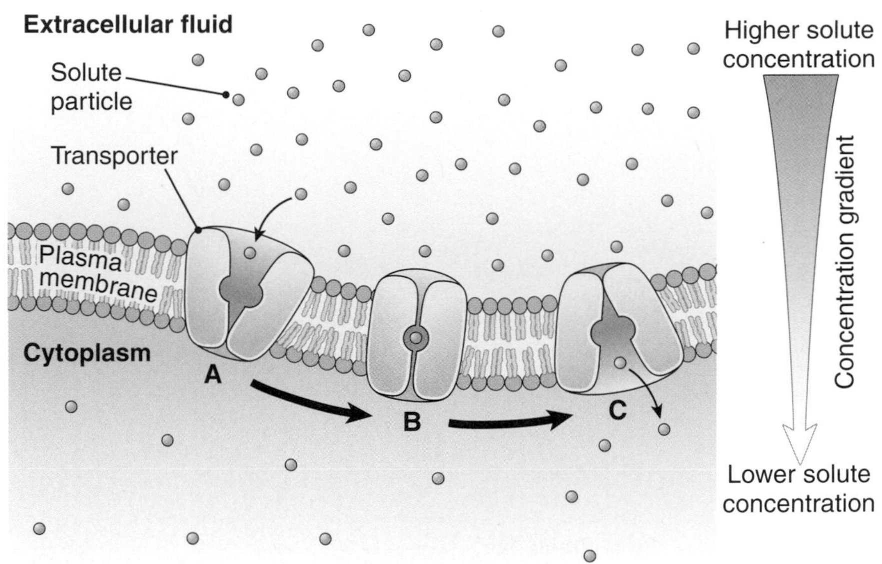

Figure 3-15 **Facilitated diffusion.** Transporters (proteins in the plasma membrane) move solute particles through a membrane from an area of higher concentration to an area of lower concentration. **(A)** A solute particle enters the transporter. **(B)** The transporter changes shape. **(C)** The transporter releases the solute particle on the other side of the membrane. *ZOOMING IN ✦* ***How would a change in the number of transporters affect the movement of a solute by facilitated diffusion?***

There are several active methods for moving large quantities of material into or out of the cell. These methods are grouped together as **bulk transport**, because of the amounts of material moved, or **vesicular transport**, because small bubbles, or vesicles, are needed for the processes.

- **Endocytosis** (en-do-si-TO-sis) is a term that describes the bulk movement of materials into the cell. There are two examples:
  - In **phagocytosis** (fag-o-si-TO-sis), relatively large particles are engulfed by the plasma membrane and moved into the cell (Fig. 3-16). Certain white blood cells carry out phagocytosis to rid the body of foreign material and dead cells. Material taken into a cell by phagocytosis is first enclosed in a vesicle made from the plasma membrane and is later destroyed by lysosomes.
  - In **pinocytosis** (pi-no-si-TO-sis), the cell membrane engulfs droplets of fluid. This is a way for large protein molecules in suspension to travel into the cell. The word *pinocytosis* means "cell drinking."
- In **exocytosis**, the cell moves materials out in vesicles (Fig. 3-17). One example of exocytosis is the export of neurotransmitters from neurons (neurotransmitters are chemicals that control the activity of the nervous system).

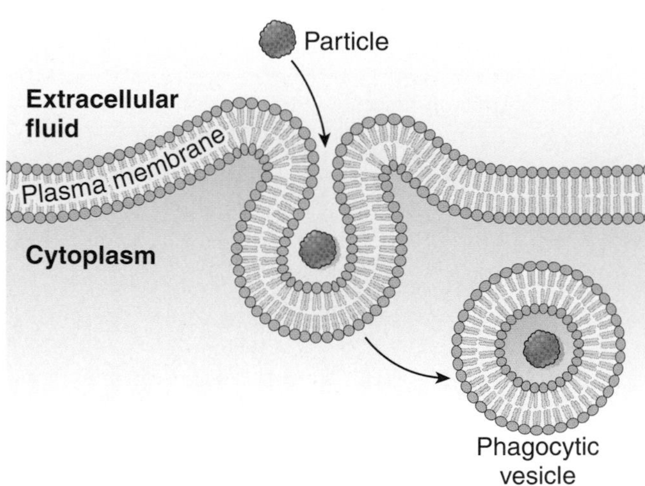

Figure 3-16 **Phagocytosis.** The plasma membrane encloses a particle from the extracellular fluid. The membrane then pinches off, forming a vesicle that carries the particle into the cytoplasm. *ZOOMING IN ✦* ***What organelle would likely help to destroy a particle taken in by phagocytosis?***

The transport methods described above are summarized in Table 3-5.

Checkpoint 3-12 Substances are constantly moving into and out of cells through the plasma membrane. What types of movement do not require cellular energy and what types of movement do require cellular energy?

How Osmosis Affects Cells

As stated earlier, water usually moves easily through the cell membrane. Therefore, for a normal fluid balance to be maintained, the fluid outside all cells must have the

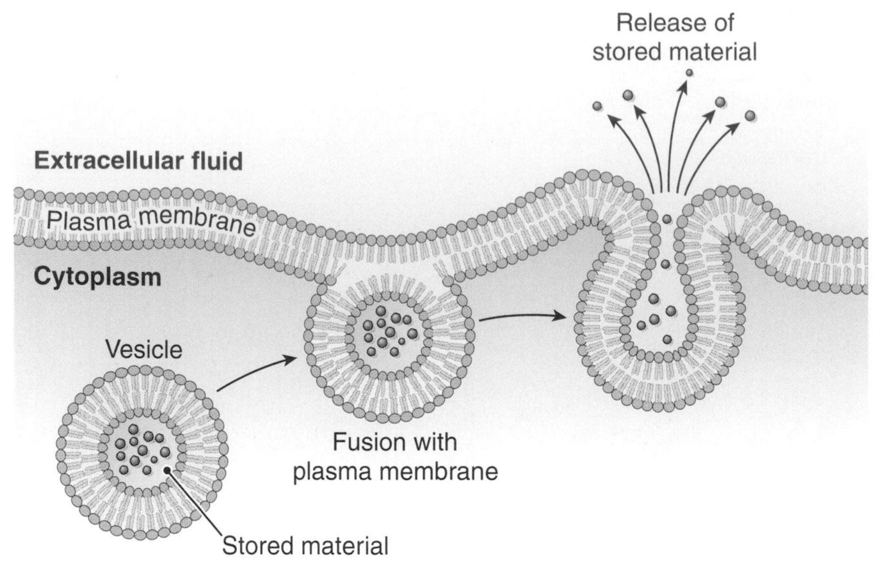

Figure 3-17 **Exocytosis.** A vesicle fuses with the plasma membrane then ruptures and releases its contents.

same concentration of dissolved substances (solutes) as the fluids inside the cells (Fig. 3-18). If not, water will move rapidly into or out of the cell by osmosis. Solutions with concentrations equal to the concentration of the cytoplasm are described as **isotonic** (i-so-TON-ik). Tissue fluids and blood plasma are isotonic for body cells. Manufactured solutions that are isotonic for the cells and can thus be used to replace body fluids include 0.9% salt, or **normal saline**, and 5% dextrose (glucose).

A solution that is less concentrated than the intracellular fluid is described as **hypotonic**. Based on the principles of osmosis already explained, a cell placed in a hypotonic solution draws water in, swells, and may burst. When a red blood cell draws in water and bursts in this way, the cell is said to undergo **hemolysis** (he-MOL-ih-sis). If a cell is placed in a **hypertonic** solution, which is more concentrated than the cellular fluid, it loses water to the surrounding fluids and shrinks, a process termed **crenation** (kre-NA-shun) (see Fig. 3-18).

Fluid balance is an important facet of homeostasis and must be properly regulated for health. You can figure out in which direction water will move through the plasma membrane if you remember the saying "water follows salt," salt meaning any dissolved material (solute). The total amount and distribution of body fluids is discussed in Chapter 21. Table 3-6 summarizes the effects of different solution concentrations on cells.

Checkpoint 3-13 The concentration of fluids in and around the cell is important in homeostasis. What term describes a fluid that is the same concentration as the fluid within the cell (intracellular fluid)? What type of fluid is less concentrated? More concentrated?

Table 3•5 Membrane Transport

PROCESS	DEFINITION	EXAMPLE
Do not require cellular energy (passive)		
Diffusion	Random movement of particles with the concentration gradient (from higher concentration to lower concentration) until they reach equilibrium	Movement of nutrients, electrolytes, gases, wastes, and other soluble materials into and out of the cell
Osmosis	Diffusion of water through a semipermeable membrane	Movement of water across the plasma membrane
Filtration	Movement of materials through a membrane under mechanical force	Movement of materials out of the blood under the force of blood pressure
Facilitated diffusion	Movement of materials across the plasma membrane along the concentration gradient using transporters to speed the process	Movement of glucose into the cells
Require cellular energy		
Active transport	Movement of materials through the plasma membrane against the concentration gradient using transporters	Transport of ions (*e.g.*, Na^+, K^+, Ca^{2+}) in the nervous system and muscular system
Endocytosis	Transport of bulk amounts of materials into the cell using vesicles	Phagocytosis, intake of large particles, as when white blood cells take in waste materials; also pinocytosis—intake of fluid
Exocytosis	Transport of bulk amounts of materials out of the cell using vesicles	Release of neurotransmitters from neurons

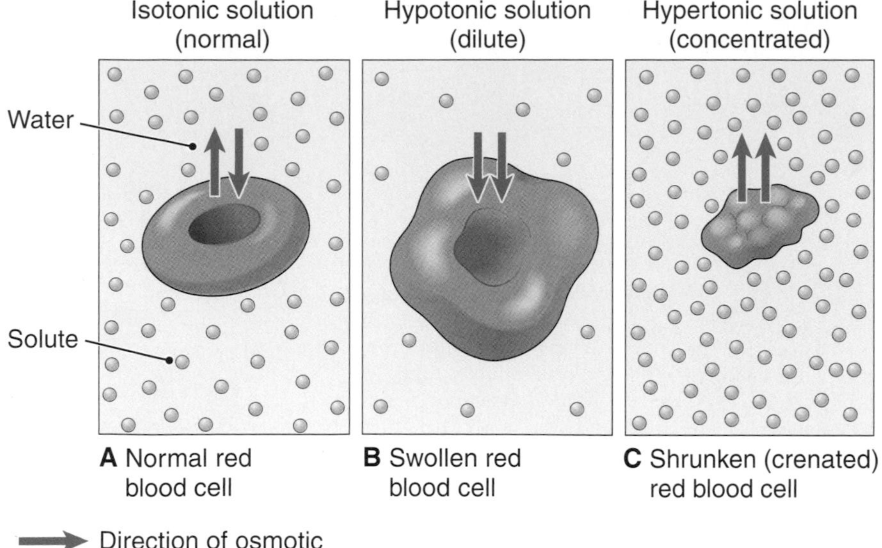

Figure 3-18 **The effect of osmosis on cells.** Water moves through a red blood cell membrane in solutions with three different concentrations of solute. **(A)** The isotonic (normal) solution has the same concentration as the cell fluid, and water moves into and out of the cell at the same rate. **(B)** A cell placed in a hypotonic (more dilute) solution draws water in, causing the cell to swell and perhaps undergo hemolysis (bursting). **(C)** The hypertonic (more concentrated) solution draws water out of the cell, causing it to shrink, an effect known as crenation. *ZOOMING IN ♦ **What would happen to red blood cells if blood lost through injury were replaced with pure water?***

Cell Aging

As cells multiply throughout life, changes occur that may lead to their damage and death. Harmful substances known as *free radicals*, produced in the course of normal metabolism, can injure cells unless these materials are destroyed. Chapter 20 covers free radicals in more detail. Lysosomes may deteriorate as they age, releasing enzymes that can harm the cell. Alteration of the genes, or **mutations**, are a natural occurrence in the process of cell division and are increased by exposure to harmful substances and radiation in the environment. Mutations usually harm cells and may lead to cancer.

As a person ages, the overall activity of the body cells slows. One example of this change is the slowing down of repair processes. A bone fracture, for example, takes considerably longer to heal in an old person than in a young person.

One theory on aging holds that cells are preprogrammed to divide only a certain number of times before they die. Support for this idea comes from the fact that cells taken from a young person divide more times when grown in the laboratory than similar cells taken from an older individual. This programmed cell death, known as *apoptosis* (ah-pop-TO-sis), is a natural part of growth and remodeling before birth in the developing embryo and in repair and remodeling of tissue throughout life (see Box 3-3, Necrosis and Apoptosis: Cellular Homicide and Suicide).

Cells and Cancer

Certain mutations (changes) in the genetic material of a cell may cause that cell to reproduce without control. Cells that normally multiply at a fast rate, such as epithelial cells, are more likely than slower-growing cells to undergo such transformations. If these altered cells do not die naturally or get destroyed by the immune system, they will continue to multiply and may spread (metastasize) to

Table 3•6 Solutions and Their Effects on Cells

TYPE OF SOLUTION	DESCRIPTION	EXAMPLES	EFFECT ON CELLS
Isotonic	Has the same concentration of dissolved substances as the fluid in the cell	0.9% salt (normal saline); 5% dextrose (glucose)	None; cell in equilibrium with its environment
Hypotonic	Has a lower concentration of dissolved substances than the fluid in the cell	Less than 0.9% salt or 5% dextrose	Cell takes in water, swells, and may burst; red blood cell undergoes hemolysis
Hypertonic	Has a higher concentration of dissolved substances than the fluid in the cell	Higher than 0.9% salt or 5% dextrose	Cell will lose water and shrink; cell undergoes crenation

Box 3-3 A Closer Look

Necrosis and Apoptosis: Cellular Homicide and Suicide

Cell death happens in two ways: by necrosis, because the cell is injured; or by apoptosis, because the cell is programmed to die. One way of remembering the difference is to think of necrosis as "cellular homicide" and apoptosis as "cellular suicide."

Necrosis disrupts the cell's normal water-balancing mechanisms and stimulates autolysis (see Box 3-1). As a result, the cell swells and its organelles break down. Finally, the cell ruptures, releasing its contents into the surrounding tissue. These contents contain digestive enzymes that damage adjacent cells, producing more injury and necrosis.

Apoptosis is an orderly, genetically programmed cell death triggered by the cell's own genes. Under the right circumstances, these "suicide genes" produce enzymes called capsases that destroy the cell swiftly and neatly. The cell shrinks, and phagocytes quickly digest it. In contrast to necrosis, apoptotic cells do not cause further chaos when they die.

Apoptosis is a normal bodily process. It is especially important during embryonic development because it removes unneeded cells, such as those from limb buds to form fingers and toes. Apoptosis also occurs after birth, as when cells subject to extreme wear and tear regularly undergo apoptosis and are replaced. For example, the cells lining the digestive tract are removed and replaced every 2 to 3 days.

other tissues, producing **cancer.** Cancer cells form tumors, which interfere with normal functions, crowding out normal cells and robbing them of nutrients. There is more information on the various types of tumors in Chapter 4.

Cancer Risk Factors

The causes of cancer are complex, involving interactions between cellular factors and the environment. Because cancer may take a long time to develop, it is often difficult to identify its cause or causes. Certain forces increase the chances of developing the disease and are considered risk factors. These include the following:

- **Heredity.** Certain types of cancer occur more frequently in some families than in others, indicating that there is some inherited predisposition to the development of cancer.
- **Chemicals.** Certain industrial and environmental chemicals are known to increase the risk of cancer. Any chemical that causes cancer is called a **carcinogen** (kar-SIN-o-jen). The most common carcinogens in our society are those present in cigarette smoke. Carcinogens are also present, both naturally and as additives, in foods. Certain drugs also may be carcinogenic.
- **Ionizing radiation.** Certain types of radiation can produce damage to cellular DNA that may lead to cancer. These include x-rays, rays from radioactive substances, and ultraviolet rays. For example, the ultraviolet rays received from exposure to the sun are very harmful to the skin.
- **Physical irritation.** Continued irritation, such as the contact of a hot pipe stem on the lip, increases cell division and thus increases the chance of mutation.
- **Diet.** It has been shown that diets high in fats and total calories are associated with an increased occurrence of certain forms of cancer. A general lack of fiber and insufficient amounts of certain fruits and vegetables in the diet can leave one susceptible to cancers of the digestive tract.
- **Viruses** have been implicated in cancers of the liver, the blood (leukemias), and lymphatic tissues (lymphomas).

Word Anatomy

Medical terms are built from standardized word parts (prefixes, roots, and suffixes). Learning the meanings of these parts can help you remember words and interpret unfamiliar terms.

WORD PART	MEANING	EXAMPLE
The Role of Cells		
cyt/o	cell	*Cytology* is the study of cells.
Microscopes		
micr/o	small	*Microscopes* are used to view structures too small to see with the naked eye.
Cell Structure		
bi-	two	The lipid *bilayer* is a double layer of lipid molecules.
-some	body	*Ribosomes* are small bodies outside the cell's nucleus that help make proteins.
chrom/o-	color	*Chromosomes* are small, threadlike bodies that stain darkly with basic dyes.

WORD PART	MEANING	EXAMPLE
Cell Structure		
end/o-	in, within	The *endoplasmic* reticulum is a network of membranes within the cytoplasm.
lys/o	loosening, dissolving, separating	*Lysosomes* are small bodies (organelles) with enzymes that dissolve materials (see also *hemolysis*).
Cell Functions		
inter-	between	*Interphase* is the stage between one cell division (mitosis) and the next.
pro-	before, in front of	*Prophase* is the first stage of mitosis.
meta-	change	*Metaphase* is the second stage of mitosis when the chromosomes change position and line up across the equator.
ana-	upward, back, again	In the *anaphase* stage of mitosis, chromosomes move to opposite sides of the cell.
tel/o-	end	*Telophase* is the last stage of mitosis.
semi-	partial, half	A *semipermeable* membrane lets some molecules pass through but not others.
phag/o	to eat, ingest	In *phagocytosis* the cell membrane engulfs large particles and moves them into the cell.
pino	to drink	In *pinocytosis* the cell membrane "drinks" (engulfs) droplets of fluid.
ex/o-	outside, out of, away from	In *exocytosis* the cell moves material out in vesicles.
iso-	same, equal	An *isotonic* solution has the same concentration as that of the cytoplasm.
hypo-	deficient, below, beneath	A *hypotonic* solution's concentration is lower than that of the cytoplasm.
hem/o	blood	*Hemolysis* is the destruction of red blood cells.
hyper-	above, over, excessive	A *hypertonic* solution's concentration is higher than that of the cytoplasm.
Cells and Cancer		
carcin/o	cancer, carcinoma	A *carcinogen* is a chemical that causes cancer.
-gen	agent that produces or originates	See preceding example.

Summary

I. The Role of Cells
1. Basic unit of life
2. Show all characteristics of life—organization, metabolism, responsiveness, homeostasis, growth, reproduction

II. Microscopes
A. Types
   1. Compound light microscope
   2. Transmission electron microscope—magnifies up to 1 million times
   3. Scanning electron microscope—gives three-dimensional image

B. Micrometer—metric unit commonly used for microscopic measurements

C. Stains—dyes used to aid in viewing cells under the microscope

III. Cell Structure
A. Plasma membrane—regulates what enters and leaves cell
   1. Phospholipid bilayer with proteins, carbohydrates, cholesterol
      a. Proteins—channels, transporters, receptors, enzymes, linkers, cell identity markers

B. Nucleus
   1. Control center of the cell
   2. Contains the chromosomes (units of heredity)
   3. Contains the nucleolus, which manufactures ribosomes

C. Cytoplasm—colloidal suspension that holds organelles
   1. Cytosol—liquid portion
   2. Organelles—structures that carry out special functions
      a. ER (endoplasmic reticulum), ribosomes, mitochondria, Golgi apparatus, lysosomes, peroxisomes, vesicles, centrioles
      b. Cilia, flagellum—surface organelles used for movement

IV. Protein synthesis
A. Nucleic acids—DNA and RNA
   1. Composed of nucleotides
      a. Each nucleotide has sugar, phosphate, nitrogen base
      b. Nitrogen bases vary, giving five nucleotides
   2. DNA
      a. Carries the genetic message
      b. Located almost entirely in the nucleus
      c. Composed of nucleotides adenine (A), guanine (G), cytosine (C), thymine (T)
      d. Double stranded by pairing of A-T, G-C, and wound into helix
   3. The role of RNA
      a. Single strand of nucleotides—A, G, C, and uracil (U)
      b. Located in the cytoplasm
      c. Translates DNA message into proteins
      d. Three types
         (1) Messenger RNA (mRNA)—transcribes the message of the DNA
         (2) Ribosomal RNA (rRNA)—makes up the ribosomes, the site of protein synthesis
         (3) Transfer RNA (tRNA)—brings amino acids to be made into proteins

V. Cell division

1. Meiosis—forms the sex cells (egg and sperm)
    a. Divides the chromosome number in half
2. Mitosis—division of somatic (body) cells
    a. Chromosomes first duplicate during interphase
    b. Division of cell into two identical daughter cells

A. Stages of mitosis—prophase, metaphase, anaphase, telophase

VI. Movement of substances across plasma membrane

A. Movement that does not require cellular energy (passive)
1. Diffusion—molecules move from area of higher concentration to area of lower concentration
2. Osmosis—diffusion of water through semipermeable membrane
    a. Osmotic pressure—measure of tendency of a solution to draw in water
3. Filtration—movement of materials through plasma membrane under mechanical force
4. Facilitated diffusion—movement of materials with aid of transporters in plasma membrane

B. Movement that requires cellular energy (active)
1. Active transport
    a. Movement of solute particles from area of lower concentration to area of higher concentration
    b. Requires transporters
2. Endocytosis—movement of bulk amounts of material into the cell in vesicles
    a. Phagocytosis—engulfing of large particles
    b. Pinocytosis—intake of droplets of fluid
3. Exocytosis—movement of bulk amounts of materials out of the cell in vesicles

C. How osmosis affects cells
1. Isotonic solution—same concentration as cell fluids; cell remains the same
2. Hypotonic solution—lower concentration than cell fluids; cell swells and may undergo hemolysis (bursting)
3. Hypertonic solution—higher concentration than cell fluids; cell undergoes crenation (shrinking)

VII. Cell aging

1. Mutations (changes) occur in genes
2. Slowing of cellular activity
3. Apoptosis—programmed cell death

VIII. Cells and cancer

1. Cancer
    a. Uncontrolled growth of cells
    b. Spread (metastasize) to other tissues

A. Cancer risk factors
1. Heredity
2. Chemicals—carcinogens
3. Ionizing radiation
4. Physical irritation
5. Diet
6. Viruses

Questions for Study and Review

Building Understanding

Fill in the blanks

1. The part of the cell that regulates what can enter or leave is the _____.
2. Distinct segments of DNA that code for specific proteins are called _____.
3. The cytosol and organelles make up the _____.
4. If Solution A has more solute and less water than Solution B, then Solution A is _____ to Solution B.
5. Mechanisms that require energy to move substances across the plasma membrane are called _____ transport mechanisms.

Matching

Match each numbered item with the most closely related lettered item.

___6. DNA duplication takes place
___7. DNA is tightly wound into chromosomes
___8. Chromosomes line up along the cell's equator
___9. Chromosomes separate and move toward opposite ends of the cell
___10. Cell membrane pinches off, dividing the cell into two new daughter cells

a. metaphase
b. anaphase
c. telophase
d. interphase
e. prophase

Multiple choice

___ 11. The main component of the plasma membrane is
a. phospholipid
b. cholesterol
c. carbohydrate
d. protein

___ 12. ATP is synthesized in the
a. nucleus
b. Golgi apparatus
c. endoplasmic reticulum
d. mitochondria

___ 13. Transcription of the DNA strand TGAAC would produce an mRNA strand with the sequence
a. CAGGU
b. ACTTG
c. CAGGT
d. ACUUG

___ 14. Somatic cells divide by the process called
a. mitosis
b. meiosis
c. crenation
d. hemolysis

___ 15. Movement of solute from a region of high concentration to one of lower concentration is called
a. exocytosis
b. diffusion
c. endocytosis
d. osmosis

Understanding Concepts

16. List the components of the plasma membrane and state a function for each.

17. Compare and contrast the following cellular components:
a. microvilli and cilia
b. nucleus and nucleolus
c. rough ER and smooth ER
d. lysosome and peroxisome
e. DNA and RNA
f. chromosome and gene

18. Describe the role of each of the following in protein synthesis: DNA, nucleotide, RNA, ribosomes, rough ER, and Golgi apparatus.

19. List and define six methods by which materials cross the cell membrane. Which of these requires cellular energy?

20. Why is the cell membrane described as selectively permeable?

21. What will happen to a red blood cell placed in a 5.0% salt solution? In distilled water?

22. Discuss the link between genetic mutation and cancer. List six risk factors associated with cancer.

Conceptual Thinking

23. Cigarette smoke paralyzes the cilia of cells lining the respiratory tract. Explain the effects of this on respiratory system function.

24. A particular type of cell manufactures a protein needed elsewhere in the body. Beginning with events in the nucleus, describe the process of making that protein and exporting it out of the cell.

25. Kidney failure causes a buildup of waste and water in the blood. A procedure called hemodialysis removes these substances from the blood. During this procedure, the patient's blood passes by a semipermeable membrane within the dialysis machine. Waste and water from the blood diffuses across the membrane into dialysis fluid on the other side. Based on this information, compare the osmotic concentration of the blood with that of the dialysis fluid.

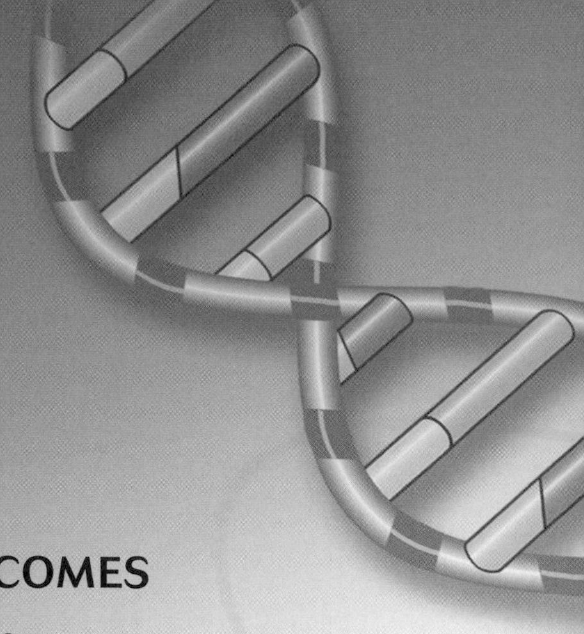

Selected Key Terms

The following terms and other boldface terms in the chapter are defined in the Glossary

adipose
areolar
benign
cartilage
chemotherapy
collagen
endocrine
epithelium
exocrine
fascia
histology
malignant
matrix
membrane
metastasis
mucosa
myelin
neoplasm
neuroglia
neuron
parietal
serosa
staging
visceral

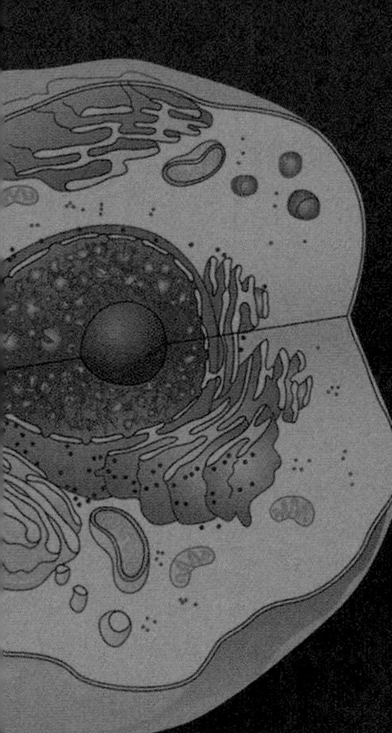

Learning Outcomes

After careful study of this chapter, you should be able to:

1. Name the four main groups of tissues and give the location and general characteristics of each
2. Describe the difference between exocrine and endocrine glands and give examples of each
3. Give examples of liquid, soft, fibrous, and hard connective tissues
4. Describe three types of epithelial membranes
5. List several types of connective tissue membranes
6. Explain the difference between benign and malignant tumors and give several examples of each type
7. List some signs of cancer
8. List six methods of diagnosing cancer
9. Describe three traditional methods of treating cancer
10. Show how word parts are used to build words related to tissues, glands, and membranes (see Word Anatomy at the end of the chapter)

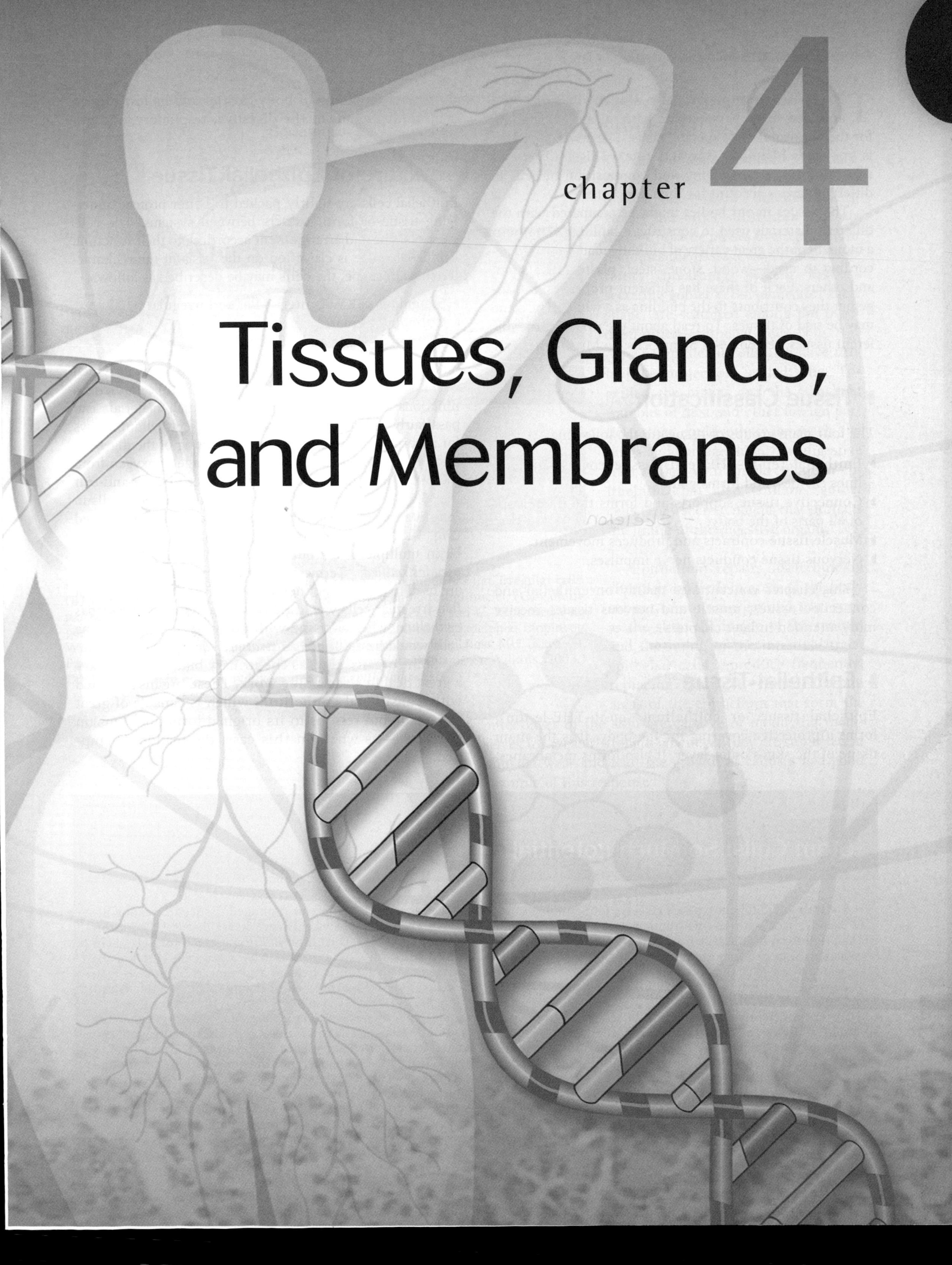

chapter 4

Tissues, Glands, and Membranes

Conceptual Thinking

23. Prolonged exposure to cigarette smoke causes damage to ciliated epithelium that lines portions of the respiratory tract. Discuss the implications of this damage.

24. The middle ear is connected to the throat by a tube called the eustachian (auditory) tube. All are lined by a continuous mucous membrane. Using this information, describe why a throat infection (pharyngitis) may lead to an ear infection (otitis media).

25. Osteogenesis imperfecta is a connective tissue disease characterized by abnormal collagen fiber synthesis. Based on the fact that collagen is the predominant fiber type in connective tissue, list some possible symptoms of this disease.

unit II

Disease and the First Line of Defense

The first chapter in this unit discusses deviation from the normal, which is the basis for disease. After a general discussion of different types of diseases, the chapter concentrates on infectious diseases and the organisms that cause them, including bacteria, viruses, fungi, protozoa, and worms. Other forms of disease are discussed in chapters on the individual body systems. The skin is the first defense against infectious organisms and other sources of injury. The properties and functions of the skin are discussed in the second chapter of this unit.

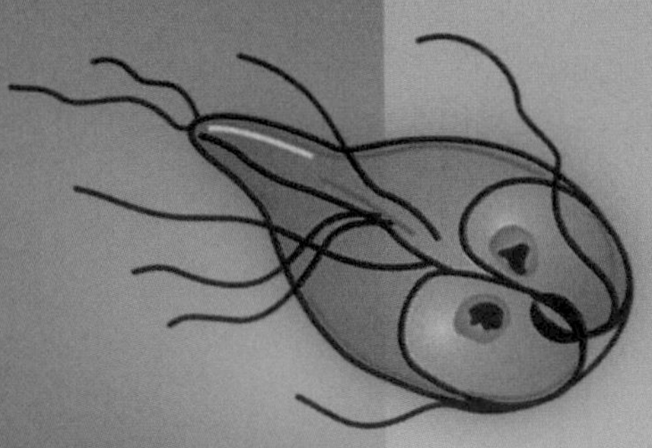

Selected Key Terms

The following terms and other boldface terms in the chapter are defined in the Glossary

acute
antisepsis
asepsis
chronic
diagnosis
disease
disinfection
epidemic
etiology
helminth
microorganism
nosocomial infection
opportunistic infection
pathogen
pathophysiology
prion
prognosis
sign
spore
sterilization
symptom
syndrome
systemic
therapy
toxin
vector

Learning Outcomes

After careful study of this chapter, you should be able to:

1. Define disease and list seven categories of disease
2. List seven predisposing causes of disease
3. Define terminology used in describing and treating disease
4. Define *complementary and alternative medicine*; cite several alternative or complementary fields of practice
5. Explain methods by which microorganisms can be transmitted from person to person
6. List four types of organisms studied in microbiology and give the characteristics of each
7. List some diseases caused by each type of microorganism
8. Define *normal flora* and explain the value of the normal flora
9. Describe the three types of bacteria according to shape
10. List several diseases in humans caused by worms
11. Give some reasons for the emergence and spread of microorganisms today
12. Describe several public health measures taken to prevent the spread of disease
13. Differentiate *sterilization, disinfection,* and *antisepsis*
14. Describe techniques included as part of body substance precautions
15. List some antimicrobial agents and describe how they work
16. Describe several methods used to identify microorganisms in the laboratory
17. Show how word parts are used to build words related to disease (see Word Anatomy at the end of the chapter)

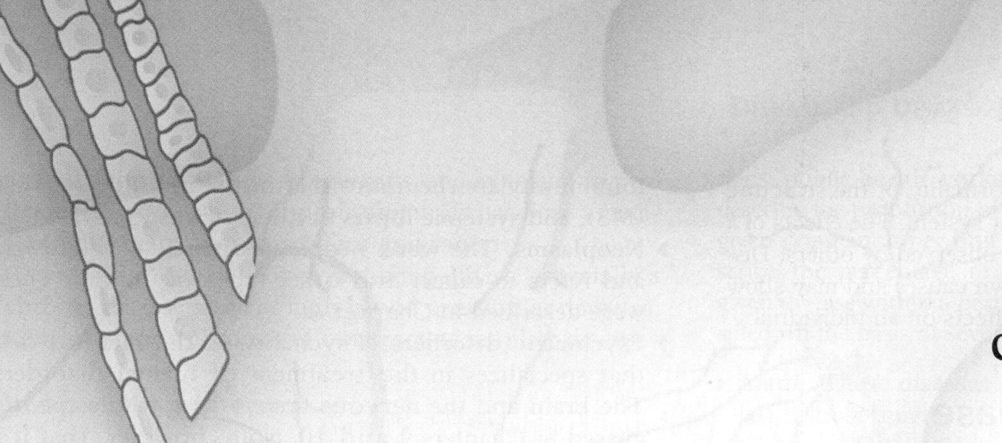

chapter 5

Disease and Disease-Producing Organisms

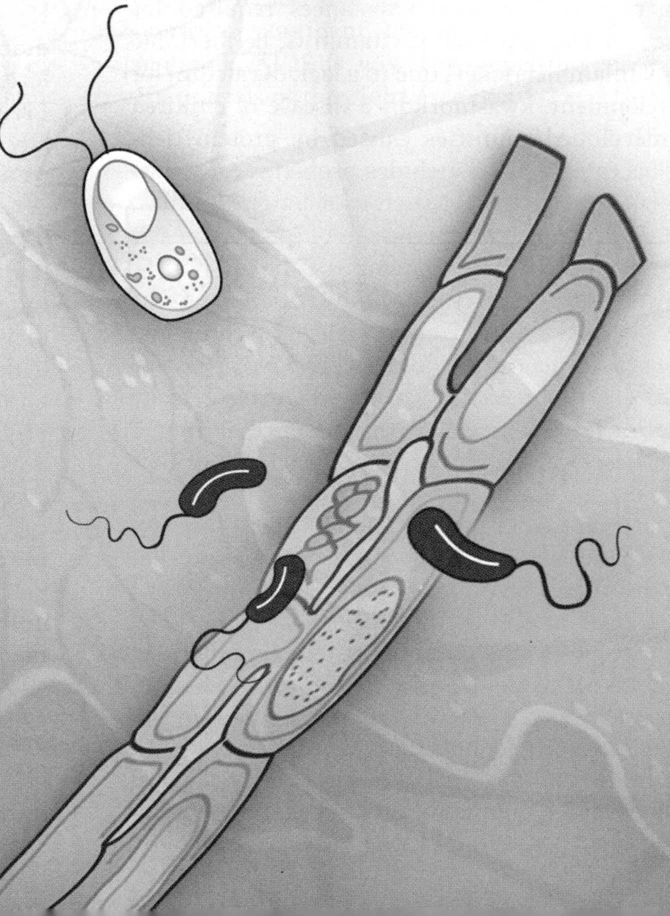

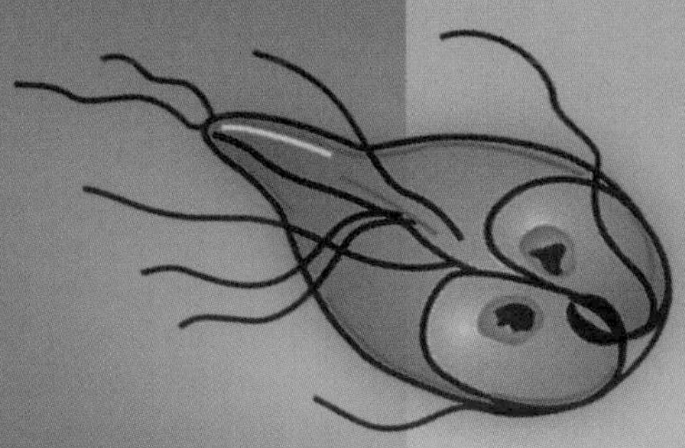

Selected Key Terms

The following terms and other boldface terms in the chapter are defined in the Glossary

alopecia
arrector pili
cicatrix
dermatitis
dermis
epidermis
erythema
exfoliation
integument
keloid
keratin
lesion
melanin
scar
sebaceous
sebum
stratum
subcutaneous
sudoriferous

Learning Outcomes

After careful study of this chapter, you should be able to:

1. Name and describe the layers of the skin
2. Describe the subcutaneous tissue
3. Give the location and function of the accessory structures of the skin
4. List the main functions of the skin
5. Summarize the information to be gained by observation of the skin
6. List the main disorders of the skin
7. Show how word parts are used to build words related to the skin (see Word Anatomy at the end of the chapter)

chapter 6

The Skin in Health and Disease

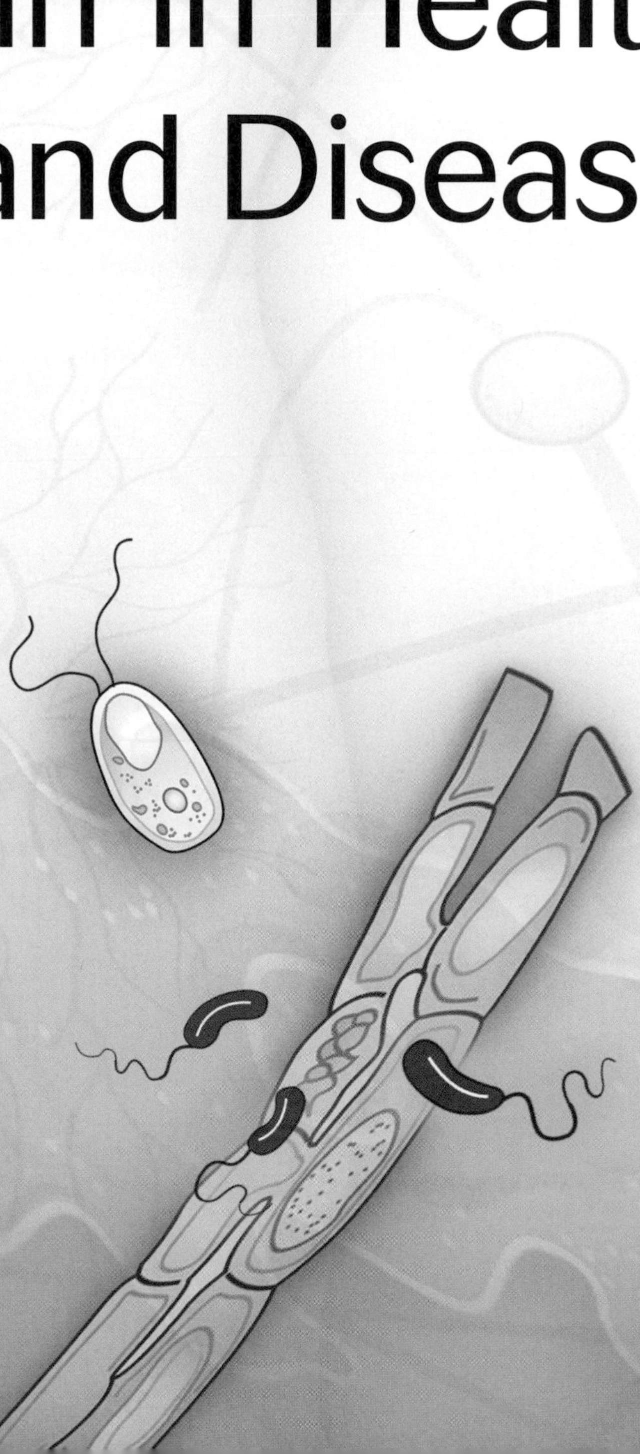

The skin is the one system that can be inspected in its entirety without requiring surgery or special equipment. The skin not only gives clues to its own health but also reflects the health of other body systems. Although the skin may be viewed simply as a membrane enveloping the body, it is far more complex than the other epithelial membranes described in Chapter 4.

The skin is associated with accessory structures, also known as appendages, which include glands, hair, and nails. Together with blood vessels, nerves, and sensory organs, the skin and its associated structures form the **integumentary** (in-teg-u-MEN-tar-e) **system.** This name is from the word integument (in-TEG-u-ment), which means "covering." The term cutaneous (ku-TA-ne-us) also refers to the skin. The functions of this system are discussed later in the chapter after a description of its structure.

Structure of the Skin

The skin consists of two layers (Fig. 6-1):

- The **epidermis** (ep-ih-DER-mis), the outermost portion, which itself is subdivided into thin layers called **strata** (STRA-tah) (sing. stratum). The epidermis is composed entirely of epithelial cells and contains no blood vessels.
- The **dermis**, or true skin, which has a framework of connective tissue and contains many blood vessels, nerve endings, and glands.

Figure 6-2 is a photograph of the skin as seen through a microscope showing the layers and some accessory structures.

Epidermis

The epidermis is the surface portion of the skin, the outermost cells of which are constantly lost through wear and tear. Because there are no blood vessels in the epidermis, the cells must be nourished by capillaries in the underlying dermis. New epidermal cells are produced in the deepest layer, which is closest to the dermis. The cells in this layer, the **stratum basale** (bas-A-le), or **stratum germinativum** (jer-min-a-TI-vum), are constantly dividing and producing daughter cells, which are then pushed upward toward the surface of the skin. As the epidermal cells die from the gradual loss of nourishment, they undergo changes. Mainly, their cytoplasm is replaced by

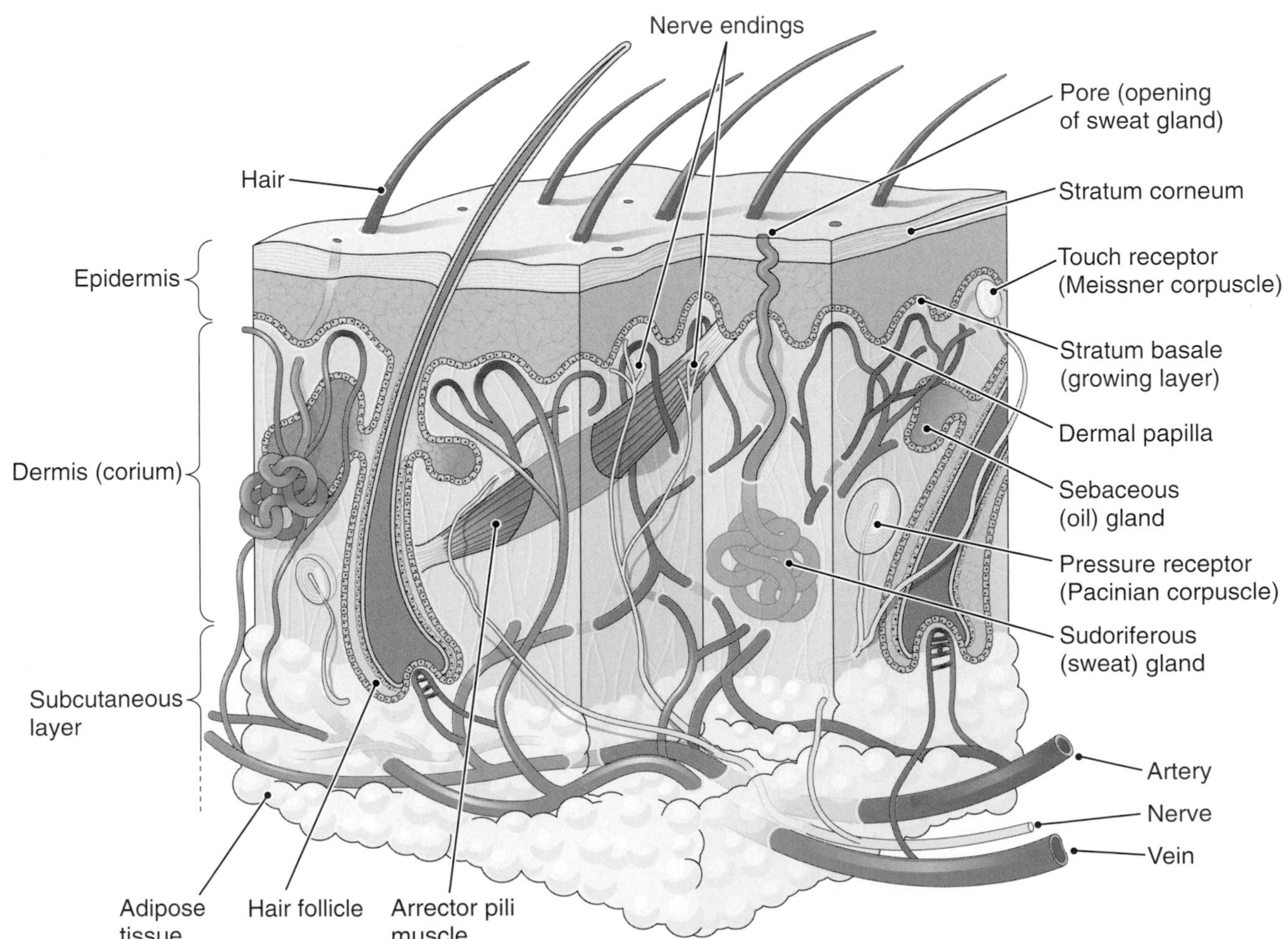

Figure 6-1 **Cross-section of the skin.**

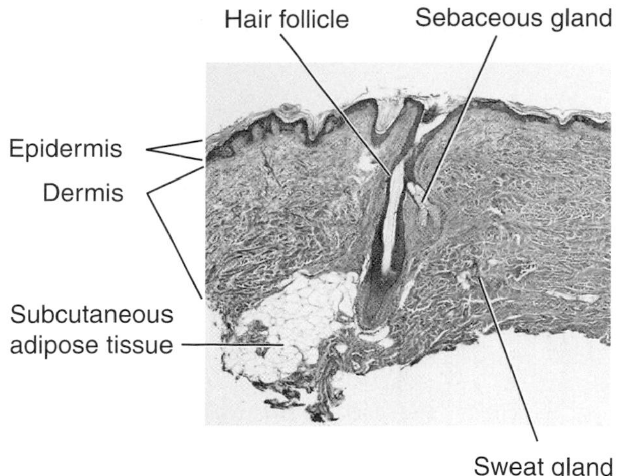

Figure 6-2 **Microscopic view of thin skin.** Tissue layers and some accessory structures are labeled. (Reprinted with permission from Cormack DH. Essential Histology. 2nd ed. Philadelphia: Lippincott Williams & Wilkins, 2001.)

large amounts of a protein called **keratin** (KER-ah-tin), which serves to thicken and protect the skin (Fig. 6-3).

By the time epidermal cells approach the surface, they have become flat, filled with keratin, and horny, forming the uppermost layer of the epidermis, the **stratum corneum** (KOR-ne-um). The stratum corneum is a protective layer and is deeper in thick skin than in thin skin. Cells at the surface are constantly being lost and replaced from below, especially in areas of the skin that are subject to wear and tear, as on the scalp, face, soles of the feet, and palms of the hands. Although this process of **exfoliation** (eks-fo-le-A-shun) occurs naturally at all times, many cosmetics companies sell products to promote exfoliation, presumably to "enliven" and "refresh" the skin.

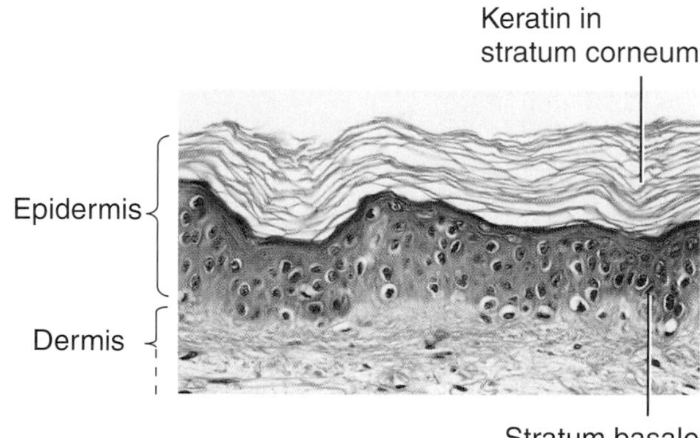

Figure 6-3 **Upper portion of the skin.** Layers of keratin in the stratum corneum are visible at the surface. Below are layers of stratified squamous epithelium making up the remainder of the epidermis. (Reprinted with permission from Cormack DH. Essential Histology. 2nd ed. Philadelphia: Lippincott Williams & Wilkins, 2001.)

Between the stratum basale and the stratum corneum there are additional layers of stratified epithelium that vary in number and quantity depending on the thickness of the skin.

Cells in the deepest layer of the epidermis produce **melanin** (MEL-ah-nin), a dark pigment that colors the skin and protects it from the harmful rays of sunlight. The cells that produce this pigment are the **melanocytes** (MEL-ah-no-sites). Irregular patches of melanin are called freckles.

Dermis

The **dermis**, the so-called "true skin," has a framework of elastic connective tissue and is well supplied with blood vessels and nerves. Because of its elasticity, the skin can stretch, even dramatically as in pregnancy, with little damage. Most of the accessory structures of the skin, including the sweat glands, the oil glands, and the hair, are located in the dermis and may extend into the subcutaneous layer under the skin.

The thickness of the dermis also varies in different areas. Some places, such as the soles of the feet and the palms of the hands, are covered with very thick layers of skin, whereas others, such as the eyelids, are covered with very thin and delicate layers. (See Box 6-1, Thick and Thin Skin: Getting a Grip on Their Differences.)

Portions of the dermis extend upward into the epidermis, allowing blood vessels to get closer to the surface cells (see Figs. 6-1 and 6-2). These extensions, or **dermal papillae**, can be seen on the surface of thick skin, such as at the tips of the fingers and toes. Here they form a distinct pattern of ridges that help to prevent slipping, such as when grasping an object. The unchanging patterns of the ridges are determined by heredity. Because they are unique to each person, fingerprints and footprints can be used for identification.

Checkpoint 6-1 The skin and all its associated structures comprise a body system. What is the name of this system?

Checkpoint 6-2 The skin itself is composed of two layers. Moving from the superficial to the deeper layer, what are the names of these two layers?

Subcutaneous Layer

The dermis rests on the **subcutaneous** (sub-ku-TA-ne-us) **layer**, sometimes referred to as the hypodermis or the superficial fascia (see Fig. 6-1). This layer connects the skin to the surface muscles. It consists of loose connective tissue and large amounts of adipose (fat) tissue. The fat serves as insulation and as a reserve supply for energy. Continuous bundles of elastic fibers connect the subcutaneous tissue with the dermis, so there is no clear boundary between the two.

Box 6-1 A Closer Look

Thick and Thin Skin: Getting a Grip on Their Differences

The skin is the largest organ in the body, weighing about 4 kg. Though it appears uniform in structure and function, its thickness in fact varies, from less than 1 mm covering the eyelids to more than 5 mm on the upper back. Many of the functional differences between skin regions reflect the thickness of the epidermis and not the skin's overall thickness. Based on epidermal thickness, skin can be categorized as **thick** (about 1 mm deep) or **thin** (about 0.1 mm deep).

Areas of the body exposed to significant wear and tear (the palms, fingertips, and bottoms of the feet and toes) are covered with thick skin. It is composed of a thick stratum corneum and an extra layer not found in thin skin, the stratum lucidum, both of which make thick skin resistant to abrasion. Thick skin is also characterized by epidermal ridges (*e.g.*, fingerprints) and numerous sweat glands, but lacks hair and sebaceous (oil) glands. These adaptations make the thick skin covering the hands and feet effective for grasping or gripping. Thick skin's dermis also contains many sensory receptors, giving the hands and feet a superior sense of touch.

Thin skin covers areas of the body not exposed to much wear and tear. It has a very thin stratum corneum and lacks a distinct stratum lucidum. Though thin skin lacks epidermal ridges and has fewer sensory receptors than thick skin, it has several specializations that thick skin does not. Thin skin is covered with hair, which may help prevent heat loss from the body. In fact, hair is most densely distributed in skin that covers regions of great heat loss—the head, axillae (armpits), and groin. Thin skin also contains numerous sebaceous glands, making it supple and free of cracks that may let infectious organisms enter.

The blood vessels that supply the skin with nutrients and oxygen and help to regulate body temperature run through the subcutaneous layer. This tissue is also rich in nerves and nerve endings, including those that supply nerve impulses to and from the dermis and epidermis. The thickness of the subcutaneous layer varies in different parts of the body; it is thinnest on the eyelids and thickest on the abdomen.

Checkpoint 6-3 What is the composition of the subcutaneous layer?

Accessory Structures of the Skin

The integumentary system includes some structures associated with the skin—glands, hair, and nails—that not only protect the skin itself but have some more generalized functions as well.

Sebaceous (Oil) Glands

The **sebaceous** (se-BA-shus) **glands** are saclike in structure, and their oily secretion, **sebum** (SE-bum), lubricates the skin and hair and prevents drying. The ducts of the sebaceous glands open into the hair follicles (Fig. 6-4 A).

Babies are born with a covering produced by these glands that resembles cream cheese; this secretion is called the **vernix caseosa** (VER-niks ka-se-O-sah), which literally means "cheesy varnish." Modified sebaceous glands, **meibomian** (mi-BO-me-an) **glands**, are associated with the eyelashes and produce a secretion that lubricates the eyes.

Blackheads consist of a mixture of dried sebum and keratin that may collect at the openings of the sebaceous glands. If these glands become infected, pimples result. If a sebaceous gland becomes blocked, a sac of accumulated sebum may form and gradually increase in size. Such a sac is referred to as a **sebaceous cyst.** Usually, it is not difficult to remove such tumorlike cysts by surgery.

Sudoriferous (Sweat) Glands

The **sudoriferous** (su-do-RIF-er-us) **glands,** or sweat glands, are coiled, tubelike structures located in the dermis and the subcutaneous tissue (see Fig. 6-4 B). Most of the sudoriferous glands function to cool the body. They release sweat, or perspiration, that draws heat from the skin as the moisture evaporates at the surface. These **eccrine** (EK-rin) type sweat glands are distributed throughout the skin. Each gland has a secretory portion and an excretory tube that extends directly to the surface and opens at a pore (see also Fig. 6-1). Because sweat contains small amounts of dissolved salts and other wastes in addition to water, these glands also serve a minor excretory function.

Present in smaller number, the **apocrine** (AP-o-krin) sweat glands are located mainly in the armpits (axillae) and groin area. These glands become active at puberty and release their secretions through the hair follicles in response to emotional stress and sexual stimulation. The apocrine glands release some cellular material in their secretions. Body odor develops from the action of bacteria in breaking down these organic cellular materials.

Several types of glands associated with the skin are modified sweat glands. These are the **ceruminous** (seh-RU-min-us) **glands** in the ear canal that produce ear wax, or **cerumen**; the **ciliary** (SIL-e-er-e) **glands** at the edges of the eyelids; and the **mammary glands.**

Checkpoint 6-4 Some skin glands produce an oily secretion called sebum. What is the name of these glands?

Checkpoint 6-5 What is the scientific name for the sweat glands?

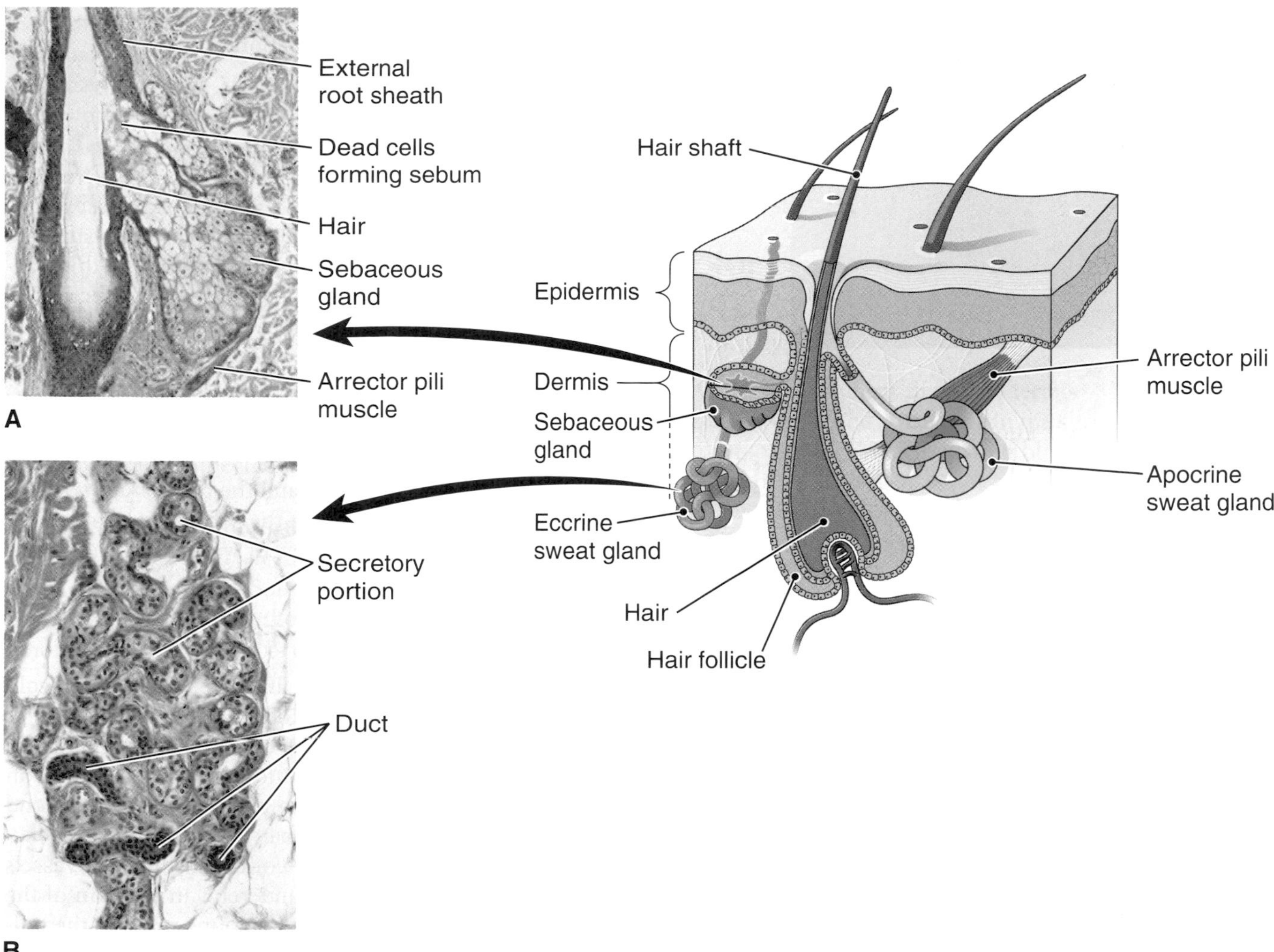

Figure 6-4 **Portion of skin showing associated glands and hair.** **(A)** A sebaceous (oil) gland and its associated hair follicle. **(B)** An eccrine (temperature-regulating) sweat gland. (A and B, Reprinted with permission from Cormack DH. Essential Histology. 2nd ed. Philadelphia: Lippincott Williams & Wilkins, 2001.) *ZOOMING IN ✦ How do the sebaceous glands and apocrine sweat glands secrete to the outside? What kind of epithelium makes up the sweat glands?*

Hair

Almost all of the body is covered with hair, which in most areas is soft and fine. Hairless regions are the palms of the hands, soles of the feet, lips, nipples, and parts of the external genital areas. Hair is composed mainly of keratin and is not living. Each hair develops, however, from living cells located in a bulb at the base of the **hair follicle**, a sheath of epithelial and connective tissue that encloses the hair (see Fig. 6-4). Melanocytes in this growth region add pigment to the developing hair. Different shades of melanin produce the various hair colors we see in the population. The part of the hair that projects above the skin is the **shaft**; the portion below the skin is the **root** of the hair.

Attached to most hair follicles is a thin band of involuntary muscle (see Fig. 6-1). When this muscle contracts, the hair is raised, forming "goose bumps" on the skin. The name of this muscle is **arrector pili** (ah-REK-tor PI-li), which literally means "hair raiser." This response is of no importance to humans but helps animals with furry coats to conserve heat. As the arrector pili contracts, it presses on the sebaceous gland associated with the hair follicle, causing the release of sebum to lubricate the skin.

Checkpoint 6-6 Each hair develops within a sheath. What is this sheath called?

Nails

Nails protect the fingers and toes and also help in grasping small objects with the hands. They are made of hard keratin produced by cells that originate in the outer layer of the epidermis (stratum corneum) (Fig. 6-5). New cells form continuously in a growth region (nail matrix) located under the proximal end of the nail, a portion called

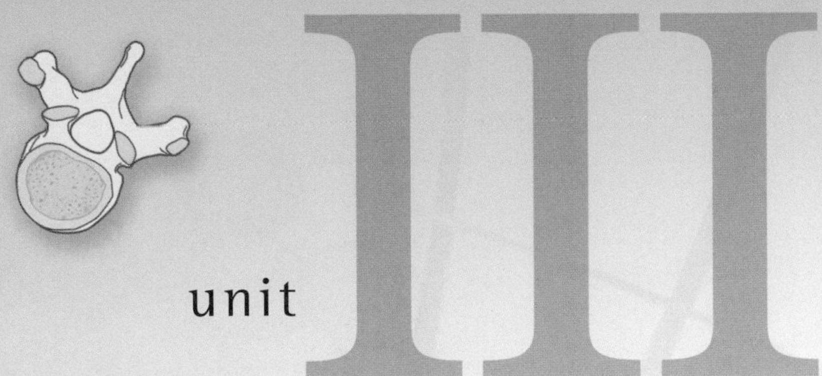

unit III

Movement and Support

This unit deals with the skeletal and muscular systems, which work together to execute movement and to support and protect vital organs. It covers the additional functions of the skeletal system in housing the blood-forming tissue and storing some minerals. The chapter on muscles describes the characteristics of all types of muscles and then concentrates on the muscles that are attached to the skeleton and how they function. The main skeletal muscles are named and located and their actions are described.

Selected Key Terms

The following terms and other boldface terms in the chapter are defined in the Glossary

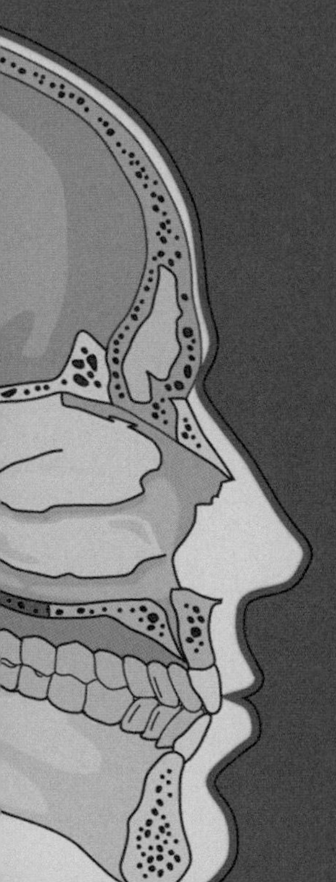

amphiarthrosis
arthritis
bursa
circumduction
diaphysis
diarthrosis
endosteum
epiphysis
fontanel
joint
osteoblast
osteoclast
osteocyte
osteon
osteopenia
osteoporosis
periosteum
resorption
skeleton
synarthrosis
synovial

Learning Outcomes

After careful study of this chapter, you should be able to:

1. List the functions of bones
2. Describe the structure of a long bone
3. Differentiate between compact bone and spongy bone with respect to structure and location
4. Differentiate between red and yellow marrow with respect to function and location
5. Name the three different types of cells in bone and describe the functions of each
6. Explain how a long bone grows
7. Name and describe various markings found on bones
8. List the bones in the axial skeleton
9. Explain the purpose of the infant fontanels
10. Describe the normal curves of the spine and explain their purpose
11. List the bones in the appendicular skeleton
12. Compare the structure of the female pelvis and the male pelvis
13. Describe five types of bone disorders
14. Name and describe eight types of fractures
15. Describe how the skeleton changes with age
16. Describe the three types of joints
17. Describe the structure of a synovial joint and give six examples of synovial joints
18. Demonstrate six types of movement that occur at synovial joints
19. Describe four types of arthritis
20. List some causes of backache
21. Show how word parts are used to build words related to the skeleton (see Word Anatomy at the end of the chapter)

chapter 7

The Skeleton: Bones and Joints

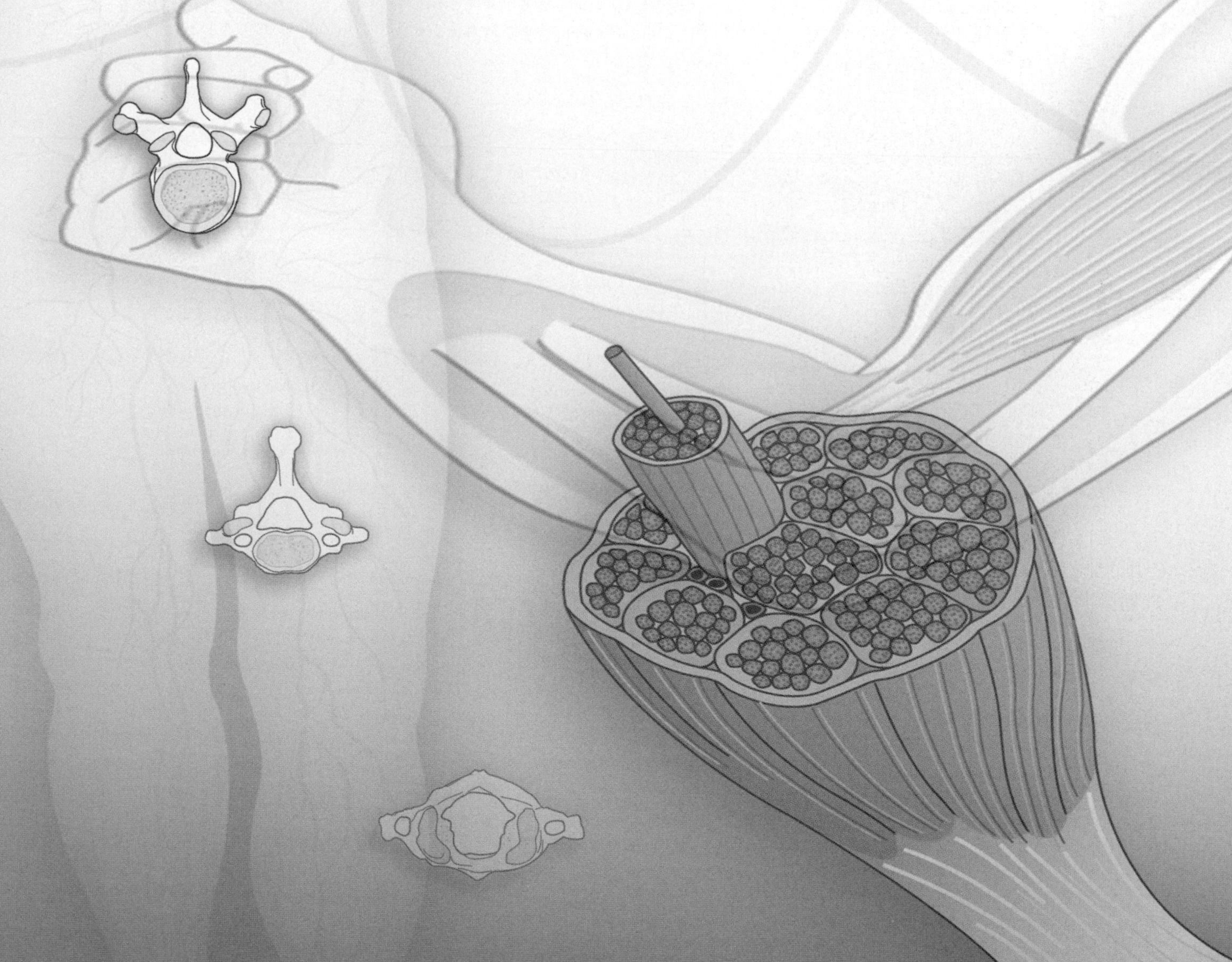

The skeleton is the strong framework on which the body is constructed. Much like the frame of a building, the skeleton must be strong enough to support and protect all the body structures. Bone tissue is the most dense form of the connective tissues described in Chapter 4. Bones work with muscles to produce movement at the joints. The bones and joints, together with supporting connective tissue, form the skeletal system.

Bones

Bones have a number of functions, several of which are not evident in looking at the skeleton:

- To serve as a firm framework for the entire body
- To protect such delicate structures as the brain and the spinal cord
- To serve as levers, working with attached muscles to produce movement
- To serve as a storehouse for calcium salts, which may be resorbed into the blood if there is not enough calcium in the diet
- To produce blood cells (in the red marrow)

Bone Structure

The complete bony framework of the body, known as the **skeleton** (Fig. 7-1), consists of 206 bones. It is divided into a central portion, the axial skeleton, and the extremities, which make up the appendicular skeleton. The individual bones in these two divisions will be described in detail later in this chapter. The bones of the skeleton can be of several different shapes. They may be flat (ribs, cranium), short (carpals of wrist, tarsals of ankle), or irregular (vertebrae, facial bones). The most familiar shape, however, is the **long bone**, the type of bone that makes up almost all of the skeleton of the arms and legs. The long narrow shaft of this type of bone is called the **diaphysis** (di-AF-ih-sis). At the center of the diaphysis is a **medullary** (MED-u-lar-e) **cavity**, which contains bone marrow. The long bone also has two irregular ends, a proximal and a distal **epiphysis** (eh-PIF-ih-sis) (Fig. 7-2).

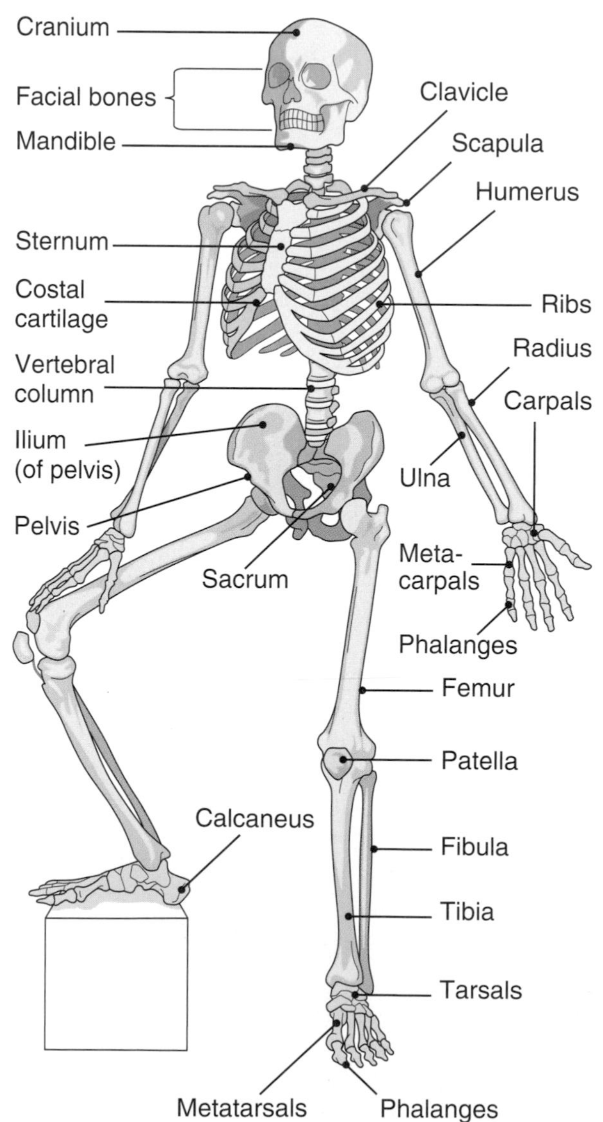

Figure 7-1 **The skeleton.** The axial skeleton is shown in yellow; the appendicular, in blue.

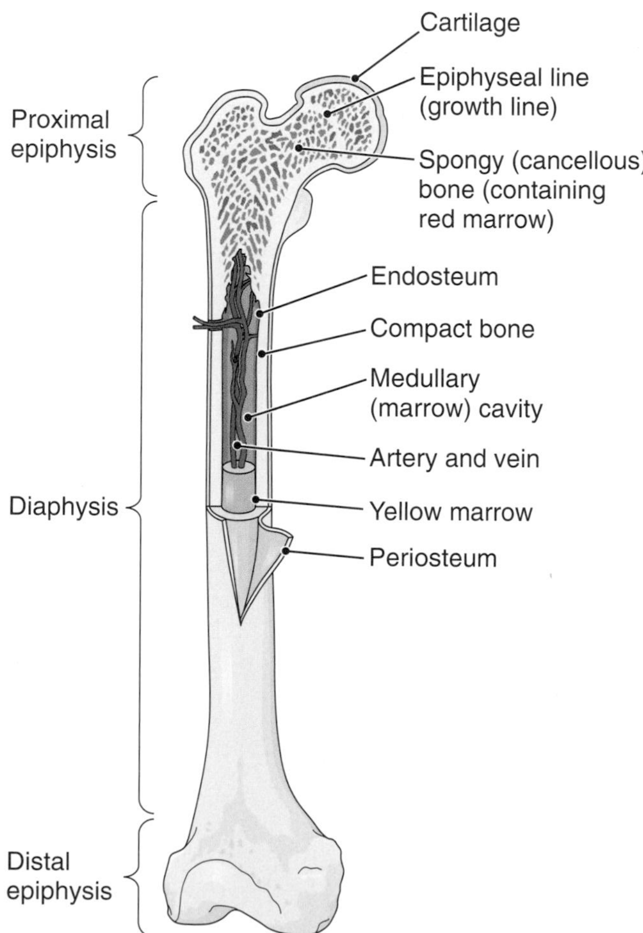

Figure 7-2 **The structure of a long bone.**

Bone Tissue Bones are not lifeless. Even though the spaces between the cells of bone tissue are permeated with stony deposits of calcium salts, the bone cells themselves are very much alive. Bones are organs, with their own system of blood vessels, lymphatic vessels, and nerves.

There are two types of bone tissue, also known as **osseous** (OS-e-us) **tissue**. One type is **compact bone**, which is hard and dense (Fig. 7-3). This tissue makes up the main shaft of a long bone and the outer layer of other bones. The cells in this type of bone are located in rings of bone tissue around a central **haversian** (ha-VER-shan) **canal** containing nerves and blood vessels. The bone cells live in spaces (lacunae) between the rings and extend out into many small radiating channels so that they can be in contact with nearby cells. Each ringlike unit with its central canal makes up a **haversian system**, also known as an **osteon** (OS-te-on) (see Fig. 7-3 B). Forming a channel across the bone, from one side of the shaft to the other, are many **perforating** (Volkmann) **canals**, which also house blood vessels and nerves.

The second type of bone tissue, called **spongy**, or **cancellous, bone**, has more spaces than compact bone. It is made of a meshwork of small, bony plates filled with red marrow. Spongy bone is found at the epiphyses (ends) of the long bones and at the center of other bones. Figure 7-4 shows a photograph of both compact and spongy tissue in a bone section.

Checkpoint 7-1 A long bone has a long, narrow shaft and two irregular ends. What are the scientific names for the shaft and the ends of a long bone?

Checkpoint 7-2 What are the two types of osseous (bone) tissue and where is each type found?

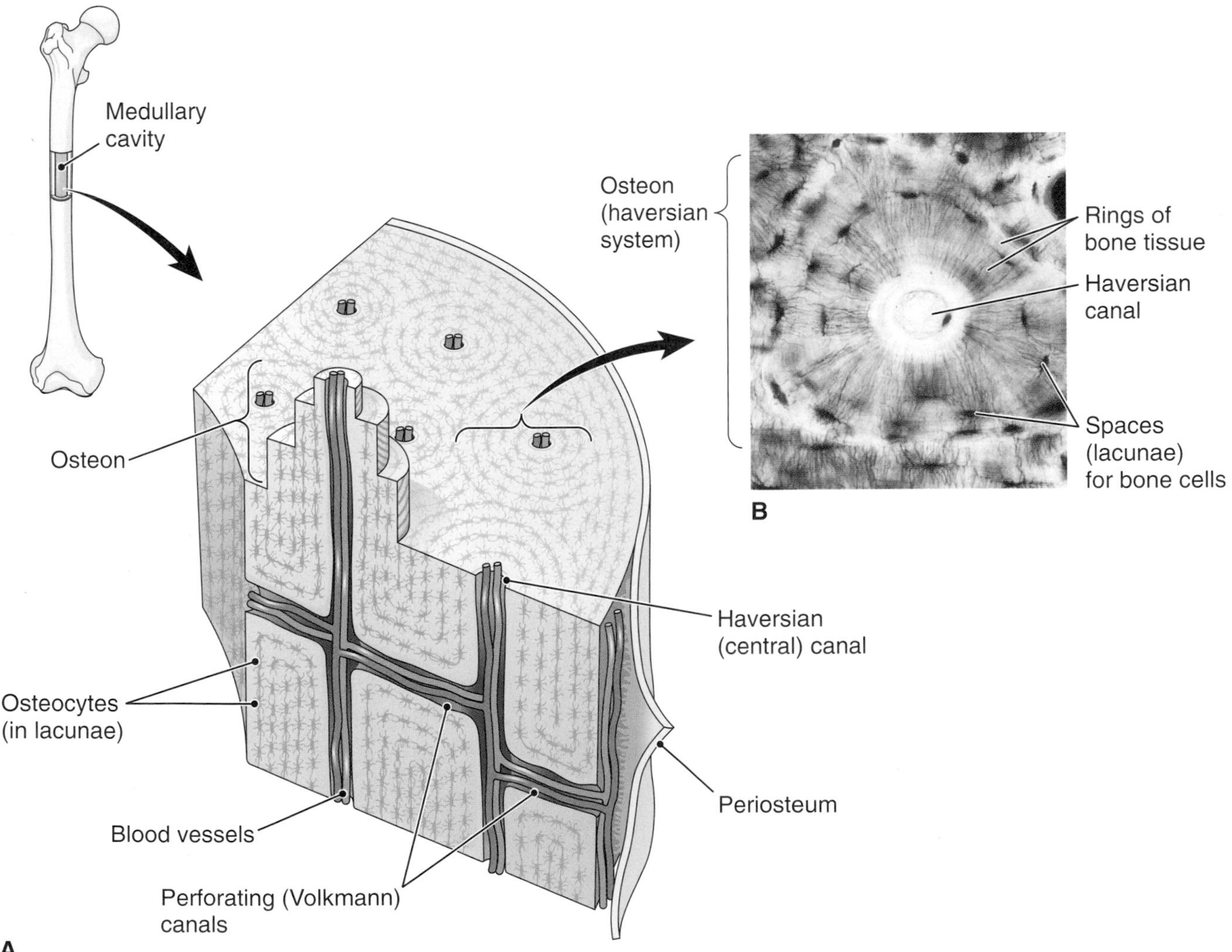

Figure 7-3 **Compact bone tissue. (A)** This section shows osteocytes (bone cells) within osteons (haversian systems). It also shows the canals that penetrate the tissue. **(B)** Microscopic view of compact bone in cross section (×300) showing a complete osteon. In living tissue, osteocytes (bone cells) reside in spaces (lacunae) and extend out into channels that radiate from these spaces. (B, Reprinted with permission from Ross MH, Kaye GI, Pawlina, W. Histology. 4th ed. Philadelphia: Lippincott Williams & Wilkins, 2003.)

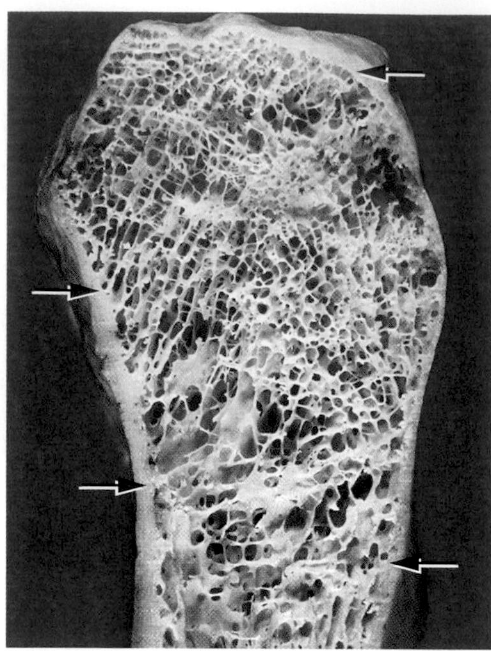

Figure 7-4 **Bone tissue, longitudinal section.** Spongy (cancellous) bone makes up most of the epiphysis (end) of this long bone, shown by the arrows. (Reprinted with permission from Ross MH, Kaye GI, Pawlina, W. Histology. 4th ed. Philadelphia: Lippincott Williams & Wilkins, 2003.)

Bone Marrow Bones contain two kinds of marrow. **Red marrow** is found at the ends of the long bones and at the center of other bones (see Fig. 7-2). Red bone marrow manufactures blood cells. **Yellow marrow** is found chiefly in the central cavities of the long bones. Yellow marrow is composed largely of fat.

Bone Membranes Bones are covered on the outside (except at the joint region) by a membrane called the **periosteum** (per-e-OS-te-um) (see Fig. 7-2). The inner layer of this membrane contains cells (osteoblasts) that are essential in bone formation, not only during growth but also in the repair of injuries. Blood vessels and lymphatic vessels in the periosteum play an important role in the nourishment of bone tissue. Nerve fibers in the periosteum make their presence known when one suffers a fracture, or when one receives a blow, such as on the shinbone. A thinner membrane, the **endosteum** (en-DOS-te-um), lines the marrow cavity of a bone; it too contains cells that aid in the growth and repair of bone tissue.

Bone Growth and Repair

During early development, the embryonic skeleton is at first composed almost entirely of cartilage. (Portions of the skull develop from fibrous connective tissue.) The conversion of cartilage to bone, a process known as **ossification**, begins during the second and third months of embryonic life. At this time, bone-building cells, called **osteoblasts** (OS-te-o-blasts), become active. First, they begin to manufacture the **matrix**, which is the material located between the cells. This intercellular substance contains large quantities of **collagen**, a fibrous protein that gives strength and resilience to the tissue. Then, with the help of enzymes, calcium compounds are deposited within the matrix.

Once this intercellular material has hardened, the cells remain enclosed within the lacunae (small spaces) in the matrix. These cells, now known as **osteocytes** (OS-te-o-sites), are still living and continue to maintain the existing bone matrix, but they do not produce new bone tissue. When bone has to be remodeled or repaired later in life, new osteoblasts develop from stem cells in the endosteum and periosteum.

One other type of cell found in bone develops from a type of white blood cell (monocyte). These large, multinucleated **osteoclasts** (OS-te-o-klasts) are responsible for the process of **resorption**, which is the breakdown of bone tissue. Resorption is necessary for remodeling and repair of bone, as occurs during growth and after injury. Bone tissue is also resorbed when its stored minerals are needed by the body.

The formation and resorption of bone tissue are regulated by several hormones. Vitamin D promotes the absorption of calcium from the intestine. Other hormones involved in these processes are produced by glands in the neck. Calcitonin from the thyroid gland promotes the uptake of calcium by bone tissue. Parathyroid hormone (PTH) from the parathyroid glands at the posterior of the thyroid causes bone resorption and release of calcium into the blood. These hormones are discussed more fully in Chapter 12.

Checkpoint 7-3 What are the three types of cells found in bone and what is the role of each?

Formation of a Long Bone In a long bone, the transformation of cartilage into bone begins at the center of the shaft during fetal development. Around the time of birth, secondary bone-forming centers, or **epiphyseal** (ep-ih-FIZ-e-al) **plates**, develop across the ends of the bones. The long bones continue to grow in length at these centers by calcification of new cartilage through childhood and into the late teens. Finally, by the late teens or early 20s, the bones stop growing in length. Each epiphyseal plate hardens and can be seen in x-ray films as a thin line, the epiphyseal line, across the end of the bone. Physicians can judge the future growth of a bone by the appearance of these lines on x-ray films.

As a bone grows in length, the shaft is remodeled so that it grows wider as the central marrow cavity increases in size. Thus, alterations in the shape of the bone are a result of the addition of bone tissue to some surfaces and its resorption from others.

The processes of bone resorption and bone formation continue throughout life, more actively in some places than in others, as bones are subjected to "wear and tear" or injuries. The bones of small children are relatively pliable because they contain a larger proportion of cartilage and are undergoing active bone formation. In elderly people, there is a slowing of the processes that continually renew bone tissue. As a result, the bones are weaker and more fragile. Elderly people also have a decreased ability to form the protein framework on which calcium salts are deposited. Fractures in elderly people heal more slowly because of these decreases in bone metabolism.

Checkpoint 7-4 As the embryonic skeleton is converted from cartilage to bone, the intercellular matrix becomes hardened. What compounds are deposited in the matrix to harden it?

Checkpoint 7-5 After birth, long bones continue to grow in length at secondary centers. What are these centers called?

Bone Markings

In addition to their general shape, bones have other distinguishing features, or **bone markings.** These markings include raised areas and depressions that help to form joints or serve as points for muscle attachments and various holes that allow the passage of nerves and blood vessels. Some of these identifying features are described next.

Projections

- **Head**—a rounded, knoblike end separated from the rest of the bone by a slender region, the neck.
- **Process**—a large projection of a bone, such as the upper part of the ulna in the forearm that creates the elbow.
- **Condyle** (KON-dile)—a rounded projection; a small projection above a condyle is an epicondyle.
- **Crest**—a distinct border or ridge, often rough, such as over the top of the hip bone.
- **Spine**—a sharp projection from the surface of a bone, such as the spine of the scapula (shoulder blade).

Depressions or Holes

- **Foramen** (fo-RA-men)—a hole that allows a vessel or a nerve to pass through or between bones. The plural is foramina (fo-RAM-ih-nah).
- **Sinus** (SI-nus)—an air space found in some skull bones.
- **Fossa** (FOS-sah)—a depression on a bone surface. The plural is fossae (FOS-se).
- **Meatus** (me-A-tus)—a short channel or passageway, such as the channel in the temporal bone of the skull that leads to the inner ear.

Examples of these and other markings can be seen on the bones illustrated in this chapter. To find out how these markings can be used in healthcare, see Box 7-1, Landmarking: Seeing With Your Fingers.

Checkpoint 7-6 Bones have a number of projections, depressions, and holes. What are some functions of these markings?

Bones of the Axial Skeleton

The skeleton may be divided into two main groups of bones (see Fig. 7-1):

- The **axial** (AK-se-al) **skeleton** consists of 80 bones and includes the bony framework of the head and the trunk.
- The **appendicular** (ap-en-DIK-u-lar) **skeleton** consists of 126 bones and forms the framework for the **extremities** (limbs) and for the shoulders and hips.

Box 7-1 **Clinical Perspectives**

Landmarking: Seeing With Your Fingers

Most body structures lie beneath the skin, hidden from view except in dissection. A technique called **landmarking** allows healthcare providers to visualize hidden structures without cutting into the patient. Bony prominences, or landmarks, can be palpated (felt) beneath the skin to serve as reference points for locating other structures. Landmarking is used during physical examinations and surgeries, when giving injections, and for many other clinical procedures. The lower tip of the sternum, the xiphoid process, is a reference point in the administration of cardiopulmonary resuscitation (CPR).

Practice landmarking by feeling for some of the other bony prominences. You can feel the joint between the mandible and the temporal bone of the skull (the temporomandibular joint, or TMJ) anterior to the ear canal as you move your lower jaw up and down. Feel for the notch in the sternum (breast bone) between the clavicles (collar bones). Approximately 4 cm below this notch you will feel a bump called the sternal angle. This prominence is an important landmark because its location marks where the trachea splits to deliver air to both lungs. Move your fingers lateral to the sternal angle to palpate the second ribs, important landmarks for locating the heart and lungs. Feel for the most lateral bony prominence of the shoulder, the acromion process of the scapula (shoulder blade). Two to three fingerbreadths down from this point is the correct injection site into the deltoid muscle of the shoulder. Place your hands on your hips and palpate the iliac crest of the hip bone. Move your hands forward until you reach the anterior end of the crest, the anterior superior iliac spine (ASIS). Feel for the part of the bony pelvis that you sit on. This is the ischial tuberosity. It and the ASIS are important landmarks for locating safe injection sites in the gluteal region.

Table 7•1 Bones of the Skeleton

REGION	BONES	DESCRIPTION
Axial Skeleton		
Skull		
Cranium	Cranial bones (8)	Chamber enclosing the brain; houses the ear and forms part of the eye socket
Facial portion	Facial bones (14)	Form the face and chambers for sensory organs
Hyoid		U-shaped bone under lower jaw; used for muscle attachments
Ossicles	Ear bones (3)	Transmit sound waves in inner ear
Trunk		
Vertebral column	Vertebrae (26)	Encloses the spinal cord
Thorax	Sternum	Anterior bone of the thorax
	Ribs (12 pair)	Enclose the organs of the thorax
Appendicular Skeleton		
Upper division		
Shoulder girdle	Clavicle	Anterior; between sternum and scapula
	Scapula	Posterior, anchors muscles that move arm
Upper extremity	Humerus	Proximal arm bone
	Ulna	Medial bone of forearm
	Radius	Lateral bone of forearm
	Carpals (8)	Wrist bones
	Metacarpals (5)	Bones of palm
	Phalanges (14)	Bones of fingers
Lower division		
Pelvis	Os coxae (2)	Join sacrum and coccyx of vertebral column to form the bony pelvis
Lower extremity	Femur	Thigh bone
	Patella	Kneecap
	Tibia	Medial bone of leg
	Fibula	Lateral bone of leg
	Tarsal bones (7)	Ankle bones
	Metatarsals (5)	Bones of instep
	Phalanges (14)	Bones of toes

We describe the axial skeleton first and then proceed to the appendicular skeleton. Table 7-1 provides an outline of all the bones included in this discussion.

Framework of the Skull

The bony framework of the head, called the **skull**, is subdivided into two parts: the cranium and the facial portion. Refer to Figures 7-5 through 7-8, which show different views of the skull, as you study the following descriptions. Color-coding of the bones will aid in identification as the skull is seen from different positions.

Cranium This rounded chamber that encloses the brain is composed of eight distinct cranial bones.

- The **frontal bone** forms the forehead, the anterior of the skull's roof, and the roof of the eye orbit (socket). The **frontal sinuses** (air spaces) communicate with the nasal cavities (see Figs. 7-7 and 7-8). These sinuses and others near the nose are described as **paranasal sinuses.**
- The two **parietal** (pah-RI-eh-tal) bones form most of the top and the side walls of the cranium.
- The two **temporal bones** form part of the sides and some of the base of the skull. Each one contains **mastoid sinuses** as well as the ear canal, the eardrum, and the entire middle and internal portions of the ear. The **mastoid process** of the temporal bone projects downward immediately behind the external part of the ear. It contains the mastoid air cells and serves as a place for muscle attachment.
- The **ethmoid** (ETH-moyd) **bone** is a light, fragile bone located between the eyes (see Fig. 7-7). It forms a part of the medial wall of the eye orbit, a small portion of the cranial floor, and most of the nasal cavity roof. It contains several air spaces, comprising some of the paranasal sinuses. A thin, platelike, downward extension of this bone (the perpendicular plate) forms much of the nasal septum, a midline partition in the nose (see Fig. 7-5 A)
- The **sphenoid** (SFE-noyd) **bone**, when seen from a superior view, resembles a bat with its wings extended. It lies at the base of the skull anterior to the temporal bones and forms part of the eye socket. The sphenoid contains a saddlelike depression, the **sella turcica** (SEL-ah TUR-sih-ka), that holds and protects the pituitary gland (see Fig. 7-7).
- The **occipital** (ok-SIP-ih-tal) **bone** forms the posterior and a part of the base of the skull. The **foramen magnum**, located at the base of the occipital bone, is a large opening through which the spinal cord communicates with the brain (see Figs. 7-6 and 7-7).

Uniting the bones of the skull is a type of flat, immovable joint known as a **suture** (SU-chur) (see Fig. 7-5). Some of the most prominent cranial sutures are the:

- Coronal (ko-RO-nal) suture, which joins the frontal bone with the two parietal bones along the coronal plane
- Squamous (SKWA-mus) suture, which joins the temporal bone to the parietal bone on the lateral surface of the cranium (named because it is in a flat portion of the skull)
- Lambdoid (LAM-doyd) suture, which joins the occipital bone with the parietal bones in the posterior cra-

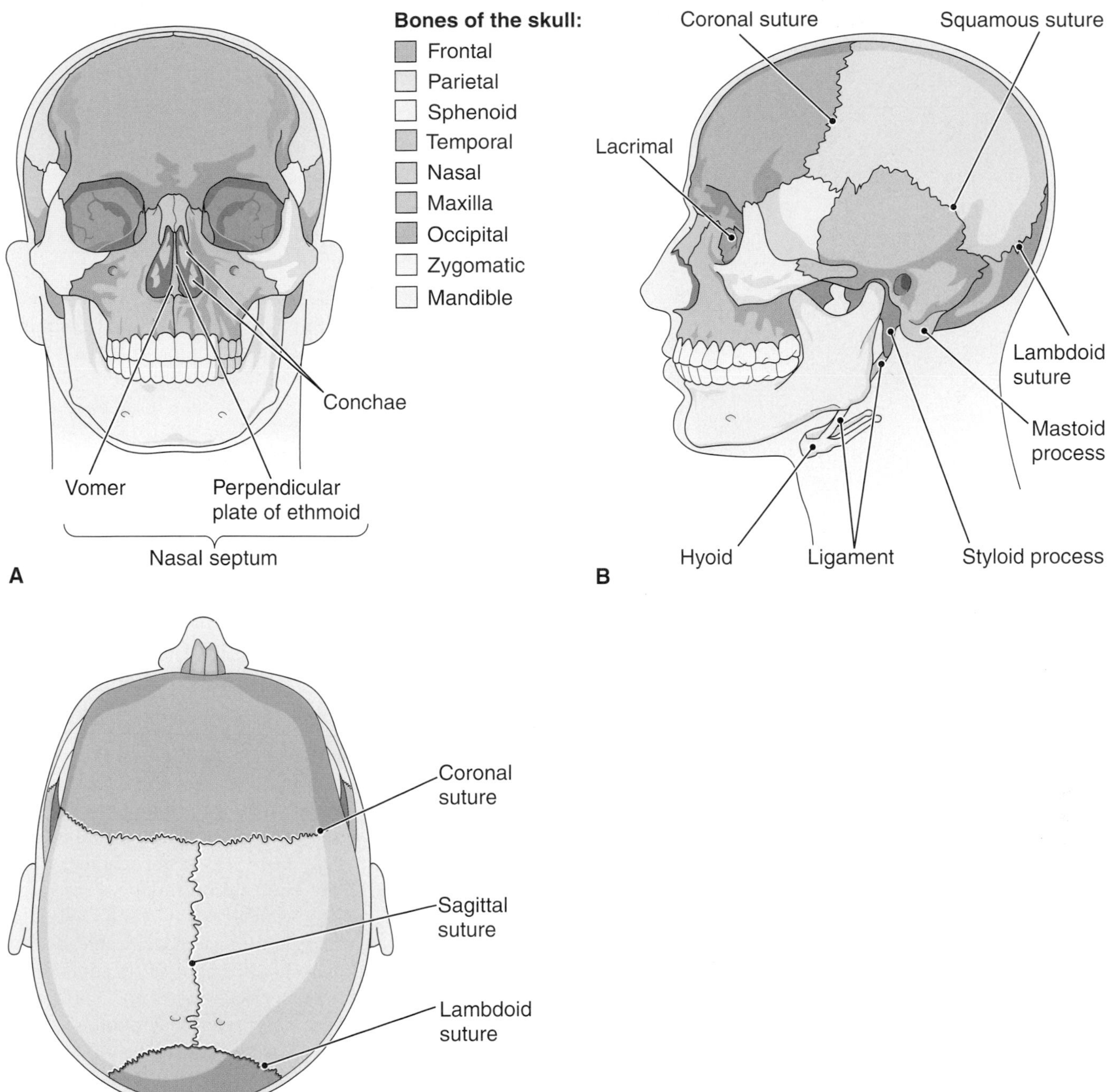

Figure 7-5 **The skull.** **(A)** Anterior view. **(B)** Left lateral view. **(C)** Superior view. *ZOOMING IN ✦ What type of joint is between bones of the skull?*

nium (named because it resembles the Greek letter lambda)

- Sagittal (SAJ-ih-tal) suture, which joins the two parietal bones along the superior midline of the cranium, along the sagittal plane

Facial Bones The facial portion of the skull is composed of 14 bones (see Fig. 7-5):

- The **mandible** (MAN-dih-bl), or lower jaw bone, is the only movable bone of the skull.
- The two **maxillae** (mak-SIL-e) fuse in the midline to form the upper jaw bone, including the front part of the hard palate (roof of the mouth). Each maxilla contains a large air space, called the **maxillary sinus**, that communicates with the nasal cavity.
- The two **zygomatic** (zi-go-MAT-ik) **bones**, one on each side, form the prominences of the cheeks.
- Two slender **nasal bones** lie side by side, forming the bridge of the nose.
- The two **lacrimal** (LAK-rih-mal) **bones**, each about the size of a fingernail, lie near the inside corner of the

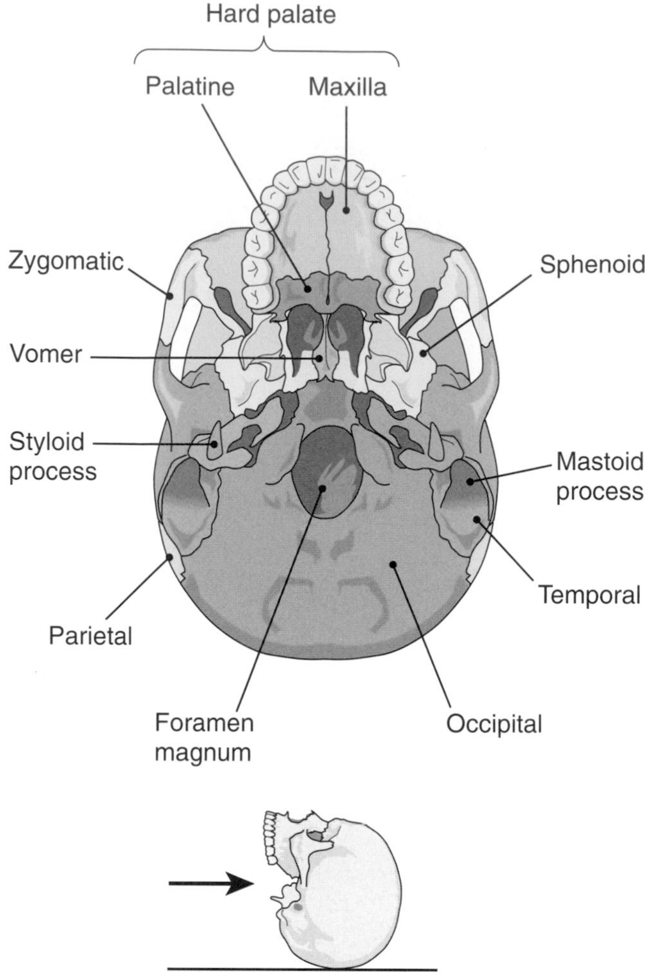

Figure 7-6 **The skull, inferior view.** The mandible (lower jaw) has been removed. *ZOOMING IN ✦ What two bones make up each side of the hard palate?*

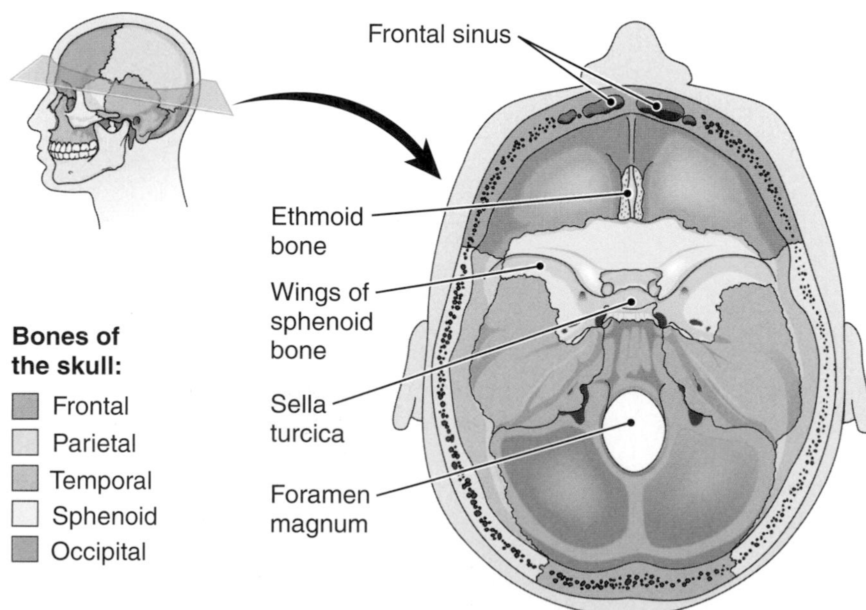

Figure 7-7 **Floor of cranium, superior view.** The internal surfaces of some of the cranial bones are visible. *ZOOMING IN ✦ What is a foramen?*

eye in the front part of the medial wall of the orbital cavity.

- The **vomer** (VO-mer), shaped like the blade of a plow, forms the lower part of the nasal septum (see Fig. 7-5 A).
- The paired **palatine** (PAL-ah-tine) **bones** form the back part of the hard palate (see Figs. 7-6 and 7-8).
- The two **inferior nasal conchae** (KON-ke) extend horizontally along the lateral wall (sides) of the nasal cavities. The paired superior and middle conchae are part of the ethmoid bone (see Figs. 7-5 A and 7-8).

In addition to the bones of the cranium and the facial bones, there are three tiny bones, or **ossicles** (OS-sik-ls), in each middle ear (see Chapter 11) and a single horseshoe, or U-shaped, bone just below the skull proper, called the **hyoid** (HI-oyd) **bone,** to which the tongue and other muscles are attached (see Fig. 7-5 B).

Openings in the base of the skull provide spaces for the entrance and exit of many blood vessels, nerves, and other structures. Projections and slightly elevated portions of the bones provide for the attachment of muscles. Some portions protect delicate structures, such as the eye orbit and the part of the temporal bone that encloses the inner portions of the ear. The sinuses provide lightness and serve as resonating chambers for the voice (which is why your voice sounds better to you as you are speaking than it sounds when you hear it played back as a recording).

Infant Skull The skull of the infant has areas in which the bone formation is incomplete, leaving so-called soft spots, properly called **fontanels** (fon-tah-NELS) (Fig. 7-9). These flexible regions allow the skull to compress and change shape during the birth process. They also allow for rapid growth of the brain during infancy. Although there are a number of fontanels, the largest and most recognizable is near the front of the skull at the junction of the two parietal bones and the frontal bone. This **anterior fontanel** usually does not close until the child is about 18 months old.

Framework of the Trunk

The bones of the trunk include the spine, or **vertebral** (VER-teh-bral), **column**, and the bones of the chest, or **thorax** (THO-raks).

Vertebral Column This bony sheath for the spinal cord is made of a series of irregularly shaped bones. These number 33 or 34 in the child, but because of fusions that occur later in the lower part of the spine, there usually are just 26 separate bones in the adult spinal column. Figures 7-10

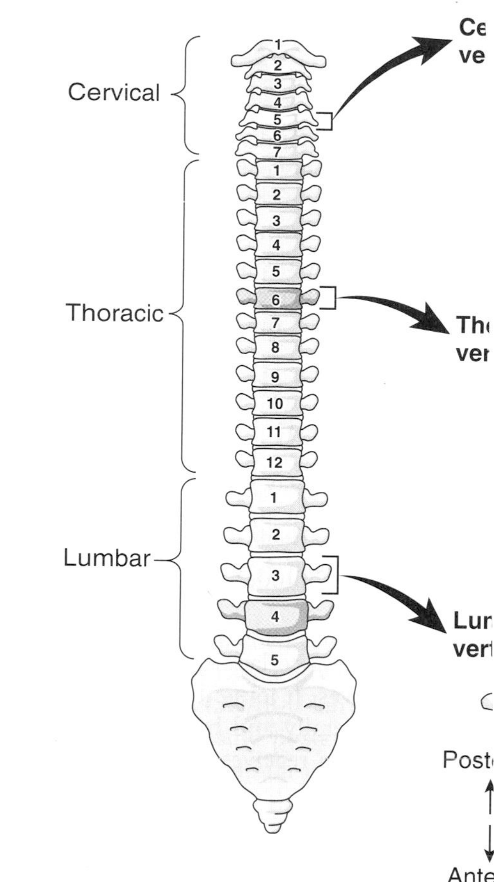

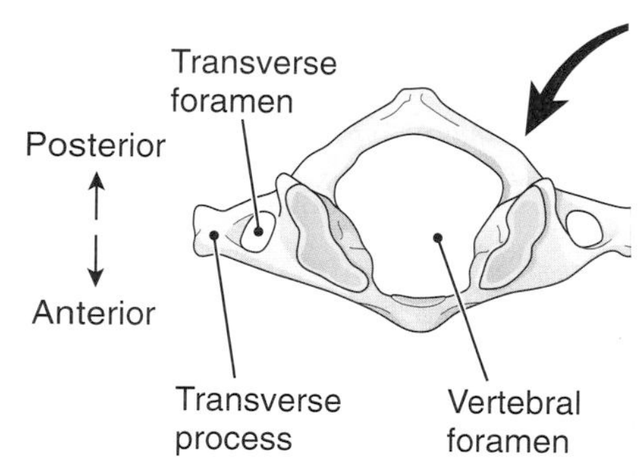

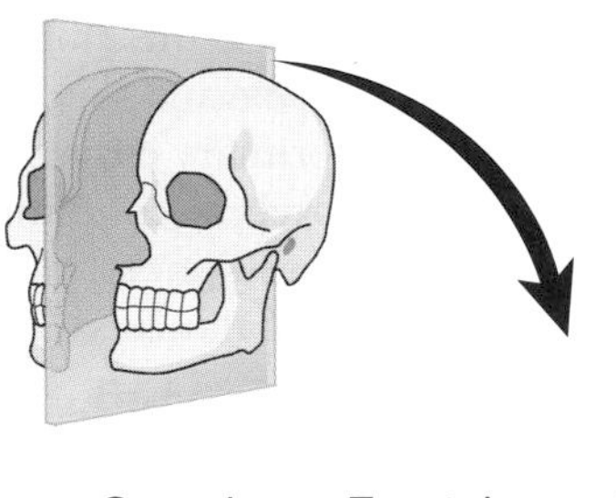

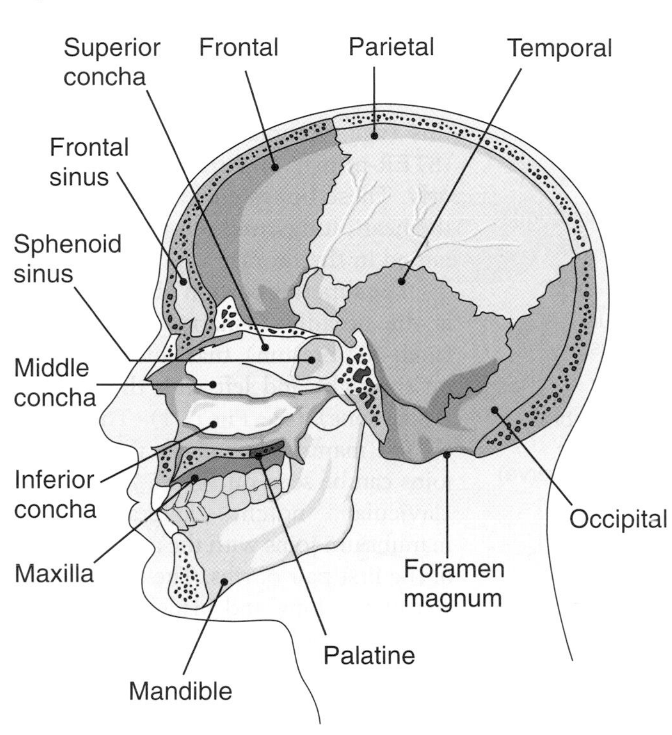

Figure 7-8 **The skull, sagittal section.**

and 7-11 show the vertebral column from lateral and anterior views.

The **vertebrae** (VER-teh-bre) have a drum-shaped **body** (centrum) located anteriorly (toward the front) that serves as the weight-bearing part; disks of cartilage between the vertebral bodies act as shock absorbers and provide flexibility (see Fig. 7-11). In the center of each vertebra is a large hole, or foramen. When all the vertebrae are linked in series by strong connective tissue bands (ligaments), these spaces form the spinal canal, a bony cylinder that protects the spinal cord. Projecting dorsally (toward the back) from the bony arch that encircles the spinal cord is the **spinous process**, which usually can be felt just under the skin of the back. Projecting laterally is a **transverse process** on each side. These processes are attachment points for muscles. When viewed from a lateral aspect, the vertebral column can be seen to have a series of **intervertebral foramina**, formed between the vertebrae as they join together, through which spinal nerves emerge as they leave the spinal cord (see Fig. 7-10).

The bones of the vertebral column are named and numbered from above downward, on the basis of location. There are five regions:

- The **cervical** (SER-vih-kal) **vertebrae**, seven in number (C1 to C7), are located in the neck (see Fig. 7-11). The first vertebra, called the **atlas**, supports the head (Fig. 7-12). (This vertebra is named for the mythologic character who was able to support the world in his hands.) When one nods the head, the skull rocks on the atlas at the occipital bone. The second cervical vertebra, the **axis** (see Fig. 7-12), serves as a pivot when the head is turned from side to side. It has an upright toothlike part, the **dens**, that projects into the atlas and serves as a pivot point. The absence of a body in these vertebrae allows for the extra movement. Only the cervical vertebrae have a hole in the tranverse process on each side (see Fig. 7-11). These **transverse foramina** accommodate blood vessels and nerves that supply the neck and head.
- The **thoracic vertebrae**, 12 in number (T1 to T12), are located in the chest. They are larger and stronger than the cervical vertebrae and each has a longer spinous process that points downward (see Fig. 7-11). The posterior ends of the 12 pairs of ribs are attached to these vertebrae.
- The **lumbar vertebrae**, five in number (L1 to L5), are located in the small of the back. They are larger and heavier than the vertebrae superior to them and can support more weight (see Fig. 7-11). All of their processes are shorter and thicker.

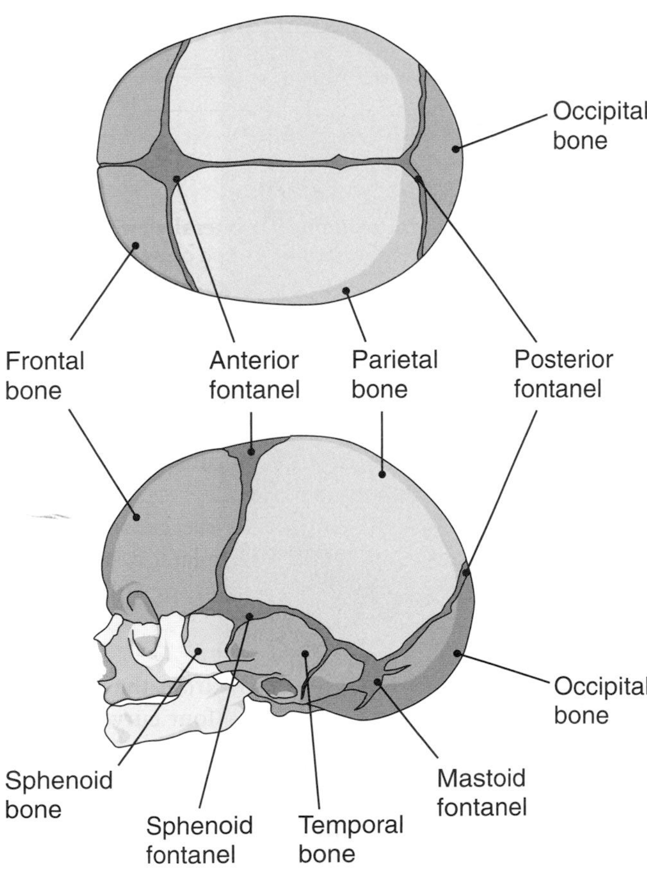

Figure 7-9 **Infant skull, showing fontanels.** *ZOOMING IN ✦ Which is the largest fontanel?*

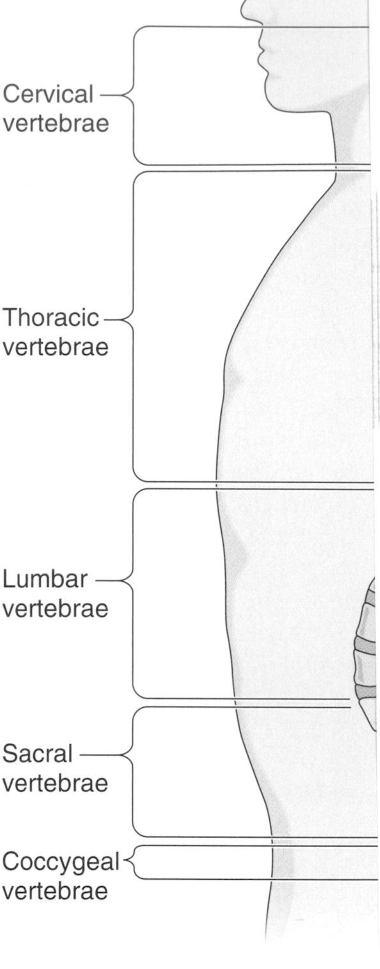

Figure 7-10 **Vertebral column, left la** *rior view, which group(s) of vertebrae forn cave curve?*

- The **sacral** (SA-kral) **vertebrae** are in the child. They eventually fuse to called the **sacrum** (SA-krum), in the tween the two hip bones, the saci posterior part of the bony pelvis.
- The **coccygeal** (kok-SIJ-e-al) **verteb** or five tiny bones in the child. Thes a single bone, the **coccyx** (KOK-sik the adult.

Curves of the Spine When viewed vertebral column can be seen to have sponding to the four groups of verteb In the fetus, the entire column is conca away from a viewer facing the fetus), a 13. This is the primary curve.

When an infant begins to assume secondary curves develop. These c (curve toward the viewer). The cerv when the head is held up at about 3

tal end of shafts of t position, ulna pops

Figure 7 supine (fa When the crosses o

2. Types of synovial joints—gliding, hinge, pivot, condyloid, saddle, ball-and-socket
3. Movement at synovial joints
   a. Angular—flexion, extension, abduction, adduction
   b. Circular—circumduction, rotation
   c. Special at forearm—supination, pronation,
   d. Special at ankle—inversion, eversion, dorsiflexion, plantar flexion

B. Disorders of Joints
1. Dislocations and sprains
2. Herniated disk—central portion of intervertebral disk projects through outer cartilage
3. Arthritis—osteoarthritis, rheumatoid arthritis, infectious arthritis, gout
4. Backache

Questions for Study and Review

Building Understanding

Fill in the blanks

1. The shaft of a long bone is called the ______.
2. The structural unit of compact bone is the ______.
3. Red bone marrow manufactures ______.
4. Bones are covered by a connective tissue membrane called ______.
5. Bone matrix is produced by ______.

Matching

Match each numbered item with the most closely related lettered item.

___ 6. A rounded bony projection
___ 7. A sharp bony prominence
___ 8. A hole through bone
___ 9. A bony depression
___ 10. An air-filled bony cavity

a. condyle
b. foramen
c. fossa
d. sinus
e. spine

Multiple choice

___ 11. On which of the following bones would the mastoid process be found?
   a. occipital bone
   b. femur
   c. temporal bone
   d. humerus

___ 12. An abnormal exaggeration of the thoracic curve is called
   a. kyphosis
   b. lordosis
   c. osteitis deformans
   d. Pott disease

___ 13. A splintered or crushed bone with multiple fractures is classified as having a(n) ______ fracture
   a. open
   b. impacted
   c. comminuted
   d. greenstick

___ 14. A joint that is freely moveable is called a(n) ______ joint.
   a. arthrotic
   b. amphiarthrotic
   c. diarthrotic
   d. synarthrotic

___ 15. Which of the following synovial joints describes the hip?
   a. gliding
   b. hinge
   c. pivot
   d. ball-and-socket

Understanding Concepts

16. List five functions of bone and describe how a long bone's structure enables it to carry out each of these functions.
17. Explain the differences between the terms in each of the following pairs:
   a. osteoblast and osteocyte
   b. periosteum and endosteum
   c. compact bone and spongy bone
   d. epiphysis and diaphysis
   e. axial skeleton and appendicular skeleton
18. Discuss the process of long bone formation during fetal development and childhood. What role does resorption play in bone formation?
19. Name the bones of the:
   a. cranium and face
   b. thoracic cavity, vertebral column, and pelvis
   c. upper and lower limbs

20. Compare and contrast osteoporosis, osteomalacia, and osteomyelitis
21. Name three effects of aging on the skeletal system.
22. What are the similarities and differences between osteoarthritis, rheumatoid arthritis, and gout?
23. Differentiate between the terms in each of the following pairs:
    a. flexion and extension
    b. abduction and adduction
    c. supination and pronation
    d. inversion and eversion
    e. circumduction and rotation
    f. dorsiflexion and plantar flexion

Conceptual Thinking

24. The vertebral bodies are much larger in the lower back than the neck. What is the functional significance of this structural difference?

25. Nine-year-old Alek is admitted into Emergency with a closed fracture of the right femur. Radiography reveals that the fracture crosses the distal epiphyseal plate. What concerns should Alek's healthcare team have about the location of his injury?

Selected Key Terms

The following terms and other boldface terms in the chapter are defined in the Glossary

acetylcholine
actin
antagonist
bursitis
fascicle
glycogen
insertion
lactic acid
motor unit
myalgia
myoglobin
myosin
neuromuscular junction
neurotransmitter
origin
oxygen debt
prime mover
spasm
synapse
synergist
tendon
tonus

Learning Outcomes

After careful study of this chapter, you should be able to:

1. Compare the three types of muscle tissue
2. Describe three functions of skeletal muscle
3. Briefly describe how skeletal muscles contract
4. List the substances needed in muscle contraction and describe the function of each
5. Define the term oxygen debt
6. Describe three compounds stored in muscle that are used to generate energy in highly active muscle cells
7. Cite the effects of exercise on muscles
8. Compare isotonic and isometric contractions
9. Explain how muscles work in pairs to produce movement
10. Compare the workings of muscles and bones to lever systems
11. Explain how muscles are named
12. Name some of the major muscles in each muscle group and describe the main function of each
13. Describe how muscles change with age
14. List the major muscular disorders
15. Show how word parts are used to build words related to the muscular system (see Word Anatomy at the end of the chapter)

chapter 8

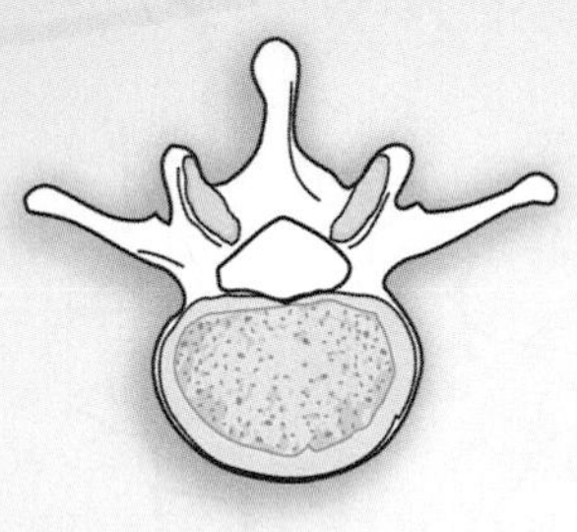

The Muscular System

Types of Muscle

There are three kinds of muscle tissue: smooth, cardiac, and skeletal muscle, as introduced in Chapter 4. After a brief description of all three types (Table 8-1), this chapter concentrates on skeletal muscle, which has been studied the most.

Smooth Muscle

Smooth muscle makes up the walls of the hollow body organs as well as those of the blood vessels and respiratory passageways. It moves involuntarily and produces the wavelike motions of peristalsis that move substances through a system. Smooth muscle can also regulate the diameter of an opening, such as the central opening of blood vessels, or produce contractions of hollow organs, such as the uterus. Smooth muscle fibers (cells) are tapered at each end and have a single, central nucleus. The cells appear smooth under the microscope because they do not contain the visible bands, or **striations**, that are seen in the other types of muscle cells. Smooth muscle may contract in response to a nerve impulse, hormonal stimulation, stretching, and other stimuli. The muscle contracts and relaxes slowly and can remain contracted for a long time.

Cardiac Muscle

Cardiac muscle, also involuntary, makes up the wall of the heart and creates the pulsing action of that organ. The cells of cardiac muscle are striated, like those of skeletal muscle. They differ in having one nucleus per cell and branching interconnections. The membranes between the cells are specialized to allow electrical impulses to travel rapidly through them, so that contractions can be better coordinated. These membranes appear as dark lines between the cells (see Table 8-1) and are called intercalated (in-TER-kah-la-ted) disks, because they are "inserted between" the cells. The electrical impulses that produce contractions of cardiac muscle are generated within the muscle itself but can be modified by nervous stimuli and hormones.

Skeletal Muscle

When viewed under the microscope, skeletal muscle cells appear heavily striated. The arrangement of protein threads within the cell that produces these striations is described later. The cells are very long and cylindrical and have multiple nuclei per cell. During development, the nuclei of these cells divide repeatedly by mitosis without division of the cell contents, resulting in a large, multinucleated cell. Such cells can contract as a large unit when stimulated. The nervous system stimulates skeletal muscle to contract, and the tissue usually contracts and relaxes rapidly. Because it is under conscious control, skeletal muscle is described as voluntary.

Skeletal muscle is so named because most of these muscles are attached to bones and produce movement at the joints. There are a few exceptions. The muscles of the abdominal wall, for example, are partly attached to other muscles, and the muscles of facial expression are attached to the

Table 8•1 Comparison of the Different Types of Muscle

	SMOOTH	CARDIAC	SKELETAL
Location	Wall of hollow organs, vessels, respiratory passageways	Wall of heart	Attached to bones
Cell characteristics	Tapered at each end, branching networks, nonstriated	Branching networks; special membranes (intercalated disks) between cells; single nucleus; lightly striated	Long and cylindrical; multinucleated; heavily striated
Control	Involuntary	Involuntary	Voluntary
Action	Produces peristalsis; contracts and relaxes slowly; may sustain contraction	Pumps blood out of heart; self-excitatory but influenced by nervous system and hormones	Produces movement at joints; stimulated by nervous system; contracts and relaxes rapidly

skin. Skeletal muscles constitute the largest amount of the body's muscle tissue, making up about 40% of the total body weight. This muscular system is composed of more than 600 individual skeletal muscles. Although each one is a distinct structure, muscles usually act in groups to execute body movements.

Checkpoint 8-1 What are the three types of muscle?

Table 8•2 Connective Tissue Layers in Skeletal Muscle

NAME OF LAYER	LOCATION
Endomysium	Around each individual muscle fiber
Perimysium	Around fascicles (bundles) of muscle fibers
Epimysium	Around entire muscle; forms the innermost layer of the deep fascia.

The Muscular System

The three primary functions of skeletal muscles are:

- Movement of the skeleton. Muscles are attached to bones and contract to change the position of the bones at a joint.
- Maintenance of posture. A steady partial contraction of muscle, known as **muscle tone**, keeps the body in position. Some of the muscles involved in maintaining posture are the large muscles of the thighs, back, neck, and shoulders as well as the abdominal muscles.
- Generation of heat. Muscles generate most of the heat needed to keep the body at 37°C (98.6°F). Heat is a natural byproduct of muscle cell metabolism. When we are cold, muscles can boost their heat output by the rapid small contractions we know of as shivering.

Checkpoint 8-2 What are the three main functions of skeletal muscle?

Structure of a Muscle

In forming whole muscles, individual muscle fibers are arranged in bundles, or **fascicles** (FAS-ih-kls), held together by fibrous connective tissue (Fig. 8-1, Table 8-2). The deepest layer of this connective tissue, the **endomysium** (en-do-MIS-e-um) surrounds the individual fibers in the fascicles. Around each fascicle is a connective tissue layer known as the **perimysium** (per-ih-MIS-e-um). The entire muscle is then encased in a tough connective tissue sheath, the **epimysium** (ep-ih-MIS-e-um), which forms the innermost layer of the **deep fascia**, the tough, fibrous sheath that encloses a muscle. (Note that all these layers are named with prefixes that describe their position added to the root *my/o*, meaning "muscle.") All of these supporting tissues merge to form the **tendon**, the band of connective tissue that attaches a muscle to a bone (see Fig. 8-1).

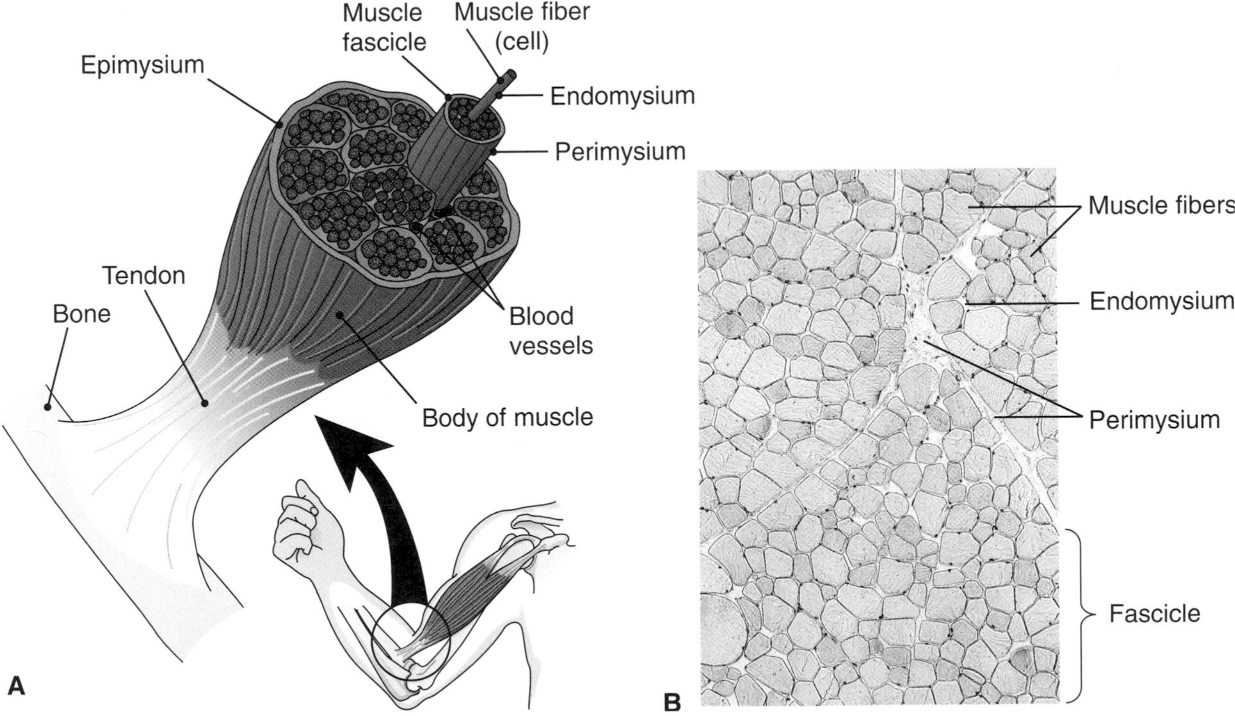

Figure 8-1 **Structure of a skeletal muscle. (A)** Structure of a muscle showing the tendon that attaches it to a bone. **(B)** Muscle tissue seen under a microscope. Portions of several fascicles are shown with connective tissue coverings. (B, Reprinted with permission from Gartner LP, Hiatt JL. Color Atlas of Histology. 3rd ed. Philadelphia: Lippincott Williams & Wilkins, 2000.) *ZOOMING IN ✦ What is the innermost layer of connective tissue in a muscle? What layer of connective tissue surrounds a fascicle of muscle fibers?*

Muscle Cells in Action

Nerve impulses coming from the brain and the spinal cord stimulate skeletal muscle fibers (see Chapter 9). Because these impulses are traveling away from the central nervous system (CNS), they are described as **motor** impulses (as contrasted to sensory impulses traveling toward the CNS), and the neurons (nerve cells) that carry these impulses are described as motor neurons. As the neuron contacts the muscle, its axon (fiber) branches to supply from a few to hundreds of individual muscle cells, or in some cases more than 1000 (Fig. 8-2).

A single neuron and all the muscle fibers it stimulates comprise a **motor unit**. Small motor units are used in fine coordination, as in movements of the eye. Larger motor units are used for maintaining posture or for broad movements, such as walking or swinging a tennis racquet.

The Neuromuscular Junction The point at which a nerve fiber contacts a muscle cell is called the **neuromuscular junction** (NMJ) (Fig. 8-3). It is here that a chemical classified as a **neurotransmitter** is released from the neuron to stimulate the muscle fiber. The specific neurotransmitter released here is **acetylcholine** (as-e-til-KO-lene), abbreviated ACh, which is found elsewhere in the body as well. A great deal is known about the events that occur at this junction, and this information is important in understanding muscle action.

The neuromuscular junction is an example of a **synapse** (SIN-aps), a point of communication between cells. Between the cells there is a tiny space, the **synaptic cleft**, across which the neurotransmitter must travel. Until its release, the neurotransmitter is stored in tiny membranous sacs, called vesicles, in the endings of the nerve fiber. Once released, the neurotransmitter crosses the synaptic cleft and attaches to receptors, which are proteins embedded in the muscle cell membrane. The membrane forms multiple folds at this point that increase surface area and hold a maximum number of receptors. The receiving membrane of the muscle cell is known as the **motor end plate**.

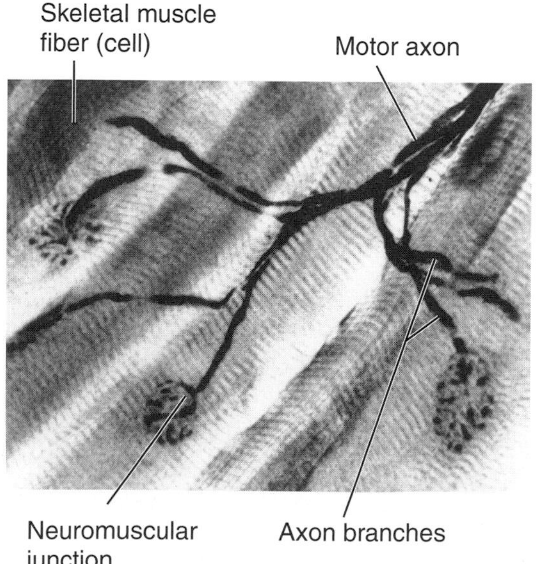

Figure 8-2 Nervous stimulation of skeletal muscle. A motor axon branches to stimulate multiple muscle fibers (cells). The point of contact between the neuron and the muscle cell is the neuromuscular junction. (Reprinted with permission from Cormack DH. Essential Histology. 2nd ed. Philadelphia: Lippincott Williams & Wilkins, 2001.)

Muscle fibers, like nerve cells, show the property of **excitability**; that is, they are able to transmit electrical current along the plasma membrane. When the muscle is stimulated at the neuromuscular junction, an electrical impulse is generated that spreads rapidly along the muscle cell membrane. This spreading wave of electrical current is called the **action potential** because it calls the muscle cell into action. Chapter 9 provides more information on synapses and the action potential.

Checkpoint 8-3 Muscles are activated by the nervous system. What is the name of the special synapse where a nerve cell makes contact with a muscle cell?

Checkpoint 8-4 What neurotransmitter is involved in the stimulation of skeletal muscle cells?

Contraction Another important property of muscle tissue is **contractility**. This is the capacity of a muscle fiber to undergo shortening and to change its shape, becoming thicker. Studies of muscle chemistry and observation of cells under the powerful electron microscope have given a concept of how muscle cells work.

These studies reveal that each skeletal muscle fiber contains many threads, or filaments, made of two kinds of proteins, called **actin** (AK-tin) and **myosin** (MI-o-sin). Filaments made of actin are thin and light; those made of myosin are thick and dark. The filaments are present in alternating bundles within the muscle cell (Fig. 8-4). It is the alternating bands of light actin and heavy myosin filaments that give skeletal muscle its striated appearance. They also give a view of what occurs when muscles contract.

Note that the actin and myosin filaments overlap where they meet, just as your fingers overlap when you fold your hands together. A contracting subunit of skeletal muscle is called a **sarcomere** (SAR-ko-mere). It consists of a band of myosin filaments and the actin filaments on each side of them (see Fig. 8-4). In movement, the myosin filaments "latch on" to the actin filaments in their overlapping region by means of many paddlelike extensions called myosin heads. In this way, the myosin heads form attachments between the actin and myosin filaments that are described as cross-bridges. Using the energy of ATP for repeated movements, the myosin heads, like the oars of a boat moving water, pull all the actin strands closer together within each sarcomere. As the overlapping filaments slide together, the

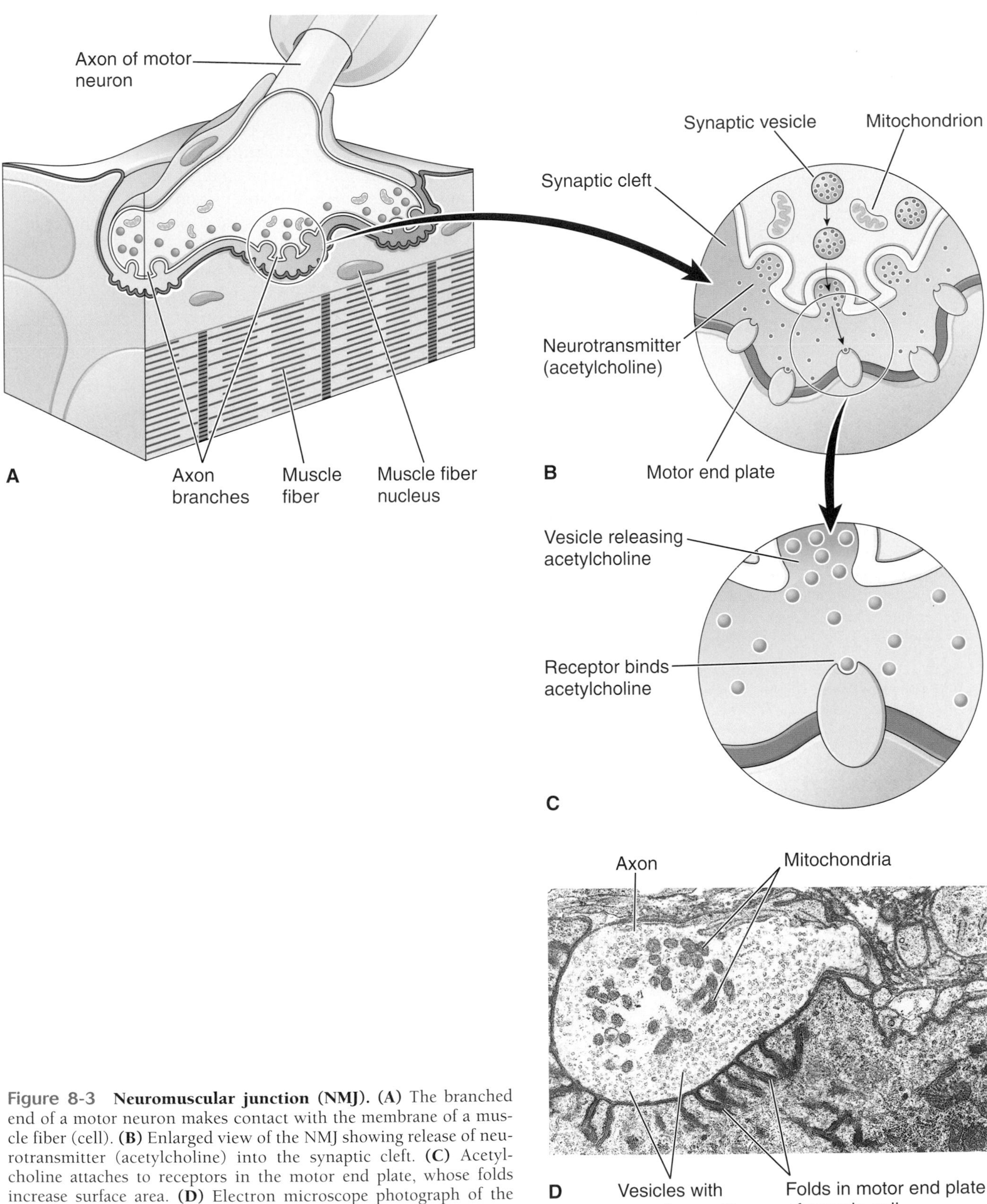

Figure 8-3 **Neuromuscular junction (NMJ). (A)** The branched end of a motor neuron makes contact with the membrane of a muscle fiber (cell). **(B)** Enlarged view of the NMJ showing release of neurotransmitter (acetylcholine) into the synaptic cleft. **(C)** Acetylcholine attaches to receptors in the motor end plate, whose folds increase surface area. **(D)** Electron microscope photograph of the neuromuscular junction. (D, Courtesy of A. Sima.)

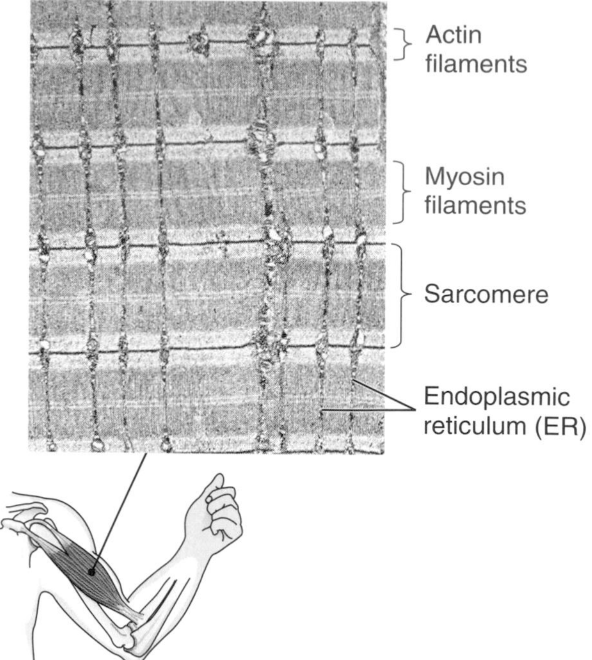

Figure 8-4 **Electron microscope photograph of skeletal muscle cell (×6500).** Actin makes up the light band and myosin makes up the dark band. The dark line in the actin band marks points where actin filaments are held together. A sarcomere is a contracting subunit of skeletal muscle. (Photomicrograph reprinted with permission from Ross MH, Kaye GI, Pawlina W. Histology. 4th ed. Philadelphia: Lippincott Williams & Wilkins, 2003.)

muscle fiber contracts, becoming shorter and thicker. Figure 8-5 shows a section of muscle as it contracts. Once the cross-bridges form, the myosin heads move the actin filaments forward, then they detach and move back to position for another "power stroke." Note that the filaments overlap increasingly as the cell contracts. (In reality, not all the myosin heads are moving at the same time. About one half are forward at any time, and the rest are preparing for another swing.) During contraction, each sarcomere becomes shorter, but the individual filaments do not change in length. As in shuffling a deck of cards, as you push the cards together, the deck becomes smaller, but the cards do not change in length.

Checkpoint 8-5 What are two properties of muscle cells that are needed for response to a stimulus?

Checkpoint 8-6 What are the filaments that interact to produce muscle contraction?

The Role of Calcium In additional to actin, myosin, and ATP, calcium is needed for muscle contraction. It enables cross-bridges to form between actin and myosin so the sliding filament action can begin. When muscles are at rest, two additional proteins called **troponin** (tro-PO-nin) and **tropomyosin** (tro-po-MI-o-sin) block the sites on actin filaments where cross-bridges can form

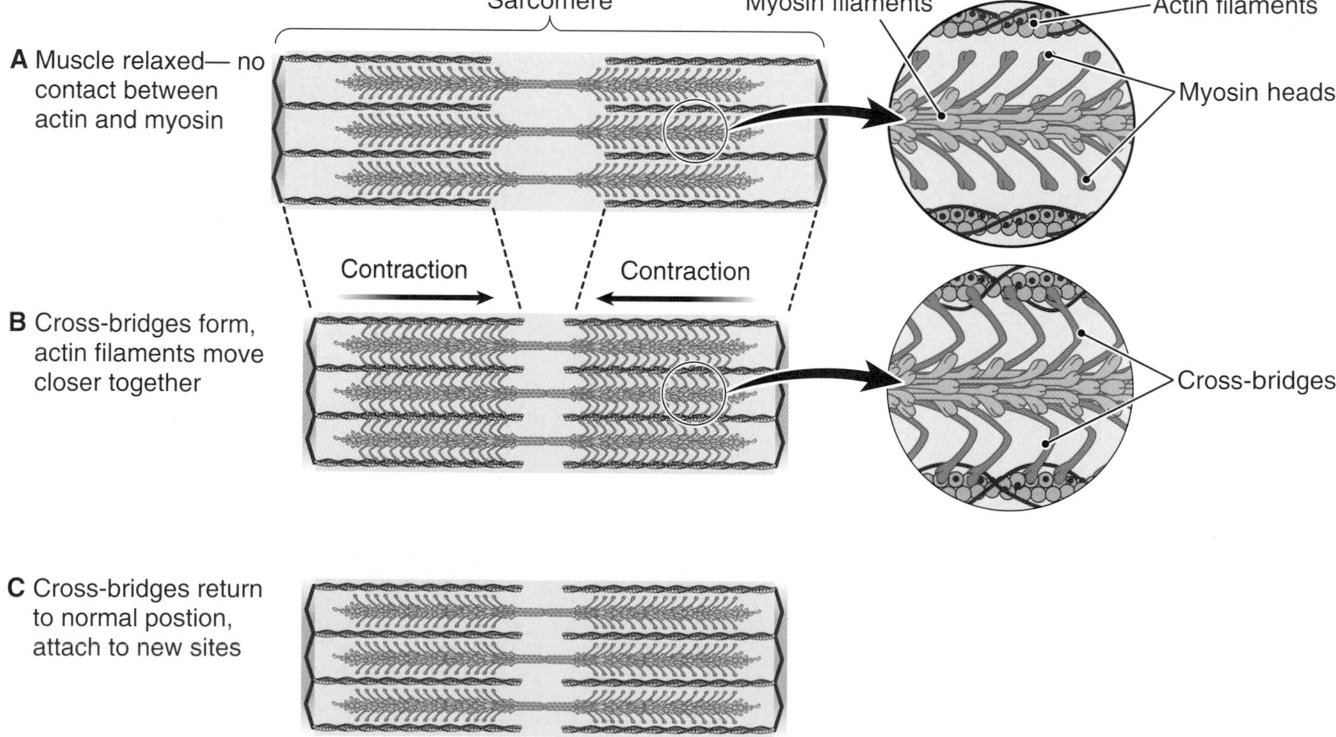

Figure 8-5 **Sliding filament mechanism of skeletal muscle contraction. (A)** Muscle is relaxed and there is no contact between the actin and myosin filaments. **(B)** Cross-bridges form and the actin filaments are moved closer together as the muscle fiber contracts. **(C)** The cross-bridges return to their original position and attach to new sites to prepare for another pull on the actin filaments and further contraction. *ZOOMING IN ✦ Do the actin or myosin filaments change in length as contraction proceeds?*

(Fig. 8-6). When calcium attaches to these proteins, they move aside, uncovering the binding sites. In resting muscles, the calcium is not available because it is stored within the endoplasmic reticulum (ER) of the muscle cell. It is released into the cytoplasm only when the cell is stimulated by a nerve fiber. Muscles relax when nervous stimulation stops and the calcium is then pumped back into the ER, ready for the next contraction.

A summary of the events in a muscle contraction is as follows:

1. Acetylcholine (ACh) is released from a neuron ending into the synaptic cleft at the neuromuscular junction
2. ACh binds to the motor end plate of the muscle and produces an action potential
3. The action potential travels to the endoplasmic reticulum (ER)
4. The endoplasmic reticulum releases calcium into the cytoplasm
5. Calcium shifts troponin and tropomyosin so that binding sites on actin are exposed
6. Myosin heads bind to actin, forming cross-bridges
7. Myosin heads pull actin filaments together within the sarcomeres and cell shortens
8. ATP is used to detach myosin heads and move them back to position for another "power stroke"
9. Muscle relaxes when stimulation ends and the calcium is pumped back into the ER

Box 8-1, Muscle Contraction and Energy, has additional details on skeletal muscle contraction.

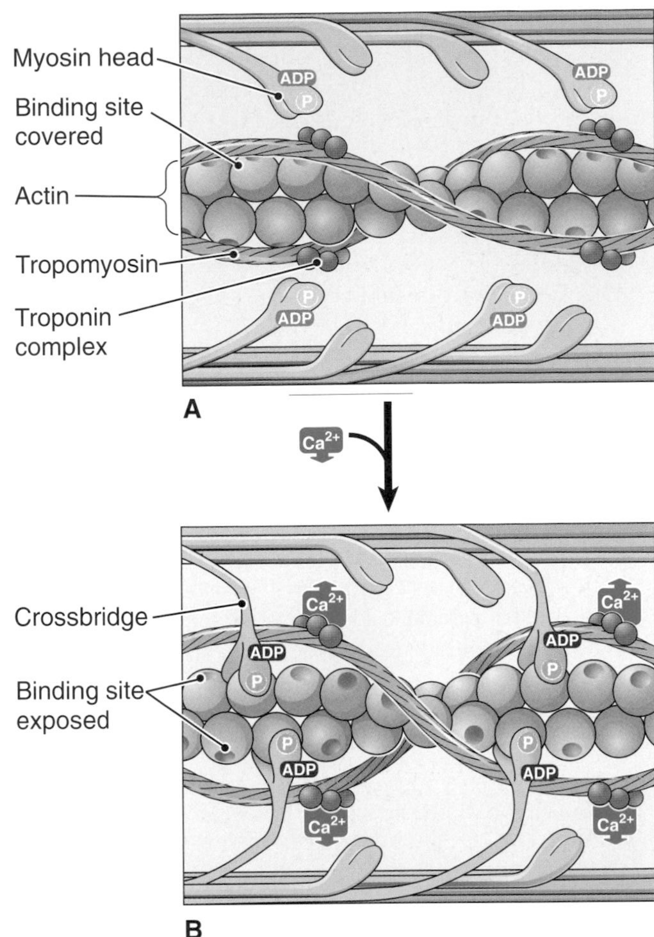

Figure 8-6 **Role of calcium in muscle contraction. (A)** Troponin and tropomyosin cover the binding sites where cross-bridges can form between actin and myosin. **(B)** Calcium shifts troponin and tropomyosin away from binding sites so cross-bridges can form.

Energy Sources

As noted earlier, all muscle contraction requires energy in the form of ATP. The source of this energy is the oxidation (commonly called "burning") of nutrients within the cells.

Box 8-1 **A Closer Look**

Muscle Contraction and Energy

When we think of muscle contraction, we might imagine a runner's rippling muscles. But muscle contraction actually occurs at a microscopic level within the sarcomere's working parts: the thick and thin filaments.

Thick filaments are composed of many myosin molecules, each shaped like two golf clubs twisted together with the myosin heads projecting away from the sarcomere's center (see Fig. 8-6). Each myosin head can bind ATP and convert it into ADP and a phosphate molecule, which remain bound. The chemical energy released during this reaction charges the myosin head, enabling it to do work.

Thin filaments' actin molecules are twisted together like two strands of beads. Each "bead" has a myosin-binding site, but the two regulatory proteins, troponin and tropomyosin, cover the binding sites when the muscle is at rest. When calcium shifts these proteins away from the binding sites, the following cycle of events occurs:

1. The charged myosin heads attach to the actin molecules and form cross-bridges between the thick and thin filaments.
2. Using their stored energy, the myosin heads pull the thin filaments to the center of the sarcomere, releasing the ADP and phosphate molecules.
3. New ATP molecules bind to the myosin heads, causing them to detach from actin and breaking the cross-bridges.
4. The myosin heads convert ATP into ADP and phosphate, which recharges them.

After death, muscles enter a stage of rigidity known as rigor mortis. This phenomenon illustrates ATP's crucial role in muscle contraction. Shortly after death, muscle cells begin to degrade. Calcium escapes into the cytoplasm, and the muscle filaments slide together. Metabolism has ceased, however, and there is no ATP to disengage the filaments, so they remain locked in a contracted state. Rigor mortis lasts about 24 hours, gradually fading as enzymes break down the muscle filaments.

To produce ATP, muscle cells must have an adequate supply of oxygen and glucose or other usable nutrient. The circulating blood constantly brings these substances to the cells, but muscle cells also store a small reserve supply of each to be used when needed, during vigorous exercise, for example. The following are compounds that store oxygen, energy, or nutrients in muscle cells:

- **Myoglobin** (mi-o-GLO-bin) stores additional oxygen. This compound is similar to the blood's hemoglobin but is located specifically in muscle cells, as indicated by the prefix *myo-* in its name.
- **Glycogen** (GLI-ko-jen) stores additional glucose. It is a polysaccharide made of multiple glucose molecules and it can be broken down into glucose when needed by the muscle cells.
- **Creatine** (KRE-ah-tin) **phosphate** stores energy. It is a compound similar to ATP, in that it has a high energy bond that releases energy when it is broken. This energy is used to make ATP for muscle contraction when the muscle cell has used up its ATP.

Checkpoint 8-7 What mineral is needed to allow actin and myosin to interact?

Checkpoint 8-8 Muscle cells obtain energy for contraction from the oxidation of nutrients. What compound is formed in oxidation that supplies the energy for contraction?

Oxygen Consumption During most activities of daily life, the tissues receive adequate oxygen, and muscles can function aerobically. During strenuous activity, however, a person may not be able to breathe in oxygen rapidly enough to meet the needs of the hard-working muscles. At first, the myoglobin, glycogen, and creatine phosphate stored in the tissues meet the increased demands, but continual exercise depletes these stores.

For a short time, glucose may be used anaerobically, that is, without the benefit of oxygen. This anaerobic process generates ATP rapidly and permits greater magnitude of activity than would otherwise be possible, as, for example, allowing sprinting instead of jogging. However, anaerobic metabolism is inefficient; it does not produce as much ATP as does metabolism in the presence of oxygen. Also, an organic acid called **lactic acid** accumulates in the cells when this alternate pathway of metabolism is used. Anaerobic metabolism can continue only until the buildup of lactic acid causes the muscles to fatigue.

Muscles operating anaerobically are in a state of **oxygen debt**. After stopping exercise, a person must continue to take in extra oxygen by continued rapid breathing (panting) until the debt is paid in full. That is, enough oxygen must be taken in to convert the lactic acid to other substances that can be metabolized further. In addition, the glycogen, myoglobin, and creatine phosphate that are stored in the cells must be replenished. The time after strenuous exercise during which extra oxygen is needed is known as the period of recovery oxygen consumption.

Checkpoint 8-9 When muscles work without oxygen, a compound is produced that causes muscle fatigue. What is the name of this compound?

Effects of Exercise

Regular exercise results in a number of changes in muscle tissue. These changes correspond to the three components of exercise: stretching, aerobics, and resistance training. When muscles are stretched, they contract more forcefully, as the internal filaments can interact over a greater length. Stretching also helps with balance and promotes flexibility at the joints. Aerobic exercise, that is, exercise that increases oxygen consumption, such as running, biking, or swimming, leads to improved endurance. Resistance training, such as weight lifting, causes muscle cells to increase in size, a condition known as hypertrophy (hi-PER-tro-fe). This change can be seen in the enlarged muscles of body-builders. Some of the changes in muscle tissue that lead to improved endurance and strength include:

- Increase in the number of capillaries in the muscle tissue, which brings more blood to the cells
- Increase in the number of mitochondria to increase production of ATP
- Increase in reserves of myoglobin, glycogen, and creatine phosphate to promote endurance

An exercise program should include all three methods—stretching, aerobic exercise, and resistance training—with periods of warm-up and cool-down before and after working out. This type of varied program is described as cross-training or interval training.

In addition to affecting muscle tissue itself, exercise causes some systemic changes. The **vasodilation** (vas-o-di-LA-shun), or widening of blood vessel diameter, that occurs during exercise allows blood to flow more easily to muscle tissue. With continued work, more blood is pumped back to the heart. The temporarily increased load on the heart strengthens the heart muscle and improves its circulation. With exercise training, the chambers of the heart gradually enlarge to accommodate more blood. The resting heart rate of a trained athlete is lower than the average rate because the heart can function more efficiently.

Regular exercise also improves breathing and respiratory efficiency. Circulation in the capillaries surrounding the alveoli (air sacs) is increased, and this brings about enhanced gas exchange. The more efficient distribution and use of oxygen delays the onset of oxygen debt. Even moderate regular exercise has the additional benefits of weight control, strengthening of the bones, decreased blood pressure, and decreased risk of heart attacks. The effects of exercise on the body are studied in the fields of

Box 8-2 **Hot Topics**

Anabolic Steroids: Winning at All Costs?

Anabolic steroids mimic the effects of the male sex hormone testosterone by promoting metabolism and stimulating growth. These drugs are legally prescribed to promote muscle regeneration and prevent atrophy from disuse after surgery. However, athletes also purchase them illegally, using them to increase muscle size and strength and improve endurance.

When steroids are used illegally to enhance athletic performance, the doses needed are large enough to cause serious side effects. They increase blood cholesterol levels, which may lead to atherosclerosis, heart disease, kidney failure, and stroke. Steroids damage the liver, making it more susceptible to disease and cancer, and suppress the immune system, increasing the risk of infection and cancer. In men, steroids cause impotence, testicular atrophy, low sperm count, infertility, and the development of female sex characteristics such as breasts (gynecomastia). In women, steroids disrupt ovulation and menstruation and produce male sex characteristics such as breast atrophy, enlargement of the clitoris, increased body hair, and deepening of the voice. In both sexes steroids increase the risk for baldness and, especially in men, cause mood swings, depression, and violence.

sports medicine and exercise physiology. Box 8-2, Anabolic Steroids: Winning at all Costs?, has information on how steroids affect muscles.

Types of Muscle Contractions

Muscle **tone** refers to a partially contracted state of the muscles that is normal even when the muscles are not in use. The maintenance of this tone, or **tonus** (TO-nus), is due to the action of the nervous system in keeping the muscles in a constant state of readiness for action. Muscles that are little used soon become flabby, weak, and lacking in tone.

In addition to the partial contractions that are responsible for muscle tone, there are two other types of contractions on which the body depends:

- **Isotonic** (i-so-TON-ik) **contractions** are those in which the tone or tension within the muscle remains the same but the muscle as a whole shortens, producing movement; that is, work is accomplished. Lifting weights, walking, running, or any other activity in which the muscles become shorter and thicker (forming bulges) are isotonic contractions.
- **Isometric** (i-so-MET-rik) **contractions** are those in which there is no change in muscle length but there is a great increase in muscle tension. Pushing against an immovable force produces an isometric contraction. For example, if you push the palms of your hands hard against each other, there is no movement, but you can feel the increased tension in your arm muscles.

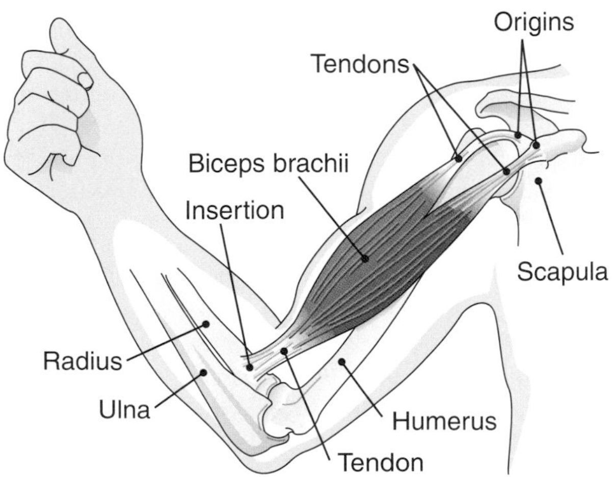

Figure 8-7 **Muscle attachments to bones.** Three attachments are shown—two origins and one insertion. *ZOOMING IN ✦ Does contraction of the biceps brachii produce flexion or extension at the elbow?*

Most movements of the body involve a combination of both isotonic and isometric contractions. When walking, for example, some muscles contract isotonically to propel the body forward, but at the same time, other muscles are contracting isometrically to keep your body in position.

The Mechanics of Muscle Movement

Most muscles have two or more points of attachment to the skeleton. The muscle is attached to a bone at each end by means of a cordlike extension called a **tendon** (Fig. 8-7). All of the connective tissue within and around the muscle merges to form the tendon, which then attaches directly to the periosteum of the bone (see Fig. 8-1). In some instances, a broad sheet called an **aponeurosis** (ap-o-nu-RO-sis) may attach muscles to bones or to other muscles.

In moving the bones, one end of a muscle is attached to a more freely movable part of the skeleton, and the other end is attached to a relatively stable part. The less movable (more fixed) attachment is called the **origin**; the attachment to the part of the body that the muscle puts into action is called the **insertion.** When a muscle contracts, it pulls on both points of attachment, bringing the more movable insertion closer to the origin and thereby causing movement of the body part. Figure 8-7 shows the action of the biceps brachii (in the upper arm) in flexing the arm at the elbow. The insertion on the radius of the forearm is brought toward the origin at the scapula of the shoulder girdle.

Checkpoint 8-10 Muscles are attached to bones by means of tendons: one attached to a less movable part of the skeleton, and one attached to a movable part. What are the names of these two attachment points?

Muscles Work Together

Many of the skeletal muscles function in pairs. A movement is performed by a muscle called the **prime mover**; the muscle that produces an opposite movement to that of the prime mover is known as the **antagonist.** Clearly, for any given movement, the antagonist must relax when the prime mover contracts. For example, when the biceps brachii at the front of the arm contracts to flex the arm, the triceps brachii at the back must relax; when the triceps brachii contracts to extend the arm, the biceps brachii must relax. In addition to prime movers and antagonists, there are also muscles that serve to steady body parts or to assist prime movers. These "helping" muscles are called **synergists** (SIN-er-jists), because they work with the prime movers to accomplish a movement.

As the muscles work together, body movements are coordinated, and a large number of complicated movements can be carried out. At first, however, the nervous system must learn to coordinate any new, complicated movement. Think of a child learning to walk or to write, and consider the number of muscles she or he uses unnecessarily or forgets to use when the situation calls for them.

Checkpoint 8-11 Muscles work together to produce movement. What is the name of the muscle that produces a movement as compared with the muscle that produces an opposite movement?

Levers and Body Mechanics

Proper body mechanics help conserve energy and ensure freedom from strain and fatigue; conversely, such ailments as lower back pain—a common complaint—can be traced to poor body mechanics. Body mechanics have special significance to healthcare workers, who are frequently called on to move patients and handle cumbersome equipment. Maintaining the body segments in correct relation to one another has a direct effect on the working capacity of the vital organs that are supported by the skeleton.

If you have had a course in physics, recall your study of levers. A lever is simply a rigid bar that moves about a fixed pivot point, the fulcrum. There are three classes of levers, which differ only in the location of the fulcrum (F), the effort (E), or force, and the resistance (R), the weight or load. In a first-class lever, the fulcrum is located between the resistance and the effort; a see-saw or a scissors is an example of this class (Fig. 8-8). The second-class lever has the resistance located between the fulcrum and the effort; a wheelbarrow or a mattress lifted at one end is an illustration of this class (Fig. 8-8 B). In the third-class lever, the effort is between the resistance and the fulcrum. A forceps or a tweezers is an example of this type of lever. The effort is applied in the center of the tool, between the fulcrum, where the pieces join, and the resistance at the tip.

The musculoskeletal system can be considered a system of levers, in which the bone is the lever, the joint is the fulcrum, and the force is applied by a muscle. An example of a first-class lever in the body is using the muscles at the back of the neck to lift the head at the joint between the occipital bone of the skull and the first cervical vertebra (atlas) (see Fig. 8-8). A second-class lever is exemplified by raising your weight to the ball of your foot (the fulcrum) using muscles of the calf.

However, there are very few examples of first- and second-class levers in the body. Most lever systems in the body are of the third-class type. A muscle usually inserts over a joint and exerts force between the fulcrum and the resistance. That is, the fulcrum is behind both the point of effort and the weight. As shown in Figure 8-8 C, when the biceps brachii flexes the forearm at the elbow, the muscle exerts its force at its insertion on the radius. The weight of the hand and forearm creates the resistance, and the fulcrum is the elbow joint, which is behind the point of effort.

By understanding and applying knowledge of levers to body mechanics, the healthcare worker can improve his or her skill in carrying out numerous clinical maneuvers and procedures.

Checkpoint 8-12 Muscles and bones work together as lever systems. Of the three classes of levers, which one represents the action of most muscles?

Skeletal Muscle Groups

The study of muscles is made simpler by grouping them according to body regions. Knowing how muscles are named can also help in remembering them. A number of different characteristics are used in naming muscles, including the following:

- Location, named for a nearby bone, for example, or for position, such as lateral, medial, internal, or external
- Size, using terms such as maximus, major, minor, longus, brevis
- Shape, such as circular (orbicularis), triangular (deltoid), trapezoid (trapezius)
- Direction of fibers, including straight (rectus) or angled (oblique)
- Number of heads (attachment points) as indicated by the suffix *-ceps*, as in biceps, triceps, quadriceps
- Action, as in flexor, extensor, adductor, abductor, levator

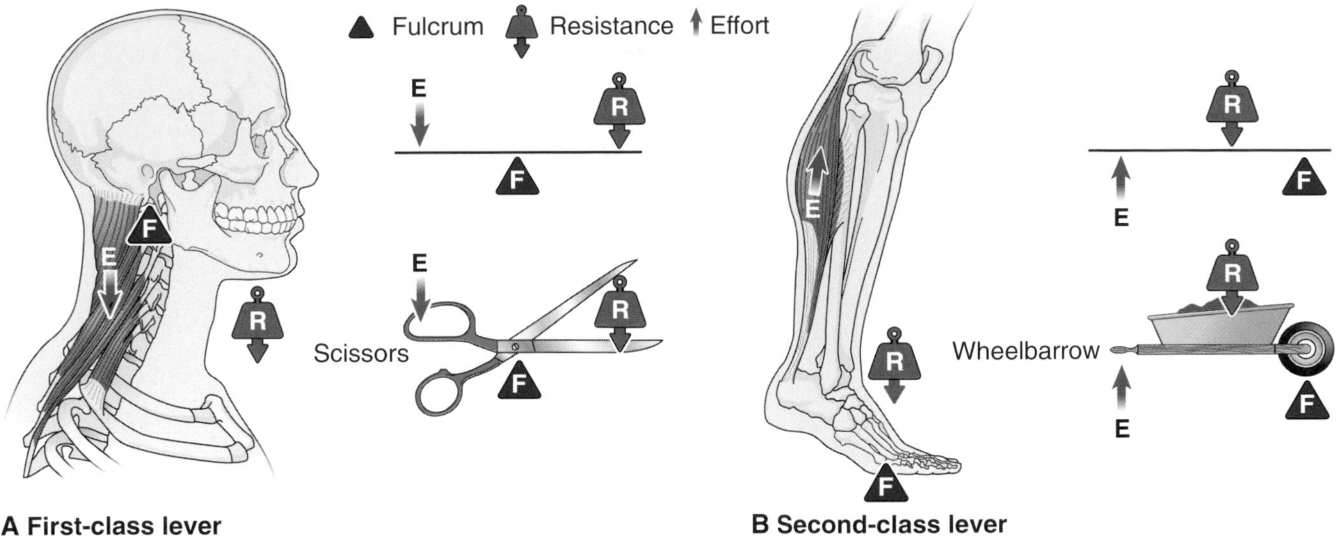

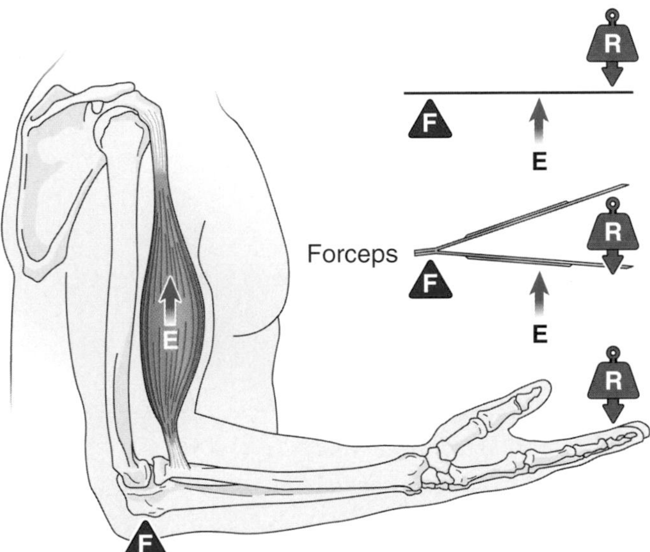

Figure 8-8 **Levers.** Three classes of levers are shown along with tools and anatomic examples that illustrate each type. R = resistance (weight); E = effort (force); F = fulcrum (pivot point).

Often, more than one feature is used in naming. Refer to Figures 8-9 and 8-10 as you study the locations and functions of some of the skeletal muscles and try to figure out why each has the name that it does. Although they are described in the singular, most of the muscles are present on both sides of the body.

Muscles of the Head

The principal muscles of the head are those of facial expression and of mastication (chewing) (Fig. 8-11, Table 8-3).

The muscles of facial expression include ring-shaped ones around the eyes and the lips, called the **orbicularis** (or-bik-u-LAH-ris) **muscles** because of their shape (think of "orbit"). The muscle surrounding each eye is called the **orbicularis oculi** (OK-u-li), whereas the muscle of the lips is the **orbicularis oris.** These muscles, of course, all have antagonists. For example, the **levator palpebrae** (PAL-pe-bre) **superioris,** or lifter of the upper eyelid, is the antagonist for the orbicularis oculi.

One of the largest muscles of expression forms the fleshy part of the cheek and is called the **buccinator** (BUK-se-na-tor). Used in whistling or blowing, it is sometimes referred to as the trumpeter's muscle. You can readily think of other muscles of facial expression: for instance, the antagonists of the orbicularis oris can produce a smile, a sneer, or a grimace. There are a number of scalp muscles by means of which the eyebrows are lifted or drawn together into a frown.

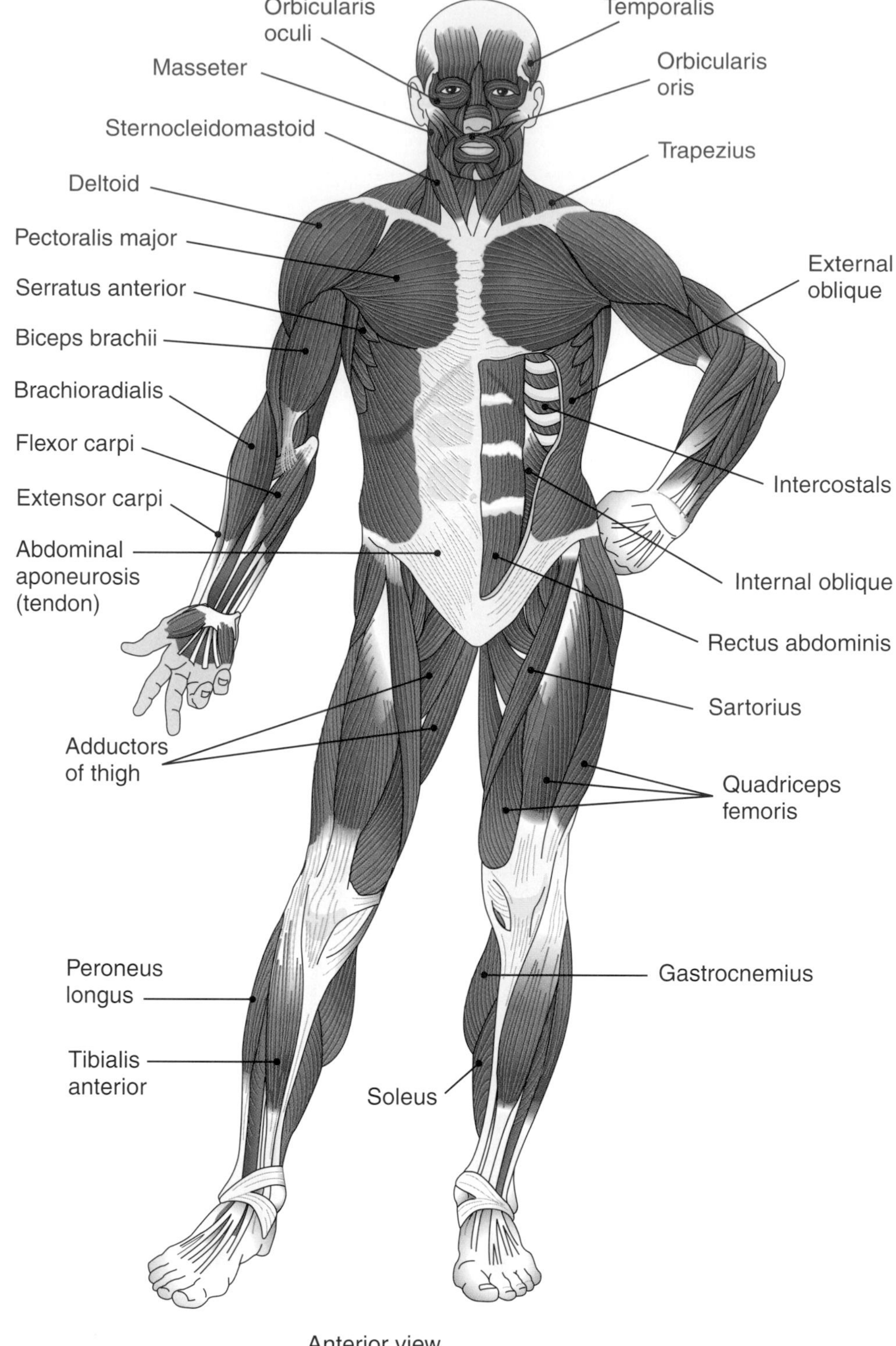

Figure 8-9 Superficial muscles, anterior view. Associated structure is labeled in parentheses.

There are four pairs of muscles of mastication, all of which insert on and move the mandible. The largest are the **temporalis** (TEM-po-ral-is), which is superior to the ear, and the **masseter** (mas-SE-ter) at the angle of the jaw.

The tongue has two groups of muscles. The first group, called the **intrinsic muscles**, is located entirely within the tongue. The second group, the **extrinsic muscles**, originates outside the tongue. It is because of these many muscles that the tongue has such remarkable flexibility and can perform so many different functions. Consider the intricate tongue motions involved in speaking, chewing, and swallowing.

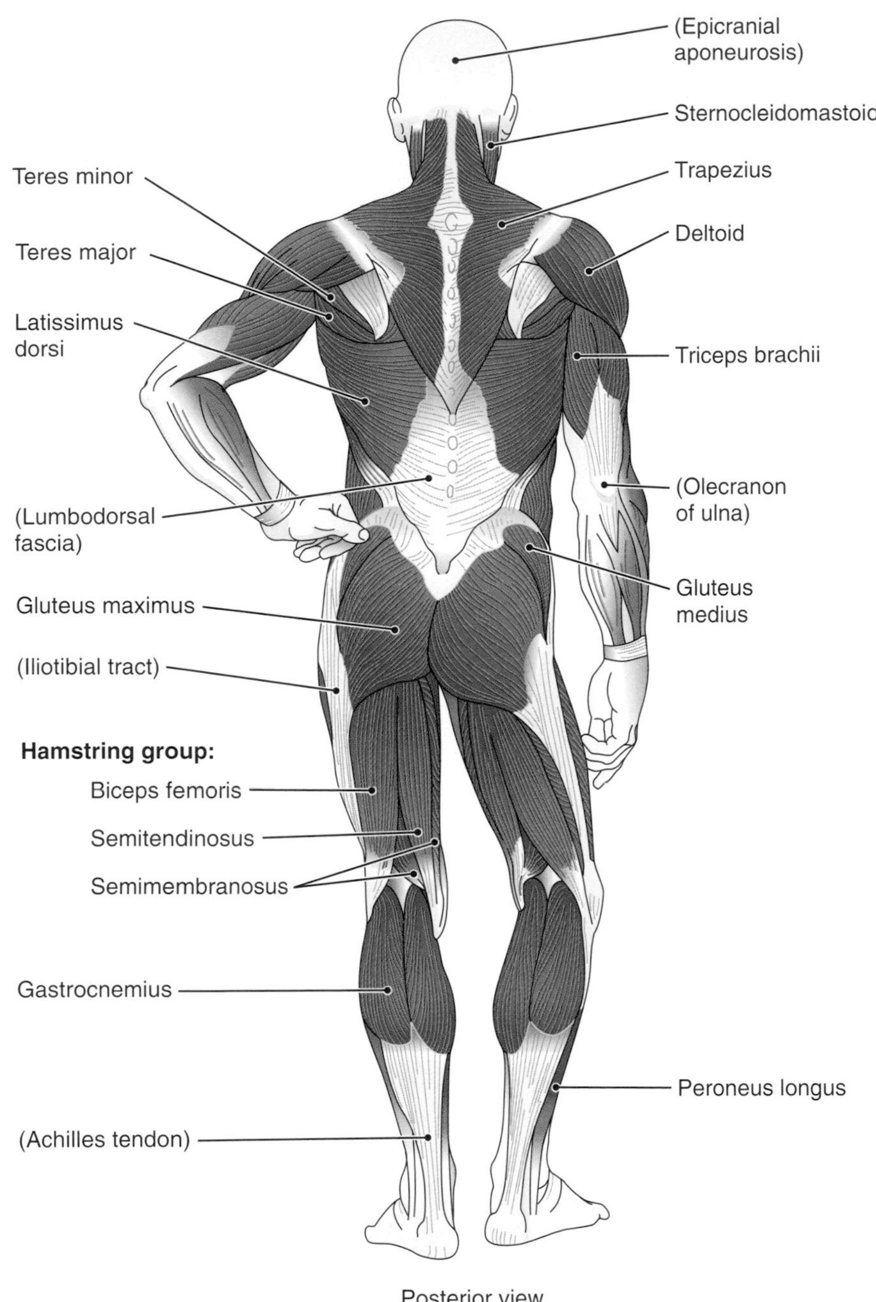

Figure 8-10 Superficial muscles, posterior view. Associated structures are labeled in parentheses.

Figure 8-11 shows some additional muscles of the face.

Muscles of the Neck

The neck muscles tend to be ribbonlike and extend up and down or obliquely in several layers and in a complex manner (Fig. 8-11, Table 8-3). The one you will hear of most frequently is the **sternocleidomastoid** (ster-no-kli-do-MAS-toyd), sometimes referred to simply as the sternomastoid. This strong muscle extends superiorly from the sternum across the side of the neck to the mastoid process. When the left and right muscles work together, they bring the head forward on the chest (flexion). Working alone, each muscle tilts and rotates the head so as to orient the face toward the side opposite that muscle. If the head is abnormally fixed in this position, the person is said to have **torticollis** (tor-tih-KOL-is), or wryneck; this condition may be due to injury or spasm of the muscle.

A portion of the trapezius muscle (described later) is located at the posterior of the neck, where it helps hold

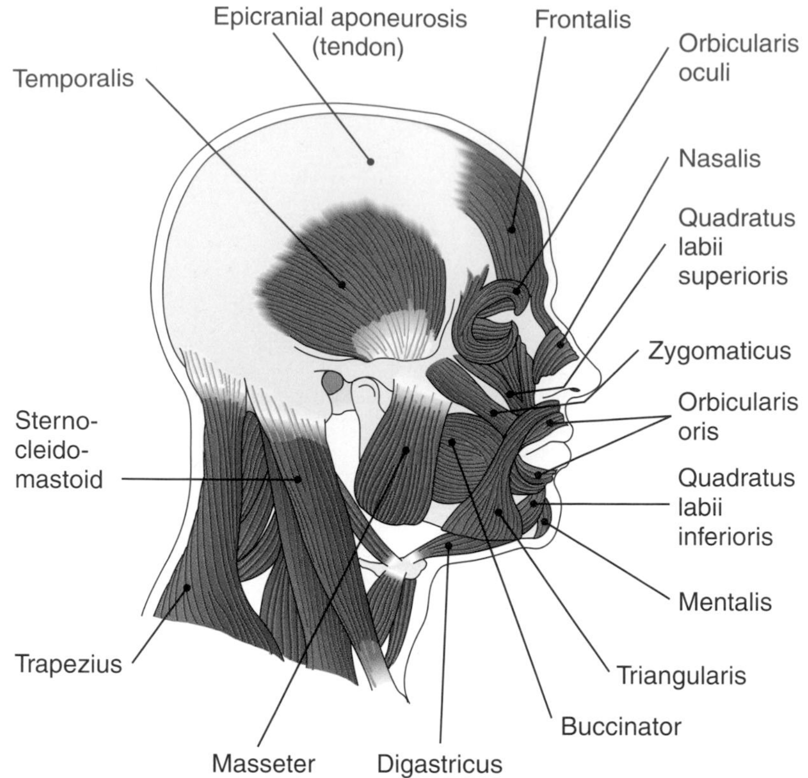

Figure 8-11 Muscles of the head. Associated structure is labeled in parentheses. *ZOOMING IN ✦ Which of the muscles in this illustration is named for a bone it is near?*

the head up (extension). Other larger deep muscles are the chief extensors of the head and neck.

Muscles of the Upper Extremities

Muscles of the upper extremities include the muscles that determine the position of the shoulder, the anterior and posterior muscles that move the arm, and the muscles that move the forearm and hand.

Table 8•3 Muscles of the Head and Neck*

NAME	LOCATION	FUNCTION
Orbicularis oculi	Encircles eyelid	Closes eye
Levator palpebrae superioris (deep muscle; not shown)	Back of orbit to upper eyelid	Opens eye
Orbicularis oris	Encircles mouth	Closes lips
Buccinator	Fleshy part of cheek	Flattens cheek; helps in eating, whistling, and blowing wind instruments
Temporalis	Above and near ear	Closes jaw
Masseter	At angle of jaw	Closes jaw
Sternocleidomastoid	Along side of neck, to mastoid process	Flexes head; rotates head toward opposite side from muscle

**These and other muscles of the face are shown in Fig. 8–11.*

Muscles That Move the Shoulder and Arm The position of the shoulder depends to a large extent on the degree of contraction of the **trapezius** (trah-PE-ze-us), a triangular muscle that covers the posterior neck and extends across the posterior shoulder to insert on the clavicle and scapula (Fig. 8-10, Table 8-4). The trapezius muscles enable one to raise the shoulders and pull them back. The upper portion of each trapezius can also extend the head and turn it from side to side.

The **latissimus** (lah-TIS-ih-mus) **dorsi** is the wide muscle of the back and lateral trunk. It originates from the vertebral spine in the middle and lower back and covers the lower half of the thoracic region, forming the posterior portion of the axilla (armpit). The fibers of each muscle converge to a tendon that inserts on the humerus. The latissimus dorsi powerfully extends the arm, bringing it down forcibly as, for example, in swimming.

A large **pectoralis** (pek-to-RAL-is) **major** is located on either side of the superior part of the chest (see Fig. 8-9). This muscle arises from the sternum, the upper ribs, and the clavicle and forms the anterior "wall" of the armpit, or axilla; it inserts on the superior part of the humerus. The pectoralis major flexes and adducts the arm, pulling it across the chest.

The **serratus** (ser-RA-tus) **anterior** is below the axilla, on the lateral part of the chest. It originates on the upper eight or nine ribs on the lateral and anterior thorax and inserts in the scapula on the side toward the vertebrae. The serratus anterior moves the scapula forward when, for example, one is pushing something. It also aids in raising the arm above the horizontal level.

The **deltoid** covers the shoulder joint and is responsible for the roundness of the upper part of the arm just inferior to the shoulder (see Figs. 8-9 and 8-10). This muscle is named for its triangular shape, which resembles the Greek letter delta. The deltoid is often used as an injection site. Arising from the shoulder girdle (clavicle and scapula), the deltoid fibers converge to insert on the lateral surface of the humerus. Contraction of this muscle abducts the arm, raising it laterally to the horizontal position.

Table 8•4 Muscles of the Upper Extremities*

NAME	LOCATION	FUNCTION
Trapezius	Posterior of neck and upper back, to clavicle and scapula	Raises shoulder and pulls it back; extends head
Latissimus dorsi	Middle and lower back, to humerus	Extends and adducts arm behind back
Pectoralis major	Superior, anterior chest, to humerus	Flexes and adducts arm across chest; pulls shoulder forward and downward
Serratus anterior	Below axilla on lateral chest to scapula	Moves scapula forward; aids in raising arm, punching, or reaching forward
Deltoid	Covers shoulder joint, to lateral humerus	Abducts arm
Biceps brachii	Anterior arm along humerus, to radius	Flexes forearm at the elbow and supinates hand
Brachioradialis	Lateral forearm from distal end of humerus to distal end of radius	Flexes forearm at the elbow
Triceps brachii	Posterior arm, to ulna	Extends forearm to straighten upper extremity
Flexor carpi groups	Anterior forearm, to hand	Flex hand
Extensor carpi groups	Posterior forearm, to hand	Extend hand
Flexor digitorum groups	Anterior forearm, to fingers	Flex fingers
Extensor digitorum groups	Posterior forearm, to fingers	Extend fingers

**These and other muscles of the upper extremities are shown in Figs. 8–9, 8–10, and 8–12.*

The shoulder joint allows for a very wide range of movement. This freedom of movement is possible because the humerus fits into a shallow socket, the glenoid cavity of the scapula. This joint requires the support of four deep muscles and their tendons, which compose the **rotator cuff**. The four muscles are the **s**upraspinatus, **i**nfraspinatus, **t**eres minor, and **s**ubscapularis, known together as SITS, based on the first letters of their names. In certain activities, such as swinging a golf club, playing tennis, or pitching a baseball, the muscles of the rotator cuff may be injured, even torn, and may require surgery for repair.

Muscles That Move the Forearm and Hand The **biceps brachii** (BRA-ke-i), located at the anterior arm along the humerus, is the muscle you usually display when you want to "flex your muscles" to show your strength (Fig. 8-12 A). It inserts on the radius and flexes the forearm. It is a supinator of the hand.

Another flexor of the forearm at the elbow is the **brachioradialis** (bra-ke-o-ra-de-A-lis), a prominent muscle of the forearm that originates at the distal end of the humerus and inserts on the distal radius.

The **triceps brachii**, located on the posterior of the arm, inserts on the olecranon of the ulna (Fig. 8-12 B). It is used to straighten the arm, as in lowering a weight from an arm curl. It is also important in pushing because it converts the arm and forearm into a sturdy rod.

Most of the muscles that move the hand and fingers originate from the radius and the ulna (see Fig. 8-12). Some of them insert on the carpal bones of the wrist, whereas others have long tendons that cross the wrist and insert on bones of the hand and the fingers.

The **flexor carpi** and the **extensor carpi muscles** are responsible for many movements of the hand. Muscles that produce finger movements are the several **flexor digitorum** (dij-e-TO-rum) and the **extensor digitorum muscles.** The names of these muscles may include bones they are near, their action, or their length, for example, longus for long and brevis for short.

Special groups of muscles in the fleshy parts of the hand are responsible for the intricate movements that can be performed with the thumb and the fingers. The thumb's freedom of movement has been one of the most useful capacities of humans.

Muscles of the Trunk

The muscles of the trunk include the muscles involved in breathing, the thin muscle layers of the abdomen, and the muscles of the pelvic floor. The following discussion also includes the deep muscles of the back that support and move the vertebral column.

Muscles of Respiration The most important muscle involved in the act of breathing is the **diaphragm.** This dome-shaped muscle forms the partition between the thoracic cavity superiorly and the abdominal cavity inferiorly (Fig. 8-13). When the diaphragm contracts, the central dome-shaped portion is pulled downward, thus enlarging the thoracic cavity from top to bottom.

The **intercostal muscles** are attached to and fill the spaces between the ribs. The external and internal intercostals run at angles in opposite directions. Contraction of the intercostal muscles serves to elevate the ribs, thus enlarging the thoracic cavity from side to side and from anterior to posterior. The mechanics of breathing are described in Chapter 18.

Checkpoint 8-13 What muscle is most important in breathing?

Muscles of the Abdomen and Pelvis The wall of the abdomen has three layers of muscle that extend from the back (dorsally) and around the sides (laterally) to the front (ventrally) (Fig. 8-14, Table 8-5). They are the **ex-**

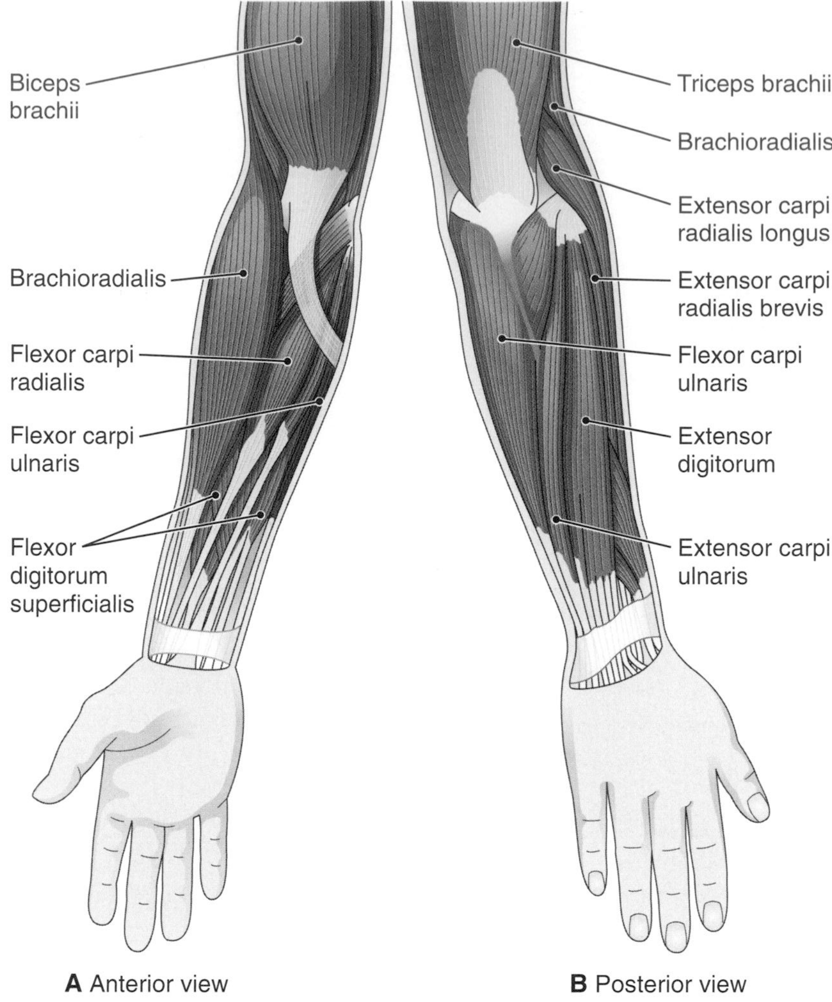

Figure 8-12 **Muscles that move the forearm and hand.**

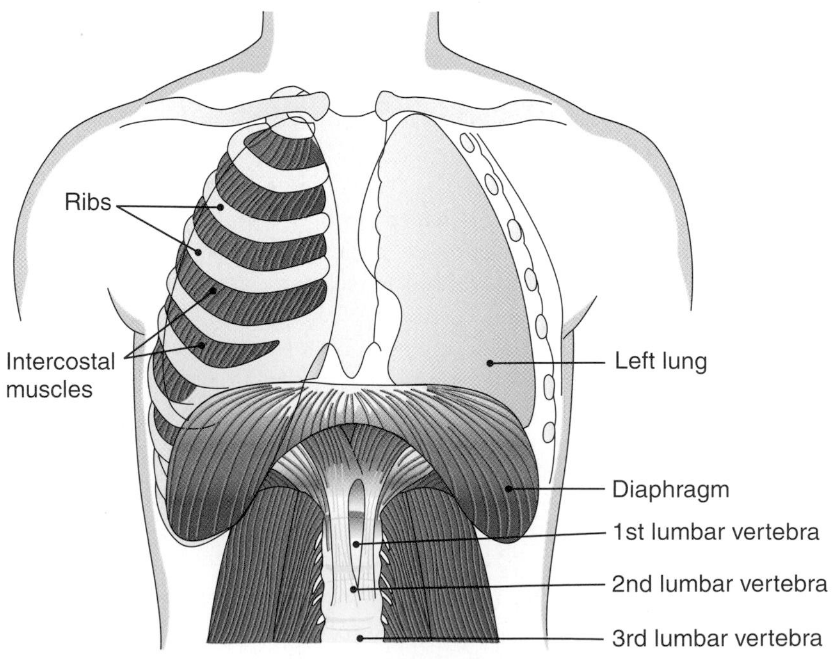

Figure 8-13 **Muscles of respiration.** Associated structures are also shown.

ternal oblique on the outside, the **internal oblique** in the middle, and the **transversus abdominis**, the innermost. The connective tissue from these muscles extends forward and encloses the vertical **rectus abdominis** of the anterior abdominal wall. The fibers of these muscles, as well as their connective tissue extensions (aponeuroses), run in different directions, resembling the layers in plywood and resulting in a strong abdominal wall. The midline meeting of the aponeuroses forms a whitish area called the **linea alba** (LIN-e-ah Al-ba), which is an important landmark on the abdomen. It extends from the tip of the sternum to the pubic joint.

These four pairs of abdominal muscles act together to protect the internal organs and compress the abdominal cavity, as in coughing, emptying the bladder (urination) and bowel (defecation), sneezing, vomiting, and childbirth (labor). The two oblique muscles and the rectus abdominis help bend the trunk forward and sideways.

The pelvic floor, or **perineum** (per-ih-NE-um), has its own form of diaphragm, shaped somewhat like a shallow dish. One of the principal muscles of this pelvic diaphragm is the **levator ani** (le-VA-tor A-ni), which acts on the rectum and thus aids in defecation. The superficial and deep muscles of the female perineum are shown in Figure 8-15 along with some associated structures.

Checkpoint 8-14 What structural feature gives strength to the muscles of the abdominal wall?

Deep Muscles of the Back The deep muscles of the back, which act on the vertebral column itself, are thick vertical masses that lie under the trapezius and latissimus dorsi. The **erector spinae** muscles make up a large group located between the sacrum and the skull. These muscles extend the spine and maintain the vertebral column in an erect posture. The muscles can be strained in lifting heavy objects if the spine is flexed while lifting. One should bend at the hip and knee in-

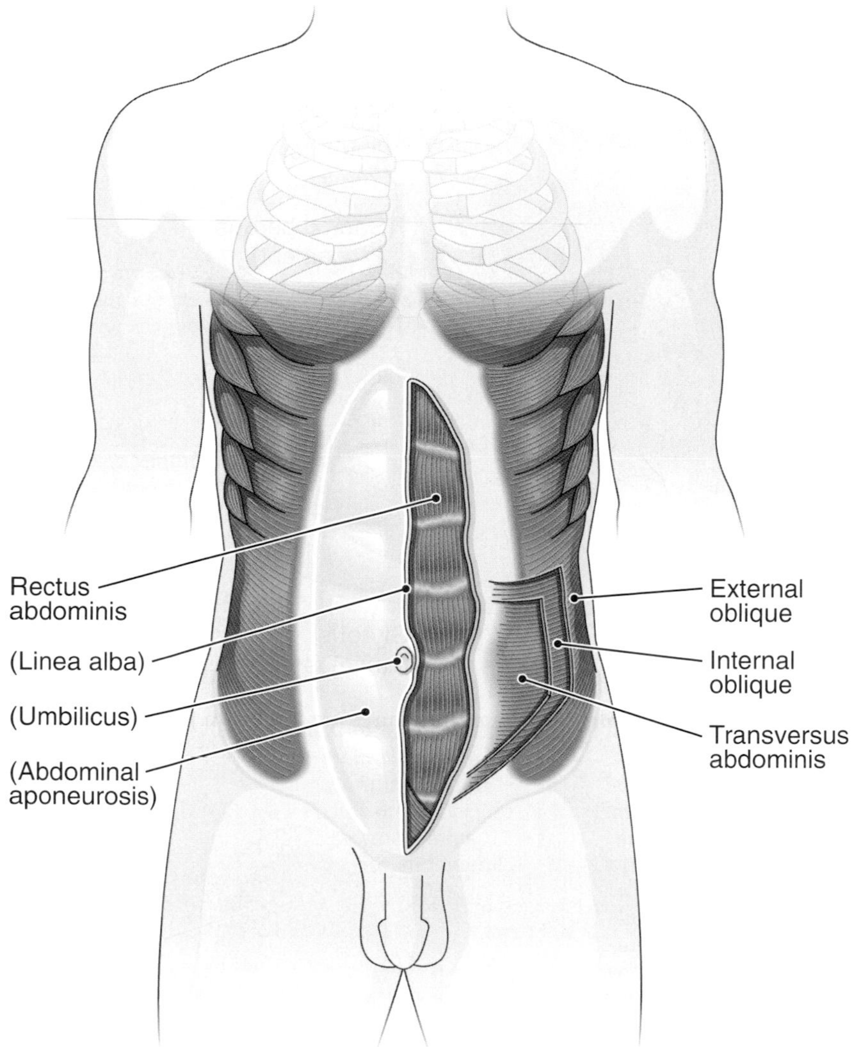

Figure 8-14 **Muscles of the abdominal wall.** Surface tissue is removed on the right side to show deeper muscles. Associated structures are labeled in parentheses.

Table 8•5 Muscles of the Trunk*

NAME	LOCATION	FUNCTION
Diaphragm	Dome-shaped partition between thoracic and abdominal cavities	Dome descends to enlarge thoracic cavity from top to bottom
Intercostals	Between ribs	Elevate ribs and enlarge thoracic cavity
Muscles of abdominal wall: External oblique, Internal oblique, Transversus abdominis, Rectus abdominis	Anterolateral abdominal wall	Compress abdominal cavity and expel substances from body; flex spinal column
Levator ani	Pelvic floor	Aids defecation
Erector spinae (deep; not shown)	Group of deep vertical muscles betweeen the sacrum and skull	Extends vertebral column to produce erect posture

**These and other muscles of the trunk are shown in Figs. 8–13, 8–14 and 8–15.*

stead and use the thigh and buttock muscles to help in lifting.

Deeper muscles in the lumbar area extend the vertebral column in that region. These deep muscles of the back are not shown in the illustrations.

Muscles of the Lower Extremities

The muscles in the lower extremities, among the longest and strongest muscles in the body, are specialized for locomotion and balance. They include the muscles that move the thigh and leg and those that control movement of the foot.

Muscles that Move the Thigh and Leg

The **gluteus maximus** (GLU-te-us MAK-sim-us), which forms much of the fleshy part of the buttock, is relatively large in humans because of its support function when a person is standing in the erect position (Fig. 8-10, Table 8-6). This muscle extends the thigh and is important in walking and running. The **gluteus medius,** which is partially covered by the gluteus maximus, abducts the thigh. It is one of the sites used for intramuscular injections.

The **iliopsoas** (il-e-o-SO-as) arises from the ilium and the bodies of the lumbar vertebrae; it crosses the anterior of the hip joint to insert on the femur (Fig. 8-16 A). It is a powerful flexor of the thigh and helps keep the trunk from falling backward when one is standing erect.

The **adductor muscles** are located on the medial part of the thigh. They arise from the pubis and ischium and insert on the femur. These strong muscles press the thighs together, as in grasping a saddle between the knees when riding a horse. They include the **adductor longus** and **adductor magnus.**

The **sartorius** (sar-TO-re-us) is a long, narrow muscle that begins at the iliac spine, winds downward and inward across the entire thigh, and ends on the upper medial surface of the tibia. It is called the tailor's muscle because it is used in crossing the legs in

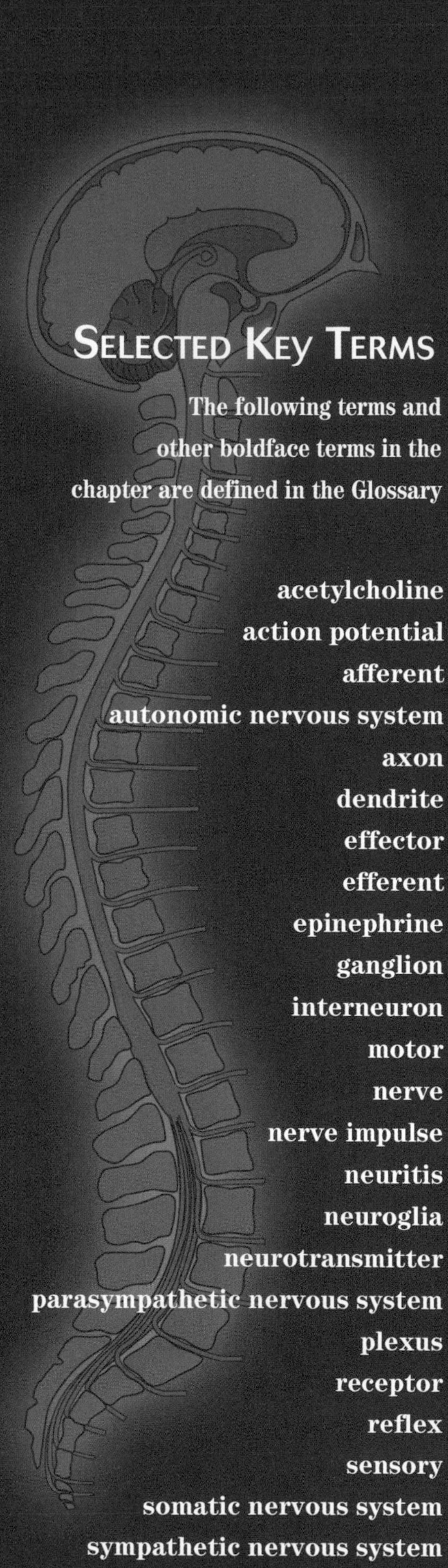

Selected Key Terms

The following terms and other boldface terms in the chapter are defined in the Glossary

acetylcholine
action potential
afferent
autonomic nervous system
axon
dendrite
effector
efferent
epinephrine
ganglion
interneuron
motor
nerve
nerve impulse
neuritis
neuroglia
neurotransmitter
parasympathetic nervous system
plexus
receptor
reflex
sensory
somatic nervous system
sympathetic nervous system
synapse
tract

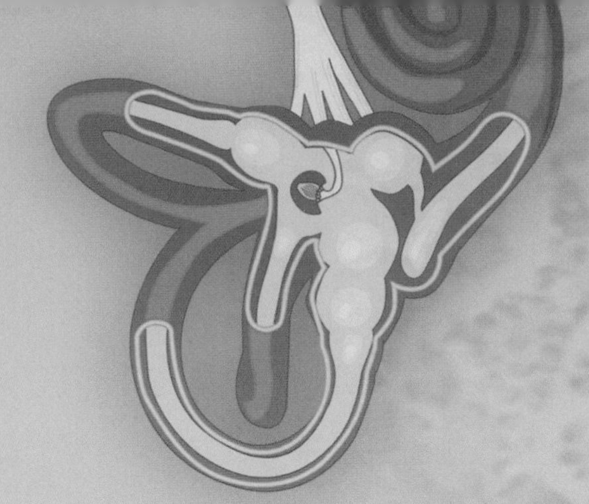

Learning Outcomes

After careful study of this chapter, you should be able to:

1. Describe the organization of the nervous system according to structure and function
2. Describe the structure of a neuron
3. Describe how neuron fibers are built into a nerve
4. Explain the purpose of neuroglia
5. Diagram and describe the steps in an action potential
6. Briefly describe the transmission of a nerve impulse
7. Explain the role of myelin in nerve conduction
8. Briefly describe transmission at a synapse
9. Define *neurotransmitter* and give several examples of neurotransmitters
10. Describe the distribution of gray and white matter in the spinal cord
11. List the components of a reflex arc
12. Define a simple reflex and give several examples of reflexes
13. Describe and name the spinal nerves and three of their main plexuses
14. Compare the location and functions of the sympathetic and parasympathetic nervous systems
15. Describe several disorders of the spinal cord and of the spinal nerves
16. Show how word parts are used to build words related to the nervous system (see Word Anatomy at the end of the chapter)

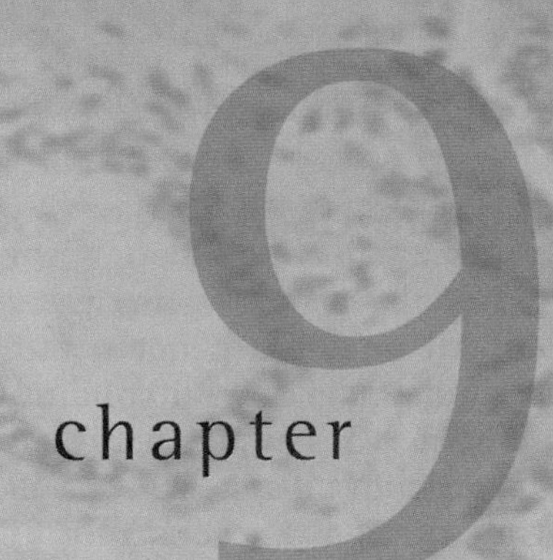

The Nervous System: The Spinal Cord and Spinal Nerves

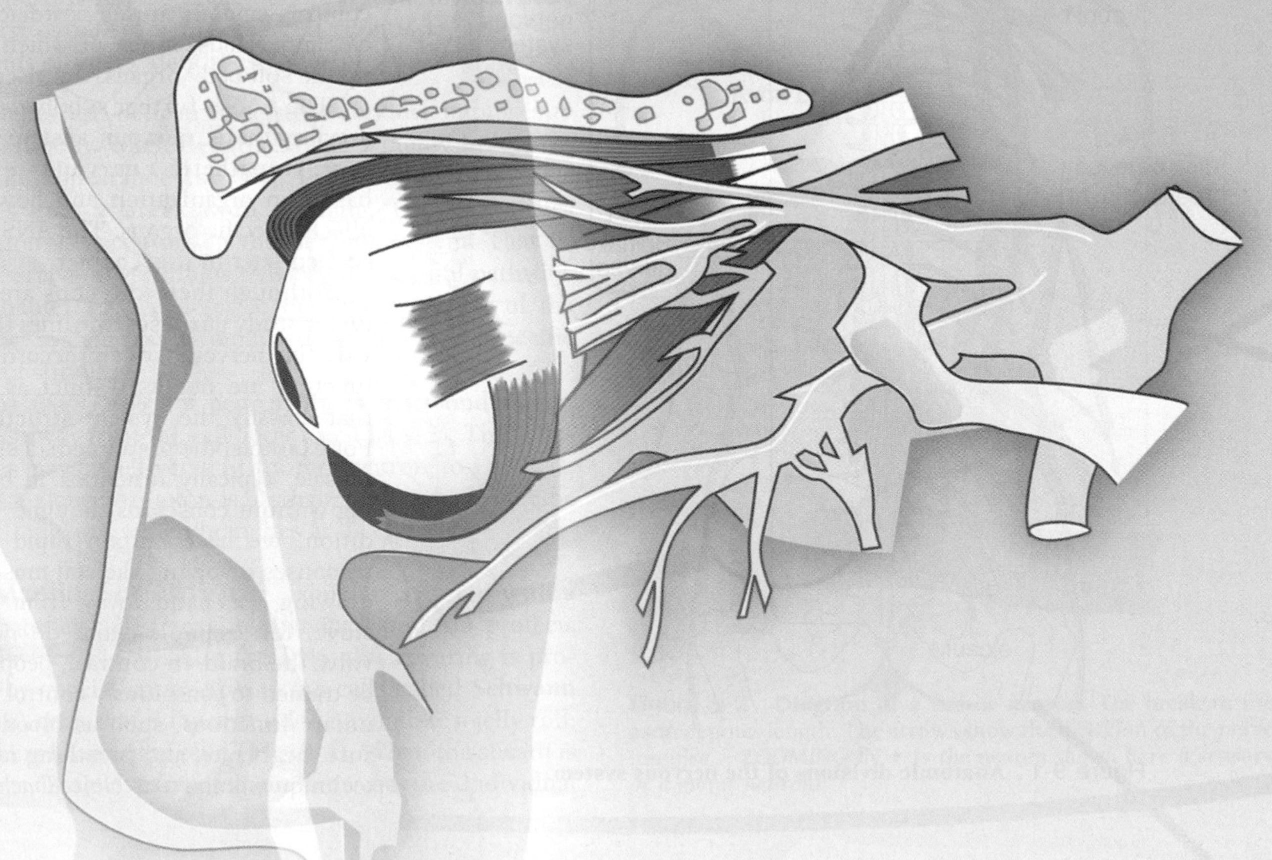

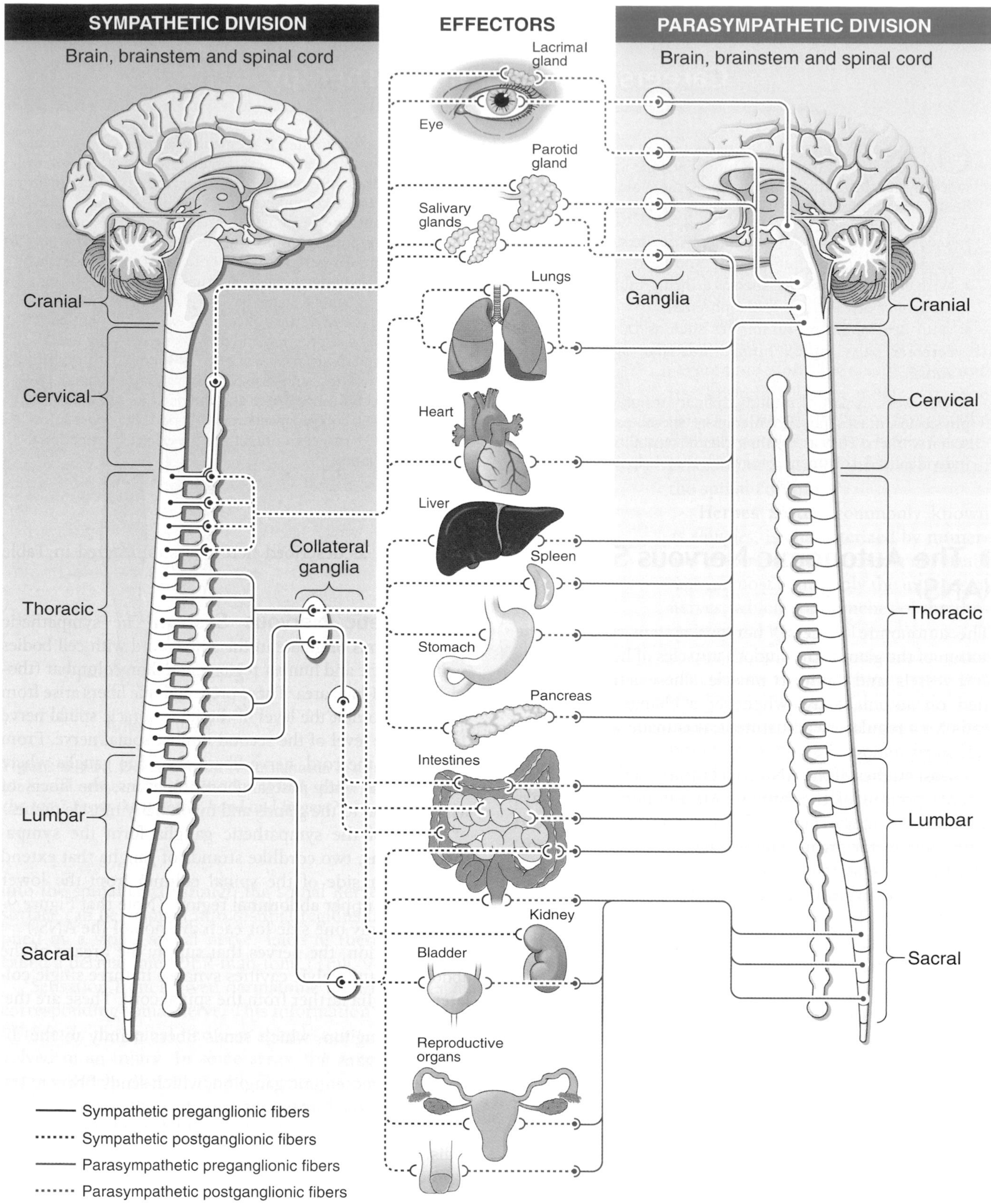

Figure 9-16 **Autonomic nervous system.** The diagram shows only one side of the body for each division. *ZOOMING IN* ✦ *Which division of the autonomic nervous system has ganglia closer to the effector organ?*

Table 9•3 Divisions of the Autonomic Nervous System

CHARACTERISTICS	DIVISIONS	
	Sympathetic Nervous System	**Parasympathetic Nervous System**
Origin of fibers	Thoracic and lumbar regions of the spinal cord; thoracolumbar	Brain stem and sacral regions of the spinal cord; craniosacral
Location of ganglia	Sympathetic chains and three single collateral ganglia (celiac, superior mesenteric, inferior mesenteric)	Terminal ganglia in or near the effector organ
Neurotransmitter	Adrenaline and noradrenaline; adrenergic	Acetylcholine; cholinergic
Effects (see Table 9-4)	Response to stress; fight-or-flight response	Reverses fight-or-flight (stress) response; stimulates some activities

Parasympathetic Nervous System The parasympathetic motor pathways begin in the **craniosacral** (kra-ne-o-SAK-ral) areas, with fibers arising from cell bodies in the brainstem (midbrain and medulla) and the lower (sacral) part of the spinal cord. From these centers, the first fibers extend to autonomic ganglia that are usually located near or within the walls of the effector organs and are called **terminal ganglia**. The pathways then continue along postganglionic neurons that stimulate the involuntary tissues.

The neurons of the parasympathetic system release the neurotransmitter acetylcholine, leading to the description of this system as **cholinergic** (activated by acetylcholine).

Functions of the Autonomic Nervous System

Most organs are supplied by both sympathetic and parasympathetic fibers, and the two systems generally have opposite effects. The sympathetic part of the ANS tends to act as an accelerator for those organs needed to meet a stressful situation. It promotes what is called the **fight-or-flight response** because in the most primitive terms, the person must decide to stay and "fight it out" with the enemy or to run away from danger. If you think of what happens to a person who is frightened or angry, you can easily remember the effects of impulses from the sympathetic nervous system:

- Increase in the rate and force of heart contractions.
- Increase in blood pressure due partly to the more effective heartbeat and partly to constriction of small arteries in the skin and the internal organs.
- Dilation of blood vessels to skeletal muscles, bringing more blood to these tissues.
- Dilation of the bronchial tubes to allow more oxygen to enter.
- Stimulation of the central portion of the adrenal gland. This produces hormones, including epinephrine, that prepare the body to meet emergency situations in many ways (see Chapter 12). The sympathetic nerves and hormones from the adrenal gland reinforce each other.
- Increase in basal metabolic rate.
- Dilation of the pupil and decrease in focusing ability (for near objects).

Table 9•4 Effects of the Sympathetic and Parasympathetic Systems on Selected Organs

Effector	Sympathetic System	Parasympathetic System
Pupils of eye	Dilation	Constriction
Sweat glands	Stimulation	None
Digestive glands	Inhibition	Stimulation
Heart	Increased rate and strength of beat	Decreased rate of beat
Bronchi of lungs	Dilation	Constriction
Muscles of digestive system	Decreased contraction (peristalsis)	Increased contraction
Kidneys	Decreased activity	None
Urinary bladder	Relaxation	Contraction and emptying
Liver	Increased release of glucose	None
Penis	Ejaculation	Erection
Adrenal medulla	Stimulation	None
Blood vessels to:		
Skeletal muscles	Dilation	Constriction
Skin	Constriction	None
Respiratory system	Dilation	Constriction
Digestive organs	Constriction	Dilation

Box 9-3 A Closer Look

Cell Receptors: Getting the Message

Neurons use neurotransmitters to communicate with other cells at synapses. Just as important, however, are the "docking sites," the receptors on the receiving (postsynaptic) cell membranes. A neurotransmitter fits into its receptor like a key in a lock. Once the neurotransmitter binds, the receptor initiates events that change the postsynaptic cell's activity. Different receptors' responses to the same neurotransmitter may vary, and a cell's response depends on the receptors it contains.

Among the many different classes of identified receptors, two are especially important and well-studied. The first is the cholinergic receptors, which bind acetylcholine (ACh). Cholinergic receptors are further subdivided into two types, each named for drugs that bind to them and mimic ACh's effects:

- Nicotinic receptors (which bind nicotine) are found on skeletal muscle cells and stimulate muscle contraction when ACh is present.
- Muscarinic receptors (which bind muscarine, a poison) are found on effector cells of the parasympathetic nervous system. ACh can either stimulate or inhibit muscarinic receptors depending on the effector organ. For example, ACh stimulates digestive organs but inhibits the heart.

The second class of receptors is the adrenergic receptors, which bind norepinephrine and epinephrine. They are found on effector cells of the sympathetic nervous system. They are further subdivided into alpha (α) and beta (β), each with several subtypes (*e.g*, α_1, α_2, β_1, and β_2). When norepinephrine (or epinephrine) binds to adrenergic receptors, it can either stimulate or inhibit, depending on the organ. For example, norepinephrine stimulates the heart and inhibits the digestive organs. With some exceptions, α_1 and β_1 receptors usually stimulate, whereas α_2 and β_2 receptors inhibit.

Some drugs block specific receptors. For example, "beta-blockers" regulate the heart in cardiac disease by preventing β_1 receptors from binding epinephrine, the neurotransmitter that increases the rate and strength of heart contractions.

The sympathetic system also acts as a brake on those systems not directly involved in the response to stress, such as the urinary and digestive systems. If you try to eat while you are angry, you may note that your saliva is thick and so small in amount that you can swallow only with difficulty. Under these circumstances, when food does reach the stomach, it seems to stay there longer than usual.

The parasympathetic part of the ANS normally acts as a balance for the sympathetic system once a crisis has passed. The parasympathetic system brings about constriction of the pupils, slowing of the heart rate, and constriction of the bronchial tubes. It also stimulates the formation and release of urine and activity of the digestive tract. Saliva, for example, flows more easily and profusely, and its quantity and fluidity increase.

Most organs of the body receive both sympathetic and parasympathetic stimulation, the effects of the two systems on a given organ generally being opposite. Table 9-4 shows some of the actions of these two systems. Box 9-3, Cell Receptors: Getting the Message, stresses the role of receptors in regulating the activities of the sympathetic and parasympathetic systems.

Checkpoint 9-15 Which division of the ANS stimulates a stress response, and which division reverses the stress response?

Word Anatomy

Medical terms are built from standardized word parts (prefixes, roots, and suffixes). Learning the meanings of these parts can help you remember words and interpret unfamiliar terms.

WORD PART	MEANING	EXAMPLE
The Nervous System as a Whole		
soma-	body	The *somatic* nervous system controls skeletal muscles that move the body.
aut/o	self	The *autonomic* nervous system is automatically controlled and is involuntary.
neur/i	nerve, nervous tissue	The *neurilemma* is the outer membrane of the myelin sheath around an axon.
-lemma	sheath	See preceding example.

WORD PART	MEANING	EXAMPLE
The Nervous System at Work		
de-	remove	*Depolarization* removes the charge on the plasma membrane of a cell.
re-	again, back	*Repolarization* restores the charge on the plasma membrane of a cell.
post-	after	The *postsynaptic* cell is located after the synapse and receives neurotransmitter from the presynaptic cell.
The Spinal Cord		
myel/o	spinal cord	*Poliomyelitis* is an infectious disease that involves the spinal cord and other parts of the CNS.
-plegia	paralysis	*Monoplegia* is paralysis of one limb.
para-	beyond	*Paraplegia* is paralysis of both lower limbs.
hemi-	half	*Hemiplegia* is paralysis of one side of the body.
tetra-	four	*Tetraplegia* is paralysis of all four limbs.

Summary

I. Role of the nervous system

A. Structural divisions—anatomic
  1. Central nervous system (CNS)—brain and spinal cord
  2. Peripheral nervous system (PNS)—spinal and cranial nerves

B. Functional divisions—physiologic
  1. Somatic nervous system—voluntary; supplies skeletal muscles
  2. Autonomic (visceral) nervous system—involuntary; supplies smooth muscle, cardiac muscle, glands

II. Neurons and their functions

A. Structure of a neuron
  1. Cell body
  2. Cell fibers
    a. Dendrite—carries impulses to cell body
    b. Axon—carries impulses away from cell body
  3. Myelin sheath
    a. Covers and protects some axons
    b. Speeds conduction
    c. Made by Schwann cells in PNS; other cells in CNS
      (1) Neurilemma—outermost layer of Schwann cell; aids axon repair
    d. White matter—myelinated tissue; gray matter—unmyelinated tissue

B. Types of neurons
  1. Sensory (afferent)—carry impulses toward CNS
  2. Motor (efferent)—carry impulses away from CNS
  3. Interneurons—in CNS

C. Nerves and tracts—bundles of neuron fibers
  1. Nerve—in peripheral nervous system
    a. Held together by connective tissue
      (1) Endoneurium—around a single fiber
      (2) Perineurium—around each fascicle
      (3) Epineurium—around whole nerve
    b. Types of nerves
      (1) Sensory (afferent) nerve—contains only fibers that carry impulses toward the CNS (from a receptor)
      (2) Motor (efferent) nerve—contains only fibers that carry impulses away from the CNS (to an effector)
      (3) Mixed nerve—contains both sensory and motor fibers
  2. Tract—in central nervous system

III. Neuroglia

  1. Nonconducting cells
  2. Protect and support nervous tissue

IV. The nervous system at work

A. Nerve impulse
  1. Potential—electrical charge on the plasma membrane of neuron
  2. Action potential
    a. Depolarization—reversal of charge
    b. Repolarization—return to normal
    c. Involves changes in concentrations of Na^+ and K^+
  3. Nerve impulse—spread of action potential along membrane
  4. Myelin sheath speeds conduction

B. Synapse—junction between neurons
  1. Nerve impulse transmitted from presynaptic neuron to postsynaptic neuron
  2. Neurotransmitter—carries impulse across synapse
  3. Receptors—in postsynaptic membrane; pick up neurotransmitters
  4. Neurotransmitter removed by diffusion, destruction by enzyme, return to presynaptic cell (reuptake)
  5. Electrical synapses—in smooth muscle, cardiac muscle, CNS

V. Spinal cord

  1. In vertebral column
  2. Ends between first and second lumbar vertebrae

A. Structure of the spinal cord
  1. H-shaped area of gray matter
  2. White matter around gray matter
    a. Ascending tracts—carry impulses toward brain
    b. Descending tracts—carry impulses away from brain

B. Reflex arc—pathway through the nervous system
  1. Components
    a. Receptor—detects stimulus

b. Sensory neuron—receptor to CNS
c. Central neuron—in CNS
d. Motor neuron—CNS to effector
e. Effector—muscle or gland that responds

2. Reflex activities—simple reflex is rapid, automatic response using few neurons
   a. Examples—stretch reflex, eye blink, withdrawal reflex
   b. Spinal reflex—coordinated in spinal cord

C. Medical procedures involving the spinal cord
   a. Lumbar puncture
   b. Administration of drugs

D. Diseases and other disorders of the spinal cord
   1. Diseases—multiple sclerosis, amyotrophic lateral sclerosis, poliomyelitis
   2. Tumors
   3. Injuries

VI. Spinal nerves—31 pairs

1. Roots
   a. Dorsal (sensory)
   b. Ventral (motor)
2. Spinal nerve—combines sensory and motor fibers (mixed nerve)

A. Branches of the spinal nerves
   1. Plexuses: networks formed by anterior branches
      a. Cervical plexus
      b. Brachial plexus
      c. Lumbosacral plexus
   2. Dermatome—region of the skin supplied by a single spinal nerve

B. Disorders of the spinal nerves—peripheral neuritis, sciatica, herpes zoster (shingles), Guillain-Barré

VII. Autonomic nervous system (visceral nervous system)

1. Involuntary
2. Controls glands, smooth muscle, heart (cardiac) muscle
3. Two motor neurons (preganglionic and postganglionic)

A. Divisions of the autonomic nervous system
   1. Sympathetic nervous system
      a. Thoracolumbar
      b. Adrenergic—uses adrenaline
      c. Synapses in sympathetic chains and three collateral ganglia (celiac, superior mesenteric, inferior mesenteric)
   2. Parasympathetic system
      a. Craniosacral
      b. Cholinergic—uses acetylcholine
      c. Synapses in terminal ganglia in or near effector organs

B. Functions of the autonomic nervous system
   1. Sympathetic—stimulates fight-or-flight (stress) response
   2. Parasympathetic—returns body to normal
   3. Usually have opposite effects on an organ

Questions for Study and Review

Building Understanding

Fill in the blanks

1. The brain and spinal cord make up the ______ nervous system.

2. Action potentials are conducted away from the neuron cell body by the ______.

3. During an action potential the flow of Na^+ into the cell causes ______.

4. In the spinal cord, sensory information travels in ______ tracts.

5. With few exceptions, the sympathetic nervous system uses the neurotransmitter ______ to act on effector organs.

Matching

Match each numbered item with the most closely related lettered item.

___ 6. Cells that carry impulses from the CNS
___ 7. Cells that carry impulses to the CNS
___ 8. Cells that carry impulses within the CNS
___ 9. Cells that detect a stimulus
___10. Cells that carry out a response to a stimulus

a. receptors
b. effectors
c. sensory neurons
d. motor neurons
e. interneurons

Multiple choice

___ 11. Skeletal muscles are voluntarily controlled by the
   a. central nervous system
   b. somatic nervous system
   c. parasympathetic nervous system
   d. sympathetic nervous system

___ 12. The cells involved in most nervous system tumors are called
   a. motor neurons
   b. sensory neurons
   c. interneurons
   d. neuroglia

___ 13. The correct order of synaptic transmission is
   a. postsynaptic neuron, synapse, and presynaptic neuron
   b. presynaptic neuron, synapse, and postsynaptic neuron

c. presynaptic neuron, postsynaptic neuron, and synapse
d. postsynaptic neuron, presynaptic neuron, and synapse

___ 14. Afferent nerve fibers enter the part of the spinal Cord called the
a.. dorsal horn
b. ventral horn
c. gray commisure
d. central canal

___ 15. The "fight-or-flight" response is promoted by the
a. sympathetic nervous system
b. parasympathetic nervous system
c. somatic nervous system
d. reflex arc

Understanding Concepts

16. Differentiate between the terms in each of the following pairs:
a. neurons and neuroglia
b. vesicle and receptor
c. gray matter and white matter
d. nerve and tract

17. Describe an action potential. How does conduction along a myelinated fiber differ from conduction along an unmyelinated fiber?

18. Discuss the structure and function of the spinal cord.

19. Explain the reflex arc using stepping on a tack as an example.

20. Describe the anatomy of a spinal nerve. How many pairs of spinal nerves are there?

21. Define a *plexus*. Name the three main spinal nerve plexuses.

22. Compare and contrast multiple sclerosis and Guillain-Barré syndrome.

23. Differentiate between the functions of the sympathetic and parasympathetic divisions of the autonomic nervous system.

Conceptual Thinking

24. Clinical depression is associated with abnormal serotonin levels. Medications that block the removal of this neurotransmitter from the synapse can control the disorder. Based on this information, is clinical depression associated with increased or decreased levels of serotonin? Explain your answer.

25. Mr. Hayward visits his dentist for a root canal and is given Novocain, a local anesthetic, at the beginning of the procedure. Novocain reduces membrane permeability to Na^+. What effect does this have on action potential?

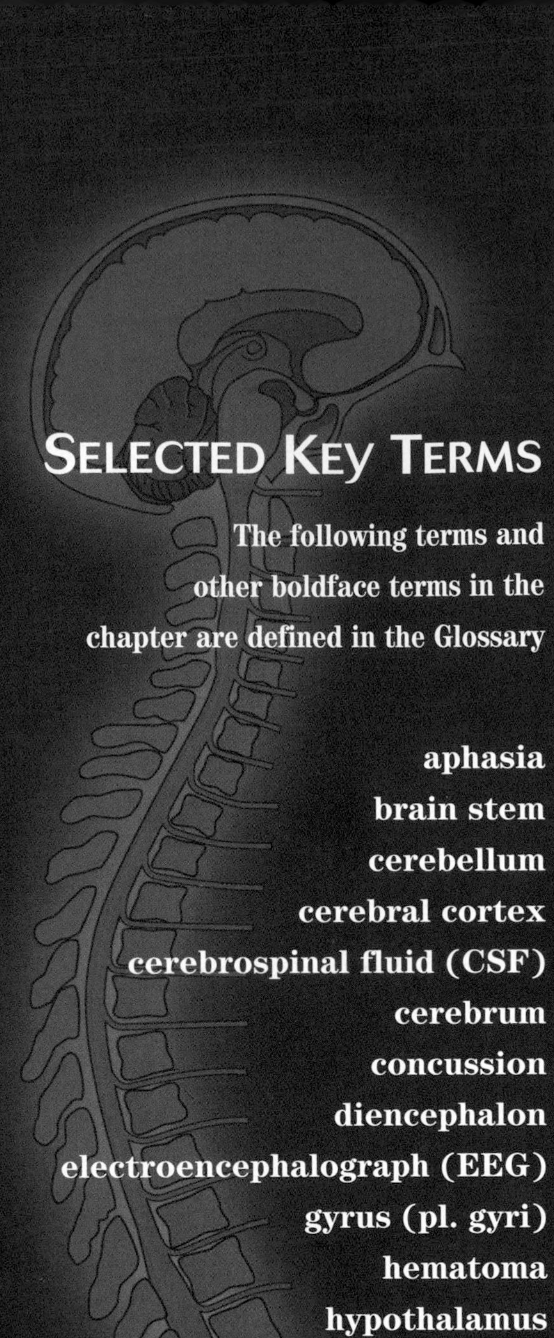

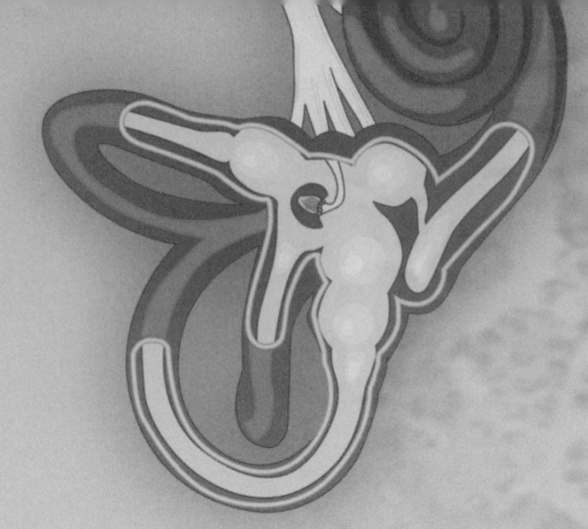

Selected Key Terms

The following terms and other boldface terms in the chapter are defined in the Glossary

aphasia
brain stem
cerebellum
cerebral cortex
cerebrospinal fluid (CSF)
cerebrum
concussion
diencephalon
electroencephalograph (EEG)
gyrus (pl. gyri)
hematoma
hypothalamus
medulla oblongata
meninges
midbrain
pons
stroke
sulcus (pl. sulci)
thalamus
ventricle

Learning Outcomes

After careful study of this chapter, you should be able to:

1. Give the location and functions of the four main divisions of the brain
2. Name and describe the three meninges
3. Cite the function of cerebrospinal fluid and describe where and how this fluid is formed
4. Name and locate the lobes of the cerebral hemispheres
5. Cite one function of the cerebral cortex in each lobe of the cerebrum
6. Name two divisions of the diencephalon and cite the functions of each
7. Locate the three subdivisions of the brain stem and give the functions of each
8. Describe the cerebellum and cite its functions
9. Name some techniques used to study the brain
10. Cite the names and functions of the 12 cranial nerves
11. List some disorders that involve the brain, its associated structures, or the cranial nerves
12. Show how word parts are used to build words related to the nervous system (see Word Anatomy at the end of the chapter)

chapter 10

The Nervous System: The Brain and Cranial Nerves

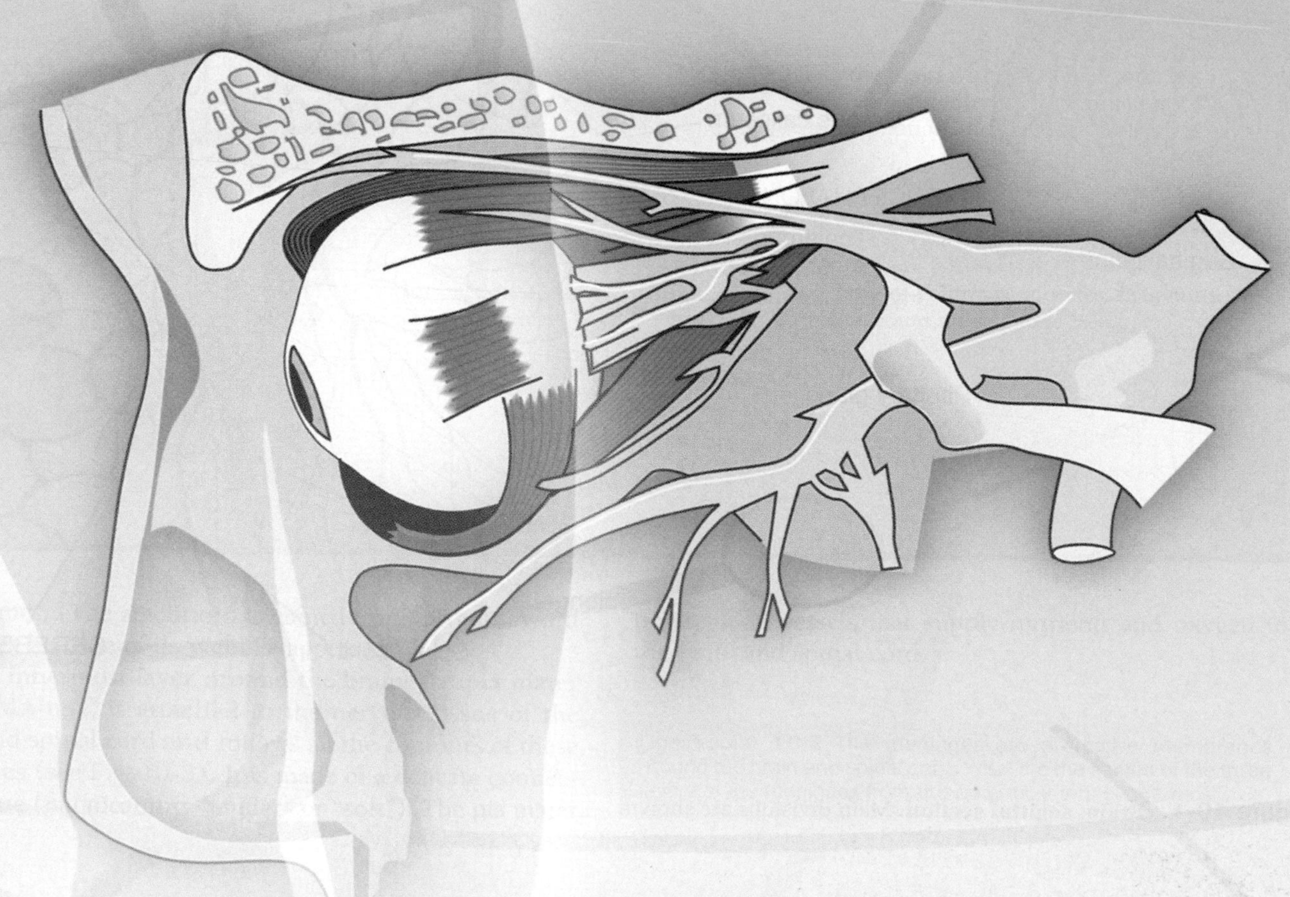

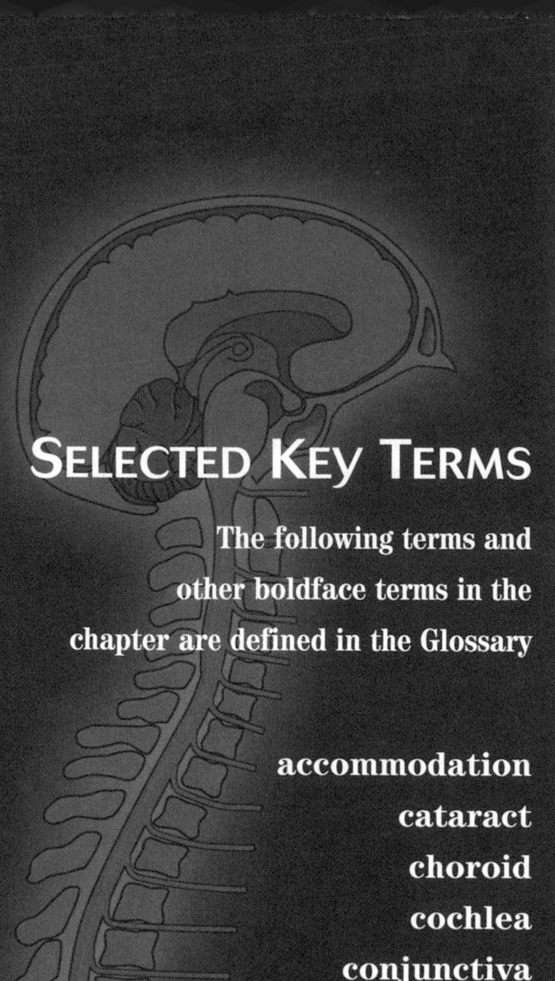

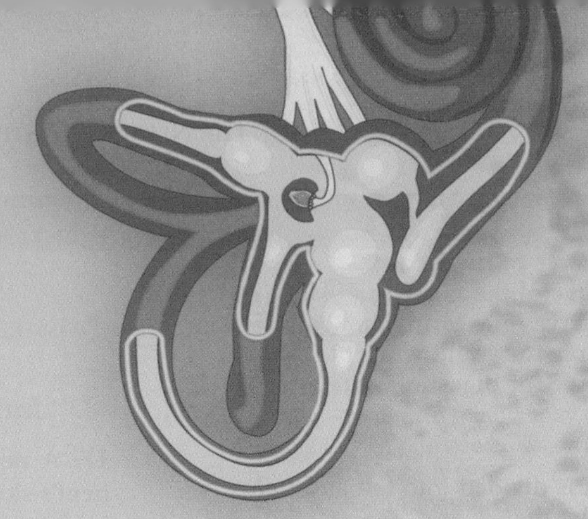

SELECTED KEY TERMS

The following terms and other boldface terms in the chapter are defined in the Glossary

accommodation
cataract
choroid
cochlea
conjunctiva
convergence
cornea
glaucoma
gustation
lacrimal apparatus
lens (crystalline lens)
olfaction
organ of Corti
ossicle
proprioceptor
refraction
retina
sclera
semicircular canal
sensory receptor
tympanic membrane
vestibule
vitreous body

LEARNING OUTCOMES

After careful study of this chapter, you should be able to:

1. Describe the function of the sensory system
2. Differentiate between the special and general senses and give examples of each
3. Describe the structure of the eye
4. List and describe the structures that protect the eye
5. Define *refraction* and list the refractive parts of the eye
6. Differentiate between the rods and the cones of the eye
7. Compare the functions of the extrinsic and intrinsic muscles of the eye
8. Describe the nerve supply to the eye
9. Describe the three divisions of the ear
10. Describe the receptor for hearing and explain how it functions
11. Compare static and dynamic equilibrium and describe the location and function of these receptors
12. Explain the function of proprioceptors
13. List several methods for treatment of pain
14. Describe sensory adaptation and explain its value
15. List some disorders of the sensory system
16. Show how word parts are used to build words related to the sensory system (see Word Anatomy at the end of the chapter)

chapter 11

The Sensory System

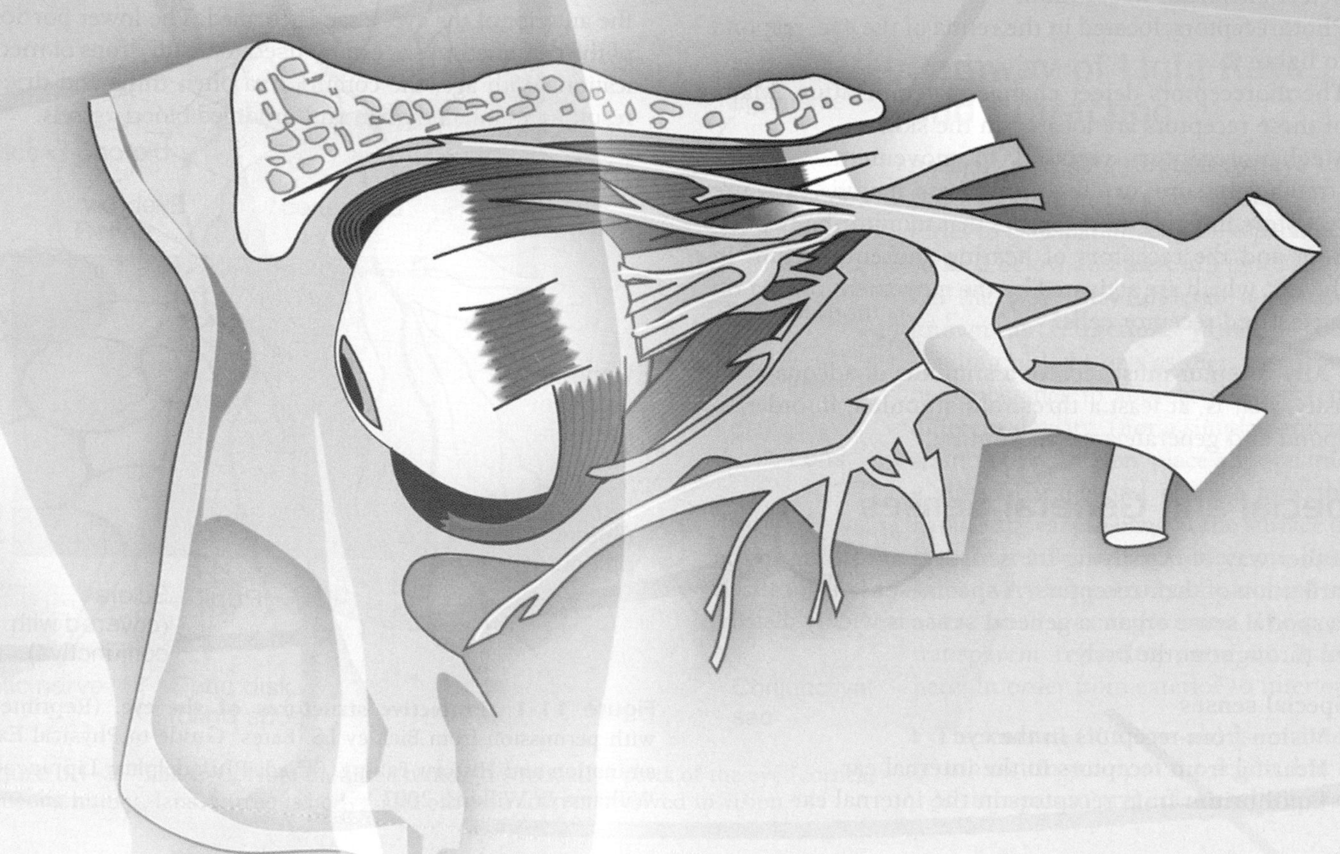

Selected Key Terms

The following terms and other boldface terms in the chapter are defined in the Glossary

endocrine
hormone
hypothalamus
pituitary (hypophysis)
prostaglandin
receptor
steroid
target tissue

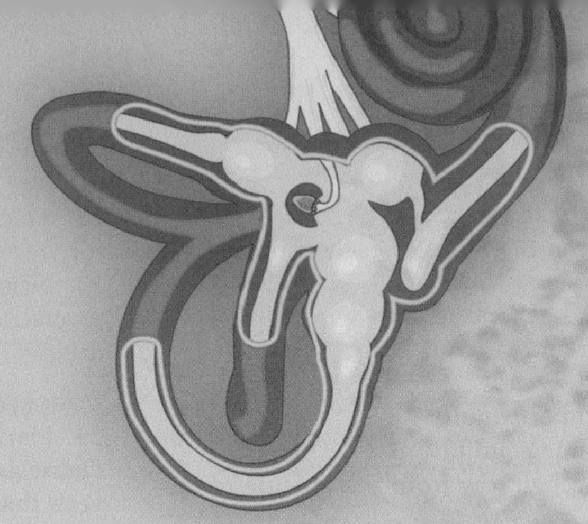

Learning Outcomes

After careful study of this chapter, you should be able to:

1. Compare the effects of the nervous system and the endocrine system in controlling the body
2. Describe the functions of hormones
3. Explain how hormones are regulated
4. Identify the glands of the endocrine system on a diagram
5. List the hormones produced by each endocrine gland and describe the effects of each on the body
6. Describe how the hypothalamus controls the anterior and posterior pituitary
7. Describe the effects of hyposecretion and hypersecretion of the various hormones
8. List tissues other than the endocrine glands that produce hormones
9. List some medical uses of hormones
10. Explain how the endocrine system responds to stress
11. Show how word parts are used to build words related to the endocrine system (see Word Anatomy at the end of the chapter)

chapter

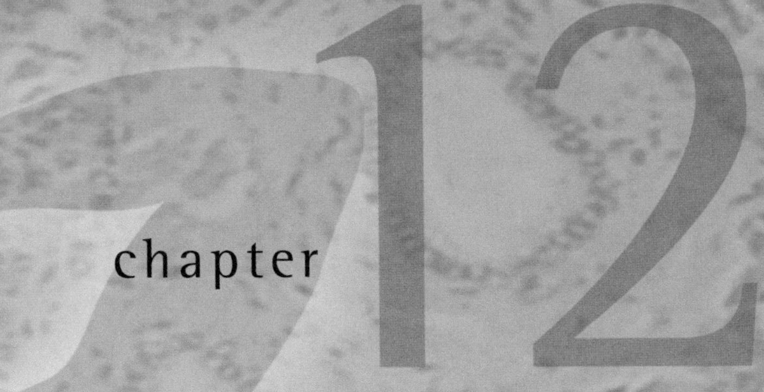

The Endocrine System: Glands and Hormones

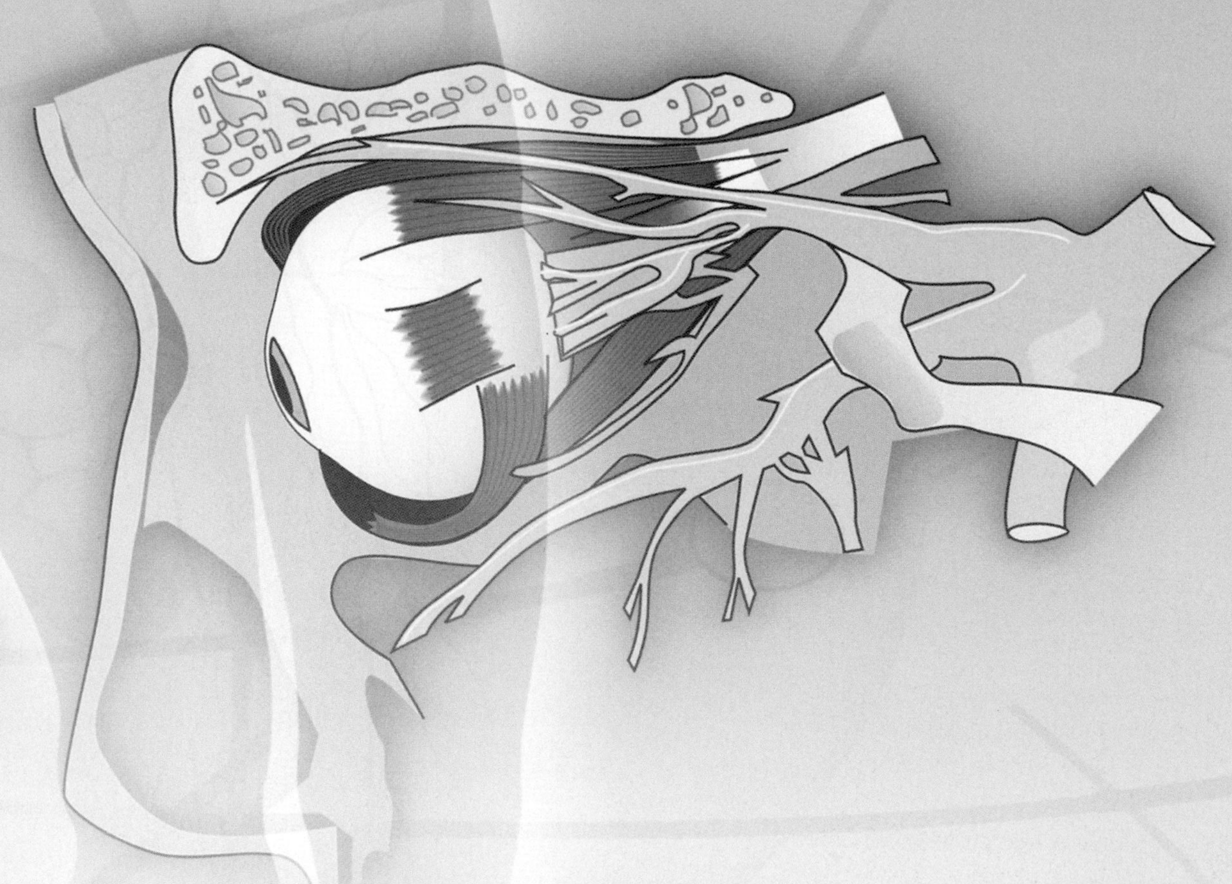

The endocrine system consists of a group of glands that produces regulatory chemicals called **hormones.** The endocrine system and the nervous system work together to control and coordinate all other systems of the body. The nervous system controls such rapid actions as muscle movement and intestinal activity by means of electrical and chemical stimuli. The effects of the endocrine system occur more slowly and over a longer period. They involve chemical stimuli only, and these chemical messengers have widespread effects on the body.

Although the nervous and endocrine systems differ in some respects, the two systems are closely related. For example, the activity of the pituitary gland, which in turn regulates other glands, is controlled by the brain's hypothalamus. The connections between the nervous system and the endocrine system enable endocrine function to adjust to the demands of a changing environment.

Hormones

Hormones are chemical messengers that have specific regulatory effects on certain cells or organs. Hormones from the endocrine glands are released directly into the bloodstream, which carries them to all parts of the body. They regulate growth, metabolism, reproduction, and behavior. Some hormones affect many tissues, for example, growth hormone, thyroid hormone, and insulin. Others affect only specific tissues. For example, one pituitary hormone, thyroid-stimulating hormone (TSH), acts only on the thyroid gland; another, adrenocorticotropic hormone (ACTH), stimulates only the outer portion of the adrenal gland.

The specific tissue acted on by each hormone is the **target tissue.** The cells that make up these tissues have **receptors** in the plasma membrane or within the cytoplasm to which the hormone attaches. Once a hormone binds to a receptor on or in a target cell, it affects cell activities, regulating the manufacture of proteins, changing the permeability of the membrane, or affecting metabolic reactions.

Hormone Chemistry

Chemically, hormones fall into two main categories:

- **Amino acid compounds.** These hormones are proteins or related compounds also made of amino acids. All hormones except those of the adrenal cortex and the sex glands fall into this category.
- **Steroids.** These hormones are types of lipids derived from the steroid cholesterol. Steroid hormones are produced by the adrenal cortex and the sex glands. Steroid hormones can be recognized by the ending *–one*, as in progesterone, testosterone.

Checkpoint 12-1 What are hormones and what are some effects of hormones?

Hormone Regulation

The amount of each hormone that is secreted is normally kept within a specific range. Negative feedback, described in Chapter 1, is the method most commonly used to regulate these levels. In negative feedback, the hormone itself (or the result of its action) controls further hormone secretion. Each endocrine gland tends to oversecrete its hormone, exerting more effect on the target tissue. When the target tissue becomes too active, there is a negative effect on the endocrine gland, which then decreases its secretory action.

We can use as an example the secretion of thyroid hormones (Fig. 12-1). As described in more detail later in the chapter, a pituitary hormone, called *thyroid-stimulating hormone* (TSH), triggers secretion of hormones from the thyroid gland located in the neck. As blood levels of these hormones rise under the effects of TSH, they act as negative feedback messengers to inhibit TSH release from the pituitary. With less TSH, the thyroid releases less hormone and blood levels drop. When hormone levels fall

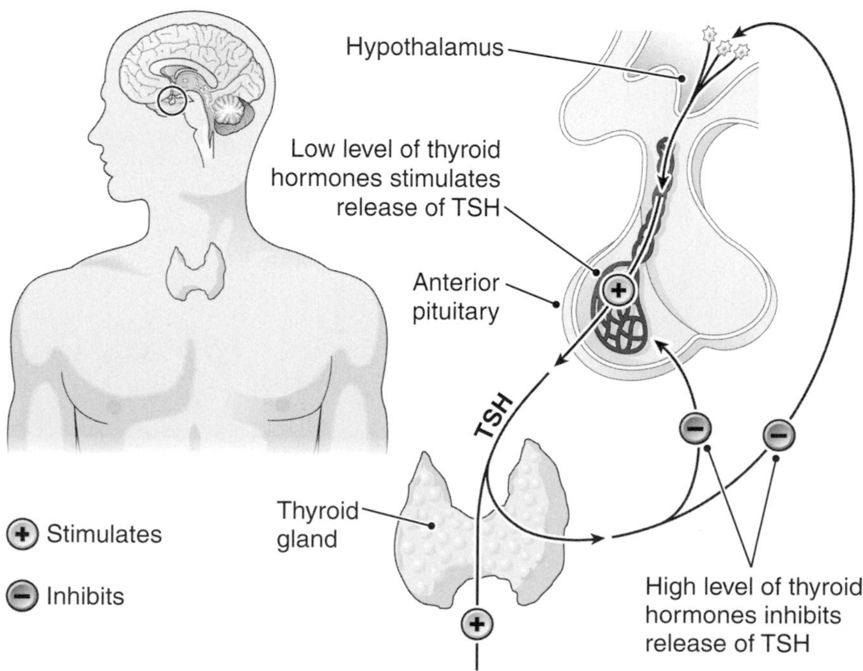

Figure 12-1 **Negative feedback control of thyroid hormones.** The anterior pituitary releases thyroid stimulating hormone (TSH) when the blood level of thyroid hormones is low. A high level of thyroid hormones inhibits release of TSH and thyroid hormone levels fall.

below the normal range, the pituitary can again begin to release TSH. This is a typical example of the kind of self-regulating system that keeps hormone levels within a set normal range.

Less commonly, some hormones are produced in response to positive feedback. In this case, response to a hormone promotes further hormone release. Examples are the action of oxytocin during labor, as described in Chapter 1, and the release of some hormones in the menstrual cycle, as described in Chapter 23.

The release of hormones may fall into a rhythmic pattern. Hormones of the adrenal cortex follow a 24-hour cycle related to a person's sleeping pattern, with the level of secretion greatest just before arising and least at bedtime. Hormones of the female menstrual cycle follow a monthly pattern.

Checkpoint 12-2 Hormones levels are normally kept within a specific range. What is the most common method used to regulate secretion of hormones?

The Endocrine Glands and Their Hormones

The remainder of this chapter deals with hormones and the tissues that produce them. Refer to Figure 12-2 to locate each of the endocrine glands as you study them. Table 12-1 summarizes the information on the endocrine glands and their hormones. Each section of the chapter also includes information on the effects of hypersecretion (oversecretion) or hyposecretion (undersecretion) of a hormone, summarized in Table 12-2.

Although most of the discussion centers on the endocrine glands, it is important to note that many tissues—other than the endocrine glands—also secrete hormones. That is, they produce substances that act on other tissues, usually at some distance from where they are produced. These tissues include the brain, digestive organs, and kidney. Some of these other tissues will be discussed later in the chapter.

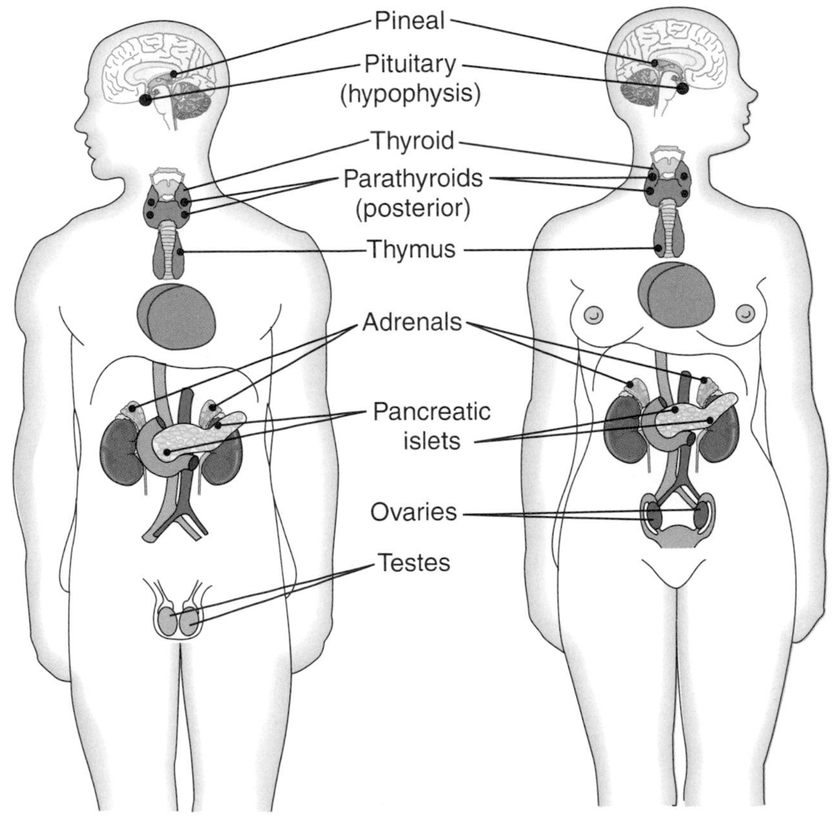

Figure 12-2 **The endocrine glands.**

The Pituitary

The **pituitary** (pih-TU-ih-tar-e), or **hypophysis** (hi-POF-ih-sis), is a small gland about the size of a cherry. It is located in a saddlelike depression of the sphenoid bone just posterior to the point where the optic nerves cross. It is surrounded by bone except where it connects with the hypothalmus of the brain by a stalk called the **infundibulum** (in-fun-DIB-u-lum). The gland is divided into two parts, the **anterior lobe** and the **posterior lobe** (Fig. 12-3).

The pituitary is often called the *master gland* because it releases hormones that affect the working of other glands, such as the thyroid, gonads (ovaries and testes), and adrenal glands. (Hormones that stimulate other glands may be recognized by the ending *-tropin,* as in *thyrotropin,* which means "acting on the thyroid gland.") However, the pituitary itself is controlled by the hypothalamus, which sends secretions and nerve impulses to the pituitary through the infundibulum (see Fig. 12-3).

Control of the Pituitary The hormones produced in the anterior pituitary are not released until chemical messengers called **releasing hormones** arrive from the hypothalamus. These releasing hormones travel to the anterior pituitary by way of a special type of circulatory pathway called a **portal system.** By this circulatory "detour," some of the blood that leaves the hypothalamus travels to capillaries in the anterior pituitary before returning to the heart. As the blood circulates through the capillaries, it delivers the hormones that stimulate the release of anterior pituitary secretions. Hypothalamic releasing hormones are indicated with the abbreviation *RH* added to an abbreviation for the name of the hormone stimulated. For example, the

Table 12•1 The Endocrine Glands and Their Hormones

GLAND	HORMONE	PRINCIPAL FUNCTIONS
Anterior pituitary	GH (growth hormone)	Promotes growth of all body tissues
	TSH (thyroid-stimulating hormone)	Stimulates thyroid gland to produce thyroid hormones
	ACTH (adrenocorticotropic hormone)	Stimulates adrenal cortex to produce cortical hormones; aids in protecting body in stress situations (injury, pain)
	PRL (prolactin)	Stimulates secretion of milk by mammary glands
	FSH (follicle-stimulating hormone)	Stimulates growth and hormone activity of ovarian follicles; stimulates growth of testes; promotes development of sperm cells
	LH (luteinizing hormone); ICSH (interstitial cell-stimulating hormone) in males	Causes development of corpus luteum at site of ruptured ovarian follicle in female; stimulates secretion of testosterone in male
Posterior pituitary	ADH (antidiuretic hormone)	Promotes reabsorption of water in kidney tubules; at high concentration stimulates constriction of blood vessels
	Oxytocin	Causes contraction of uterine muscle; causes ejection of milk from mammary glands
Thyroid	Thyroxine (T_4) and triiodothyronine(T_3)	Increases metabolic rate, influencing both physical and mental activities; required for normal growth
	Calcitonin	Decreases calcium level in blood
Parathyroids	Parathyroid hormone (PTH)	Regulates exchange of calcium between blood and bones; increases calcium level in blood
Adrenal medulla	Epinephrine and norephinephrine	Increases blood pressure and heart rate; activates cells influenced by sympathetic nervous system plus many not affected by sympathetic nerves
Adrenal cortex	Cortisol (95% of glucocorticoids)	Aids in metabolism of carbohydrates, proteins, and fats; active during stress
	Aldosterone (95% of mineralocorticoids)	Aids in regulating electrolytes and water balance
	Sex hormones	May influence secondary sexual characteristics
Pancreatic islets	Insulin	Needed for transport of glucose into cells; required for cellular metabolism of foods, especially glucose; decreases blood sugar levels
	Glucagon	Stimulates liver to release glucose, thereby increasing blood sugar levels
Testes	Testosterone	Stimulates growth and development of sexual organs (testes, penis) plus development of secondary sexual characteristics, such as hair growth on body and face and deepening of voice; stimulates maturation of sperm cells
Ovaries	Estrogens (*e.g.*, estradiol)	Stimulates growth of primary sexual organs (uterus, tubes) and development of secondary sexual organs, such as breasts, plus changes in pelvis to ovoid, broader shape
	Progesterone	Stimulates development of secretory parts of mammary glands; prepares uterine lining for implantation of fertilized ovum; aids in maintaining pregnancy
Thymus	Thymosin	Promotes growth of T cells active in immunity
Pineal	Melatonin	Regulates mood, sexual development, and daily cycles in response to the amount of light in the environment

releasing hormone that controls growth hormone is GH-RH.

Two anterior pituitary hormones are also regulated by inhibiting hormones (IH) from the hypothalamus. Inhibiting hormones suppress both growth hormone, which stimulates growth and metabolism, and prolactin, which stimulates milk production in the mammary glands. These inhibiting hormones are abbreviated GH-IH (growth hormone-inhibiting hormone) and PIH (prolactin-inhibiting hormone)

The two hormones of the posterior pituitary (antidiuretic hormone, or ADH, and oxytocin) are actually produced in the hypothalamus and stored in the posterior pituitary. Their release is controlled by nerve impulses that travel over pathways (tracts) between the hypothalamus and the posterior pituitary.

Table 12•2 Disorders Associated with Endocrine Dysfunction

HORMONE	EFFECTS OF HYPERSECRETION	EFFECTS OF HYPOSECRETION
Growth hormone	Gigantism (children), acromegaly (adults)	Dwarfism (children)
Antidiuretic hormone	Syndrome of inappropriate antidiuretic hormone (SIADH)	Diabetes insipidus
Aldosterone	Aldosteronism	Addison disease
Cortisol	Cushing syndrome	Addison disease
Thyroid hormone	Graves disease, thyrotoxicosis	Infantile hypothyroidism (cretinism) in children; myxedema in adults
Insulin	Hypoglycemia	Diabetes mellitus
Parathyroid hormone	Bone degeneration	Tetany (muscle spasms)

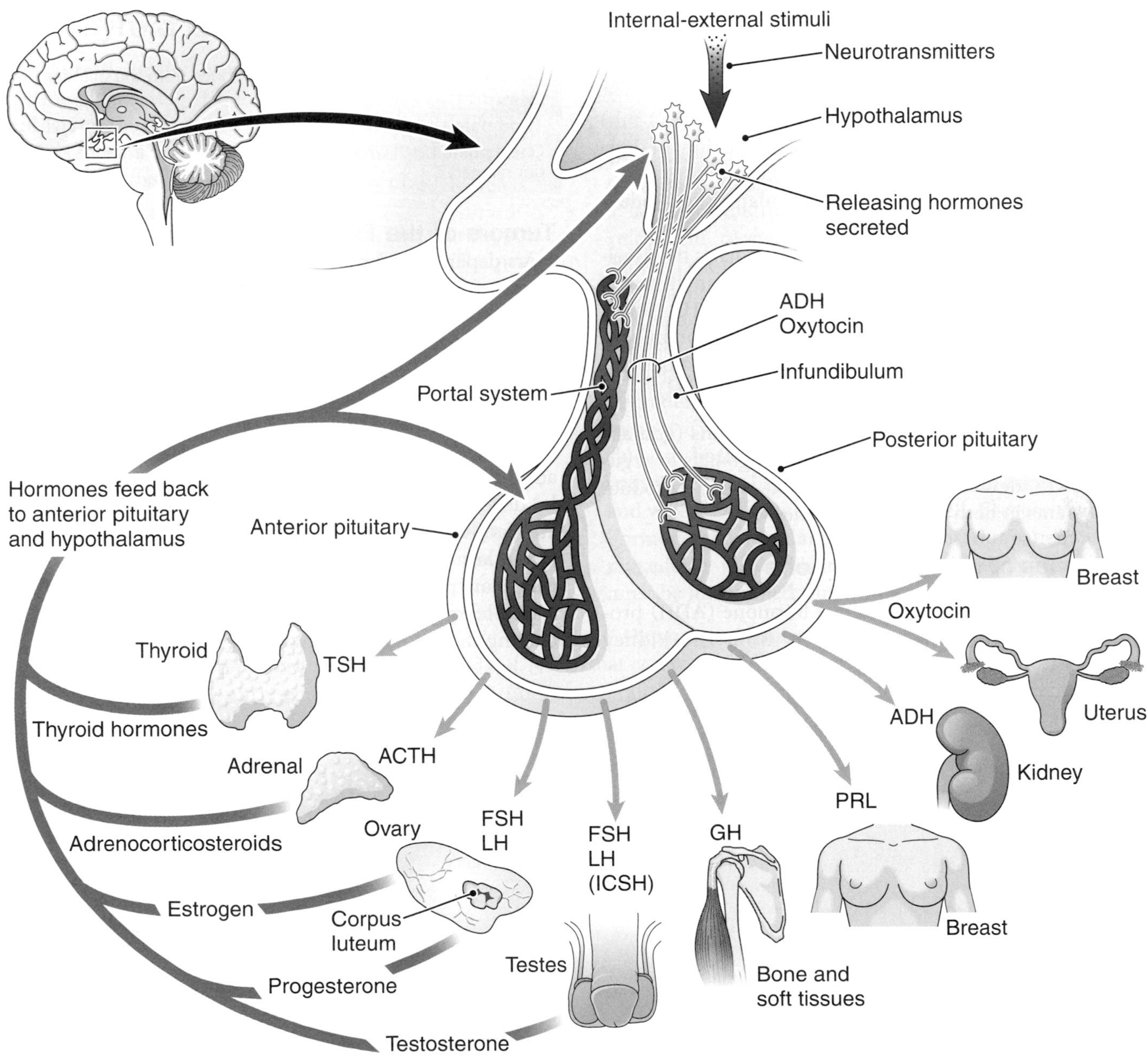

Figure 12-3 **The hypothalamus, pituitary gland, and target tissues.** Arrows indicate the hormones' target issues and feedback pathways. *ZOOMING IN ✦ What two structures does the infundibulum connect?*

Questions for Study and Review

Building Understanding

Fill in the blanks

1. Chemical messengers carried by the blood are called ______.
2. The part of the brain that regulates endocrine activity is the ______.
3. Red blood cell production in the bone marrow is stimulated by ______.
4. A hormone produced by the heart is ______.
5. Local hormones active in promoting inflammation are ______.

Matching

Match each numbered item with the most closely related lettered item.

___ 6. A disorder caused by overproduction of growth hormone in the adult.
___ 7. A disorder caused by underproduction of parathyroid hormone.
___ 8. A disorder caused by underproduction of thyroid hormone.
___ 9. A disorder caused by overproduction of growth hormone in the child.
___ 10. A disorder caused by underproduction of antidiuretic hormone.

a. cretinism
b. gigantism
c. tetany
d. diabetes insipidus
e. acromegaly

Multiple choice

___ 11. A target tissue responds to a hormone only if it has the appropriate
a. amino acid
b. transporter
c. ion channel
d. receptor

___ 12. Uterine contractions and milk ejection are promoted by
a. prolactin
b. oxytocin
c. estrogen
d. luteinizing hormone

___ 13. The principal hormone that increases the metabolic rate in body cells is
a. thyroxine
b. triiodothyronine
c. aldosterone
d. progesterone

___ 14. Epinephrine and norepinephrine are released by the
a. adrenal cortex
b. adrenal medulla
c. kidneys
d. pancreas

___ 15. Sleep-wake cycles are regulated by the
a. pituitary
b. thyroid
c. thymus
d. pineal

Understanding Concepts

16. With regard to regulation, what are the main differences between the nervous system and the endocrine system?
17. Explain how the hypothalamus and pituitary gland regulate certain endocrine glands. Use the thyroid as an example.
18. Name the two divisions of the pituitary gland. List the hormones released from each division and describe the effects of each.
19. Compare and contrast the following hormones:
    a. calcitonin and parathyroid hormone
    b. cortisol and aldosterone
    c. insulin and glucagon
    d. testosterone and estrogen
20. Describe the anatomy of the following endocrine glands:
    a. thyroid
    b. pancreas
    c. adrenals
21. Compare and contrast the following diseases:
    a. myxedema and Graves disease
    b. type I diabetes and type II diabetes
    c. Addison disease and Cushing syndrome
22. Name the hormone released by the thymus gland; by the pineal body. What are the effects of each?
23. List several hormones released during stress. What is the relationship between prolonged stress and disease?

Conceptual Thinking

24. Danielle M. (13-year-old female Caucasian) is rushed to the hospital after collapsing at school. She is disoriented, dehydrated, and hyperglycemic. What endocrine disorder does Danielle have? Explain her symptoms. What is the best way to treat this disease?
25. Mr. Jefferson has rheumatoid arthritis, which is being treated with glucocorticoids. During a recent checkup, his doctor notices that Mr. Jefferson's face is "puffy" and his arms are bruised. Why does the doctor decide to lower his patient's glucocorticoid dosage?

unit V

Circulation and Body Defense

The chapters in this unit discuss the systems that move materials through the body. The blood is the main transport medium. It circulates through the cardiovascular system, consisting of the heart and the blood vessels. The lymphatic system, in addition to other functions, helps to balance body fluids by bringing substances from the tissues back to the heart. Components of the blood and the lymphatic system are involved in body defenses against infection as part of the immune system.

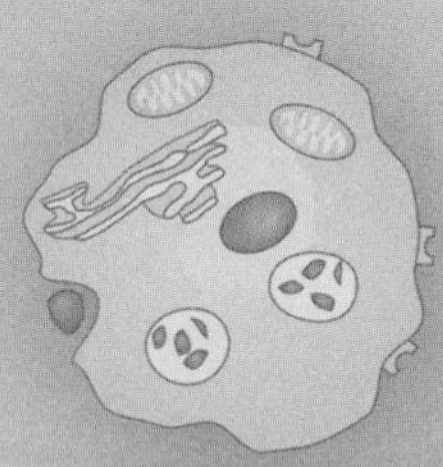

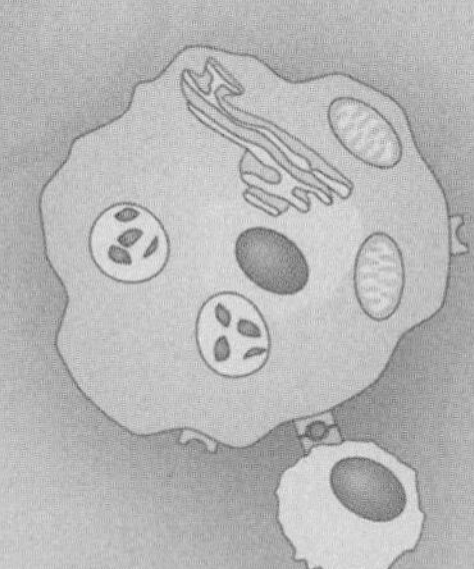

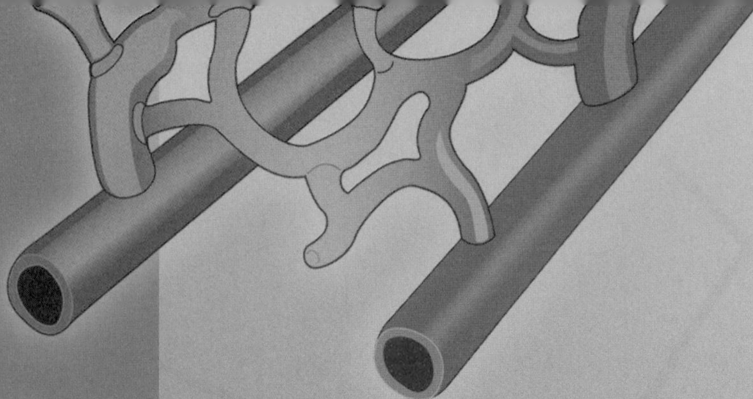

Selected Key Terms

The following terms and other boldface terms in the chapter are defined in the Glossary

agglutination
anemia
antigen
antiserum
centrifuge
coagulation
cryoprecipitate
erythrocyte
fibrin
hematocrit
hemoglobin
hemolysis
hemorrhage
hemostasis
leukemia
leukocyte
megakaryocyte
plasma
platelet (thrombocyte)
serum
thrombocytopenia
transfusion

Learning Outcomes

After careful study of this chapter, you should be able to:

1. List the functions of the blood
2. List the main ingredients in plasma
3. Describe the formation of blood cells
4. Name and describe the three types of formed elements in the blood and give the function of each
5. Characterize the five types of leukocytes
6. Define *hemostasis* and cite three steps in hemostasis
7. Briefly describe the steps in blood clotting
8. Define *blood type* and explain the relation between blood type and transfusions
9. List the possible reasons for transfusions of whole blood and blood components
10. Define *anemia* and list the causes of anemia
11. Define *leukemia* and name the two types of leukemia
12. Describe several forms of clotting disorders
13. Specify the tests used to study blood
14. Show how word parts are used to build words related to the blood (see Word Anatomy at the end of the chapter)

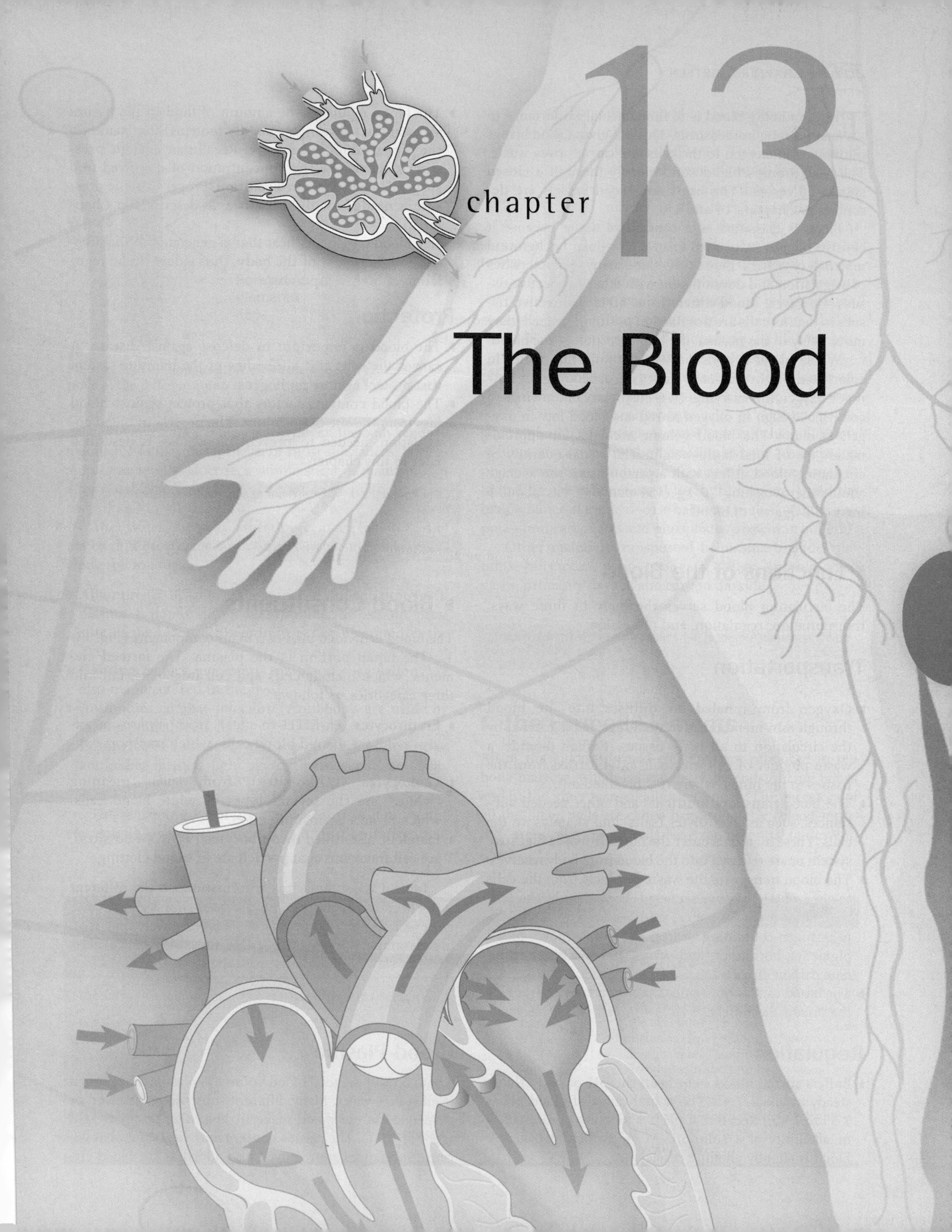

chapter 13

The Blood

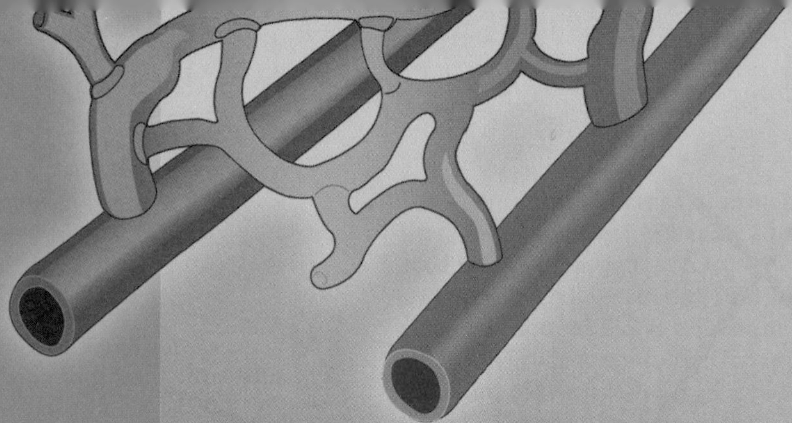

Selected Key Terms

The following terms and other boldface terms in the chapter are defined in the Glossary

arrhythmia
atherosclerosis
atrium
bradycardia
coronary
coronary thrombosis
diastole
echocardiograph
electrocardiography
endocardium
epicardium
fibrillation
infarct
ischemia
murmur
myocardium
pacemaker
pericardium
plaque
septum
stenosis
systole
tachycardia
valve
ventricle

Learning Outcomes

After careful study of this chapter, you should be able to:

1. Describe the three layers of the heart wall
2. Describe the structure of the pericardium and cite its functions
3. Compare the functions of the right and left sides of the heart
4. Name the four chambers of the heart and compare their functions
5. Name the valves at the entrance and exit of each ventricle and cite the function of the valves
6. Briefly describe blood circulation through the myocardium
7. Briefly describe the cardiac cycle
8. Name and locate the components of the heart's conduction system
9. Explain the effects of the autonomic nervous system on the heart rate
10. List and define several terms that describe variations in heart rates
11. Explain what produces the two main heart sounds
12. Describe several common types of heart disease
13. List five actions that can be taken to minimize the risk of heart disease
14. Briefly describe four methods for studying the heart
15. Describe several approaches to the treatment of heart disease
16. Show how word parts are used to build words related to the heart (see Word Anatomy at the end of the chapter)

chapter 14

The Heart and Heart Disease

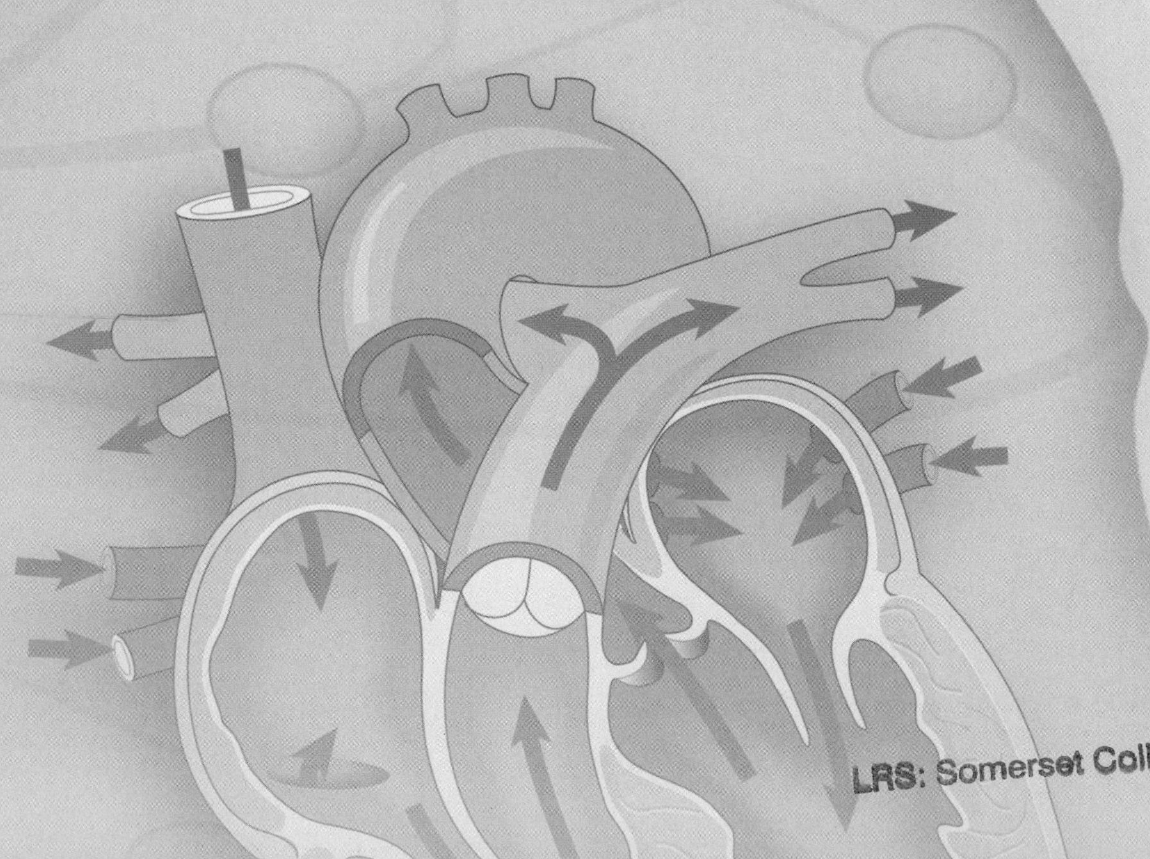

Circulation and the Heart

The next two chapters investigate how the blood delivers oxygen and nutrients to the cells and carries away the waste products of cell metabolism. The continuous one-way circuit of blood through the body in the blood vessels is known as the **circulation**. The prime mover that propels blood throughout the body is the **heart**. This chapter examines the structure and function of the heart to lay the foundation for the detailed discussion of blood vessels that follows.

The importance of the heart has been recognized for centuries. Strokes (the contractions) of this pump average about 72 per minute and are carried on unceasingly for the whole of a lifetime. The beating of the heart is affected by the emotions, which may explain the frequent references to it in song and poetry. However, the vital functions of the heart and its disorders are of more practical concern.

Location of the Heart

The heart is slightly bigger than a person's fist. This organ is located between the lungs in the center and a bit to the left of the midline of the body (Fig. 14-1). It occupies most of the mediastinum, the central region of the thorax. The heart's **apex**, the pointed, inferior portion, is directed toward the left. The broad, superior **base** is the area of attachment for the large vessels carrying blood into and out of the heart.

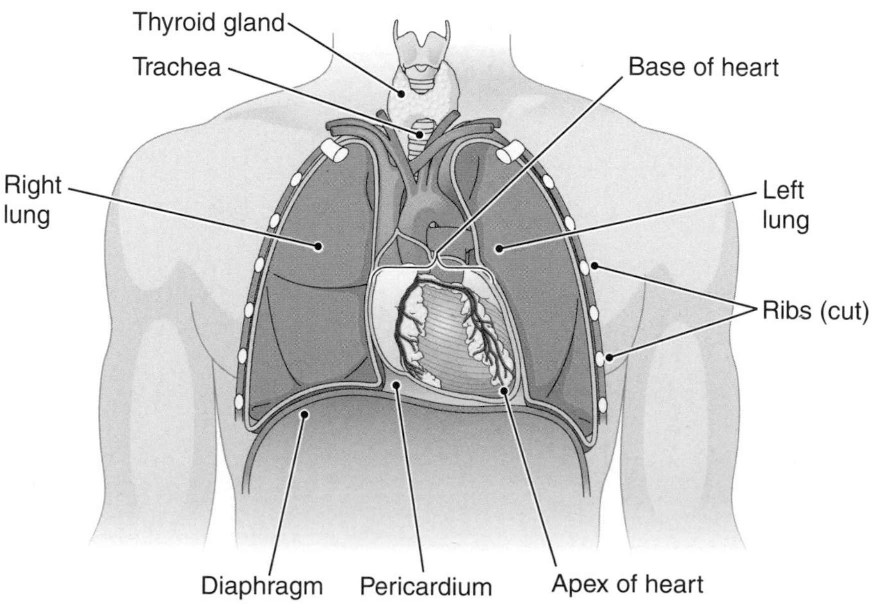

Thyroid gland
Trachea
Base of heart
Right lung
Left lung
Ribs (cut)
Diaphragm
Pericardium
Apex of heart

Figure 14-1 **The heart in position in the thorax (anterior view).** *ZOOMING IN ✦ Why is the left lung smaller than the right lung?*

Structure of the Heart

The heart is a hollow organ, with walls formed of three different layers. Just as a warm coat might have a smooth lining, a thick and bulky interlining, and an outer layer of a third fabric, so the heart wall has three tissue layers (Fig. 14-2, Table 14-1). Starting with the innermost layer, these are as follows:

- The **endocardium** (en-do-KAR-de-um) is a thin, smooth layer of epithelial cells that lines the heart's interior. The endocardium provides a smooth surface for easy flow as blood travels through the heart. Extensions of this membrane cover the flaps (cusps) of the heart valves.
- The **myocardium** (mi-o-KAR-de-um), the heart muscle, is the thickest layer and pumps blood through the vessels. Cardiac muscle's unique structure is described in more detail next.
- The **epicardium** (ep-ih-KAR-de-um) is a serous membrane that forms the thin, outermost layer of the heart wall.

The Pericardium

The **pericardium** (per-ih-KAR-de-um) is the sac that encloses the heart (Fig. 14-2, Table 14-2). The formation of the pericardial sac was described and illustrated in chapter 4 under a discussion of membranes (see Fig. 4-9). The outermost and heaviest layer of this sac is the fibrous pericardium. Connective tissue anchors this pericardial layer to the diaphragm, located inferiorly; the sternum, located anteriorly; and to other structures surrounding the heart, thus holding the heart in place. A serous membrane lines this fibrous sac and folds back at the base to cover the heart's surface. Anatomically, the outer layer of this serous membrane is called the parietal layer, and the inner layer is the visceral layer, also known as the epicardium, as previously noted. A thin film of fluid between these two layers reduces friction as the heart moves within the pericardium. Normally the visceral and parietal layers are very close together, but fluid may accumulate in the region between them, the pericardial cavity, under certain disease conditions.

Checkpoint 14-1 What are the names of the innermost, middle, and outermost layers of the heart?

Checkpoint 14-2 What is the name of the sac that encloses the heart?

Table 14•1 Layers of the Heart Wall

LAYER	LOCATION	DESCRIPTION	FUNCTION
Endocardium	Innermost layer of the heart wall	Thin, smooth layer of epithelial cells	Lines the interior of the chambers and covers the heart valves
Myocardium	Middle layer of the heart wall	Thick layer of cardiac muscle	Contracts to pump blood into the arteries
Epicardium	Outermost layer of the heart wall	Thin serous membrane	Covers the heart and forms the visceral layer of the serous pericardium

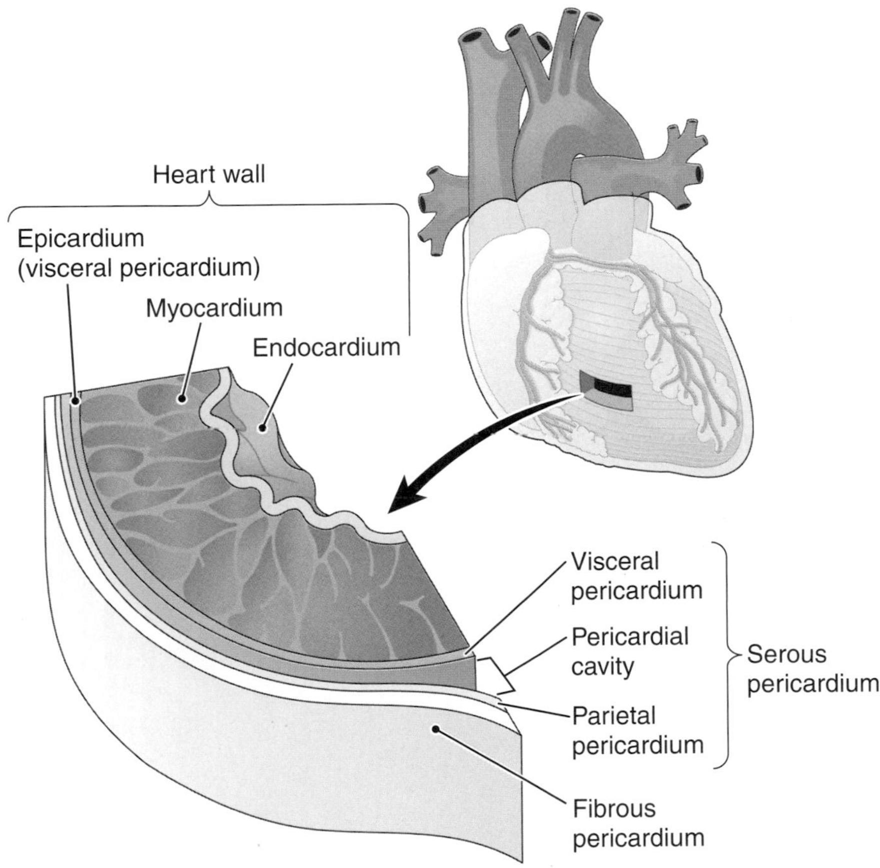

Figure 14-2 **Layers of the heart wall and pericardium.** The serous pericardium covers the heart and lines the fibrous pericardium. *ZOOMING IN ✦ Which layer of the heart wall is the thickest?*

Table 14•2 Layers of the Pericardium

LAYER	LOCATION	DESCRIPTION	FUNCTION
Fibrous pericardium	Outermost layer	Fibrous sac	Encloses and protects the heart; anchors heart to surrounding structures
Serous pericardium	Between the fibrous pericardium and the myocardium	Doubled membranous sac with fluid between layers	Fluid reduces friction within the pericardium as the heart functions
Parietal layer	Lines the fibrous pericardium	Serous membrane	Forms the outer layer of the serous pericardium
Visceral layer	Surface of the heart	Serous membrane	Forms the inner layer of the serous pericardium; also called the epicardium

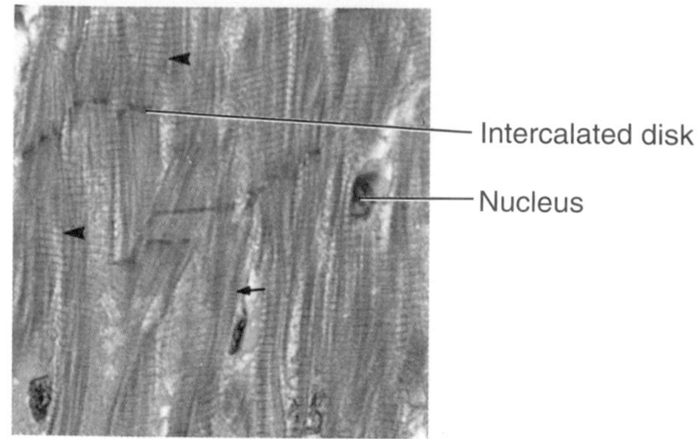

Figure 14-3 Cardiac muscle tissue viewed under the microscope (×540). The sample shows light striations (arrowheads), intercalated disks, and branching fibers (arrow). (Reprinted with permission from Gartner LP, Hiatt JL. Color Atlas of Histology. 3rd ed. Philadelphia: Lippincott Williams & Wilkins, 2000.)

Special Features of the Myocardium

Cardiac muscle cells are lightly striated (striped) based on alternating actin and myosin filaments, as seen in skeletal muscle cells (see Chapter 8). Unlike skeletal muscle cells, however, cardiac muscle cells have a single nucleus instead of multiple nuclei. Also, cardiac muscle tissue is involuntarily controlled. There are specialized partitions between cardiac muscle cells that show faintly under a microscope (Fig. 14-3). These **intercalated** (in-TER-cah-la-ted) **disks** are actually modified plasma membranes that firmly attach adjacent cells to each other but allow for rapid transfer of electrical impulses between them. The adjective *intercalated* is from Latin and means "inserted between."

Another feature of cardiac muscle tissue is the branching of the muscle fibers (cells). These fibers are interwoven so that the stimulation that causes the contraction of one fiber results in the contraction of a whole group. The intercalated disks and the branching cellular networks allow cardiac muscle cells to contract in a coordinated manner.

Divisions of the Heart

Healthcare professionals often refer to the *right heart* and the *left heart*, because the human heart is really a double pump (Fig. 14-4). The right side pumps blood low in oxygen to the lungs through the **pulmonary circuit**. The left side pumps oxygenated blood to the remainder of the body through the **systemic circuit**. Each side of the heart is divided into two chambers.

Four Chambers The upper chambers on the right and left sides, the **atria** (A-tre-ah), are mainly blood-receiving chambers (Fig. 14-5, Table 14-3). The lower chambers on the right and left side, the **ventricles** (VEN-trih-klz) are forceful pumps. The chambers, listed in the order in which blood flows through them, are as follows:

1. The **right atrium** (A-tre-um) is a thin-walled chamber that receives the blood returning from the body tissues. This blood, which is low in oxygen, is carried in veins, the blood vessels leading back to the heart from the body tissues. The superior vena cava brings blood

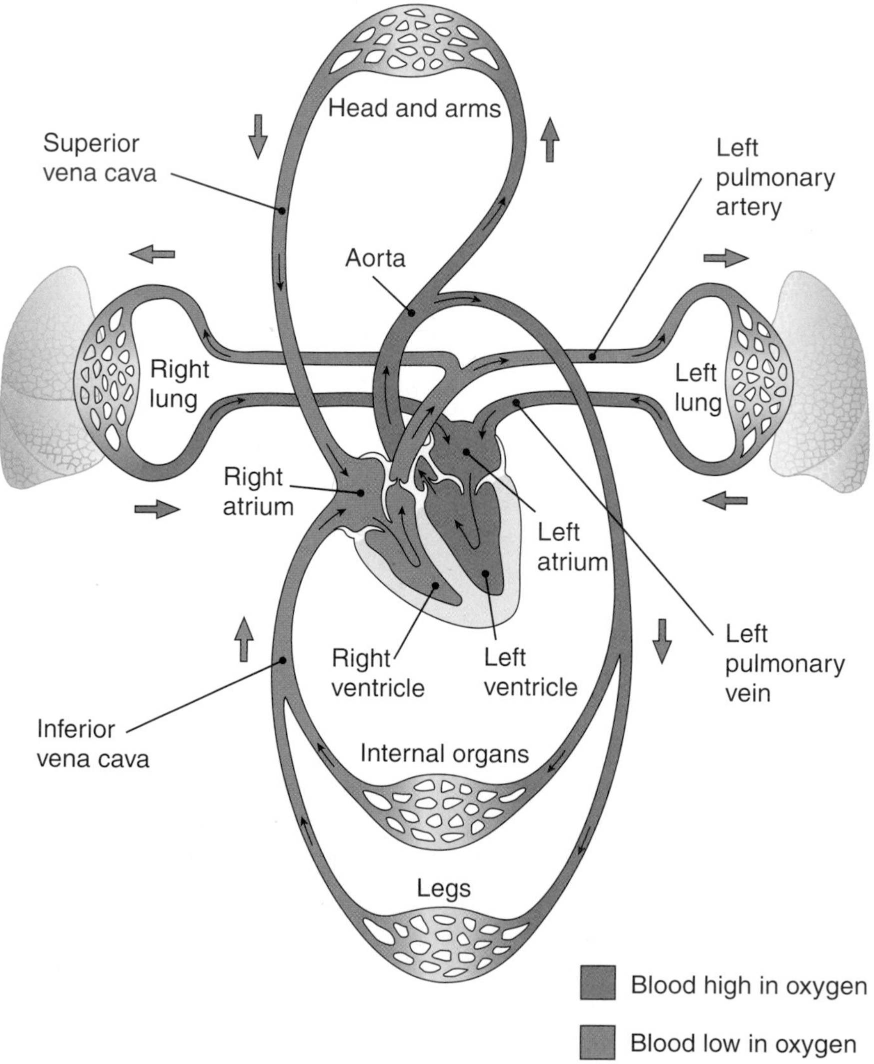

Figure 14-4 The heart as a double pump. The right side of the heart pumps blood through the pulmonary circuit to the lungs to be oxygenated; the left side of the heart pumps blood through the systemic circuit to all other parts of the body. *ZOOMING IN ✦ What vessel carries blood into the systemic circuit?*

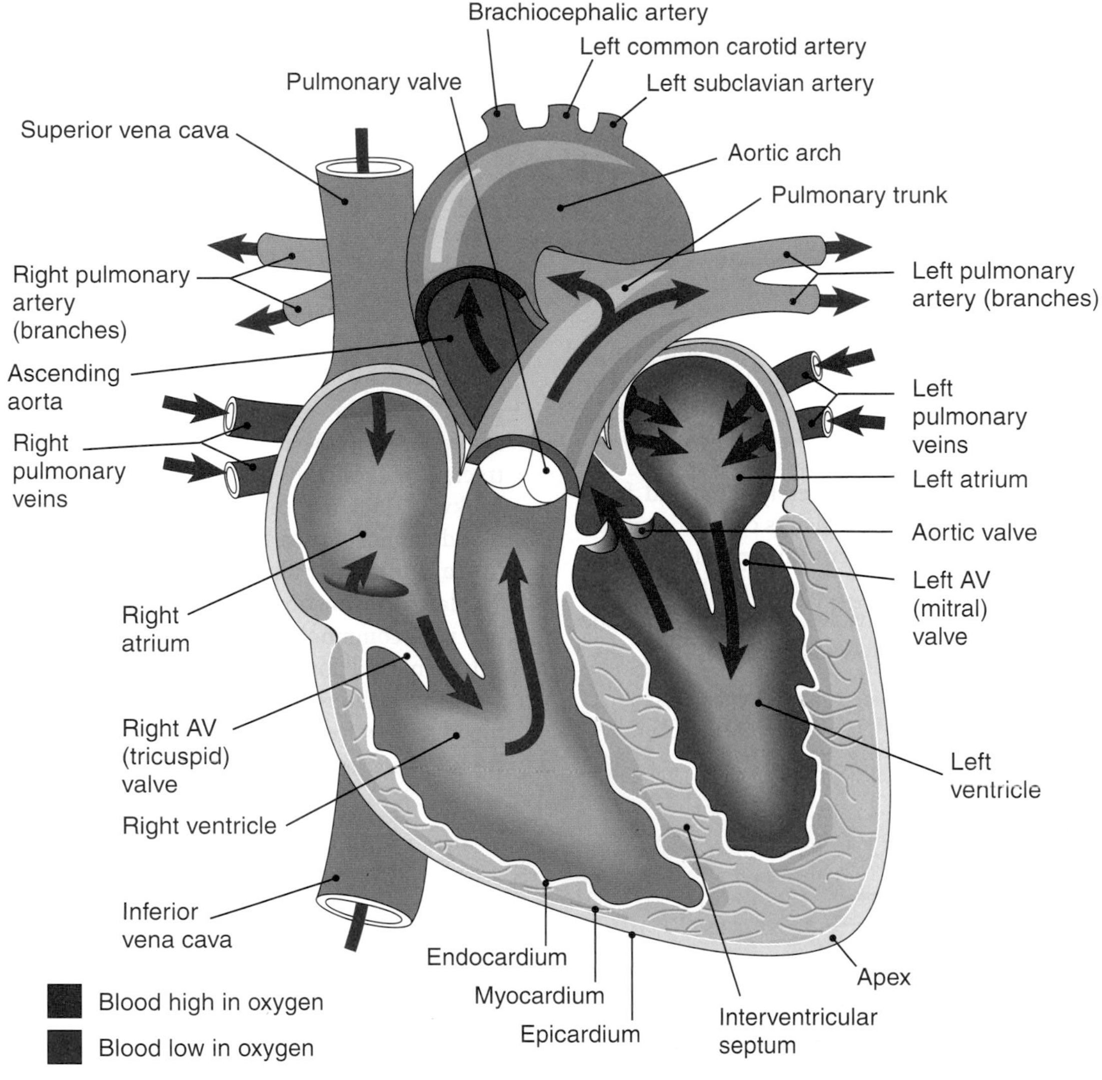

Figure 14-5 **The heart and great vessels.** *ZOOMING IN ✦ Which heart chamber has the thickest wall?*

from the head, chest, and arms; the inferior vena cava delivers blood from the trunk and legs. A third vessel that opens into the right atrium brings blood from the heart muscle itself, as described later in this chapter.

2. The **right ventricle** pumps the venous blood received from the right atrium to the lungs. It pumps into a large pulmonary trunk, which then divides into right and left pulmonary arteries, which branch to the lungs. An artery is a vessel that takes blood from the heart to the tissues. Note that the pulmonary arteries

Table 14•3 Chambers of the Heart

CHAMBER	LOCATION	FUNCTION
Right atrium	Upper right chamber	Receives blood from the vena cavae and the coronary sinus; pumps blood into the right ventricle
Right ventricle	Lower right chamber	Receives blood from the right atrium and pumps blood into the pulmonary artery, which carries blood to the lungs to be oxygenated
Left atrium	Upper left chamber	Receives oxygenated blood coming back to the heart from the lungs in the pulmonary veins; pumps blood into the left ventricle
Left ventricle	Lower left chamber	Receives blood from the left atrium and pumps blood into the aorta to be carried to tissues in the systemic circuit

passes through the heart twice in making a trip from the heart's right side through the pulmonary circuit to the lungs and back to the heart's left side to start on its way through the systemic circuit. Although Figure 14-7 follows the path of a single drop of blood in sequence through the heart, the heart's two sides function in unison to pump blood through both circuits at the same time.

Checkpoint 14-4 What is the purpose of valves in the heart?

Blood Supply to the Myocardium

Only the endocardium comes into contact with the blood that flows through the heart chambers. Therefore, the myocardium must have its own blood vessels to provide oxygen and nourishment and to remove waste products. Together, these blood vessels provide the **coronary** (KOR-o-na-re) **circulation**. The main arteries that supply blood to the muscle of the heart are the right and left coronary arteries (Fig. 14-8), named because they encircle the heart like a crown. These arteries, which are the first to branch off the aorta, arise just above the cusps of the aortic valve and branch to all regions of the heart muscle. They receive blood when the heart relaxes because the aortic valve must be closed to expose the entrance to these vessels (Fig. 14-9). After passing through capillaries in the myocardium, blood drains into a system of cardiac veins that brings blood back toward the right atrium. Blood finally collects in the **coronary sinus**, a dilated vein that opens into the right atrium near the inferior vena cava (see Fig. 14-8).

Checkpoint 14-5 The myocardium must have its own vascular system to supply it with blood. What name is given to this blood supply to the myocardium?

Function of the Heart

Although the heart's right and left sides are separated from each other, they work together. Blood is squeezed through the chambers by a heart muscle contraction that begins in the thin-walled upper chambers, the atria, and is followed by a contraction of the thick muscle of the lower chambers, the ventricles. This active phase is called **systole** (SIS-to-le), and in each case, it is followed by a resting period known as **diastole** (di-AS-to-le). One complete sequence of heart contraction and relaxation is called the **cardiac cycle** (Fig. 14-10). Each cardiac cycle represents a single heartbeat. At rest, one cycle takes an average of 0.8 seconds.

The contraction phase of the cardiac cycle begins with contraction of both atria, which forces blood through the AV valves into the ventricles. The atrial walls are thin, and their contractions are not very powerful. However, they do improve the heart's efficiency by forcing blood into the ventricles before these lower chambers contract. Atrial contraction is completed at the time ventricular contraction begins. Thus, a resting phase (diastole) begins in the atria at the same time that a contraction (systole) begins in the ventricles.

After the ventricles have contracted, all chambers are relaxed for a short period as they fill with blood. Then another cycle begins with an atrial contraction followed by a ventricular contraction. Although both upper and lower chambers

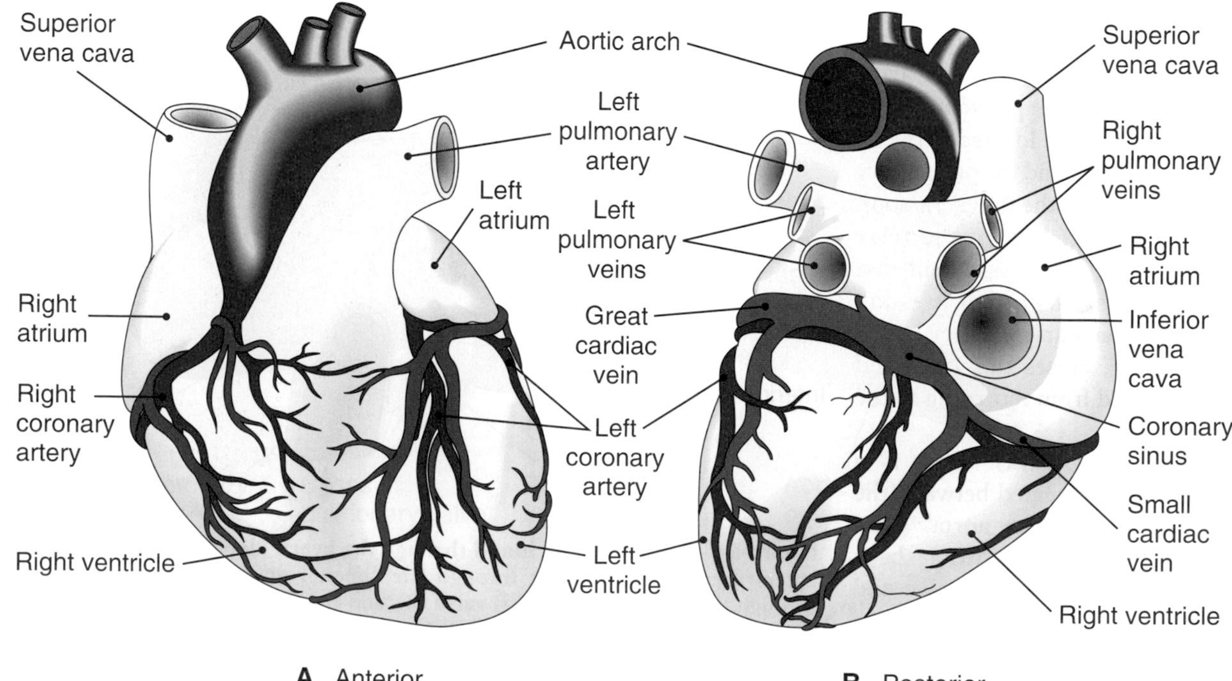

Figure 14-8 Blood vessels that supply the myocardium. Coronary arteries and cardiac veins are shown. **(A)** Anterior view. **(B)** Posterior view.

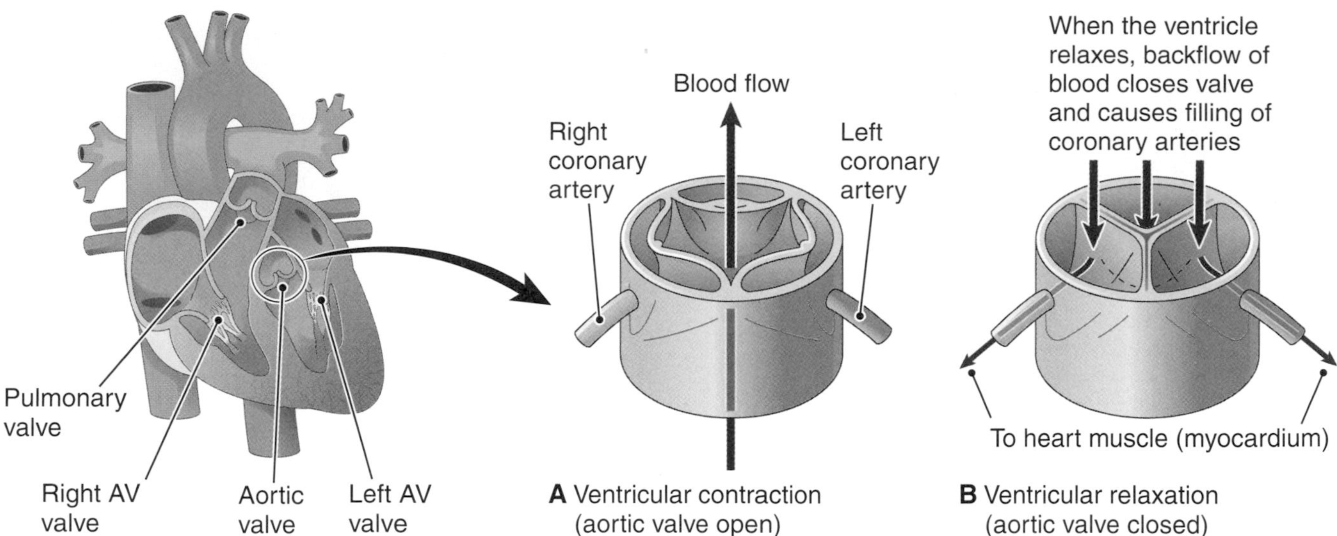

Figure 14-9 **Opening of coronary arteries in the aortic valve (anterior view). (A)** When the left ventricle contracts, the aortic valve opens. The valve cusps prevent filling of the coronary arteries. **(B)** When the left ventricle relaxes, backflow of blood closes the aortic valve and the coronary arteries fill. (Modified with permission from Moore KL, Dalley AF. Clinically Oriented Anatomy. 4th ed. Baltimore: Lippincott Williams & Wilkins, 1999.)

have a systolic and diastolic phase in each cardiac cycle, discussions of heart function usually refer to these phases as they occur in the ventricles, because these chambers contract more forcefully and drive blood into the arteries.

Cardiac Output

A unique property of heart muscle is its ability to adjust the strength of contraction to the amount of blood received. When the heart chamber is filled and the wall stretched (within limits), the contraction is strong. As less blood enters the heart, contractions become less forceful. Thus, as more blood enters the heart, as occurs during exercise, the muscle contracts with greater strength to push the larger volume of blood out into the blood vessels (see Box 14-1, Cardiac Reserve).

The volume of blood pumped by each ventricle in 1 minute is termed the **cardiac output** (CO). It is the product of the **stroke volume** (SV)—the volume of blood ejected from the ventricle with each beat—and the **heart rate** (HR)—the number of times the heart beats per minute. To summarize:

$$CO = HR \times SV$$

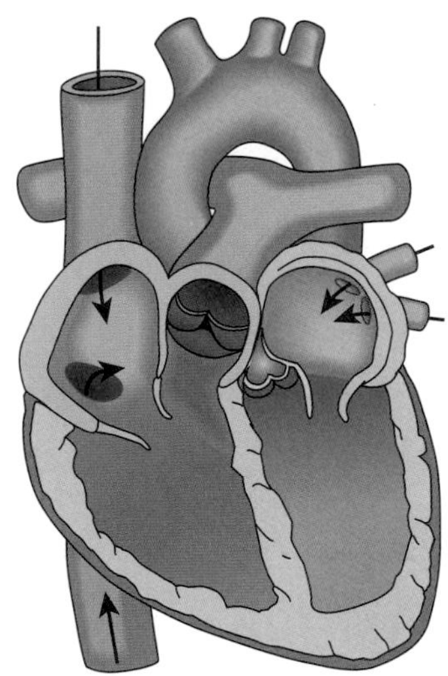

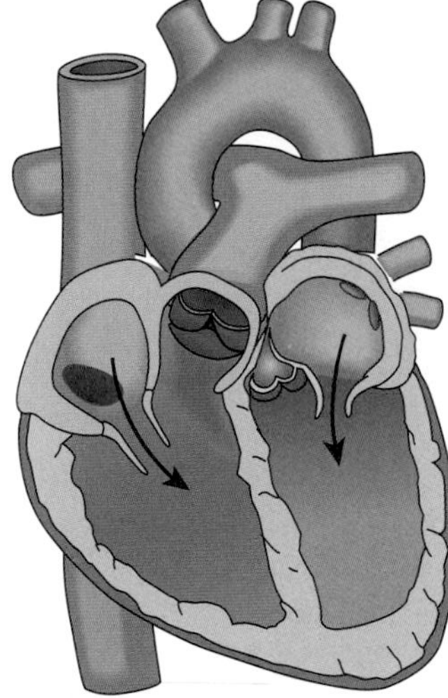

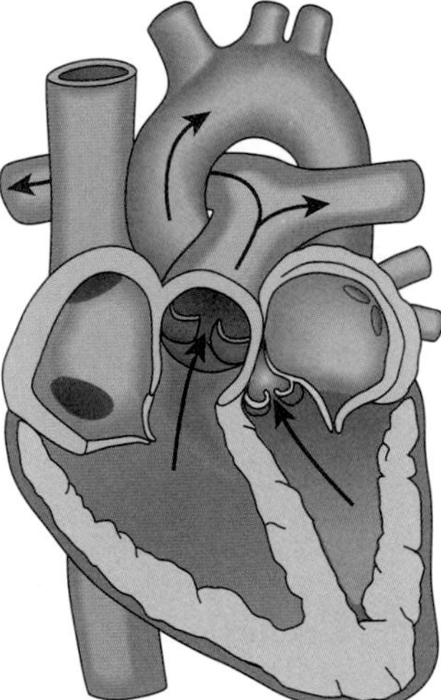

Diastole
Atria fill with blood, which begins to flow into ventricles as soon as their walls relax.

Atrial systole
Contraction of atria pumps blood into the ventricles.

Ventricular systole
Contraction of ventricles pumps blood into aorta and pulmonary arteries.

Figure 14-10 **The cardiac cycle.** *ZOOMING IN ✦ When the ventricles contract, what valves close? What valves open?*

Box 14-1 A Closer Look

Cardiac Reserve: Extra Output When Needed

Like many other organs, the heart has great reserves of strength. The cardiac reserve is a measure of how many times more than average the heart can produce when needed. Based on a heart rate of 75 beats/minute and a stroke volume of 70 ml/beat, the average cardiac output for an adult at rest is about 5 L/minute. This means that at rest, the heart pumps the equivalent of the total blood volume each minute.

During mild exercise, this volume might double and even double again during strenuous exercise. For most people the cardiac reserve is 4 to 5 times the resting output. This increase in cardiac output is achieved by an increase in either stroke volume, heart rate, or both. In athletes exercising vigorously, the ratio may reach 6 to 7 times. In contrast, those with heart disease may have little or no cardiac reserve. They may be fine at rest but quickly become short of breath or fatigued when exercising or even when carrying out the simple tasks of daily living.

Cardiac reserve can be measured using an exercise stress test that measures cardiac output while the patient walks on a treadmill or pedals an exercise bicycle. The exercise becomes more and more strenuous until the patient's peak cardiac output (cardiac reserve) is reached.

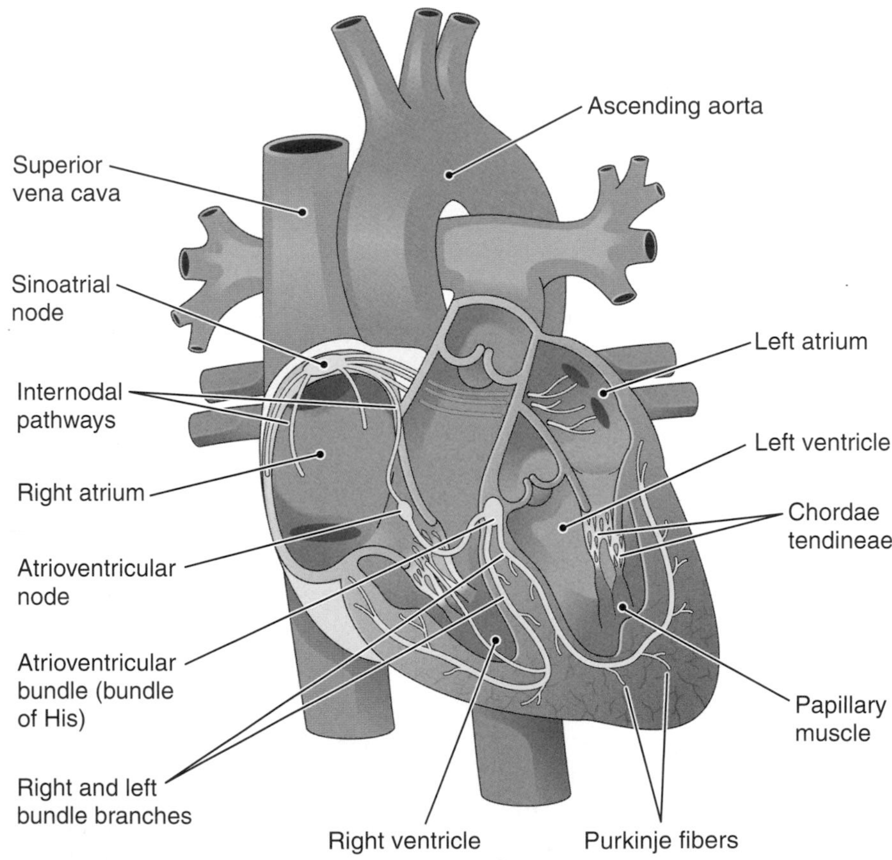

Figure 14-11 Conduction system of the heart. The sinoatrial (SA) node, the atrioventricular (AV) node, and specialized fibers conduct the electrical energy that stimulates the heart muscle to contract. *ZOOMING IN ✦ What parts of the conduction system do the internodal pathways connect?*

Checkpoint 14-6 The cardiac cycle consists of an alternating pattern of contraction and relaxation. What name is given to the contraction phase? To the relaxation phase?

Checkpoint 14-7 Cardiac output is the amount of blood pumped by each ventricle in 1 minute. What two factors determine cardiac output?

The Heart's Conduction System

Like other muscles, the heart muscle is stimulated to contract by a wave of electrical energy that passes along the cells. This action potential is generated by specialized tissue within the heart and spreads over structures that form the heart's conduction system (Fig. 14-11). Two of these structures are tissue masses called **nodes**, and the remainder consists of specialized fibers that branch through the myocardium.

The **sinoatrial** (SA) node is located in the upper wall of the right atrium in a small depression described as a sinus. This node initiates the heartbeats by generating an action potential at regular intervals. Because the SA node sets the rate of heart contractions, it is commonly called the **pacemaker**. The second node, located in the interatrial septum at the bottom of the right atrium, is called the **atrioventricular** (AV) node.

The **atrioventricular bundle**, also known as the **bundle of His**, is located at the top of the interventricular septum. It has branches that extend to all parts of the ventricular walls. Fibers travel first down both sides of the interventricular septum in groups called the right and left bundle branches. Smaller **Purkinje** (pur-KIN-je) **fibers**, also called *conduction myofibers*, then travel in a branching network throughout the myocardium of the ventricles. Intercalated disks allow the rapid flow of impulses throughout the heart muscle.

The Conduction Pathway The order in which impulses travel through the heart is as follows:

1. The sinoatrial node generates the electrical impulse that begins the heartbeat (see Fig. 14-11).
2. The excitation wave travels throughout the muscle of each atrium, causing the atria to contract. At the same time, impulses also travel directly to the AV node by means of fibers in the wall of the atrium that make up the **internodal pathways**.
3. The atrioventricular node is stimulated. A relatively slower rate of conduction through the AV node allows time for the atria to contract and complete the filling of the ventricles before the ventricles contract.
4. The excitation wave travels rapidly through the bundle of His and then throughout the ventricular walls by means of the bundle branches and Purkinje fibers. The entire ventricular musculature contracts almost at the same time.

A normal heart rhythm originating at the SA node is termed a **sinus rhythm**. As a safety measure, a region of the conduction system other than the sinoatrial node can generate a heartbeat if the sinoatrial node fails, but it does so at a slower rate.

Checkpoint 14-8 The heartbeat is started by a small mass of tissue in the upper right atrium. This structure is commonly called the pacemaker, but what is its scientific name?

Control of the Heart Rate

Although the heart's fundamental beat originates within the heart itself, the heart rate can be influenced by the nervous system, hormones and other factors in the internal environment.

The autonomic nervous system (ANS) plays a major role in modifying the heart rate according to need (Fig. 14-12). Sympathetic nervous system stimulation increases the heart rate. During a fight-or-flight response, the sympathetic nerves can boost the cardiac output two to three times the resting value. Sympathetic fibers increase the contraction rate by stimulating the SA and AV nodes. They also increase the contraction force by acting directly on the fibers of the myocardium. These actions translate into increased cardiac output. Parasympathetic stimulation decreases the heart rate to restore homeostasis. The parasympathetic nerve that supplies the heart is the vagus nerve (cranial nerve X). It slows the heart rate by acting on the SA and AV nodes.

These ANS influences allow the heart to meet changing needs rapidly. The heart rate is also affected by substances circulating in the blood, including hormones, ions, and drugs. Regular exercise strengthens the heart and increases the amount of blood ejected with each beat. Consequently, the circulatory needs of the body at rest can be met with a lower heart rate. Trained athletes usually have a low resting heart rate.

Variations in Heart Rates

- **Bradycardia** (brad-e-KAR-de-ah) is a relatively slow heart rate of less than 60 beats/ minute. During rest and sleep, the heart may beat less than 60 beats/minute, but the rate usually does not fall below 50 beats/minute.
- **Tachycardia** (tak-e-KAR-de-ah) refers to a heart rate of more than 100 beats/minute. Tachycardia is normal during exercise or stress but may also occur under abnormal conditions.
- **Sinus arrhythmia** (ah-RITH-me-ah) is a regular variation in heart rate caused by changes in the rate and depth of breathing. It is a normal phenomenon.
- **Premature beat**, also called *extrasystole*, is a beat that comes before the expected normal beat. In healthy people, they may be initiated by caffeine, nicotine, or psychological stresses. They are also common in people with heart disease.

Heart Sounds

The normal heart sounds are usually described by the syllables "lubb" and "dupp." The first, "lubb," is a longer,

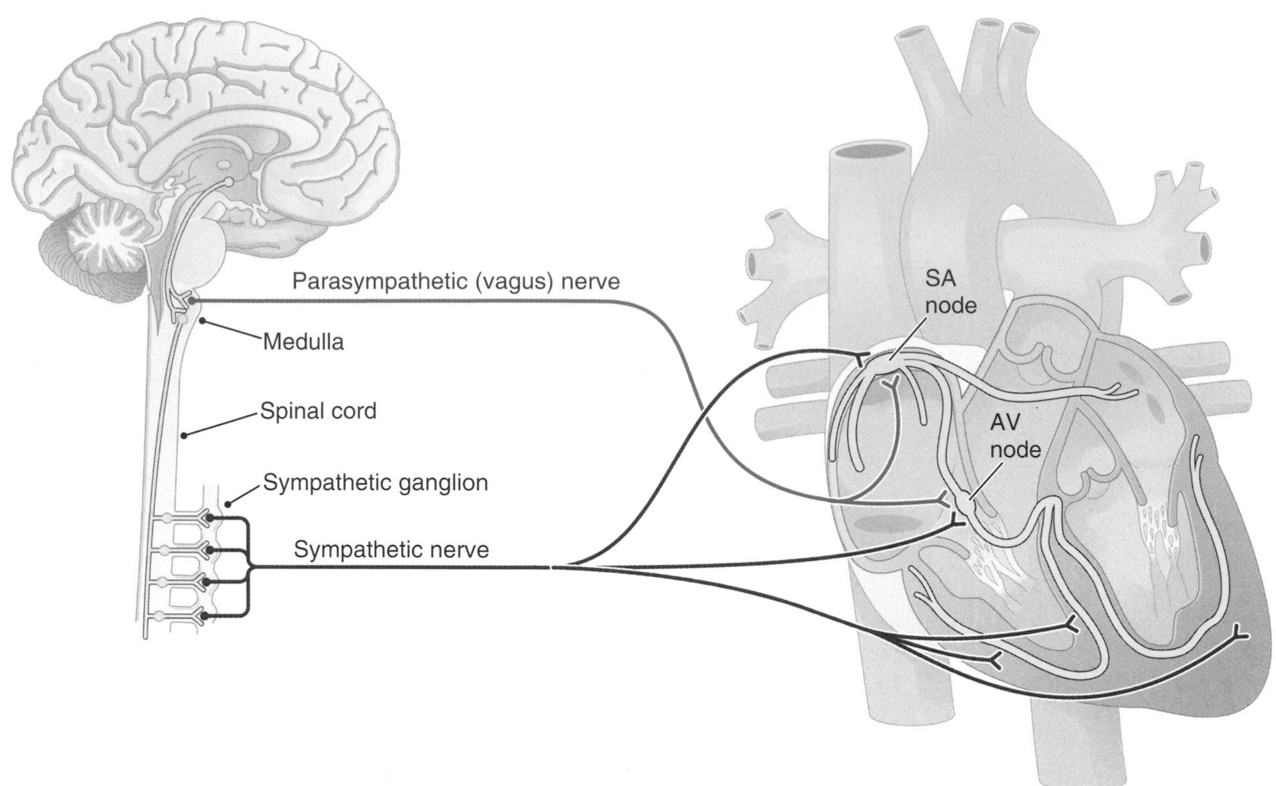

Figure 14-12 **Autonomic nervous system regulation of the heart.** The ANS affects the rate and force of heart contractions. *ZOOMING IN ✦ What parts of the conduction system does the autonomic nervous system affect?*

lower-pitched sound that occurs at the start of ventricular systole. It is probably caused by a combination of events, mainly closure of the atrioventricular valves. This action causes vibrations in the blood passing through the valves and in the tissue surrounding the valves. The second, or "dupp," sound is shorter and sharper. It occurs at the beginning of ventricular relaxation and is caused largely by sudden closure of the semilunar valves.

Murmurs An abnormal sound is called a **murmur** and is usually due to faulty action of a valve. For example, if a valve fails to close tightly and blood leaks back, a murmur is heard. Another condition giving rise to an abnormal sound is the narrowing (stenosis) of a valve opening.

The many conditions that can cause abnormal heart sounds include congenital (birth) defects, disease, and physiologic variations. An abnormal sound caused by any structural change in the heart or the vessels connected with the heart is called an **organic murmur.** Certain normal sounds heard while the heart is working may also be described as murmurs, such as the sound heard during rapid filling of the ventricles. To differentiate these from abnormal sounds, they are more properly called **functional murmurs.**

Checkpoint 14-9 What system exerts the main influence on the rate and strength of heart contractions?

Checkpoint 14-10 What is a heart murmur?

Heart Disease

Diseases of the heart and circulatory system are the most common causes of death in industrialized countries. Few people escape having some damage to the heart and blood vessels in a lifetime.

Classifications of Heart Disease

There are many ways of classifying heart disease. The heart's anatomy forms the basis for one grouping of heart pathology:

- **Endocarditis** (en-do-kar-DI-tis) means "inflammation of the lining of the heart." Endocarditis may involve the lining of the chambers, but the term most commonly refers to inflammation of the endocardium on the valves and valvular disease.
- **Myocarditis** (mi-o-kar-DI-tis) is inflammation of heart muscle.
- **Pericarditis** (per-ih-kar-DI-tis) refers to inflammation of the serous membrane on the heart surface as well as that lining the pericardial sac.

These inflammatory diseases are often caused by infection, but may also be secondary to other types of respiratory or systemic diseases.

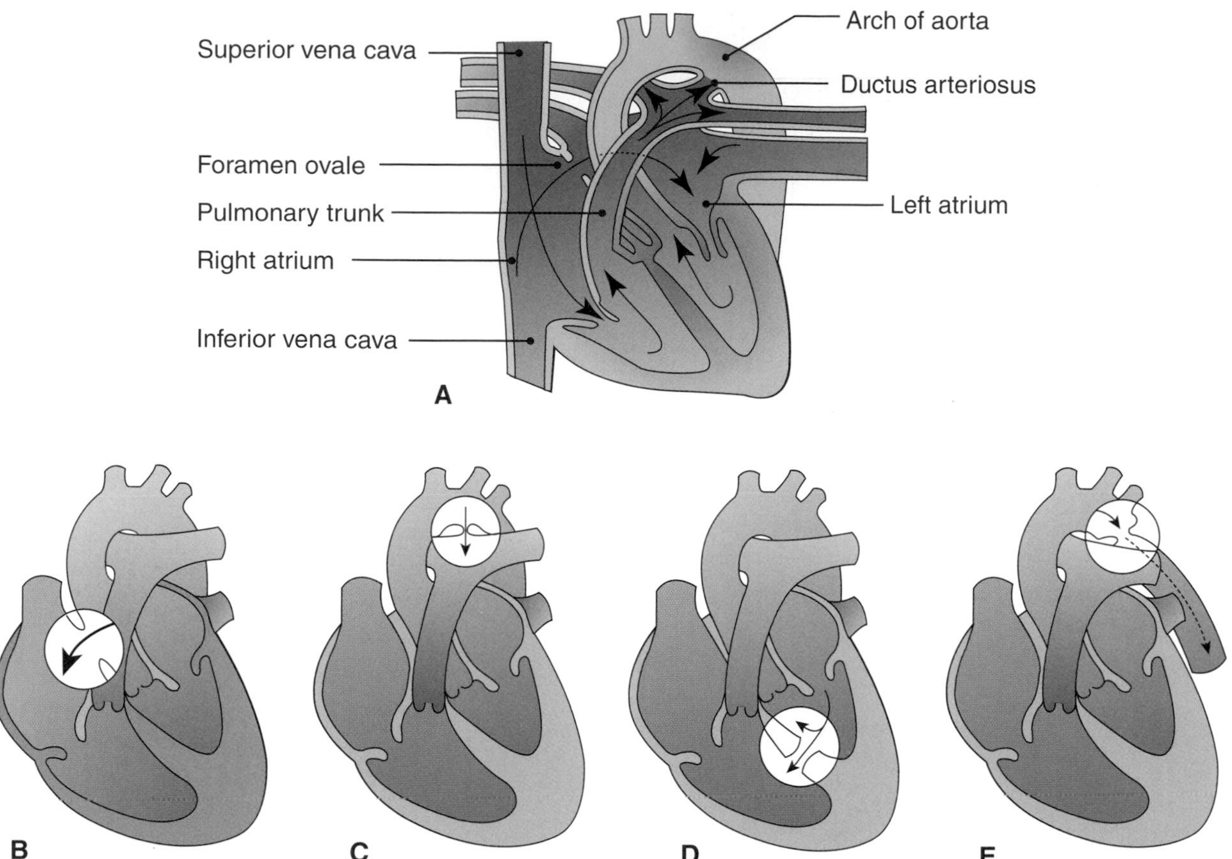

Figure 14-13 **Congenital heart defects. (A)** Normal fetal heart showing the foramen ovale and ductus arteriosus. **(B)** Persistence of the foramen ovale results in an atrial septal defect. **(C)** Persistence of the ductus arteriosus (patent ductus arteriosus) forces blood back into the pulmonary artery. **(D)** A ventricular septal defect. **(E)** Coarctation of the aorta restricts outward blood flow in the aorta. (Reprinted with permission from Porth CM. Pathophysiology. 7th ed. Philadelphia: Lippincott Williams & Wilkins, 2004.)

Another classification of heart disease is based on causative factors:

- **Congenital heart disease** is a condition present at birth.
- **Rheumatic** (ru-MAT-ik) **heart disease** originates with an attack of rheumatic fever in childhood or in youth.
- **Coronary artery disease** involves the walls of the blood vessels that supply the heart muscle.
- **Heart failure** is caused by deterioration of the heart tissues and is frequently the result of long-standing disorders, such as high blood pressure.

Congenital Heart Disease

Congenital heart diseases often are the result of defects in fetal development. Two of these disorders represent the abnormal persistence of structures that are part of the normal fetal circulation (Fig. 14-13 A). Because the lungs are not used until a child is born, the fetus has some adaptations that allow blood to bypass the lungs. The fetal heart has a small hole, the foramen ovale (for-A-men o-VAL-e), in the septum between the right and left atria. This opening allows some blood to flow directly from the right atrium into the left atrium, thus bypassing the lungs. Failure of the foramen ovale to close is one cause of an abnormal opening known as an **atrial septal defect** (see Fig. 14-13 B).

The ductus arteriosus (ar-te-re-O-sus) in the fetus is a small blood vessel that connects the pulmonary artery and the aorta so that some blood headed toward the lungs will enter the aorta instead. The ductus arteriosus normally closes on its own once the lungs are in use. Persistence of the vessel after birth is described as **patent** (open) **ductus arteriosus** (see Fig. 14-13 C).

The most common single congenital heart defect is a hole in the septum between the two ventricles, a disorder known as **ventricular septal defect** (see Fig. 14-13 D).

In each of the above defects, part of the heart's left side output goes back to the lungs instead of out to the body. A small defect remaining from the foramen ovale or a small patent ductus may cause no difficulty and is often not diagnosed until an adult is examined for other cardiac problems. More serious defects greatly increase the left ventricle's work and may lead to heart failure. In addition, ventricular septal defect creates high blood pressure in the lungs, which damages lung tissue.

Other congenital defects that tax the heart involve restriction of outward blood flow. **Coarctation** (ko-ark-TA-shun) **of the aorta** is a localized narrowing of the aortic arch (see Fig. 14-13 E). Another example is obstruction or narrowing of the pulmonary trunk that prevents blood from passing in sufficient quantity from the right ventricle to the lungs.

In many cases, several congenital heart defects occur together. The most common combination is that of four specific defects known as the **tetralogy of Fallot**. So-called "blue babies" commonly have this disorder. The blueness, or **cyanosis** (si-ah-NO-sis), of the skin and mucous membranes is caused by a relative lack of oxygen. (See Chap. 18 for other causes of cyanosis.)

In recent years, it has become possible to remedy many congenital defects by heart surgery, one of the more spectacular advances in modern medicine. A patent ductus arteriosus may also respond to drug treatment. During fetal life, prostaglandins (hormones) keep the ductus arteriosus open. Drugs that inhibit prostaglandins can promote closing of the duct after birth.

Checkpoint 14-11 What is congenital heart disease?

Rheumatic Heart Disease

A certain type of streptococcal infection, the type that causes "strep throat," is indirectly responsible for rheumatic fever and rheumatic heart disease. The toxin produced by these streptococci causes a normal immune response. However, in some cases, the initial infection may be followed some 2 to 4 weeks later by rheumatic fever, a generalized inflammatory disorder with marked swelling of the joints. The antibodies formed to combat the toxin are believed to cause this disease. These antibodies may also attack the heart valves, producing a condition known as *rheumatic endocarditis*. The heart valves, particularly the mitral valve, become inflamed, and the normally flexible valve cusps thicken and harden. The mitral valve may not open sufficiently (mitral stenosis) to allow enough blood into the ventricle or may not close effectively, allowing blood to return to the left atrium (mitral regurgitation). Either condition interferes with blood flow from the left atrium into the left ventricle, causing pulmonary congestion, an important characteristic of mitral heart disease. The incidence of rheumatic heart disease has declined with antibiotic treatment of streptococcal infections. However, children who do not receive adequate diagnosis and treatment are subject to developing the disease.

Checkpoint 14-12 What types of organisms cause rheumatic fever?

Coronary Artery Disease

Like vessels elsewhere in the body, the coronary arteries that supply the heart muscle, can undergo degenerative changes with time. The lumen (space) inside the vessel may gradually narrow because of a progressive deposit of fatty material known as **plaque** (PLAK) in the lining of the vessels, usually the arteries. This process, called **atherosclerosis** (ath-er-o-skleh-RO-sis), causes thickening and hardening of the vessels with a loss of elasticity (Fig. 14-14). The *athero* part of the name means "gruel," because of the porridge-like material that adheres to the vessel walls. The vessels' narrowing leads to **ischemia** (is-KE-me-ah), a lack of blood supply to the areas fed by those arteries. Degenerative changes in the arterial wall also may cause the inside vascular surface to become roughened, promoting blood clot (thrombus) formation. (see Fig. 14-14 C).

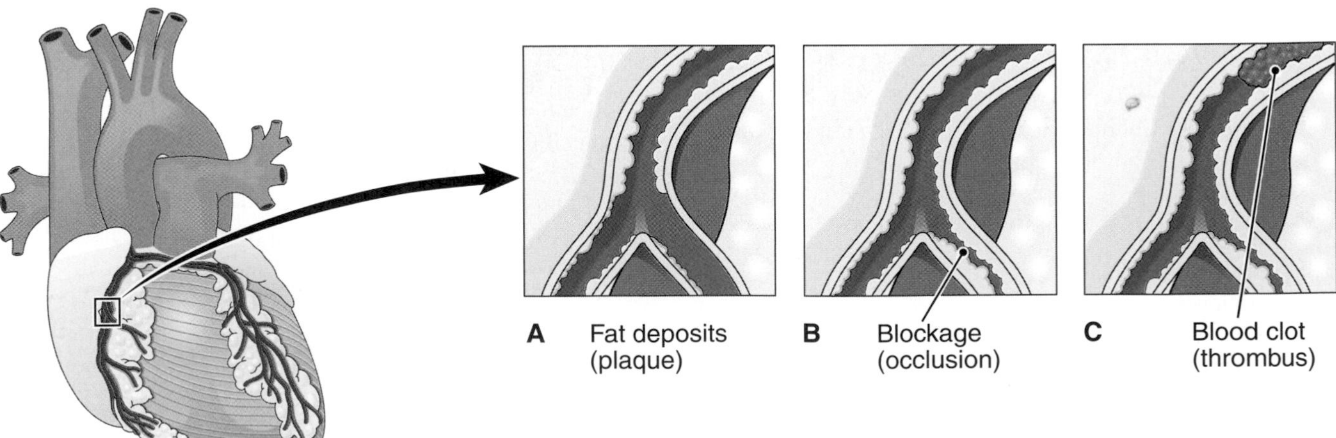

Figure 14-14 Coronary atherosclerosis. (A) Fat deposits (plaque) narrow an artery, leading to ischemia (lack of blood supply). **(B)** Plaque causes blockage (occlusion) of a vessel. **(C)** Formation of a blood clot (thrombus) in a vessel leads to myocardial infarction (MI).

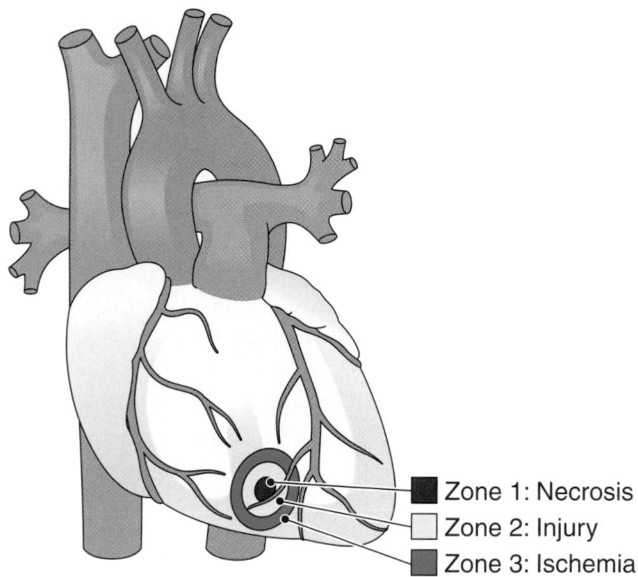

Figure 14-15 **Myocardial infarction (MI).** (Reprinted with permission from Cohen BJ. Medical Terminology. 4th ed. Philadelphia: Lippincott Williams & Wilkins, 2004.)

Myocardial Infarction In the heart, thrombus formation results in a life-threatening condition known as **coronary thrombosis**. Sudden **occlusion** (ok-LU-zhun), or closure, of a coronary vessel with complete obstruction of blood flow is commonly known as a *heart attack*. Because the area of tissue damaged in a heart attack is described as an **infarct** (IN-farkt), the medical term for a heart attack is **myocardial infarction** (MI) (Fig. 14-15). The oxygen-deprived tissue will eventually undergo necrosis (death). The symptoms of MI commonly include the abrupt onset of severe, constricting chest pain that may radiate to the left arm, back, neck or jaw. Patients may experience shortness of breath, sweating, nausea, vomiting, or pain in the epigastric region, which can be mistaken for indigestion. They may feel weak, restless, or anxious and the skin may be pale, cool and moist.

The outcome of a myocardial infarction depends largely on the extent and location of the damage. Many people die within the first hour after onset of symptoms, but prompt, aggressive treatment can improve outcomes. Medical personnel make immediate efforts to relieve chest pain, stabilize the heart rhythm, and reopen the blocked vessel. Complete and prolonged lack of blood to any part of the myocardium results in tissue necrosis and weakening of the heart wall.

Angina Pectoris Inadequate blood flow to the heart muscle causes a characteristic discomfort, called **angina pectoris** (an-JI-nah PEK-to-ris), felt in the region of the heart and in the left arm and shoulder. Angina pectoris may be accompanied by a feeling of suffocation and a general sensation of forthcoming doom. Coronary artery disease is a common cause of angina pectoris, although the condition has other causes as well.

Abnormalities of Heart Rhythm Coronary artery disease or myocardial infarction often results in an abnormal rhythm of the heartbeat, or **arrhythmia** (ah-RITH-me-ah). Extremely rapid but coordinated contractions, numbering up to 300 per minute, are described as **flutter**. An episode of rapid, wild, and uncoordinated heart muscle contractions is called **fibrillation** (fih-brih-LA-shun), which may involve the atria only or both the atria and the ventricles. Ventricular fibrillation is a serious disorder because there is no effective heartbeat. It must be corrected by a **defibrillator**, a device that generates a strong electrical current to discharge all the cardiac muscle cells at once, allowing a normal rhythm to resume.

An interruption of electric impulses in the heart's conduction system is called **heart block**. The seriousness of this condition depends on how completely the impulses are blocked. It may result in independent beating of the chambers if the ventricles respond to a second pacemaker.

Treatment of Heart Attacks The death rate for heart attacks is high when treatment is delayed. Initial treatment involves cardiopulmonary resuscitation (CPR) and defibrillation at the scene when needed. The American Heart Association is adding training in the use of the **automated external defibrillator** (AED) to the basic course in CPR. The AED detects fatal arrhythmia and automatically delivers the correct preprogrammed shock. Work is underway to place machines in shopping centers, sports venues, and other public settings.

Prompt transport by paramedics who are able to monitor the heart and give emergency drugs helps people to survive and reach a hospital. The next step is to restore blood flow to the ischemic areas by administering **thrombolytic** (throm-bo-LIT-ik) **drugs**, which act to dissolve the clots blocking the coronary arteries. Therapy must be given promptly to prevent permanent heart muscle damage. In many cases, a pulmonary artery catheter (tube) is put in place to monitor cardiac function and response to medication.

Supportive care includes treatment of chest pain with intravenous (IV) morphine. Healthcare workers monitor heart rhythm and give medications to maintain a functional rhythm. Oxygen is given to improve heart muscle function. Some patients require surgery, such as angioplasty to reopen vessels or a vascular graft to bypass damaged vessels; others may need an artificial pacemaker to maintain a normal heart rhythm.

Recovery from a heart attack and resumption of a normal lifestyle is often possible if the patient follows his or her prescribed drug therapy plan and takes steps to reduce cardiac risk factors.

Checkpoint 14-13 Narrowing or blockage of the vessels that supply the heart muscle causes coronary artery disease. What degenerative process commonly causes narrowing of these vessels?

Heart Failure

Heart failure is a condition in which the heart is unable to pump sufficient blood to supply the tissues with oxygen and nutrients. The heart's chambers enlarge to contain more blood than the stretched fibers are able to pump. Blood backs up into the lungs, increasing blood pressure in the lungs. The ventricular muscles do not get enough blood, decreasing their ability to contract. Additional mechanisms cause the retention of fluid, leading to the name *congestive heart failure* (CHF). In an attempt to increase blood flow, the nervous system increases contraction of smooth muscle in the blood vessels, increasing blood pressure. Soon there is an accumulation of fluids in the lungs, liver, abdomen, and legs. People can live with compensated heart failure by attention to diet, drug therapy, and a balance of activity and rest.

The Heart in the Elderly

There is much individual variation in the way the heart ages, depending on heredity, environmental factors, diseases, and personal habits. However, some of the changes that may occur with age are as follows. The heart becomes smaller, and there is a decrease in the strength of heart muscle contraction. The valves become less flexible, and incomplete closure may produce an audible murmur. By 70 years of age, the cardiac output may decrease by as much as 35%. Damage within the conduction system can produce abnormal rhythms, including extra beats, rapid atrial beats, and slowing of ventricular rate. Temporary failure of the conduction system (heart block) can cause periodic loss of consciousness. Because of the decrease in the reserve strength of the heart, elderly people are often limited in their ability to respond to physical or emotional stress.

Prevention of Heart Disease

Prevention of heart ailments is based on identification of cardiovascular risk factors and modification of those factors that can be changed. Risk factors that cannot be modified include the following:

- Age. The risk of heart disease increases with age.
- Gender. Until middle age, men have greater risk than women. Women older than 50 years or past menopause have risk equal to that of males.
- Heredity. Those with immediate family members with heart disease are at greater risk.
- Body type, particularly the hereditary tendency to deposit fat in the abdomen or on the chest surface, increases risk.

Risk factors that can be changed include the following:

- Smoking, which leads to spasm and hardening of the arteries. These arterial changes result in decreased blood flow and poor supply of oxygen and nutrients to heart muscle.
- Physical inactivity. Lack of exercise weakens the heart muscle and decreases the efficiency of the heart. It also decreases the efficiency of the skeletal muscles, which further taxes the heart.
- Weight over the ideal increases risk.
- Saturated fat in the diet. Elevated fat levels in the blood lead to blockage of the coronary arteries by plaque (see Box 14-2, Lipoproteins).
- High blood pressure (hypertension) damages heart muscle.
- Diabetes and gout. Both diseases cause damage to small blood vessels.

Efforts to prevent heart disease should include having regular physical examinations and minimizing the controllable risk factors.

Box 14-2 **Clinical Perspectives**

Lipoproteins: What's the Big DL?

Although cholesterol has received a lot of bad press in recent years, it is a necessary substance in the body. It is found in bile salts needed for digestion of fats, in hormones, and in the plasma membrane of the cell. However, high levels of cholesterol in the blood have been associated with atherosclerosis and heart disease.

It now appears that the total amount of blood cholesterol is not as important as the form in which it occurs. Cholesterol is transported in the blood in combination with other lipids and with protein, forming compounds called lipoproteins. These compounds are distinguished by their relative density. High-density lipoprotein (HDL) is about one-half protein, whereas low-density lipoprotein (LDL) has a higher proportion of cholesterol and less protein. VLDLs, or very-low-density lipoproteins, are substances that are converted to LDLs.

LDLs carry cholesterol from the liver to the tissues, making it available for membrane or hormone synthesis. HDLs remove cholesterol from the tissues, such as the walls of the arteries, and carry it back to the liver for reuse or disposal. Thus, high levels of HDLs indicate efficient removal of arterial plaques, whereas high levels of LDLs suggest that arteries will become clogged.

Diet is an important factor in regulating lipoprotein levels. Saturated fatty acids (found primarily in animal fats) raise LDL levels, while unsaturated fatty acids (found in most vegetable oils) lower LDL levels and stimulate cholesterol excretion. Thus, a diet lower in saturated fat and higher in unsaturated fat may reduce the risk of atherosclerosis and heart disease. Other factors that affect lipoprotein levels include cigarette smoking, coffee drinking, and stress, which raise LDL levels, and exercise, which lowers LDL levels.

Heart Studies

Experienced listeners can gain much information about the heart using a **stethoscope** (STETH-o-skope). This relatively simple instrument is used to convey sounds from within the patient's body to an examiner's ear.

The **electrocardiograph** (**ECG** or **EKG**) is used to record electrical changes produced as the heart muscle contracts. (The abbreviation EKG comes from the German spelling of the word.) The ECG may reveal certain myocardial injuries. Electrodes (leads) placed on the skin surface pick up electrical activity, and the ECG tracing, or electrocardiogram, represents this activity as **waves.** The P wave represents the activity of the atria; the QRS and T waves represent the activity of the ventricles (Fig. 14-16). Changes in the waves and the intervals between them are used to diagnose heart damage and arrhythmias.

Many people with heart disease undergo **catheterization** (kath-eh-ter-i-ZA-shun). In right heart catheterization, an extremely thin tube (catheter) is passed through the veins of the right arm or right groin and then into the right side of heart. A **fluoroscope** (flu-OR-o-scope), an instrument for examining deep structures with x-rays, is used to show the route taken by the catheter. The tube is passed all the way through the pulmonary valve into the large lung arteries. Blood samples are obtained along the way for testing, and pressure readings are taken.

In left heart catheterization, a catheter is passed through an artery in the left groin or arm to the heart. Dye can then be injected into the coronary arteries to map damage to the vessels. The tube may also be passed through the aortic valve into the left ventricle for studies of pressure and volume in that chamber.

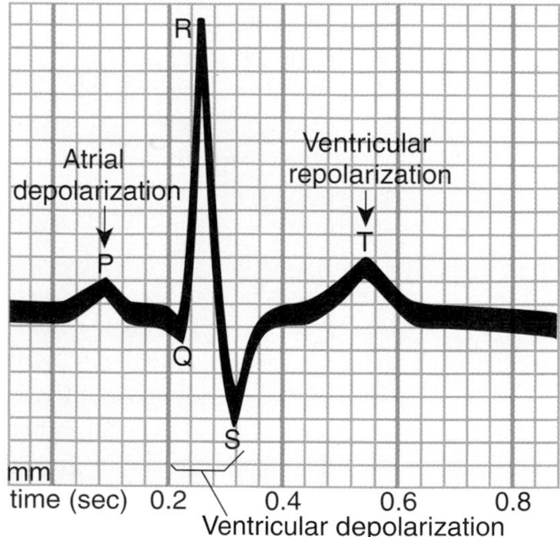

Figure 14-16 **Normal ECG tracing.** The tracing shows a single cardiac cycle. What is the length of the cardiac cycle shown in this diagram? *ZOOMING IN ✦ What is the length of the cardiac cycle shown in this diagram?*

Ultrasound consists of sound waves generated at a frequency above the range of sensitivity of the human ear. In **echocardiography** (ek-o-kar-de-OG-rah-fe), also known as *ultrasound cardiography,* high-frequency sound waves are sent to the heart from a small instrument on the surface of the chest. The ultrasound waves bounce off the heart and are recorded as they return, showing the heart in action. Movement of the echoes is traced on an electronic instrument called an *oscilloscope* and recorded on film. (The same principle is employed by submarines to detect ships.) The method is safe and painless, and it does not use x-rays. It provides information on the size and shape of heart structures, on cardiac function, and on possible heart defects.

Checkpoint 14-14 What do ECG and EKG stand for?

Treatment of Heart Disease

Heart specialists employ medical and surgical approaches to the treatment of heart disease, often in combination.

Medications

One of the oldest drugs for heart treatment, and still the most important drug for many patients, is **digitalis** (dij-ih-TAL-is). This agent, which slows and strengthens heart muscle contractions, is obtained from the leaf of the foxglove, a plant originally found growing wild in many parts of Europe. Foxglove is now cultivated to ensure a steady supply of digitalis for medical purposes.

Several forms of **nitroglycerin** are used to relieve angina pectoris. This drug dilates (widens) the vessels in the coronary circulation and improves the blood supply to the heart.

Beta-adrenergic blocking agents ("beta-blockers") control sympathetic stimulation of the heart. They reduce the rate and strength of heart contractions, thus reducing the heart's oxygen demand. Propanolol is one example.

Antiarrhythmic agents (*e.g.,* quinidine) are used to regulate the rate and rhythm of the heartbeat.

Slow calcium-channel blockers aid in the treatment of coronary heart disease and hypertension by several mechanisms. They may dilate vessels, control the force of heart contractions, or regulate conduction through the atrioventricular node. Their actions are based on the fact that calcium ions must enter muscle cells before contraction can occur.

Anticoagulants (an-ti-ko-AG-u-lants) are valuable drugs for some heart patients. They may be used to prevent clot formation in patients with damage to heart valves or blood vessels or in patients who have had a myocardial infarction. **Aspirin** (AS-pir-in), chemically known as acetylsalicylic (a-SE-til-sal-ih-sil-ik) acid (ASA), is an inexpensive and time-tested drug for pain and inflammation that reduces blood clotting by interfering with platelet activity. A small daily dose of aspirin is recommended for patients with angina pectoris, those who have suffered a myocardial infarction, and those who have undergone surgery to open or bypass narrowed coronary arteries. It is contraindicated for people with bleeding disorders or gastric ulcers, because aspirin irritates the lining of the stomach.

Correction of Arrhythmias

If the SA node fails to generate a normal heartbeat or there is some failure in the cardiac conduction system, an electric, battery-operated **artificial pacemaker** can be employed (Fig. 14-17). This device, implanted under the skin, supplies regular impulses to stimulate the heartbeat. The site of implantation is usually in the left chest area. A pacing wire (lead) from the pacemaker is then passed into the heart through a vessel and lodged in the heart. The lead may be fixed in an atrium or a ventricle (usually on the right side). A dual chamber pacemaker has a lead in each chamber to coordinate beats between the atrium and ventricle. Some pacemakers operate at a set rate; others can be set to stimulate a beat only when the heart fails to do so on its own. Another type of pacemaker adjusts its pacing rate in response to changing activity, as during exercise. This rather simple device has saved many people whose hearts cannot beat effectively alone. In an emergency, a similar stimulus can be supplied to the heart muscle through electrodes placed externally on the chest wall.

In cases of chronic ventricular fibrillation, a battery-powered device can be implanted in the chest to restore a normal rhythm. The device detects a rapid abnormal rhythm and delivers a direct shock to the heart. The restoration of a normal heartbeat either by electric shock or drugs, is called *cardioversion*, and this device is known as an implantable cardioverter-defibrillator (ICD). A lead wire from the defibrillator is placed in the right ventricle through the pulmonary artery. In cases of severe tachycardia, tissue that is causing the disturbance can be destroyed by surgery or catheterization.

Heart Surgery

The heart-lung machine makes many operations on the heart and other thoracic organs possible. There are several types of machines in use, all of which serve as temporary substitutes for the patient's heart and lungs. The machine siphons off the blood from the large vessels entering the heart on the right side, so that no blood passes through the heart and lungs. While in the machine, the blood is oxygenated, and carbon dioxide is removed chemically. The blood is also "defoamed," or rid of air bubbles, which could fatally obstruct blood vessels. The machine then pumps the processed blood back into the general circulation through a large artery. Modern advances have enabled cardiac surgeons to perform certain procedures without bypassing the circulation, immobilizing part of the heart while it continues to beat.

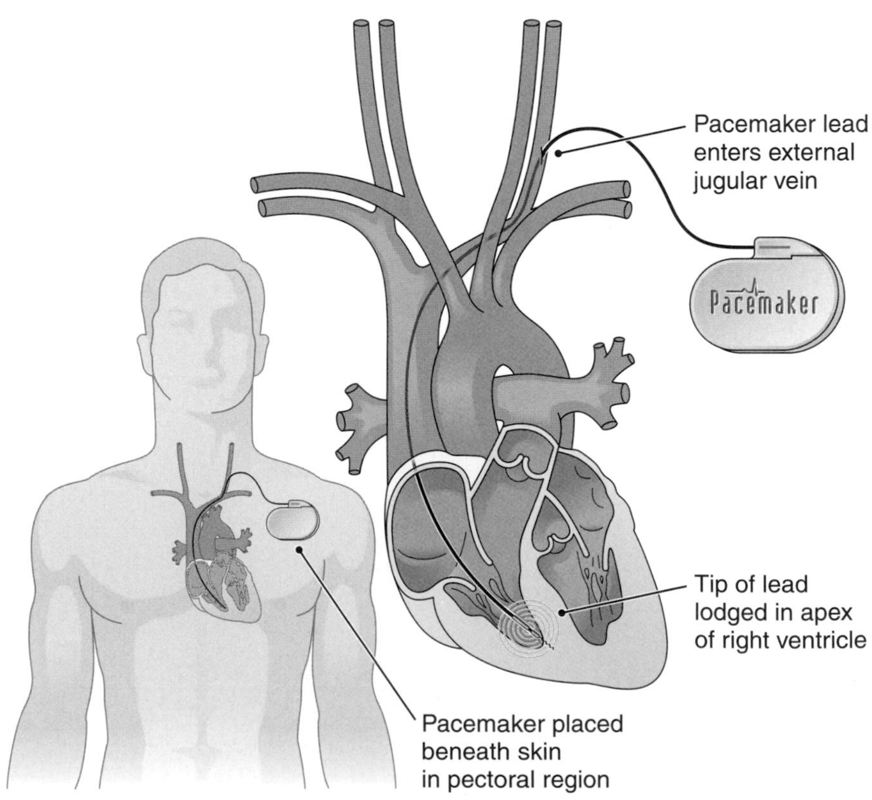

Figure 14-17 Placement of an artificial pacemaker. The lead is placed in an atrium or ventricle (usually on the right side). A dual chamber pacemaker has a lead in both chambers. (Reprinted with permission from Cohen BJ. Medical Terminology. 4th ed. Philadelphia: Lippincott Williams & Wilkins, 2004.)

Coronary artery bypass graft (CABG) to relieve obstruction in the coronary arteries is a common and often successful treatment (Fig. 14-18). While the damaged coronary arteries remain in place, healthy segments of blood vessels from other parts of the patient's body are grafted onto the vessels to bypass any obstructions. Usually, parts of the saphenous vein (a superficial vein in the leg) or the mammary artery in the chest are used.

Sometimes, as many as six or seven segments are required to establish an adequate blood supply. The mortality associated with this operation is low, and most patients are able to return to a nearly normal lifestyle after recovery from the surgery. The effectiveness of this procedure diminishes over a period of years, however, owing to blockage of the replacement vessels.

Less invasive surgical procedures include the technique of **angioplasty** (AN-je-o-plas-te), which is used to open restricted arteries in the heart and other areas of the body. In coronary angioplasty, a fluoroscope guides a catheter with a balloon to the affected area (Fig. 14-19). There, the

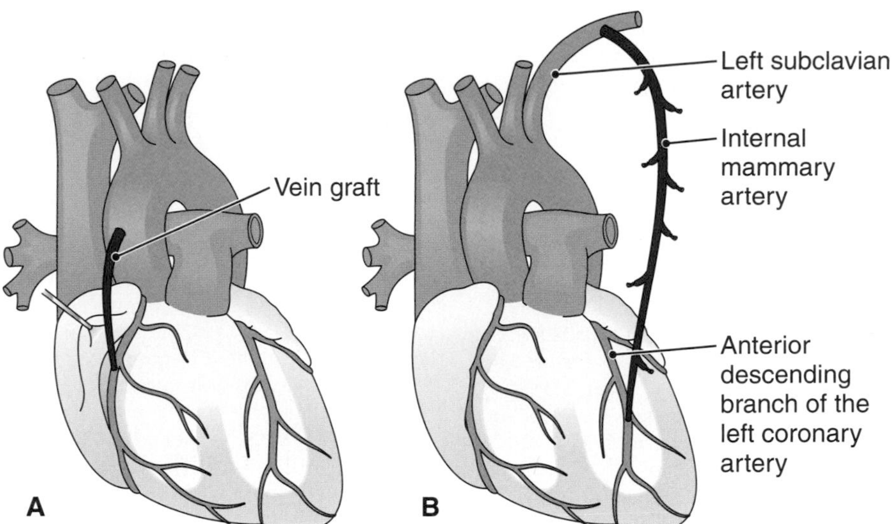

Figure 14-18 **Coronary artery bypass graft (CABG). (A)** This graft uses a segment of the saphenous vein to carry blood from the aorta to a part of the right coronary artery that is distal to the occlusion. **(B)** The mammary artery is grafted to bypass an obstruction in the left anterior descending (LAD) artery. (Reprinted with permission from Cohen BJ. Medical Terminology. 4th ed. Philadelphia: Lippincott Williams & Wilkins, 2004.)

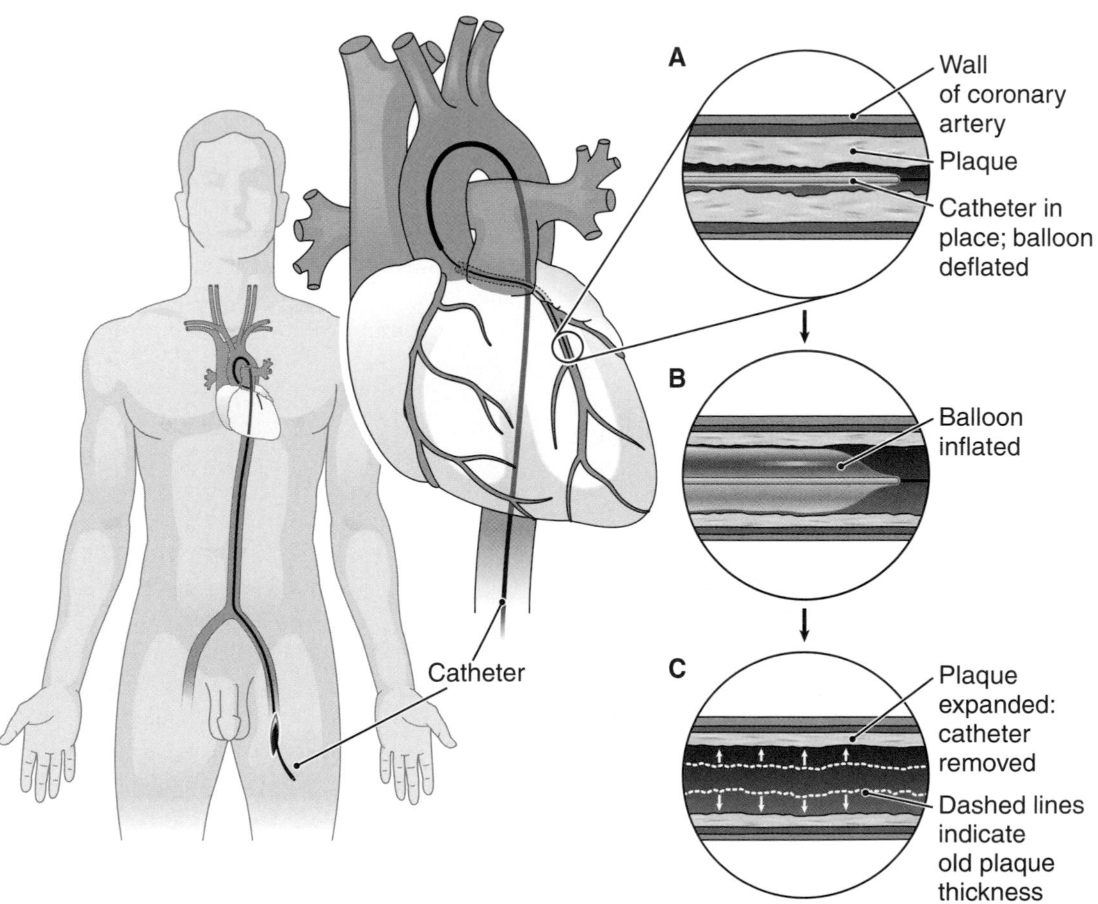

Figure 14-19 **Coronary angioplasty (PTCA). (A)** A guide catheter is threaded into the coronary artery. **(B)** A balloon catheter is inserted through the occlusion and inflated. **(C)** The balloon is inflated and deflated until plaque is flattened and the vessel is opened. (Reprinted with permission from Cohen BJ. Medical Terminology. 4th ed. Philadelphia: Lippincott Williams & Wilkins, 2004.)

Box 14-3 **Hot Topics**

Artificial Hearts: Saving Lives With Technology

More than 2000 Americans receive a heart transplant each year. Because, unfortunately, the number of individuals waiting to receive a transplant far exceeds the number of donor hearts available, researchers are inventing alternate technologies.

The ventricular assist device (VAD) is a mechanical pump that helps a patient's damaged heart to pump blood. The device is surgically implanted into a patient's chest or abdomen and connected to either the left or right ventricle. Powered by an external battery connected to it by a thin wire, the VAD pulls blood from the ventricle and pumps it to the aorta (in the case of a left VAD) or the pulmonary artery (in the case of a right VAD). These devices were first designed to help a patient survive until a suitable donor heart could be found, but a permanent model has recently been approved for use in the United States.

More than thirty years ago, researchers began experimenting with total artificial hearts, which are designed to completely replace a patient's damaged heart. The best known of these pumps is the Jarvik-7, an air-driven pump that required tubes and wires to remain connected through the skin to a large external unit. Unfortunately, all of the patients who received this device died of complications shortly after surgery and testing was discontinued. Today, researchers are experimenting with a new completely self-contained artificial heart that uses a wireless rechargeable external battery. A computer implanted in the abdomen closely monitors and controls the heart's pumping speed. If the experiments are successful, total artificial hearts may become a real alternative for patients who would otherwise die waiting for a heart transplant.

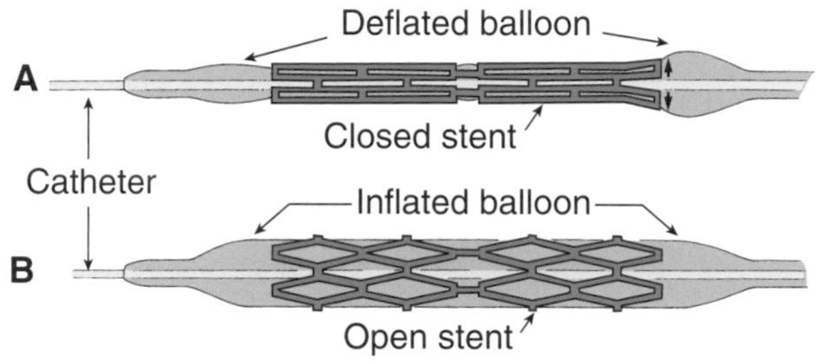

Figure 14-20 **Intracoronary artery stent. (A)** Stent closed, before the balloon is inflated. **(B)** The balloon is inflated to open the stent. The stent will remain expanded after the balloon is deflated and removed. (Reprinted with permission from Smeltzer SC, Bare BG. Brunner and Suddarth's Textbook of Medical-Surgical Nursing. 9th ed. Philadelphia: Lippincott Williams & Wilkins, 2000.)

balloon is inflated to break up the blockage in the coronary artery, thus restoring effective circulation to the heart muscle. To prevent repeated blockage, a small tube called a **stent** may be inserted in the vessel to keep it open (Fig. 14-20).

Diseased valves may become so deformed and scarred from endocarditis that they are ineffective and often obstructive. In most cases, there is so much damage that **valve replacement** is the best treatment. Substitute valves made of a variety of natural and artificial materials have been used successfully.

The news media have given considerable attention to the **surgical transplantation** of human hearts and sometimes of lungs and hearts together. This surgery is done in specialized centers and is available to some patients with degenerative heart disease who are otherwise in good health. Tissues of the recently deceased donor and of the recipient must be as closely matched as possible to avoid rejection.

Efforts to replace a damaged heart with a completely artificial heart have not met with long term success so far. There are devices available, however, to assist a damaged heart in pumping during recovery from heart attack or while a patient is awaiting a donor heart (see Box 14-3, Artificial Hearts).

Checkpoint 14-15 What technique is used to open a restricted coronary artery with a balloon catheter?

Word Anatomy

Medical terms are built from standardized word parts (prefixes, roots, and suffixes). Learning the meanings of these parts can help you remember words and interpret unfamiliar terms.

WORD PART	MEANING	EXAMPLE
Structure of the Heart		
cardi/o	heart	The *myocardium* is the heart muscle.
pulmon/o	lung	The *pulmonary* circuit carries blood to the lungs.

WORD PART	MEANING	EXAMPLE
Function of the Heart		
sin/o	sinus	The *sinoatrial* node is in a space (sinus) in the wall of the right atrium.
brady-	slow	*Bradycardia* is a slow heart rate.
tachy-	rapid	*Tachycardia* is a rapid heart rate.
Heart Disease		
cyan/o	blue	*Cyanosis* is a bluish discoloration of the skin due to lack of oxygen.
sten/o	narrowing, closure	*Stenosis* is a narrowing of a structure, such as a valve.
scler/o	hard	In *atherosclerosis*, vessels harden with fatty, gruel-like (ather/o) material that deposits on vessel walls.
isch-	suppression	Narrowing of blood vessels leads to *ischemia*, a lack of blood (-emia) supply to tissues.
Heart Studies		
steth/o	chest	A *stethoscope* is used to listen to body sounds, such as those heard through the wall of the chest.
Treatment of Heart Disease		
angi/o	vessel	*Angioplasty* is used to reshape vessels that are narrowed by disease.
-plasty	molding, surgical formation	See preceding example.

Summary

I. Circulation and the heart—heart contractions drive blood through the blood vessels

A. Location of the heart
 1. In mediastinum
 2. Slightly left of the midline; apex pointed toward left

II. Structure of the heart

 1. Endocardium—thin inner layer of epithelium
 2. Myocardium—thick muscle layer
 3. Epicardium—thin outer layer of serous membrane
  a. Also called visceral pericardium

A. Pericardium—sac that encloses the heart
 1. Outer layer fibrous
 2. Inner layers—parietal and visceral serous membranes

B. Special features of myocardium
 1. Lightly striated
 2. Intercalated disks
 3. Branching of fibers

C. Divisions of the heart
 1. Two sides divided by septa
 2. Four chambers
  a. Atria—left and right receiving chambers
  b. Ventricles—left and right pumping chambers
 1. Four valves—prevent backflow of blood
  a. Right atrioventricular (AV) valve—tricuspid
  b. Left atrioventricular valve—mitral or bicuspid
  c. Pulmonic (semilunar) valve—at entrance to pulmonary artery
  d. Aortic (semilunar) valve—at entrance to aorta

D. Blood supply to the myocardium
 1. Coronary arteries—first branches of aorta; fill when heart relaxes
 2. Coronary sinus—collects venous blood from heart and empties into right atrium

III. Function of the heart

 1. Cardiac cycle
  a. Diastole—relaxation phase
  b. Systole—contraction phase

A. Cardiac output—volume pumped by each ventricle per minute
 1. Stroke volume—amount pumped with each beat
 2. Heart rate—number of beats per minute

B. Heart's conduction system
 1. Sinoatrial node (pacemaker)—at top of right atrium
 2. Atrioventricular node—between atria and ventricles
 3. Atrioventricular bundle (bundle of His)—at top of interventricular septum
  a. Bundle branches—right and left, on either side of septum
  b. Purkinje fibers—branch through myocardium of ventricles

C. Control of the heart rate
 1. Autonomic nervous system
  a. Sympathetic system—speeds heart rate
  b. Parasympathetic system—slows heart rate through vagus nerve
 2. Others—hormones, ions, drugs

3. Variations in heart rates
   a. Bradycardia—slower rate than normal; less than 60 beats/minute
   b. Tachycardia—faster rate than normal; more than 100 beats/minute
   c. Sinus arrhythmia—related to breathing changes
   d. Premature beat—extrasystole

D. Heart sounds
1. Normal
   a. "Lubb"—occurs at closing of atrioventricular valves
   b. "Dupp"—occurs at closing of semilunar valves
2. Abnormal—murmur

IV. Heart disease

A. Classification of heart disease
1. Anatomic classification—endocarditis, myocarditis, pericarditis
2. Causal classification

B. Congenital heart diseases—present at birth
1. Failure of fetal lung bypasses to close
   a. Atrial septal defect
   b. Patent ductus arteriosus
2. Ventricular septal defect
3. Narrowing of aorta or pulmonary artery
4. Tetralogy of Fallot

C. Rheumatic heart disease—results from a type of streptococcal infection
1. Mitral stenosis—valve cusps do not open
2. Mitral regurgitation—valve cusps do not close

D. Coronary artery disease
1. Characteristics
   a. Atherosclerosis—thickening and hardening of arteries with plaque
   b. Ischemia—lack of blood to area fed by blocked arteries
   c. Coronary occlusion—closure of coronary arteries, as by a thrombus (clot)
   d. Infarct—area of damaged tissue
   e. Angina pectoris—pain caused by lack of blood to heart muscle
   f. Abnormal rhythm—arrhythmia
      (1) Flutter—rapid, coordinated beats
      (2) Fibrillation—rapid, uncoordinated contractions of heart muscle
      (3) Heart block—interruption of electric conduction
2. Treatment of heart attacks—CPR, defibrillation, thrombolytic drugs, monitoring, good health habits

E. Heart failure—due to hypertension, disease, malnutrition, anemia, age

V. The heart in the elderly

1. Individual variations in how heart ages
2. Common variations include:
   a. Decrease in heart size, strength of muscle contraction, flexibility of values, cardiac output
   b. Abnormal rhythms, temporary failure of conduction system

VI. Prevention of heart ailments

1. Risk factors
2. Preventive measures—physical examination, proper diet, quitting smoking, regular exercise, control of chronic illness

VII. Heart studies

1. Stethoscope—used to listen to heart sounds
2. Electrocardiograph (ECG, EKG)—records electrical activity as waves
3. Catheterization—thin tube inserted into heart for blood samples, pressure readings, and other tests
4. Fluoroscope—examines deep tissue with x-rays; used to guide catheter
5. Echocardiography—uses ultrasound to record pictures of heart in action

VIII. Treatment of heart disease

A. Medications—examples are digitalis, nitroglycerin, beta-adrenergic blocking agents, antiarrhythmic agents, slow channel calcium-channel blockers, anticoagulants

B. Correction of arrhythmia
1. Artificial pacemakers—electronic devices implanted under skin to regulate heartbeat
2. Implantable cardioverter-defibrillator (ICD)
3. Destruction of abnormal tissue

C. Heart surgery
1. Bypass—vessels grafted to detour blood around blockage
2. Angioplasty—balloon catheter used to open blocked arteries
   a. Stents used to keep vessels open
3. Valve replacement
4. Heart transplantation
5. Artificial hearts

Questions for Study and Review

Building Understanding

Fill in the blanks

1. The central thoracic region that contains the heart is the ______.

2. The layer of the heart responsible for pumping blood is called the______.

3. The heart beat is initiated by electrical impulses from the______.

4. Lack of blood to a tissue fed by blocked arteries is called ______.

5. Pain caused by lack of blood to heart muscle is called ______.

Matching

Match each numbered item with the most closely related lettered item.

___ 6. receives deoxygenated blood from the body
___ 7. receives oxygenated blood from the lungs
___ 8. sends deoxygenated blood to the lungs
___ 9. sends oxygenated blood to the body

a. right atrium
b. left atrium
c. right ventricle
d. left ventricle

Multiple choice

___ 10. Rapid transfer of electrical signals between cardiac muscle cells is promoted by
a. the striated nature of the cells
b. branching of the cells
c. the abundance of mitochondria within the cells
d. intercalated disks between the cells

___ 11. The upper chambers of the heart are separated by the
a. intercalated disk
b. interatrial septum
c. interventricular septum
d. ductus arteriosus

___ 12. One complete sequence of heart contraction and relaxation is called the
a. systole
b. diastole
c. cardiac cycle
d. cardiac output

___ 13. A medication that reduces the rate and strength of heart contractions by lowering sympathetic tone is called a(n)
a. anticoagulant
b. antiarrhythmic agent
c. slow calcium-channel blocker
d. beta-adrenergic blocking agent

___ 14. The ductus arteriosus shunts blood away from the
a. lungs and towards the aorta
b. lungs and towards the superior vena cava
c. aorta and towards the lungs
d. away from the superior vena cava and towards the lungs

___ 15. A regular variation in heart rate due to changes in the rate and depth of breathing is called a
a. murmur
b. cyanosis
c. sinus arrhythmia
d. stent

Understanding Concepts

16. Differentiate between the terms in each of the following pairs:
a. pulmonary and systemic circuit
b. coronary artery and coronary sinus
c. serous pericardium and fibrous pericardium
d. systole and diastole

17. Explain the purpose of the four heart valves and describe their structure and location. What prevents the valves from opening backwards?

18. Trace a drop of blood from the superior vena cava to the lungs and then from the lungs to the aorta.

19. Describe the order in which electrical impulses travel through the heart. What is an interruption of these impulses in the conduction system of the heart called?

20. Compare the effects of the sympathetic and parasympathetic nervous systems on the working of the heart.

21. Compare and contrast the following disease conditions:
a. endocarditis and pericarditis
b. tachycardia and bradycardia
c. functional murmur and organic murmur
d. flutter and fibrillation
e. atrial and ventricular septal defect

22. What part does infection play in rheumatic heart disease?

23. List some age-related changes to the heart.

Conceptual Thinking

24. Jim's father has recently passed away following a massive myocardial infarction. At 45 years old, Jim is frightened that he may suffer the same fate. What can Jim do to lower his risk of heart disease? What risk factors can he not change?

25. Three month-old Hannah R. is brought to the doctor by her parents. They have noticed that when she cries she becomes breathless and turns blue. The doctor examines Hannah and notices that she is lethargic, small for her age, and has a loud mitral valve murmur. With this information, explain the cause of Hannah's symptoms.

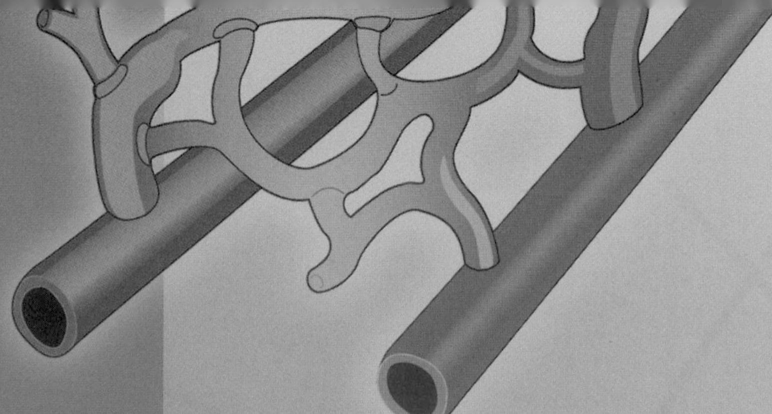

Selected Key Terms

The following terms and other boldface terms in the chapter are defined in the Glossary

anastomosis
aneurysm
aorta
arteriole
artery
atherosclerosis
capillary
embolus
endarterectomy
endothelium
hemorrhage
hypertension
hypotension
ischemia
phlebitis
pulse
shock
sinusoid
sphygmomanometer
thrombus
varicose vein
vasoconstriction
vasodilation
vein
vena cava
venous sinus
venule

Learning Outcomes

After careful study of this chapter, you should be able to:

1. Differentiate among the five types of blood vessels with regard to structure and function
2. Compare the pulmonary and systemic circuits relative to location and function
3. Name the four sections of the aorta and list the main branches of each section
4. Define *anastomosis.* Cite the function of anastomoses and give several examples
5. Compare superficial and deep veins and give examples of each type
6. Name the main vessels that drain into the superior and inferior venae cavae
7. Define *venous sinus* and give several examples of venous sinuses
8. Describe the structure and function of the hepatic portal system
9. Explain the forces that affect exchange across the capillary wall
10. Describe the factors that regulate blood flow
11. Define *pulse* and list factors that affect pulse rate
12. List the factors that affect blood pressure
13. Explain how blood pressure is commonly measured
14. List reasons why hypertension should be controlled
15. List some disorders that involve the blood vessels
16. List steps in first aid for hemorrhage
17. List four types of shock
18. Show how word parts are used to build words related to the blood vessels and circulation (see Word Anatomy at the end of the chapter)

chapter 15

Blood Vessels and Blood Circulation

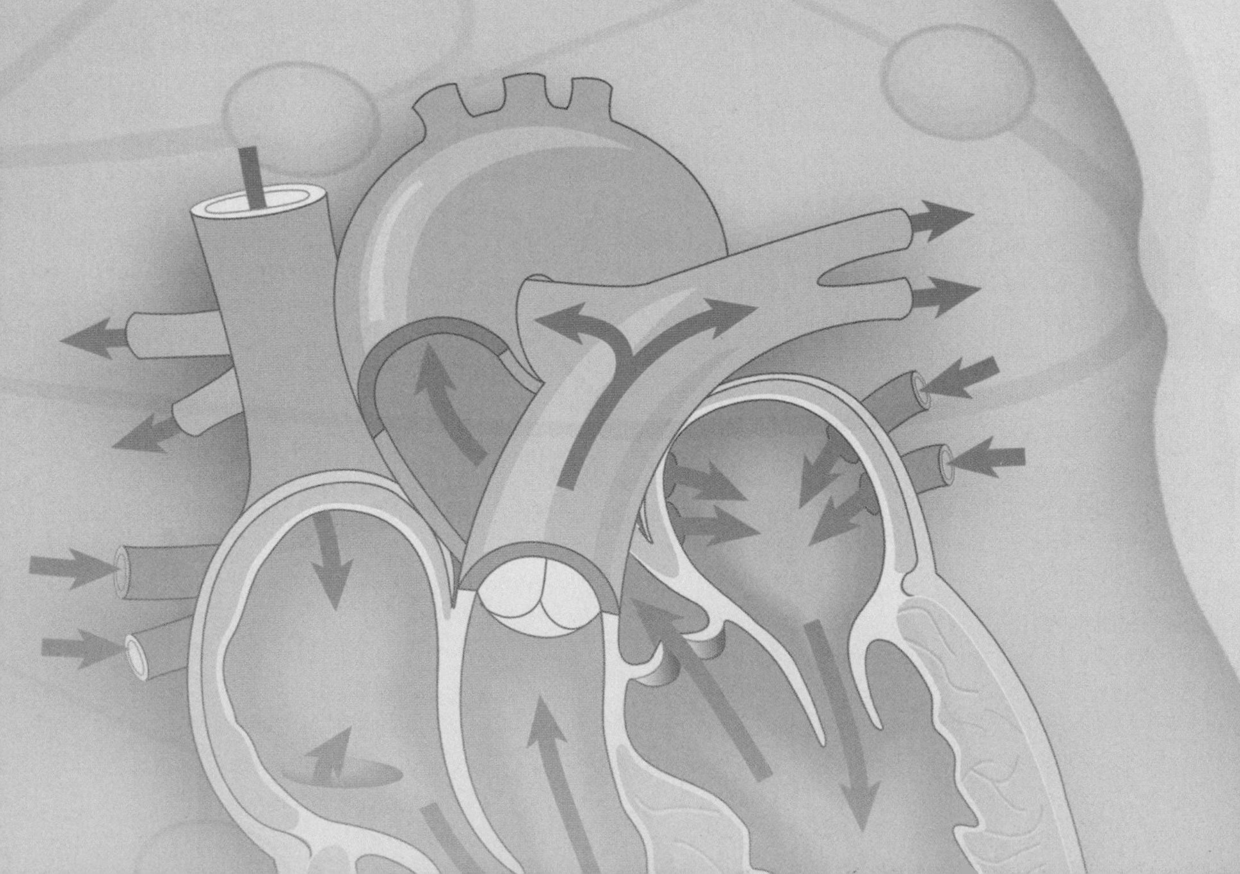

The blood vessels, together with the four chambers of the heart, form a closed system in which blood is carried to and from the tissues. Although whole blood does not leave the vessels, components of the plasma and tissue fluids can be exchanged through the walls of the tiniest vessels, the capillaries.

The vascular system is easier to understand if you refer to the appropriate illustrations in this chapter as the vessels are described. When this information is added to what you already know about the blood and the heart, a picture of the cardiovascular system as a whole will emerge.

Blood Vessels

Blood vessels may be divided into five groups, named below according to the sequence of blood flow from the heart:

- **Arteries** carry blood away from the heart and toward the tissues. The heart's ventricles pump blood into the arteries.
- **Arterioles** (ar-TE-re-olz) are small subdivisions of the arteries. They carry blood into the capillaries.
- **Capillaries** are tiny, thin-walled vessels that allow for exchanges between systems. These exchanges occur between the blood and the body cells and between the blood and the air in the lung tissues. The capillaries connect the arterioles and venules.
- **Venules** (VEN-ulz) are small vessels that receive blood from the capillaries and begin its transport back toward the heart.
- **Veins** are vessels formed by the merger of venules. They continue the transport of blood until it is returned to the heart

Checkpoint 15-1 What are the five types of blood vessels?

Blood Circuits

The vessels together may be subdivided into two groups, or circuits: pulmonary and systemic. Figure 15-1 shows the vessels in these two circuits; the anatomic relation of the circuits to the heart is shown in Chapter 14's Figure 14-4.

The Pulmonary Circuit The **pulmonary circuit** delivers blood to the lungs where carbon dioxide is eliminated and oxygen is replenished. The pulmonary vessels that carry blood to and from the lungs include the following:

- The pulmonary artery and its branches, which carry blood from the right ventricle to the lungs
- The capillaries in the lungs, through which gases are exchanged
- The pulmonary veins, which carry blood back to the left atrium

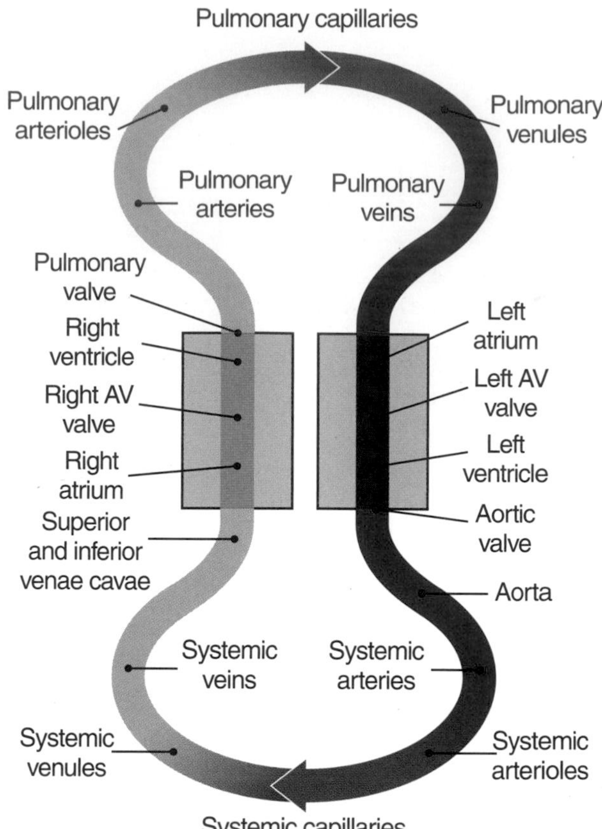

Figure 15-1 Blood flow in a closed system of vessels. Oxygen content changes as blood flows through the capillaries. *ZOOMING IN ✦ Judging from color coding, which vessels pick up oxygen? Which vessels release oxygen?*

The pulmonary vessels differ from those in the systemic circuit in that the pulmonary arteries carry blood that is *low* in oxygen, and the pulmonary veins carry blood that is *high* in oxygen. All the remaining arteries carry highly oxygenated blood, and all remaining veins carry blood that is low in oxygen.

The Systemic Circuit The **systemic** (sis-TEM-ik) **circuit** serves the rest of the body. These vessels supply nutrients and oxygen to all the tissues and carry waste materials away from the tissues for disposal. The systemic vessels include the following:

- The **aorta** (a-OR-tah), which receives blood from the left ventricle and then branches into the systemic arteries carrying blood to the tissues
- The systemic capillaries, through which materials are exchanged
- The systemic veins, which carry blood back toward the heart. The venous blood flows into the right atrium of the heart through the superior vena cava and inferior vena cava.

Checkpoint 15-2 What are the two blood circuits and what areas does each serve?

Vessel Structure

The arteries have thick walls because they must be strong enough to receive blood pumped under pressure from the heart's ventricles (Fig. 15-2). The three tunics (coats) of the arteries resemble the three tissue layers of the heart:

- The innermost membrane of simple, flat epithelial cells makes up the **endothelium** (en-do-THE-le-um), forming a smooth surface over which the blood flows easily.
- The middle and thickest layer is made of smooth (involuntary) muscle, which is under the control of the autonomic nervous system.
- An outer tunic is made of a supporting connective tissue.

Elastic tissue between the layers of the arterial wall allows these vessels to stretch when receiving blood and then return to their original size. The amount of elastic tissue diminishes as the arteries branch and become smaller.

The small subdivisions of the arteries, the arterioles, have thinner walls in which there is little elastic connective tissue but relatively more smooth muscle. The autonomic nervous system controls this involuntary muscle. The vessels become narrower (constrict) when the muscle contracts and widen (dilate) when the muscle relaxes. In this manner, the arterioles regulate the amount of blood that enters the various tissues at a given time. Change in the diameter of the arterioles is also a major factor in blood pressure control.

The microscopic capillaries that connect arterioles and venules have the thinnest walls of any vessels: one cell layer. The capillary walls are transparent and are made of smooth, squamous epithelial cells that are a continuation of the lining of the arteries. The thinness of these walls allows for exchanges between the blood and the body cells and between the lung tissue and the outside air. The capillary boundaries are the most important center of activity for the entire circulatory system. Their function is explained later in this chapter (see also Box 15-1).

The smallest veins, the venules, are formed by the union of capillaries, and their walls are only slightly thicker than those of the capillaries. As the venules merge to form veins, the smooth muscle in the vessel walls becomes thicker and the venules begin to acquire the additional layers found in the larger vessels.

The walls of the veins have the same three layers as those of the arteries. However, the middle smooth muscle tunic is relatively thin in the veins. A vein wall is much

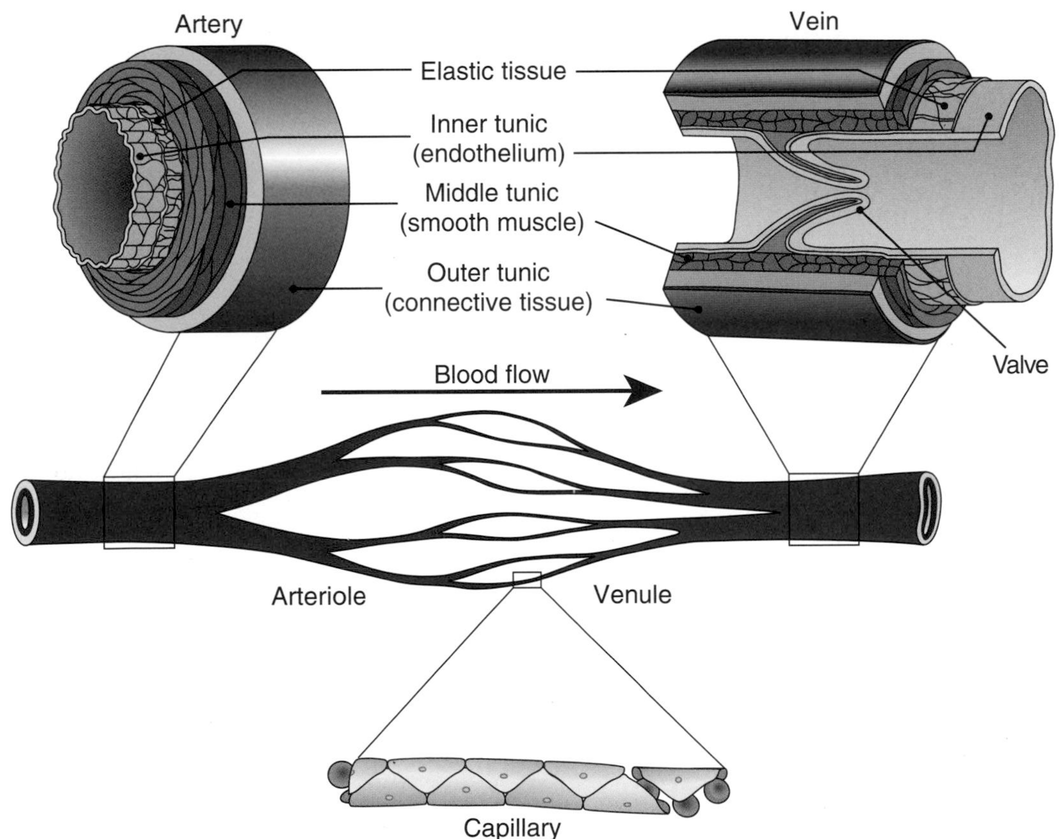

Figure 15-2 **Sections of small blood vessels.** Drawings show the thick wall of an artery, the thin wall of a vein, and the single-layered wall of a capillary. A venous valve also is shown. The arrow indicates the direction of blood flow. *ZOOMING IN ✦ Which vessels have valves that control blood flow?*

Box 15-1 A Closer Look

Capillaries: The Body's Free Trade Zones

The exchange of substances between body cells and the blood occurs along about 50,000 miles (80,000 kilometers) of capillaries. Rates of exchange vary because, based on their structure, different types of capillaries vary in permeability.

Continuous capillaries are the most common type and are found in muscle, connective tissue, the lungs, and the central nervous system (CNS). These capillaries are composed of a continuous layer of endothelial cells. Adjacent cells are loosely attached to each other, with small openings called intercellular clefts between them. Although continuous capillaries are the least permeable, water and small molecules can diffuse easily through their walls. Large molecules, such as plasma proteins and blood cells, cannot. In certain regions of the body, like the CNS, adjacent endothelial cells are joined tightly together, making the capillaries impermeable to many substances (see Box 10-1 in Chapter 10, The Blood Brain Barrier: Access Denied).

Fenestrated (FEN-es-tra-ted) capillaries are much more permeable than continuous capillaries, because they have many holes, or fenestrations, in the endothelium. These sieve-like capillaries are permeable to water and solutes as large as peptides. In the digestive tract, fenestrated capillaries permit rapid absorption of water and nutrients into the bloodstream. In the kidneys, they permit rapid filtration of blood plasma, the first step in urine formation.

Discontinuous capillaries, or sinusoids, are the most permeable. In addition to fenestrations, they have large spaces between endothelial cells that allow the exchange of water, large solutes, such as plasma proteins, and even blood cells. Sinusoids are found in the liver and red bone marrow, for example. Albumin, clotting factors, and other proteins formed in the liver enter the bloodstream through sinusoids. In red bone marrow, newly formed blood cells travel through sinusoids to join the bloodstream.

thinner than the wall of a comparably sized artery. These vessels also have less elastic tissue between the layers. As a result, the blood within the veins is carried under much lower pressure. Because of their thinner walls, the veins are easily collapsed. Only slight pressure on a vein by a tumor or other mass may interfere with return blood flow.

Most veins are equipped with one-way valves that permit blood to flow in only one direction: toward the heart (see Fig. 15-2). Such valves are most numerous in the veins of the extremities. Figure 15-3 is a cross-section of an artery and a vein as seen through a microscope.

Checkpoint 15-3 What type of tissue makes up the middle layer of arteries and veins, and how is this tissue controlled?

Checkpoint 15-4 How many cell layers make up the wall of a capillary?

Systemic Arteries

The systemic arteries begin with the aorta, the largest artery, which measures about 2.5 cm (1 inch) in diameter. This vessel receives blood from the left ventricle then travels downward through the body, branching to all organs.

The Aorta and Its Parts

The aorta ascends toward the right from the left ventricle. Then it curves posteriorly and to the left. It continues downward posterior to the heart and just anterior to the vertebral column, through the diaphragm, and into the abdomen (Figs. 15-4 and 15-5). The aorta is one continuous artery, but it may be divided into sections:

- The **ascending aorta** is near the heart and inside the pericardial sac.
- The **aortic arch** curves from the right to the left and also extends posteriorly.
- The **thoracic aorta** lies just anterior to the vertebral col-

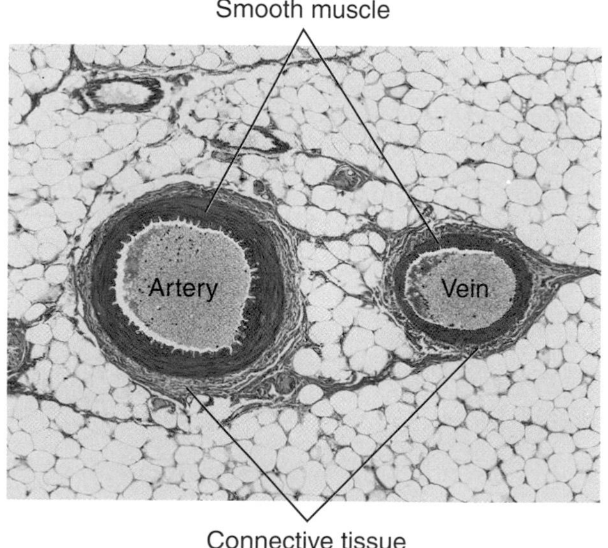

Figure 15-3 Cross-section of an artery and vein. The smooth muscle and connective tissue of the vessels are visible in this photomicrograph. (Reprinted with permission from Cormack DH. Essential Histology. 2nd ed. Philadelphia: Lippincott Williams & Wilkins, 2001.) *ZOOMING IN ✦ Which type of vessel shown has a thicker wall?*

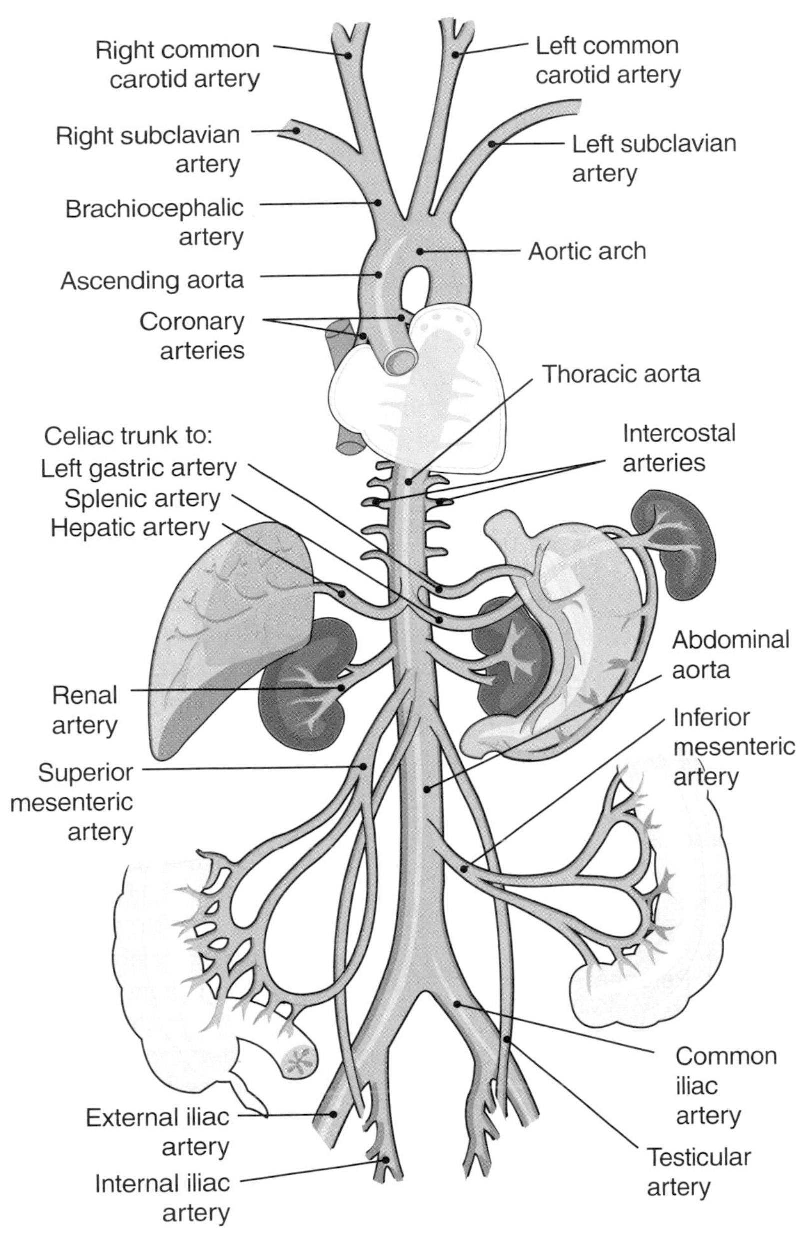

Figure 15-4 The aorta and its branches. *ZOOMING IN ✦ How many brachiocephalic arteries are there?*

umn posterior to the heart and in the space behind the pleura.

- The **abdominal aorta** is the longest section of the aorta, spanning the abdominal cavity.

The thoracic and abdominal aorta together make up the descending aorta.

Branches of the Ascending Aorta and Aortic Arch

The first, or ascending, part of the aorta has two branches near the heart, called the **left** and **right coronary arteries,** which supply the heart muscle. These form a crown around the heart's base and give off branches to all parts of the myocardium.

The arch of the aorta, located immediately beyond the ascending aorta, divides into three large branches.

- The **brachiocephalic** (brak-e-o-seh-FAL-ik) **artery** is a short vessel that supplies the arm and the head on the right side. After extending upward somewhat less than 5 cm (2 inches), it divides into the **right subclavian** (sub-KLA-ve-an) **artery**, which extends under the right clavicle (collar bone) and supplies the right upper extremity (arm), and the **right common carotid** (kah-ROT-id) **artery**, which supplies the right side of the neck, head and brain. Note that the brachiocephalic artery is unpaired.
- The **left common carotid artery** extends upward from the highest part of the aortic arch. It supplies the left side of the neck and the head.
- The **left subclavian artery** extends under the left clavicle and supplies the left upper extremity. This is the last branch of the aortic arch.

Branches of the Thoracic Aorta

The thoracic aorta supplies branches to the chest wall, **esophagus** (e-SOF-ah-gus), and bronchi (the subdivisions of the trachea), and their treelike subdivisions in the lungs. There are usually 9 to 10 pairs of **intercostal** (in-ter-KOS-tal) **arteries** that extend between the ribs, sending branches to the muscles and other structures of the chest wall.

Branches of the Abdominal Aorta

As in the case of the thoracic aorta, there are unpaired branches extending anteriorly and paired arteries extending laterally. The unpaired vessels are large arteries that supply the abdominal viscera. The most important of these visceral branches are as follows:

- The **celiac** (SE-le-ak) **trunk** is a short artery about 1.25 cm (1/2 inch) long that subdivides into three branches: the **left gastric artery** goes to the stomach, the **splenic** (SPLEN-ik) **artery** goes to the spleen, and the **hepatic** (heh-PAT-ik) **artery** carries oxygenated blood to the liver.
- The **superior mesenteric** (mes-en-TER-ik) **artery**, the largest of these branches, carries blood to most of the small intestine and to the first half of the large intestine.
- The much smaller **inferior mesenteric artery,** located below the superior mesenteric artery and near the end

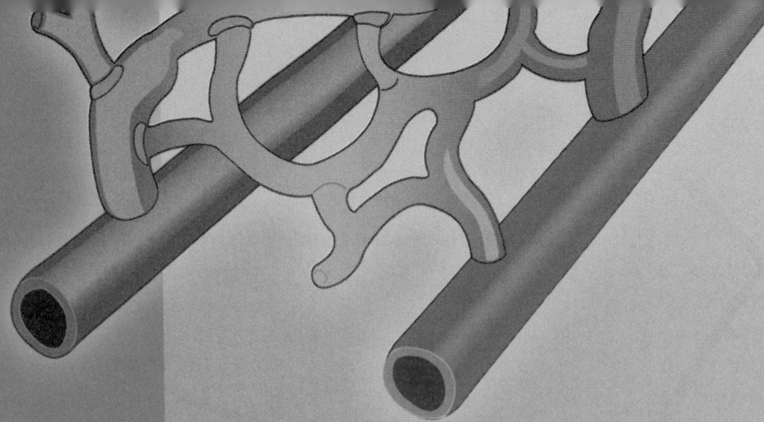

Selected Key Terms

The following terms and other boldface terms in the chapter are defined in the Glossary

adenoids
chyle
lacteal
lymph
lymphadenitis
lymphadenopathy
lymphangitis
lymphatic duct
lymph node
spleen
thymus
tonsil

Learning Outcomes

After careful study of this chapter, you should be able to:

1. List the functions of the lymphatic system
2. Explain how lymphatic capillaries differ from blood capillaries
3. Name the two main lymphatic ducts and describe the area drained by each
4. List the major structures of the lymphatic system and give the locations and functions of each
5. Describe the composition and function of the reticuloendothelial system
6. Describe the major lymphatic system disorders
7. Show how word parts are used to build words related to the lymphatic system (see Word Anatomy at the end of the chapter)

chapter 16

The Lymphatic System and Lymphoid Tissue

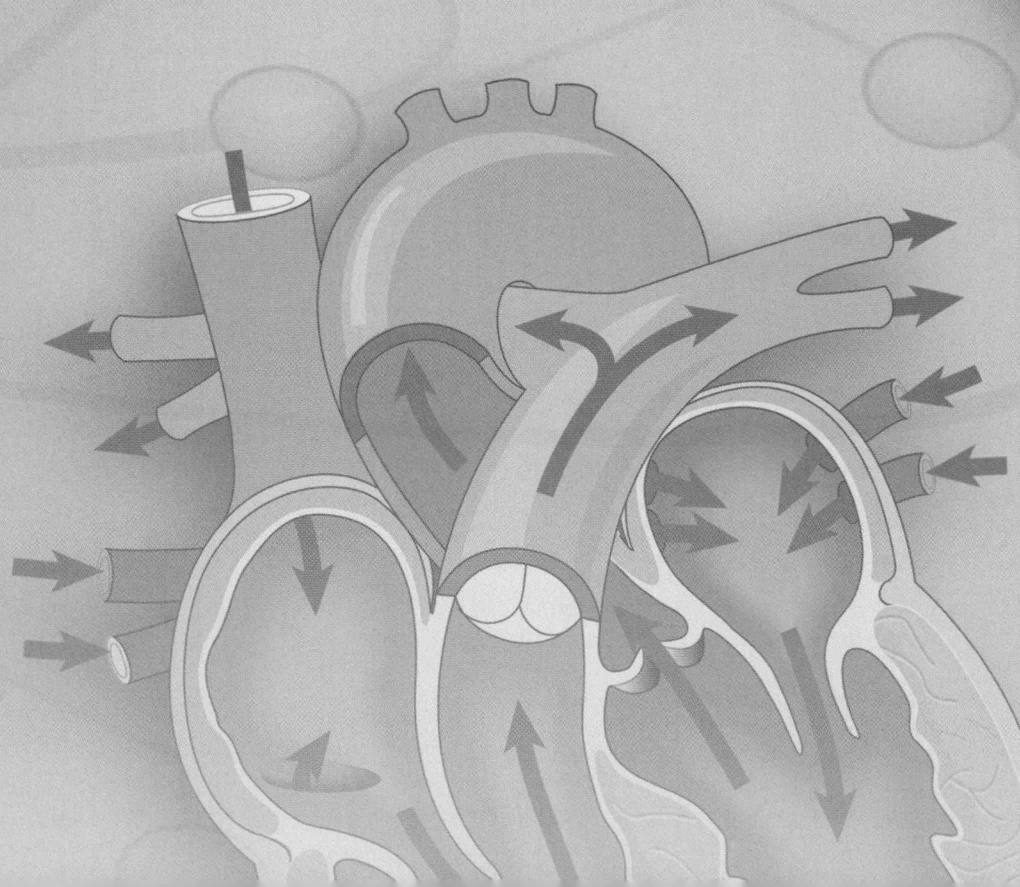

The Lymphatic System

The lymphatic system is a widespread system of tissues and vessels. Its organs are not in continuous order, but are scattered throughout the body, and it services almost all regions. Only bone tissue, cartilage, epithelium and the central nervous system are not in direct communication with this system.

Functions of the Lymphatic System

The functions of the lymphatic system are just as varied as its locations. These functions fall into three categories:

- **Fluid balance**. As blood circulates through the capillaries in the tissues, water and dissolved substances are constantly exchanged between the bloodstream and the interstitial (in-ter-STISH-al) fluids that bathe the cells. Ideally, the volume of fluid that leaves the blood should be matched by the amount that returns to the blood. However, there is always a slight excess of fluid left behind in the tissues. In addition, some proteins escape from the blood capillaries and are left behind. This fluid and protein would accumulate in the tissues if not for a second drainage pathway through lymphatic vessels (Fig. 16-1).

  In addition to the blood-carrying capillaries, the tissues also contain microscopic lymphatic capillaries. These small vessels pick up excess fluid and protein left behind in the tissues (Fig. 16-2). The capillaries then drain into larger vessels, which eventually return these materials to the venous system near the heart.

  The fluid that circulates in the lymphatic system is called **lymph** (limf), a clear fluid similar in composition to interstitial fluid. Although lymph is formed from the components of blood plasma, it differs from the plasma in that it has much less protein.
- **Protection from infection**. The lymphatic system is an important component of the immune system, which fights infection. One group of white blood cells, the lymphocytes, can live and multiply in the lymphatic system, where they attack and destroy foreign organisms. Lymphoid tissue scattered throughout the body filters out pathogens, other foreign matter and cellular debris in body fluids. More will be said about the lymphocytes and immunity in Chapter 17.
- **Absorption of fats**. Following the chemical and mechanical breakdown of food in the digestive tract, most nutrients are absorbed into the blood through intestinal capillaries. Many digested fats, however, are too large to enter the blood capillaries and are instead absorbed into lymphatic capillaries. These fats are added to the blood when lymph joins the bloodstream. The topic of digestion is covered in Chapter 19.

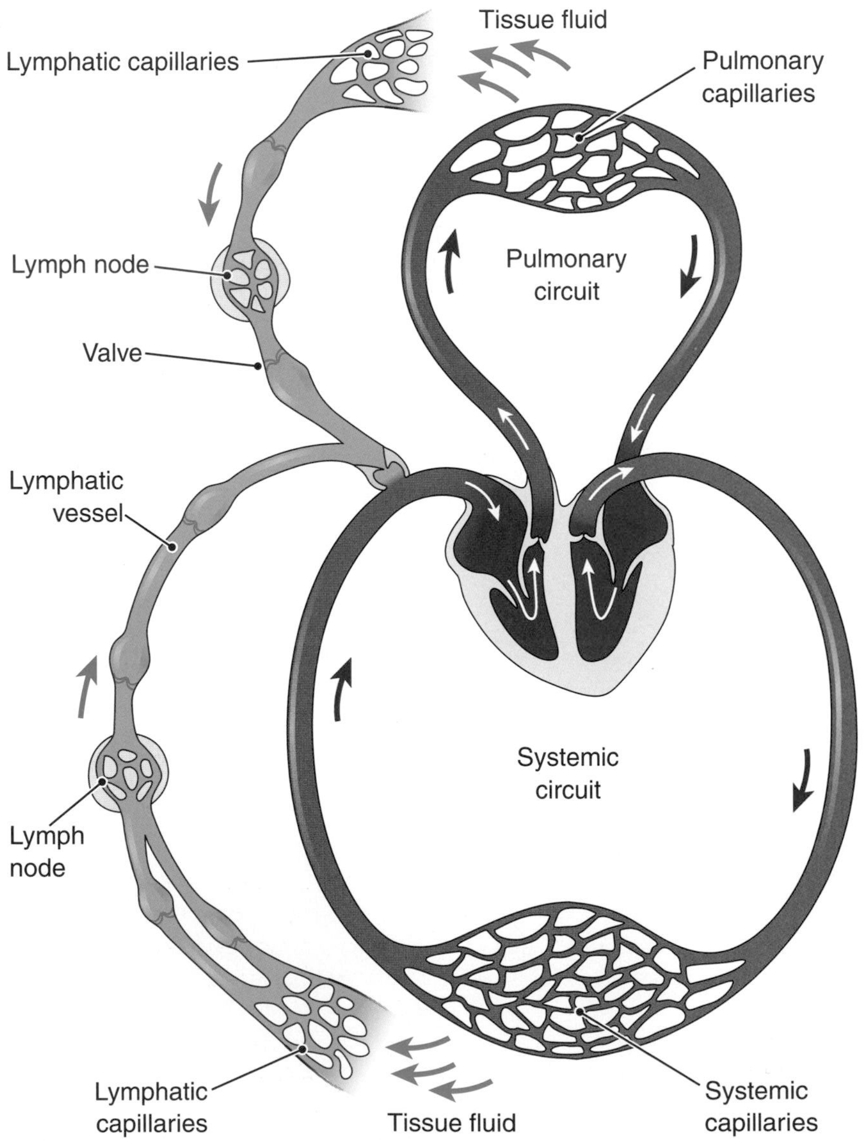

Checkpoint 16-1 What are three functions of the lymphatic system?

Figure 16-1 **The lymphatic system in relation to the cardiovascular system.** Lymphatic vessels pick up fluid in the tissues and return it to the blood in vessels near the heart. *ZOOMING IN ✦ What type of blood vessel receives lymph collected from the body?*

Lymphatic Circulation

Lymph travels through a network of small and large channels that are in some ways similar to the blood vessels.

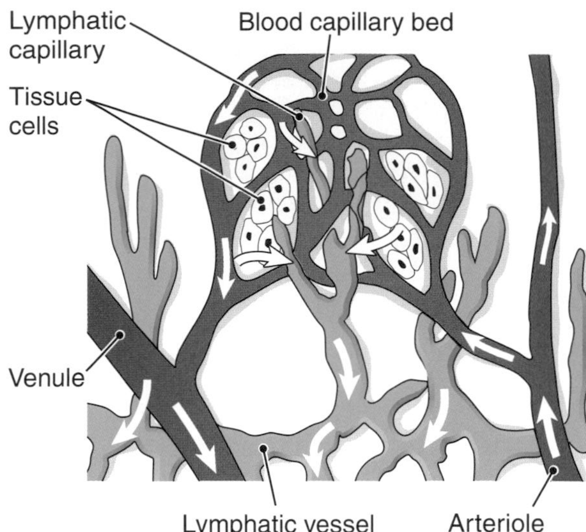

Figure 16-2 **Pathway of lymphatic drainage in the tissues.** Lymphatic capillaries are more permeable than blood capillaries and can pick up fluid and proteins left in the tissues as blood leaves the capillary bed to travel back toward the heart.

However, the system is not a complete circuit. It is a one-way system that begins in the tissues and ends when the lymph joins the blood (see Fig. 16-1).

Lymphatic Capillaries

The walls of the lymphatic capillaries resemble those of the blood capillaries in that they are made of one layer of flattened (squamous) epithelial cells. This thin layer, also called *endothelium*, allows for easy passage of soluble materials and water (Fig. 16-3). The gaps between the endothelial cells in the lymphatic capillaries are larger than those of the blood capillaries. The lymphatic capillaries are thus more permeable, allowing for easier entrance of relatively large protein particles. The proteins do not move back out of the vessels because the endothelial cells overlap slightly, forming one-way valves to block their return.

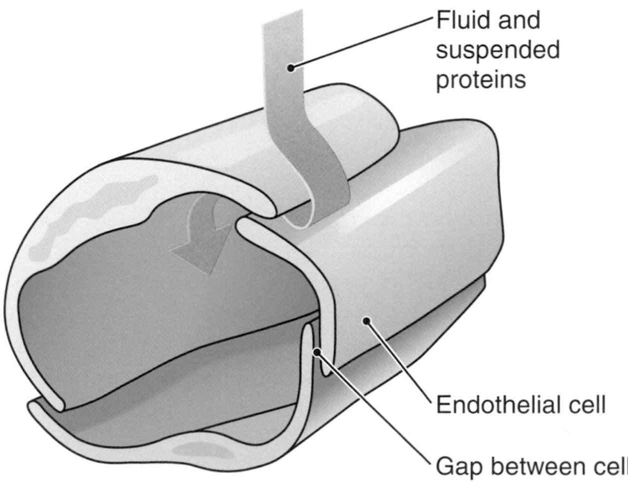

Figure 16-3 **Structure of a lymphatic capillary.** Fluid and proteins can enter the capillary with ease through gaps between the endothelial cells. Overlapping cells act as valves to prevent the material from leaving.

Unlike the blood capillaries, the lymphatic capillaries arise blindly; that is, they are closed at one end and do not form a bridge between two larger vessels. Instead, one end simply lies within a lake of tissue fluid, and the other communicates with a larger lymphatic vessel that transports the lymph toward the heart (see Figs. 16-1 and 16-2).

Some specialized lymphatic capillaries located in the lining of the small intestine absorb digested fats. Fats taken into these **lacteals** (LAK-te-als) are transported in the lymphatic vessels until the lymph is added to the blood. More information on the role of the lymphatic system in digestion is found in Chapter 19.

Checkpoint 16-2 What are two differences between blood capillaries and lymphatic capillaries?

Lymphatic Vessels

The lymphatic vessels are thin walled and delicate and have a beaded appearance because of indentations where valves are located (see Fig. 16-1). These valves prevent back flow in the same way as do those found in some veins.

Lymphatic vessels (Fig. 16-4) include **superficial** and **deep** sets. The surface lymphatics are immediately below the skin, often lying near the superficial veins. The deep vessels are usually larger and accompany the deep veins.

Lymphatic vessels are named according to location. For example, those in the breast are called **mammary** lymphatic vessels, those in the thigh are called **femoral** lymphatic vessels, and those in the leg are called **tibial** lymphatic vessels. At certain points, the vessels drain through lymph nodes, small masses of lymphatic tissue that filter the lymph. The nodes are in groups that serve a particular region. For example, nearly all the lymph from the upper extremity and the breast passes through the **axillary lymph nodes**, whereas lymph from the lower extremity passes through the **inguinal nodes**. Lymphatic vessels carrying lymph away from the regional nodes eventually drain into one of two terminal vessels, the right lymphatic duct or the thoracic duct, both of which empty into the bloodstream.

The Right Lymphatic Duct The **right lymphatic duct** is a short vessel, approximately 1.25 cm (1/2 inch) long, that receives only the lymph that comes from the superior right quadrant of the body: the right side of the head, neck, and thorax, as well as the right upper extremity. It empties into the right subclavian vein near the heart (see Fig. 16-4 B). Its opening into this vein is

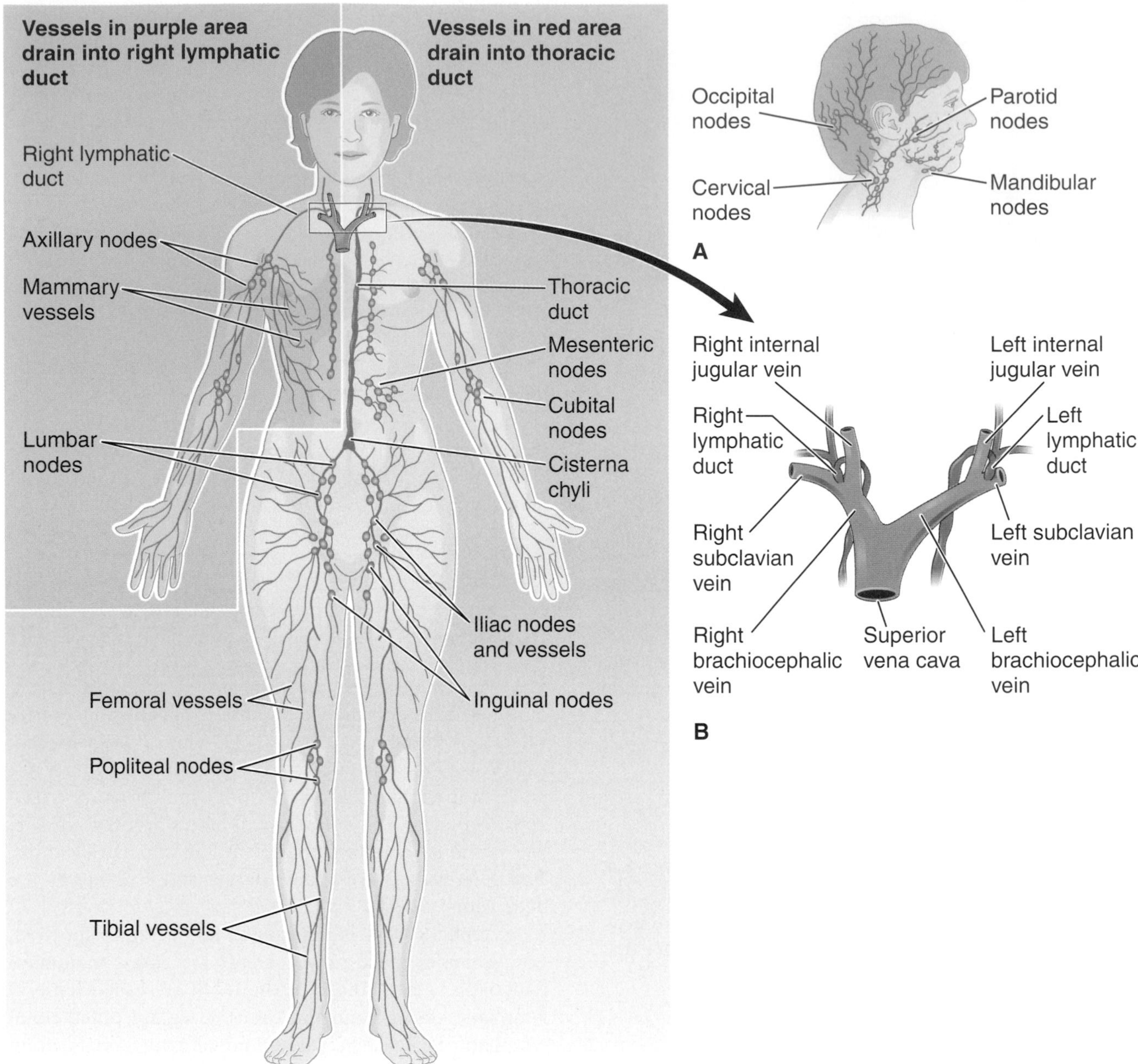

Figure 16-4 **Vessels and nodes of the lymphatic system.** **(A)** Lymph nodes and vessels of the head. **(B)** Drainage of right lymphatic duct and thoracic duct into subclavian veins.

guarded by two pocket-like semilunar valves to prevent blood from entering the duct. The rest of the body is drained by the thoracic duct.

The Thoracic Duct The **thoracic duct**, or left lymphatic duct, is the larger of the two terminal vessels, measuring approximately 40 cm (16 inches) in length. As shown in Figure 16-4, the thoracic duct receives lymph from all parts of the body except those superior to the diaphragm on the right side. This duct begins in the posterior part of the abdominal cavity, inferior to the attachment of the diaphragm. The first part of the duct is enlarged to form a cistern, or temporary storage pouch, called the **cisterna chyli** (sis-TER-nah KI-li). **Chyle** (kile) is the milky fluid that drains from the intestinal lacteals, and is formed by the combination of fat globules and lymph. Chyle passes through the intestinal lymphatic vessels and the lymph nodes of the mesentery (membrane around the intestines), finally entering the cisterna chyli. In addition to chyle, all the lymph from below the diaphragm empties into the cisterna chyli, passing through the various clusters of lymph nodes. The thoracic duct then carries this lymph into the bloodstream.

The thoracic duct extends upward through the diaphragm and along the posterior wall of the thorax into the base of the neck on the left side. Here, it receives the left jugular lymphatic vessels from the head and neck, the left subclavian vessels from the left upper extremity, and other lymphatic vessels from the thorax and its parts. In addition to the valves along the duct, there are two valves at its opening into the left subclavian vein to prevent the passage of blood into the duct.

Checkpoint 16-3 What are the two main lymphatic vessels?

Movement of Lymph

The segments of lymphatic vessels located between the valves contract rhythmically, propelling the lymph along. The contraction rate is related to the volume of fluid in the vessel—the more fluid, the more rapid the contractions.

Lymph is also moved by the same mechanisms that promote venous return of blood to the heart. As skeletal muscles contract during movement, they compress the lymphatic vessels and drive lymph forward. Changes in pressures within the abdominal and thoracic cavities caused by breathing aid the movement of lymph during passage through these body cavities. Box 16-1 describes what happens when lymph does not flow properly.

Lymphoid Tissue

Lymphoid (LIM-foyd) **tissue** is distributed throughout the body and makes up the specialized organs of the lymphatic system. The lymph nodes have already been described relative to describing lymphatic circulation, but these tissues and other components of the lymphatic system are discussed in greater detail in the next section.

Lymph Nodes

The lymph nodes, as noted, are designed to filter the lymph once it is drained from the tissues (Fig. 16-5). They are also sites where lymphocytes of the immune system multiply and work to combat foreign organisms. The lymph nodes are small, rounded masses varying from pinhead size to as long as 2.5 cm (1 inch). Each has a fibrous connective tissue capsule from which partitions (trabeculae) extend into the substance of the node. At various points in the node's surface, afferent lymphatic vessels pierce the capsule to carry lymph into the node. An indented area called the **hilum** (HI-lum) is the exit point for efferent lymphatic vessels carrying lymph out of the node. At this region, other structures, including blood vessels and nerves, connect with the node.

Each node is subdivided into lymph-filled spaces (sinuses) and cords of lymphatic tissue. Pulplike nodules in the outer region, or cortex, have germinal centers where certain immune lymphocytes multiply. The inner region, the medulla, has populations of immune cells, including lymphocytes and macrophages (phagocytes) along open channels that lead into the efferent vessels.

Lymph nodes are seldom isolated. As a rule, they are massed together in groups, varying in number from 2 or 3 to well over 100. Some of these groups are placed deeply, whereas others are superficial. The main groups include the following:

- **Cervical nodes**, located in the neck in deep and superficial groups, drain various parts of the head and neck. They often become enlarged during upper respiratory infections.
- **Axillary nodes**, located in the axillae (armpits), may become enlarged after infections of the upper extremi-

Box 16-1 Clinical Perspectives

Lymphedema: When Lymph Stops Flowing

Fluid balance in the body requires appropriate distribution of fluid among the cardiovascular system, lymphatic system, and the tissues. **Edema** occurs when the balance is tipped toward excess fluid in the tissues. Often, edema is due to heart failure. However, blockage of lymphatic vessels (and the resulting fluid accumulation in the subcutaneous tissues) can cause another form of edema called **lymphedema**. The clinical hallmark of lymphedema is chronic swelling of an arm or leg, whereas heart failure usually causes swelling of both legs.

Lymphedema may be either primary or secondary. Primary lymphedema is a rare congenital condition caused by abnormal development of lymphatic vessels. Secondary lymphedema, or acquired lymphedema, can develop as a result of trauma to a limb, surgery, radiation therapy, or infection of the lymphatic vessels (lymphangitis). One of the most common causes of lymphedema is the removal of axillary lymph nodes during mastectomy (breast removal), which disrupts lymph flow from the adjacent arm. Lymphedema may also occur following prostate surgery.

Therapies that encourage the flow of fluid through the lymphatic vessels are useful in treating lymphedema. These therapies may include elevation of the affected limb, manual lymphatic drainage through massage, light exercise, and firm wrapping of the limb to apply compression. In addition, changes in daily habits can lessen the effects of lymphedema. For example, further blockage of lymph drainage can be prevented by wearing loose clothing and jewelry, carrying a purse or handbag on the unaffected arm, and sitting with legs uncrossed. Lymphangitis requires the use of appropriate antibiotics. Prompt treatment is necessary because, in addition to swelling, other complications include poor wound healing, skin ulcers, and increased risk of infection.

Matching

Match each numbered item with the most closely related lettered item.

___ 6. Inflammation of lymphatic vessels
___ 7. Inflammation of lymph nodes
___ 8. Fluid retention due to obstruction of lymph vessels
___ 9. Tumor that occurs in lymphoid tissue

a. lymphoma
b. lymphangitis
c. lymphedema
d. lymphadenitis

Multiple choice

___ 10. Compared to plasma, lymph contains much less
a. fat
b. protein
c. carbohydrate
d. water

___ 11. Lymph from the lower extremities returns to the cardiovascular system via the
a. cisterna chyli
b. right lymphatic duct
c. thymus
d. thoracic duct

___ 12. Macrophages and monocytes found throughout the body make up the
a. tonsils
b. Peyer patches
c. reticuloendothelial system
d. appendix

___ 13. The hallmark clinical sign of infectious mononucleosis is:
a. splenomegaly
b. lymphadenopathy
c. lymphangitis
d. edema

Understanding Concepts

14. How does the structure of lymphatic capillaries correlate with their function? List some differences between lymphatic and blood capillaries.
15. Describe three mechanisms that propel lymph through the lymphatic vessels.
16. Trace a globule of fat from a lacteal in the small intestine to the right atrium.
17. Describe the structure of a typical lymph node.
18. State the location of the spleen and list several of its functions.
19. Describe two forms of lymphoma.

Conceptual Thinking

20. Explain the absence of arteries in the lymphatic circulatory system.

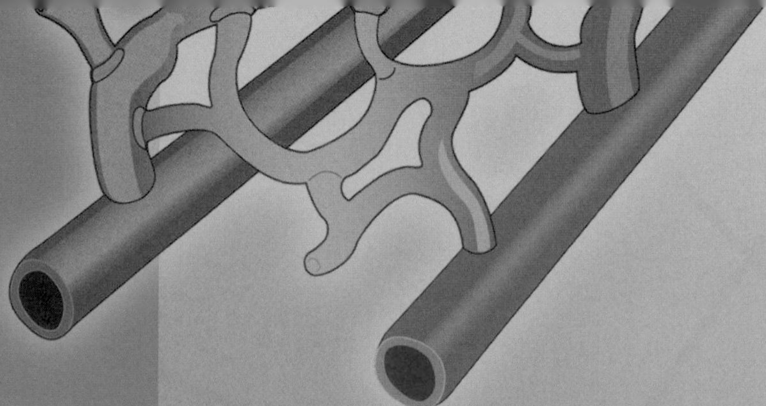

Selected Key Terms

The following terms and other boldface terms in the chapter are defined in the Glossary

allergy
anaphylaxis
antibody
antigen
antiserum
attenuated
autoimmunity
B cell
complement
gamma globulin
immunity
immunization
immunodeficiency
inflammation
interferon
interleukin
lymphocyte
macrophage
plasma cell
T cell
toxin
toxoid
transplantation
vaccine

Learning Outcomes

After careful study of this chapter, you should be able to:

1. List the factors that determine the occurrence of infection
2. Differentiate between nonspecific and specific body defenses and give examples of each
3. Briefly describe the inflammatory reaction
4. List several types of inborn immunity
5. Define *antigen* and *antibody*
6. Compare T cells and B cells with respect to development and type of activity
7. Explain the role of macrophages in immunity
8. Describe some protective effects of an antigen-antibody reaction
9. Differentiate between naturally acquired and artificially acquired immunity
10. Differentiate between active and passive immunity
11. Define the term *vaccine* and give several examples of vaccines
12. Define the term *immune serum* and give several examples of immune sera
13. List several disorders of the immune system
14. Explain the possible role of the immune system in preventing cancer
15. Explain the role of the immune system in tissue transplantation
16. Show how word parts are used to build words related to body defenses, immunity, and vaccines (see Word Anatomy at the end of the chapter)

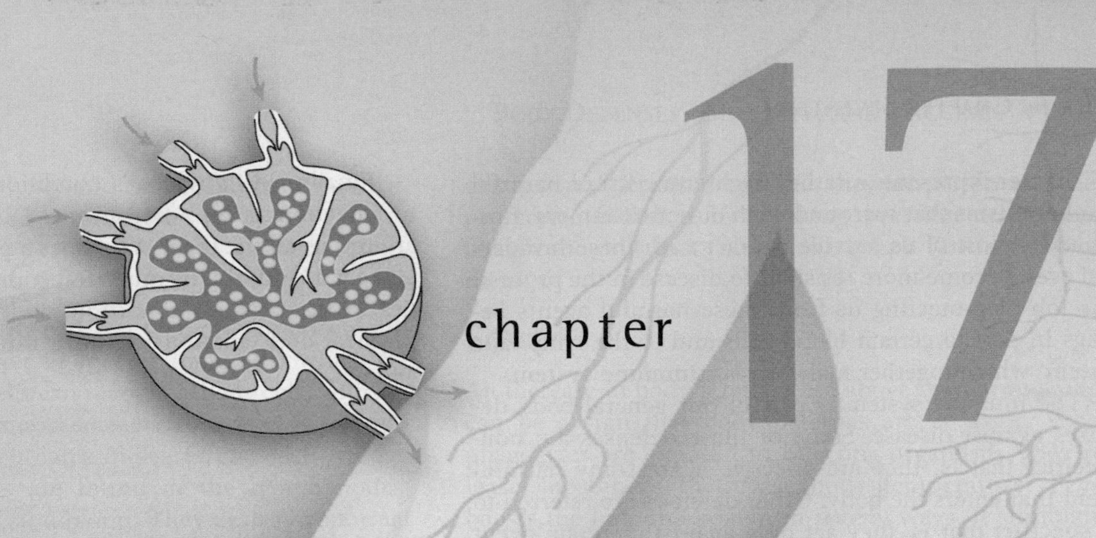

chapter 17

Body Defenses, Immunity, and Vaccines

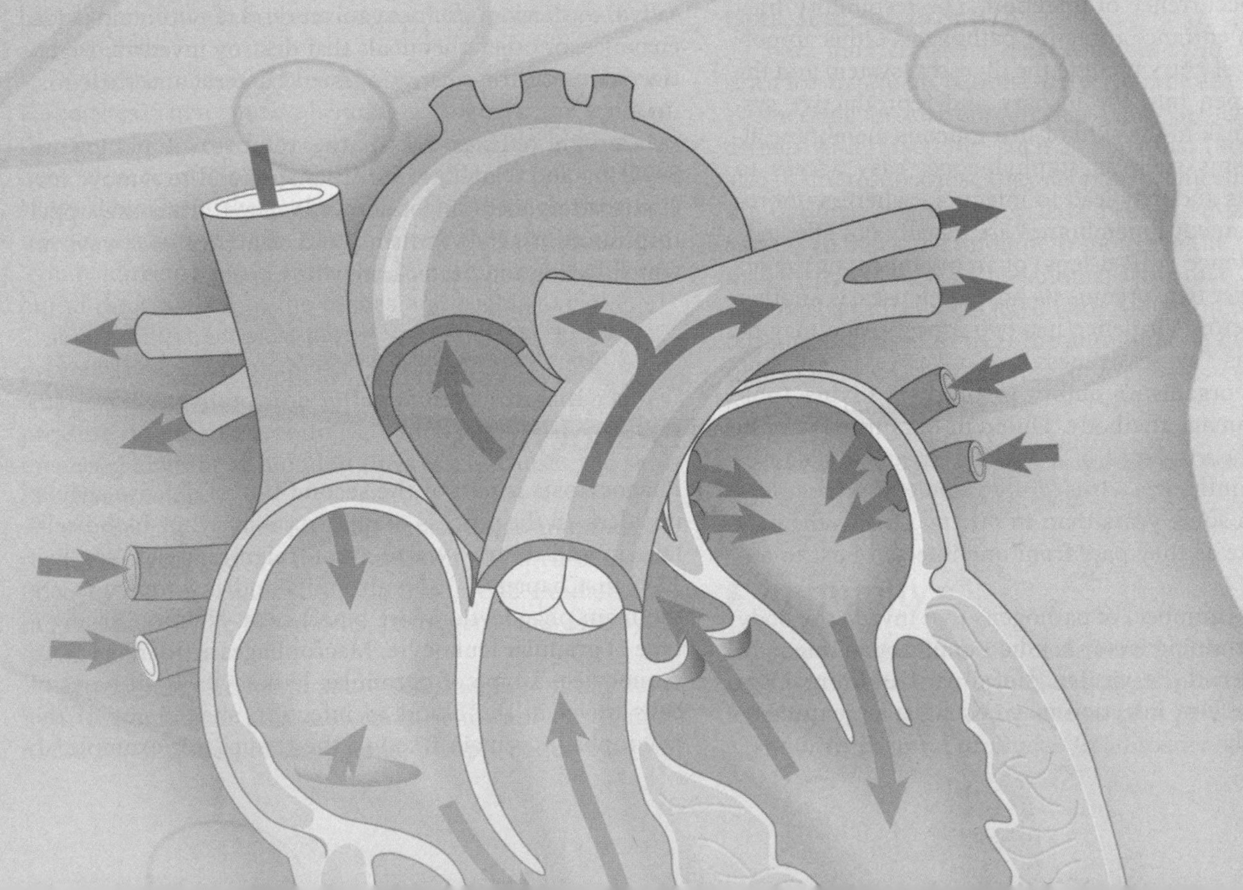

Selected Key Terms

The following terms and other boldface terms in the chapter are defined in the Glossary

alveolus (pl., alveoli)
asthma
bronchiole
bronchus (pl., bronchi)
chemoreceptor
compliance
diaphragm
emphysema
epiglottis
epistaxis
hemoglobin
hilum
hypercapnia
hypoxia
larynx
lung
mediastinum
pharynx
phrenic nerve
pleura
pneumothorax
respiration
surfactant
trachea
ventilation

Learning Outcomes

After careful study of this chapter, you should be able to:

1. Define *respiration* and describe the three phases of respiration
2. Name and describe all the structures of the respiratory system
3. Explain the mechanism for pulmonary ventilation
4. List the ways in which oxygen and carbon dioxide are transported in the blood
5. Describe nervous and chemical controls of respiration
6. Give several examples of altered breathing patterns
7. List and define four conditions that result from inadequate breathing
8. Describe several types of respiratory infection
9. Describe some allergic responses that affect the respiratory system
10. Name the diseases involved in chronic obstructive pulmonary disease (COPD)
11. Describe some disorders that involve the pleura
12. Describe equipment used to treat respiratory disorders
13. Show how word parts are used to build words related to respiration (see Word Anatomy at the end of the chapter)

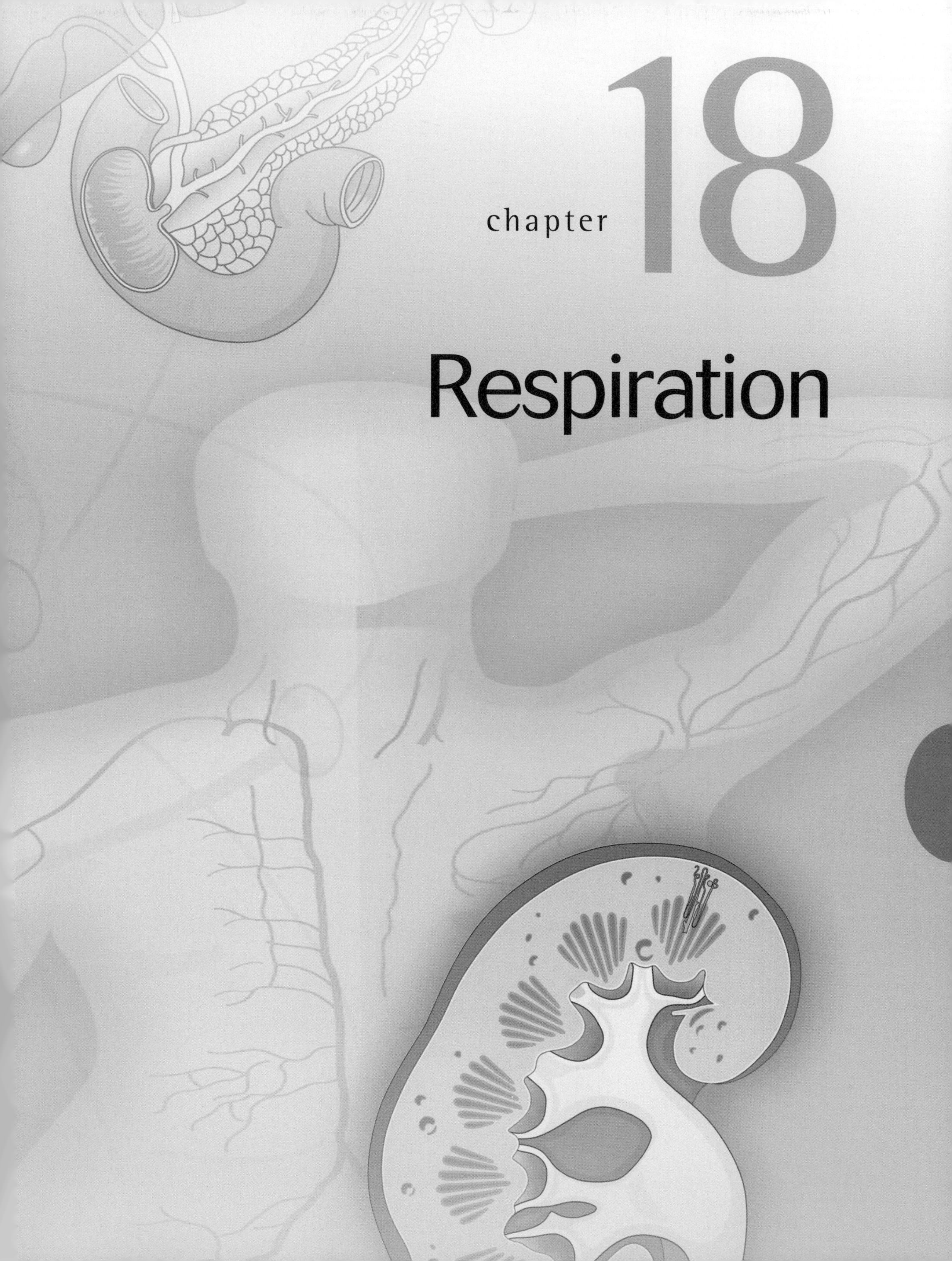

chapter 18

Respiration

Phases of Respiration

Most people think of respiration simply as the process by which air moves into and out of the lungs, that is, *breathing*. By scientific definition, respiration is the process by which oxygen is obtained from the environment and delivered to the cells. Carbon dioxide is transported to the outside in a reverse pathway (Fig. 18-1).

Respiration includes three phases:

- **Pulmonary ventilation,** which is the exchange of air between the atmosphere and the air sacs (alveoli) of the lungs. This is normally accomplished by the inhalation and exhalation of breathing.
- **External exchange of gases**, which occurs in the lungs as oxygen (O_2) diffuses from the air sacs into the blood and carbon dioxide (CO_2) diffuses out of the blood to be eliminated.
- **Internal exchange of gases**, which occurs in the tissues as oxygen diffuses from the blood to the cells, whereas carbon dioxide passes from the cells into the blood.

Gas exchange requires close association of the respiratory system with the circulatory system, as the circulating blood is needed to transport oxygen to the cells and transport carbon dioxide back to the lungs.

The term *respiration* is also used to describe a related process that occurs at the cellular level. In **cellular respiration,** oxygen is taken into a cell and used in the breakdown of nutrients with the release of energy. Carbon dioxide is the waste product of cellular respiration (see Chapter 20's discussion of metabolism).

Checkpoint 18-1 What are the three phases of respiration?

The Respiratory System

The respiratory system is an intricate arrangement of spaces and passageways that conduct air into the lungs

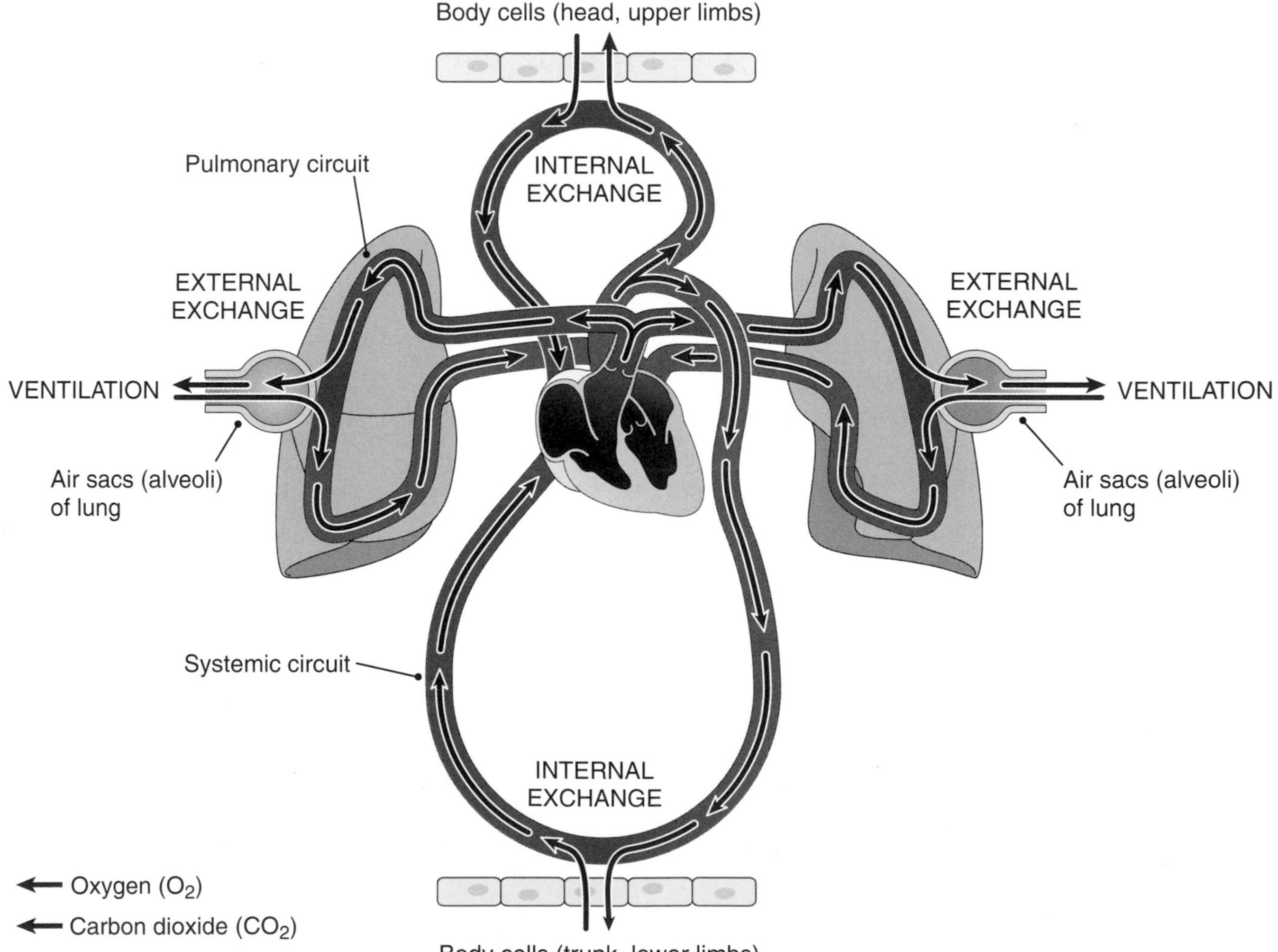

Figure 18-1 **Overview of respiration.** In ventilation, gases are moved into and out of the lungs. In external exchange, gases move between the air sacs (alveoli) of the lungs and the blood. In internal exchange, gases move between the blood and body cells. The circulation transports gases in the blood.

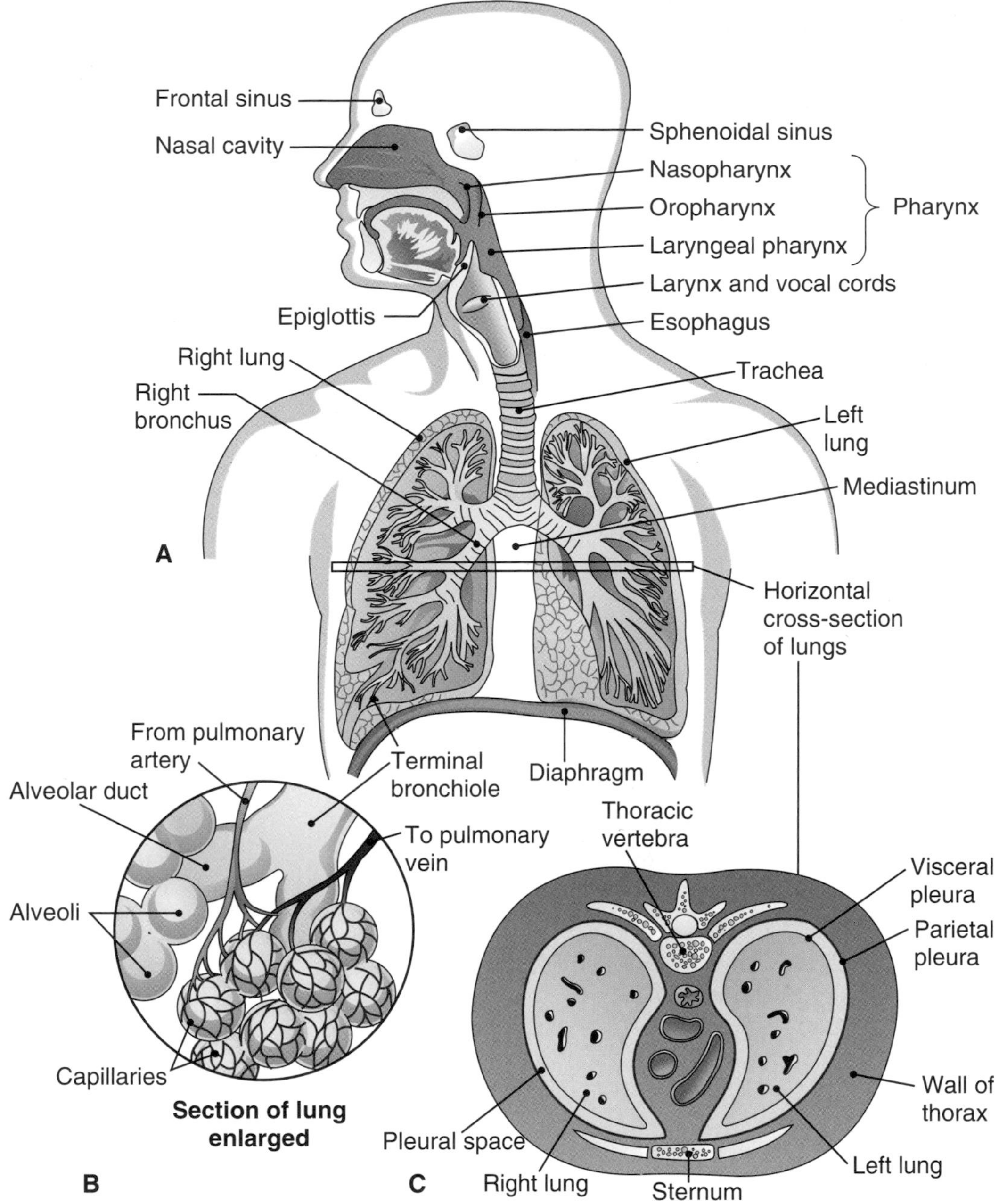

Figure 18-2 The respiratory system. (A) Overview. **(B)** Enlarged section of lung tissue showing the relationship between the alveoli (air sacs) of the lungs and the blood capillaries. **(C)** A transverse section through the lungs. *ZOOMING IN ✦ What organ is located in the medial depression of the left lung?*

(Fig. 18-2). These spaces include the **nasal cavities;** the **pharynx** (FAR-inks), which is common to the digestive and respiratory systems; the voice box, or **larynx** (LAR-inks); the windpipe, or **trachea** (TRA-ke-ah); and the **lungs** themselves, with their conducting tubes and air sacs. The entire system might be thought of as a pathway for air between the atmosphere and the blood.

The Nasal Cavities

Air enters the body through the openings in the nose called the **nostrils**, or **nares** *(NA-reze)* (sing. naris). Immediately inside the nostrils, located between the roof of the mouth and the cranium, are the two spaces known as the **nasal cavities.** These two spaces are separated from each other by a partition, the **nasal septum.** The superior portion of the septum is formed by a thin plate of the ethmoid bone that extends downward, and the inferior portion is formed by the vomer (see Fig. 7-5 A in Chapter 7). An anterior extension of the septum is made of hyaline cartilage. The septum and the walls of the nasal cavity are covered with mucous membrane. On the lateral walls of each nasal cavity are three projections called the **conchae** (KONG-ke) (see Figs. 7-5 A and 7-8 in Chapter 7). The shell-like conchae greatly increase the surface area of the mucous membrane over which air travels on its way through the nasal cavities.

The mucous membrane lining the nasal cavities contains many blood vessels that deliver heat and moisture. The cells of this membrane secrete a large amount of fluid—up to 1 quart each day. The following changes are produced in the air as it comes in contact with the lining of the nose:

- Foreign bodies, such as dust particles and pathogens, are filtered out by the hairs of the nostrils or caught in the surface mucus.
- Air is warmed by blood in the well-vascularized mucous membrane.
- Air is moistened by the liquid secretion.

To allow for these protective changes to occur, it is preferable to breathe through the nose rather than through the mouth.

The **sinuses** are small cavities lined with mucous membrane in the skull bones. They are resonating chambers for the voice and lessen the weight of the skull. The sinuses communicate with the nasal cavities, and they are highly susceptible to infection.

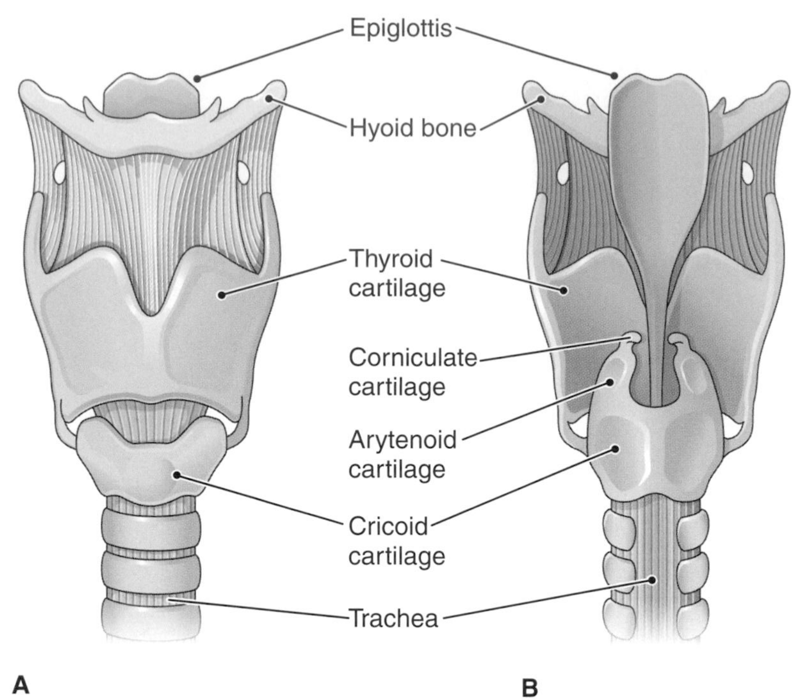

Figure 18-3 **The larynx. (A)** Anterior view. **(B)** Posterior view.

Checkpoint 18-2 What happens to air as it passes over the nasal mucosa?

The Pharynx

The muscular **pharynx,** or throat, carries air into the respiratory tract and carries foods and liquids into the digestive system (see Fig. 18-2). The superior portion, located immediately behind the nasal cavity, is called the **nasopharynx** (na-zo-FAR-inks); the middle section, located posterior to the mouth, is called the **oropharynx** (o-ro-FAR-inks); and the most inferior portion is called the **laryngeal** (lah-RIN-je-al) **pharynx.** This last section opens into the larynx toward the anterior and into the esophagus toward the posterior.

The Larynx

The **larynx,** commonly called the *voice box* (Fig. 18-3), is located between the pharynx and the trachea. It has a framework of cartilage, part of which is the thyroid cartilage that protrudes in the front of the neck. The projection formed by the thyroid cartilage is commonly called the *Adam's apple* because it is considerably larger in the male than in the female.

Folds of mucous membrane used in producing speech are located on both sides at the superior portion of the larynx. These are the vocal folds, or **vocal cords** (Fig. 18-4), which vibrate as air flows over them from the lungs. Variations in the length and tension of the vocal cords and the distance between them regulate the pitch of sound. The amount of air forced over them regulates volume. A difference in the size of the larynx and the vocal cords is what accounts for the difference between adult male and female voices. In general, a man's larynx is larger than a woman's. His vocal cords are thicker and longer, so they vibrate more slowly, resulting in a lower range of pitch. Muscles of the pharynx, tongue, lips, and face also are used to form clear pronunciations. The mouth, nasal cavities, paranasal sinuses, and the pharynx all serve as resonating chambers for speech, just as does the cabinet for an audio speaker.

The space between the vocal cords is called the **glottis** (GLOT-is). This is somewhat open during normal breathing but widely open during forced breathing (see Fig. 18-4). The little leaf-shaped cartilage that covers the larynx during swallowing is called the **epiglottis** (ep-ih-GLOT-is). The glottis and epiglottis help keep food and liquids out of the remainder of the respiratory tract. As the larynx moves upward and forward during swallowing, the epiglottis moves downward, covering the opening into the larynx. You can feel the larynx move upward toward the epiglottis during this process by placing the flat ends of your fingers on your larynx as you swallow. Muscles in the larynx assist in keeping foreign materials out of the respiratory tract by closing the glottis during swallowing. Muscles also close the glottis when one holds his or her breath and strains, as to defecate or lift a heavy weight.

The Trachea

The **trachea**, commonly called the *windpipe,* is a tube that extends from the inferior edge of the larynx to the upper part of the chest superior to the heart. The trachea's purpose is to conduct air between the larynx and the lungs.

A framework of separate cartilages reinforces the trachea and keeps it open. These cartilages, each shaped somewhat like a tiny horseshoe or the letter C, are found along the trachea's entire length. The open sections in the cartilages are lined up at their posterior so that the esophagus can expand into this region during swallowing.

Checkpoint 18-3 What are the scientific names for the throat, voice box, and windpipe?

Checkpoint 18-4 What are the three regions of the pharynx?

The Bronchi

At its inferior end, the trachea divides into two primary, or main-stem, **bronchi** (BRONG-ki), which enter the lungs (see Fig. 18-2). The right bronchus is considerably larger in diameter than the left and extends downward in a more vertical direction. Therefore, if a foreign body is inhaled, it is likely to enter the right lung. Each bronchus enters the lung at a notch or depression called the **hilum** (HI-lum). Blood vessels and nerves also connect with the lung in this region.

The Lining of the Air Passageways The trachea, bronchi, and other conducting passageways of the respiratory tract are lined with a special type of epithelium (Fig. 18-5). Basically, it is simple columnar epithelium, but the cells are arranged in such a way that they appear stratified. The tissue is thus described as *pseudostratified,* meaning "falsely stratified." These epithelial cells have cilia to filter out impurities and to create fluid movement within the conducting tubes. The cilia beat to drive impurities toward the throat, where they can be swallowed or eliminated by coughing, sneezing, or blowing the nose.

Checkpoint 18-5 The cells that line the respiratory passageways help to keep impurities out of the lungs. What feature of these cells enables them to filter impurities and move fluids?

The Lungs

The **lungs** are the organs in which gas diffusion takes place through the extremely thin and delicate lung tissues (see Fig. 18-2). The two lungs are set side by side in the thoracic (chest) cavity. Between them are the heart, the great blood vessels, and other organs of the **mediastinum** (me-de-as-TI-num), the space between the lungs, including the esophagus, trachea, and lymph nodes.

On its medial side, the left lung has an indentation that accommodates the heart. The right lung is subdivided by fissures into three lobes; the left lung is divided into two lobes. Each lobe is then further subdivided into segments and then lobules. These subdivisions correspond to subdivisions of the bronchi as they branch throughout the lungs.

Each primary bronchus enters the lung at the hilum and immediately subdivides. The right bronchus divides into three secondary bronchi, each of which enters one of the three lobes of the right lung. The left bronchus gives rise to two secondary bronchi, which enter the two lobes of the left lung. Because the bronchial subdivisions resemble the branches of a tree, they have been given the common name *bronchial tree.* The bronchi subdivide again and again, becoming progressively smaller as they branch through lung tissue.

The smallest of these conducting tubes are called **bronchioles** (BRONG-ke-oles). The bronchi contain small

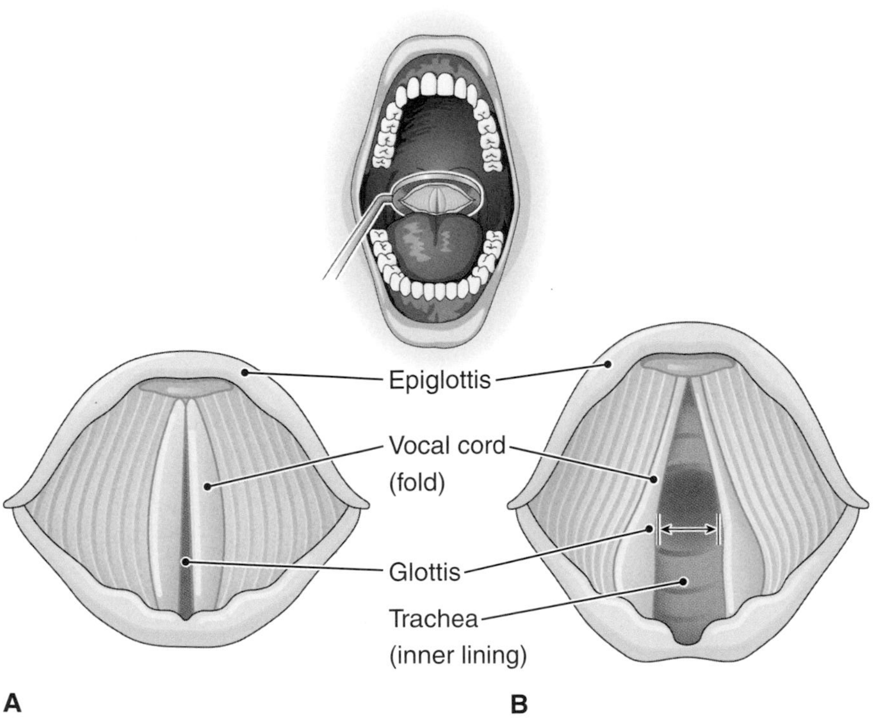

Figure 18-4 **The vocal cords, superior view. (A)** The glottis in closed position. **(B)** The glottis in open position. *ZOOMING IN ✦ What cartilage is named for its position above the glottis?*

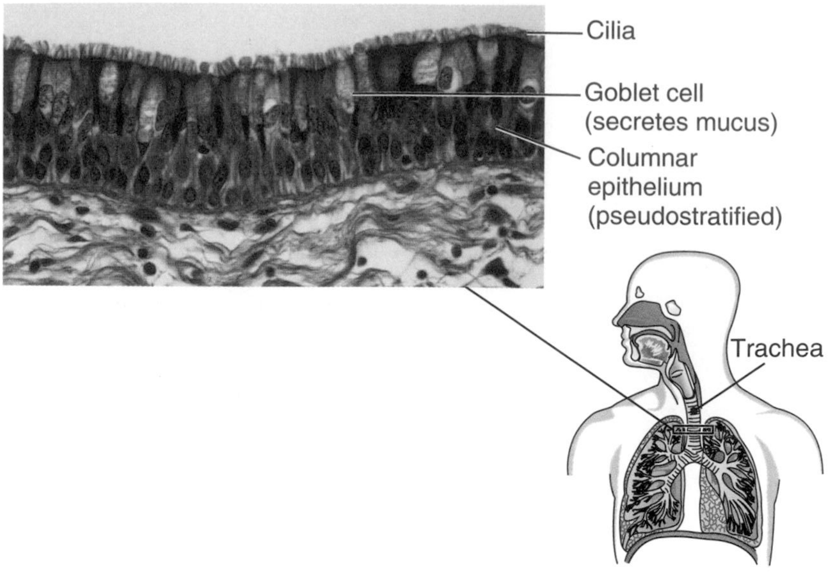

Figure 18-5 **Microscopic view of ciliated epithelium.** Ciliated epithelium lines the respiratory passageways, as shown here in the trachea. (Micrograph reprinted with permission from Cormack DH. Essential Histology. 2nd ed. Philadelphia: Lippincott Williams & Wilkins, 2001.)

bits of cartilage, which give firmness to their walls and hold the passageways open so that air can pass in and out easily. As the bronchi become smaller, however, the cartilage decreases in amount. In the bronchioles, there is no cartilage at all; what remains is mostly smooth muscle, which is under the control of the autonomic (involuntary) nervous system.

The Alveoli At the end of the **terminal bronchioles,** the smallest subdivisions of the bronchial tree, there are clusters of tiny air sacs in which most gas exchange takes place. These sacs are known as **alveoli** (al-VE-o-li) (sing. alveolus) (see Fig. 18-2). The wall of each alveolus is made of a single-cell layer of squamous (flat) epithelium. This thin wall provides easy passage for the gases entering and leaving the blood as the blood circulates through the millions of tiny capillaries covering the alveoli.

Certain cells in the alveolar wall produce **surfactant** (sur-FAK-tant), a substance that reduces the surface tension ("pull") of the fluids that line the alveoli. This surface action prevents collapse of the alveoli and eases expansion of the lungs.

There are about 300 million alveoli in the human lungs. The resulting surface area in contact with gases approximates 60 square meters (some books say even more). This area is equivalent, as an example, to the floor surface of a classroom that measures about 24 by 24 feet. As with many other systems in the body, there is great functional reserve; we have about three times as much lung tissue as is minimally necessary to sustain life. Because of the many air spaces, the lung is light in weight; normally, a piece of lung tissue dropped into a glass of water will float. Figure 18-6 shows a microscopic view of lung tissue.

The pulmonary circuit brings blood to and from the lungs. In the lungs, blood passes through the capillaries around the alveoli, where gas exchange takes place.

The Lung Cavities and Pleura

The lungs occupy a considerable portion of the thoracic cavity, which is separated from the abdominal cavity by the muscular partition known as the **diaphragm.** A continuous doubled sac, the **pleura,** covers each lung. The two layers of the pleura are named according to location. The portion of the pleura that is attached to the chest wall is the **parietal pleura,** and the portion that is attached to the surface of the lung is called the **visceral pleura.** Each closed sac completely surrounds the lung, except in the place where the bronchus and blood vessels enter the lung, a region known as the *root* of the lung.

Between the two layers of the pleura is the **pleural space** containing a thin film of fluid that lubricates the membranes. The effect of this fluid is the same as between two flat pieces of glass joined by a film of water; that is, the surfaces slide easily on each other but strongly resist separation. Thus, the lungs are able to move and enlarge effortlessly in response to changes in the thoracic volume that occur during breathing.

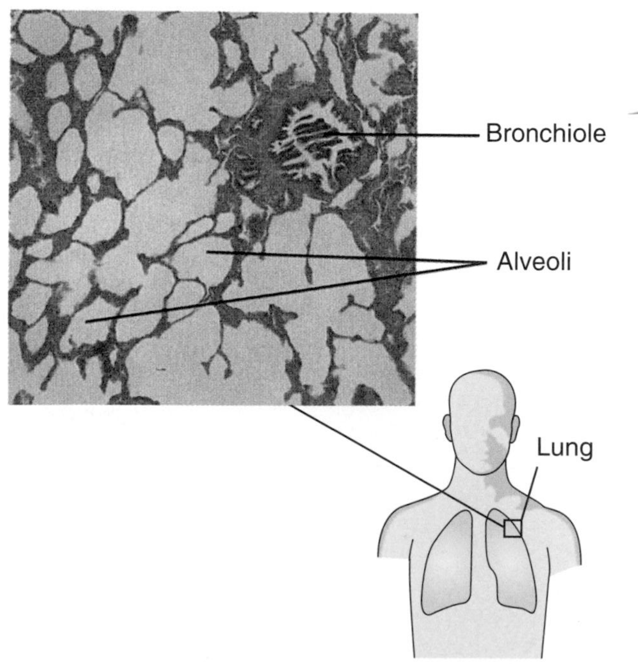

Figure 18-6 **Lung tissue viewed through a microscope.** (Micrograph courtesy of Dana Morse Bittus and BJ Cohen.)

Checkpoint 18-6 In what structures does gas exchange occur in the lung?

Checkpoint 18-7 What is the name of the membrane that encloses the lung?

The Process of Respiration

Respiration involves ventilation of the lungs, exchange of gases, and their transport in the blood. Respiratory needs are met by central and peripheral controls of breathing.

Pulmonary Ventilation

Ventilation is the movement of air into and out of the lungs, normally accomplished by breathing. There are two phases of ventilation (Fig. 18-7):

- **Inhalation**, or inspiration, is the drawing of air into the lungs.
- **Exhalation**, or expiration, is the expulsion of air from the lungs.

In **inhalation**, the active phase of breathing, respiratory muscles contract to enlarge the thoracic cavity. During quiet breathing, the movement of the diaphragm accounts for most of the increase in thoracic volume. The diaphragm is a strong, dome-shaped muscle attached to the body wall around the base of the rib cage. The contraction and flattening of the diaphragm cause a piston-like downward motion that increases the vertical dimension of the chest. Other muscles that participate in breathing are the external and internal intercostal muscles. These muscles run at different angles in two layers between the ribs. As the external intercostals contract for inhalation, they lift the rib cage upward and outward. Put the palms of your hands on either side of the rib cage to feel this action as you inhale. During forceful inhalation, the rib cage is moved further up and out by contraction of muscles in the neck and chest wall.

As the thoracic cavity increases in size, gas pressure within the cavity decreases. This phenomenon follows a law in physics stating that when the volume of a given amount of gas increases, the pressure of the gas decreases. Conversely, when the volume decreases, the pressure increases. If you blow air into a tight balloon that does not expand very much, the gas particles are in close contact and will hit the wall of the balloon frequently, creating greater pressure (Fig. 18-8). If you tap this balloon, it will spring back to its original shape. When you blow into a soft balloon that expands easily under pressure, the gas particles spread out into a larger area and will not hit the balloon's wall as often. If you tap the balloon, your finger will make an indentation. Thus, pressure in the chest cavity drops as the thorax expands. When the pressure drops to slightly below the air pressure outside the lungs, air is drawn into the lungs, as by suction.

The ease with which one can expand the lungs and thorax is called **compliance**. Normal elasticity of the lung tissue, aided by surfactant, allows the lungs to expand under pressure and fill adequately with air during inhalation. Compliance is decreased when the lungs resist expansion. Conditions that can decrease compliance include diseases that damage or scar lung tissue, fluid accumulation in the lungs, deficiency of surfactant, and interference with the action of breathing muscles.

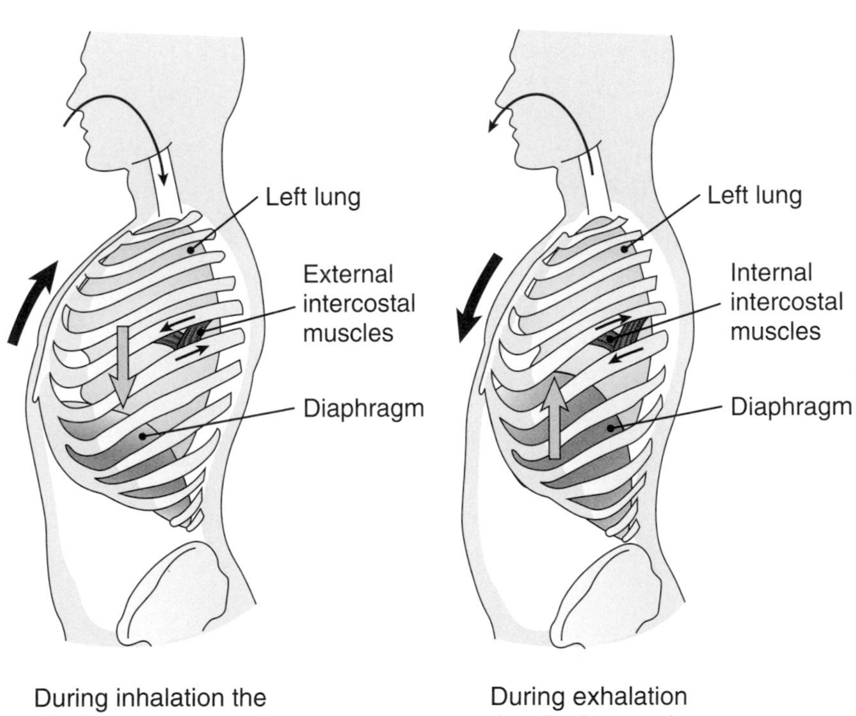

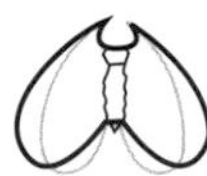

A. Action of rib cage in inhalation

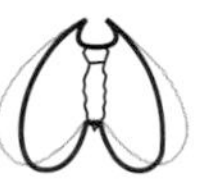

B. Action of rib cage in exhalation

Figure 18-7 **Pulmonary ventilation. (A)** Inhalation. **(B)** Exhalation. *ZOOMING IN ✦ What muscles are located between the ribs?*

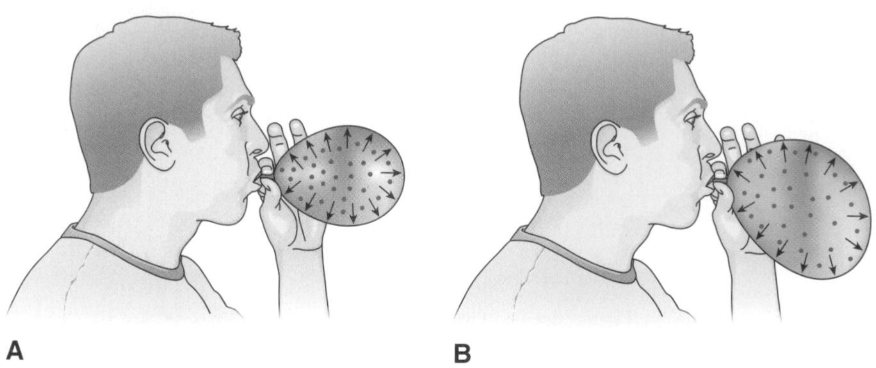

Figure 18-8 The relationship of gas pressure to volume. (A) Inflation of a stiff balloon creates strong air pressure against the wall of the balloon. **(B)** The same amount of air in a soft balloon spreads out into the available space, resulting in lower gas pressure. *ZOOMING IN ✦ What happens to gas pressure as the volume of its container increases?*

Air enters the respiratory passages and flows through the ever-dividing tubes of the bronchial tree. As the air traverses this route, it moves more and more slowly through the great number of bronchial tubes until there is virtually no forward flow as it reaches the alveoli. The incoming air mixes with the residual air remaining in the respiratory passageways, so that the gases soon are evenly distributed. Each breath causes relatively little change in the gas composition of the alveoli, but normal continuous breathing ensures the presence of adequate oxygen and the removal of carbon dioxide.

In **exhalation,** the passive phase of breathing, the respiratory muscles relax, allowing the ribs and diaphragm to return to their original positions. The lung tissues are elastic and recoil to their original size during exhalation. Surface tension within the alveoli aids in this return to resting size. During forced exhalation, the internal intercostal muscles contract, pulling the bottom of the rib cage in and down. The muscles of the abdominal wall contract, pushing the abdominal viscera upward against the relaxed diaphragm.

Table 18-1 gives the definitions and average values for some of the breathing volumes and capacities that are important in evaluating respiratory function. A lung *capacity* is a sum of volumes. These same values are shown on a graph as they might appear on a tracing made by a **spirometer** (spi-ROM-eh-ter), an instrument for recording lung volumes (Fig. 18-9). The tracing is a **spirogram** (SPI-ro-gram).

Checkpoint 18-8 What are the two phases of breathing? Which is active and which is passive?

Table 18•1 Lung Volumes and Capacities

VOLUME	DEFINITION	AVERAGE VALUE (mL)
Tidal volume	The amount of air moved into or out of the lungs in quiet, relaxed breathing	500
Residual volume	The volume of air that remains in the lungs after maximum exhalation	1200
Inspiratory reserve volume	The additional amount that can be breathed in by force after a normal inhalation	2600
Expiratory reserve volume	The additional amount that can be breathed out by force after a normal exhalation	900
Vital capacity	The volume of air that can be expelled from the lungs by maximum exhalation after maximum inhalation	4000
Functional residual capacity	The amount of air remaining in the lungs after normal exhalation	2100
Total lung capacity	The total volume of air that can be contained in the lungs after maximum inhalation	5200

Gas Exchange

External exchange is the movement of gases between the alveoli and the capillary blood in the lungs (see Fig. 18-1). The barrier that separates alveolar air from the blood is composed of the alveolar wall and the capillary wall, both of which are extremely thin. This respiratory membrane is not only very thin, it is also moist. The moisture is important because the oxygen and carbon dioxide must go into solution before they can diffuse across the membrane. Recall that **diffusion** refers to the movement of molecules from an area in which they are in higher concentration to an area in which they are in lower concentration. Therefore, the relative concentrations of a gas on the two sides of a membrane determine the direction of diffusion. Normally, inspired air contains about 21% oxygen and 0.04% carbon dioxide; expired air has only 16% oxygen and 3.5% carbon dioxide. These values illustrate that a two-way diffusion takes place through the walls of the alveoli and capillaries (Fig. 18-10).

Internal exchange takes place between the blood and the tissues. In metabolism, the cells constantly consume oxygen and produce carbon dioxide. Based on relative concentrations of these gases, oxygen diffuses out of the blood and carbon dioxide enters.

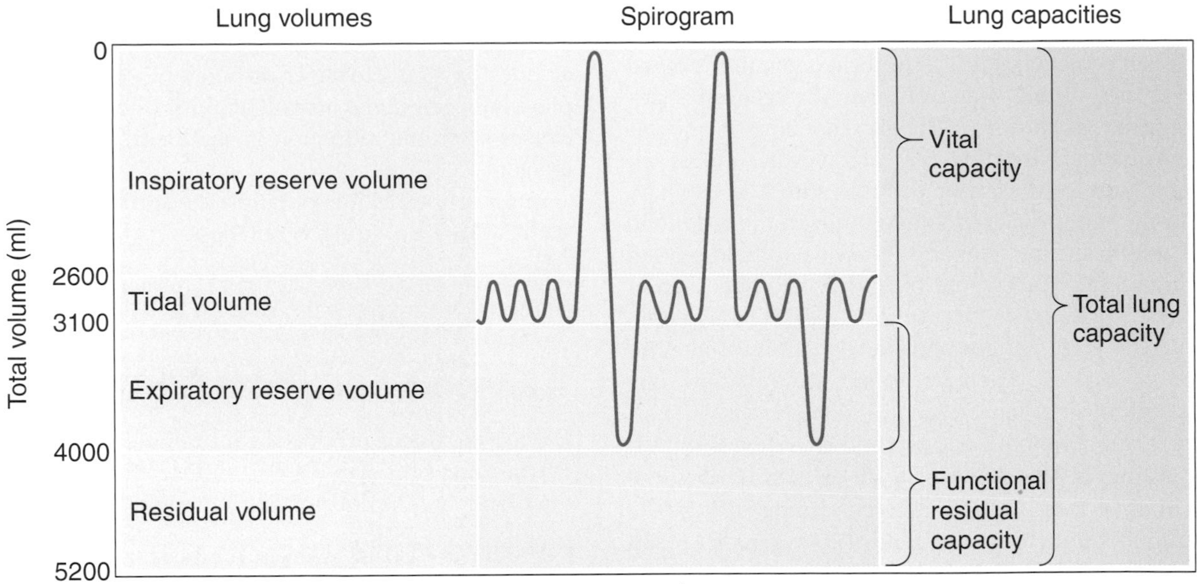

Figure 18-9 A spirogram. The tracing of lung volumes is made with a spirometer. *ZOOMING IN ✦ What lung volume cannot be measured with a spirometer?*

At this point, blood returning from the tissues and entering the lung capillaries through the pulmonary circuit is relatively low in oxygen and high in carbon dioxide. Again, the blood will pick up oxygen and give up carbon dioxide. After a return to the left side of the heart, it starts once more on its route through the systemic circuit.

> **Checkpoint 18-9** Gases move between the alveoli and the blood by the process of diffusion. What is the definition of diffusion?

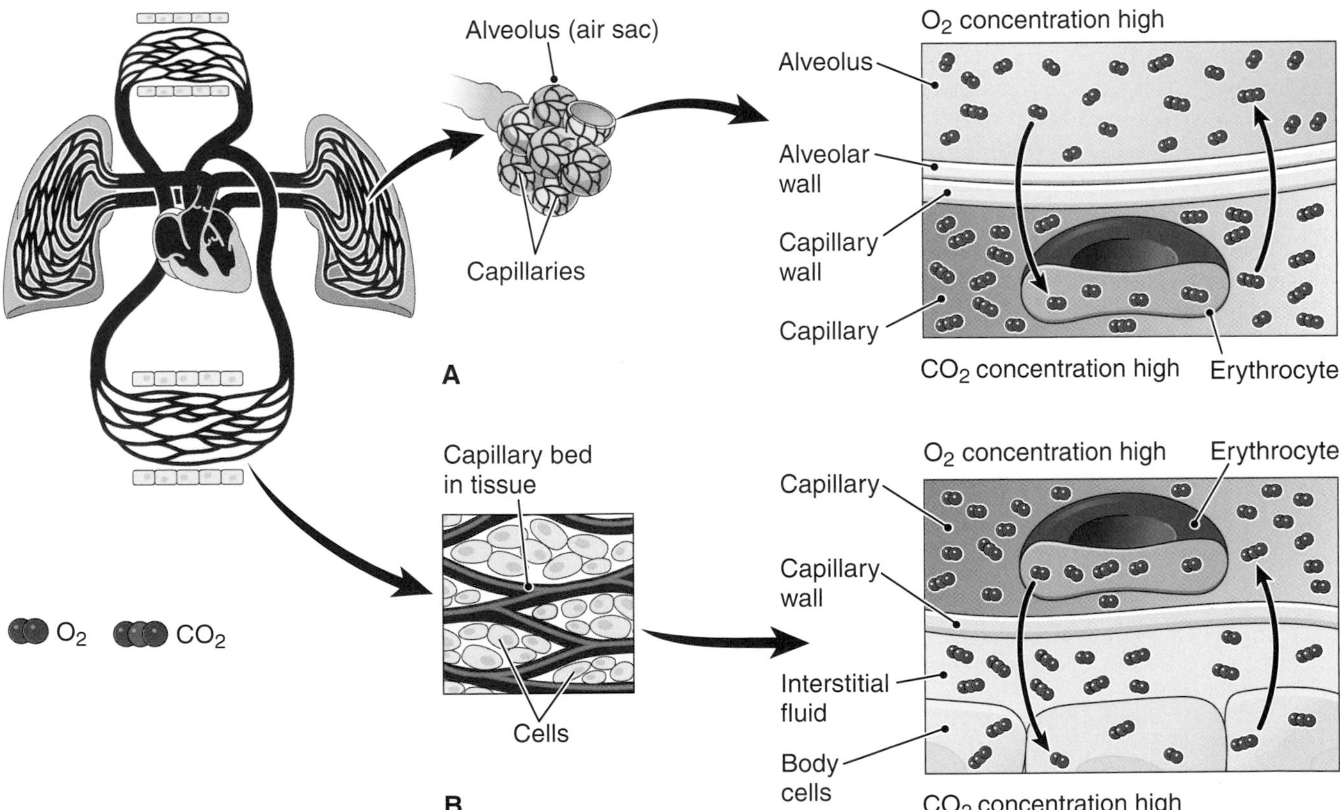

Figure 18-10 Gas exchange. (A) External exchange between the alveoli and the blood. Oxygen diffuses into the blood and carbon dioxide diffuses out, based on concentrations of the two gases in the alveoli and in the blood. **(B)** Internal exchange between the blood and the cells. Oxygen diffuses out of the blood and into tissues, while carbon dioxide diffuses from the cells into the blood.

Transport of Oxygen

A very small percentage (1.5%) of the oxygen in the blood is carried in solution in the plasma. (Oxygen does dissolve in water, as shown by the fact that aquatic animals get their oxygen from water.) However, almost all (98.5%) of the oxygen that diffuses into the capillary blood in the lungs binds to **hemoglobin** in the red blood cells. If not for hemoglobin and its ability to hold oxygen in the blood, the heart would have to work much harder to supply enough oxygen to the tissues. The hemoglobin molecule is a large protein with four small iron-containing "heme" regions. Each heme portion can bind one molecule of oxygen.

Oxygenated blood (in systemic arteries and pulmonary veins) is 97% saturated with oxygen. That is, the total hemoglobin in the red cells is holding 97% of the maximum amount that it can hold. Deoxygenated blood (in systemic veins and pulmonary arteries) is usually about 70% saturated with oxygen. This 27% difference represents the oxygen that has been taken up by the cells. Note, however, that even blood that is described as deoxygenated still has a reserve of oxygen. Even under conditions of high oxygen consumption, as in vigorous exercise, for example, the blood is never totally depleted of oxygen.

In clinical practice, gas concentrations are expressed as pressure in millimeters of mercury (mmHg), as is blood pressure. Because air is a mixture of gases, each gas exerts only a portion of the total pressure, or a **partial pressure** (P). The partial pressures of oxygen and carbon dioxide are symbolized as Po_2 and Pco_2 respectively.

To enter the cells, oxygen must separate from hemoglobin. Normally, the bond between oxygen and hemoglobin is easily broken, and oxygen is released as blood travels into areas where the oxygen concentration is relatively low. Cells are constantly using oxygen in metabolism and obtaining fresh supplies by diffusion from the blood.

The poisonous gas, carbon monoxide (CO) at low partial pressure binds with hemoglobin at the same sites as does oxygen. However, it binds more tightly and displaces oxygen. Even a small amount of carbon monoxide causes a serious reduction in the blood's ability to carry oxygen.

For an interesting variation on normal gas transport, see Box 18-1 on liquid ventilation.

Checkpoint 18-10 What substance in red blood cells carries almost all of the oxygen in the blood?

Transport of Carbon Dioxide

Carbon dioxide is produced continuously in the tissues as a byproduct of metabolism. It diffuses from the cells into the blood and is transported to the lungs in three ways:

- About 10% is dissolved in the plasma and in the fluid within red blood cells. (Carbonated beverages are examples of water in which CO_2 is dissolved.)
- About 15% is combined with the protein portion of hemoglobin and plasma proteins.
- About 75% is transported as an ion, known as a **bicarbonate ion**, which is formed when carbon dioxide undergoes a chemical change after it dissolves in blood fluids.

The bicarbonate ion is formed slowly in the plasma but much more rapidly inside the red blood cells, where an enzyme called **carbonic anhydrase** (an-HI-drase) increases the speed of the reaction. The bicarbonate formed in the red blood cells moves to the plasma and then is carried to the lungs. In the lungs, the process is reversed as bicarbonate reenters the red blood cells and releases carbon dioxide for diffusion into the alveoli and exhalation. For those with a background in chemistry, the equation for these reactions follows. The arrows going in both directions signify that the reactions are reversible. The

Box 18-1 **Clinical Perspectives**

Liquid Ventilation: Breath in a Bottle

Researchers have been attempting for years to develop a fluid that could transport high concentrations of oxygen in the body. Such a fluid could substitute for blood in transfusions or be used to carry oxygen into the lungs. Early work on liquid ventilation climaxed in the mid-1960s when a pioneer in this field submerged a laboratory mouse in a beaker of fluid and the animal survived total immersion for more than 10 minutes. The fluid was a synthetic substance that could hold as much oxygen as does air.

A newer version of this fluid, a fluorine-containing chemical known as PFC, has been tested to ventilate the collapsed lungs of premature babies. In addition to delivering oxygen to the lung alveoli, it also removes carbon dioxide. The fluid is less damaging to delicate lung tissue than is air, which has to be pumped in under higher pressure. Others who might benefit from liquid ventilation include people whose lungs have been damaged by infection, inhaled toxins, asthma, emphysema, and lung cancer, but more clinical research is required. Scientists are also investigating whether liquid ventilation could be used to deliver drugs directly to lung tissue.

upper arrows describe what happens as CO_2 enters the blood; the lower arrows indicate what happens as CO_2 is released from the blood to be exhaled from the lungs.

$$\underset{\text{carbon dioxide}}{CO_2} + \underset{\text{water}}{H_2O} \rightleftarrows \underset{\text{carbonic acid}}{H_2CO_3} \rightleftarrows \underset{\text{hydrogen ion}}{H^+} + \underset{\text{bicarbonate ion}}{HCO_3^-}$$

Carbon dioxide is important in regulating the blood's pH (acid–base balance). As a bicarbonate ion is formed from carbon dioxide in the plasma, a hydrogen ion (H^+) is also produced. Therefore, the blood becomes more acidic as the amount of carbon dioxide in the blood increases to yield more hydrogen and bicarbonate ions. The exhalation of carbon dioxide shifts the blood's pH more toward the alkaline (basic) range. The bicarbonate ion is also an important buffer in the blood, acting chemically to help keep the pH of body fluids within a steady range of 7.35 to 7.45.

Checkpoint 18-11 What is the main form in which carbon dioxide is carried in the blood?

Regulation of Respiration

Centers in the central nervous system control the fundamental respiratory pattern. This pattern is modified by special receptors that detect changes in the blood's chemical composition.

Nervous Control Regulation of respiration is a complex process that must keep pace with moment-to-moment changes in cellular oxygen requirements and carbon dioxide production. Regulation depends primarily on a respiratory control center located partly in the medulla and partly in the pons of the brain stem. The control center's main part, located in the medulla, sets the basic pattern of respiration. This pattern can be modified by centers in the pons. These areas continuously regulate breathing, so that levels of oxygen, carbon dioxide, and acid are kept within normal limits.

From the respiratory center in the medulla, motor nerve fibers extend into the spinal cord. From the cervical (neck) part of the cord, these nerve fibers continue through the **phrenic** (FREN-ik) **nerve** (a branch of the vagus nerve) to the diaphragm. The diaphragm and the other respiratory muscles are voluntary in the sense that they can be regulated consciously by messages from the higher brain centers, notably the cerebral cortex. It is possible for a person to deliberately breathe more rapidly or more slowly or to hold his or her breath and not breathe at all for a while. In a short time, however, the respiratory center in the brain stem will override the voluntary desire to not breathe, and breathing will resume. Most of the time, we breathe without thinking about it, and the respiratory center is in control.

Checkpoint 18-12 What part of the brain stem sets the basic pattern of respiration?

Checkpoint 18-13 What is the name of the motor nerve that controls the diaphragm?

Chemical Control Of vital importance in the control of respiration are **chemoreceptors** (ke-mo-re-SEP-tors) which, like the receptors for taste and smell, are sensitive to chemicals dissolved in body fluids. The chemoreceptors that regulate respiration are located centrally (near the brain stem) and peripherally (in arteries).

The central chemoreceptors are on either side of the brain stem near the medullary respiratory center. These receptors respond to the CO_2 level in circulating blood, but the gas acts indirectly. CO_2 is capable of diffusing through the capillary blood-brain barrier. It dissolves in CSF (the fluid in and around the brain) and separates into hydrogen ion and bicarbonate ion, as explained previously. It is the presence of hydrogen ion and its effect in lowering pH that actually stimulates the central chemoreceptors. The rise in blood CO_2 level, known as **hypercapnia** (hi-per-KAP-ne-ah), thus triggers ventilation.

The peripheral chemoreceptors that regulate respiration are found in structures called the *carotid* and *aortic bodies*. The carotid bodies are located near the bifurcation (forking) of the common carotid arteries in the neck, whereas the aortic bodies are located in the aortic arch. These bodies contain sensory neurons that respond mainly to a decrease in oxygen supply. They are not usually involved in regulating breathing, because they don't act until oxygen drops to a very low level. Because there is usually an ample reserve of oxygen in the blood, carbon dioxide has the most immediate effect in regulating respiration at the level of the central chemoreceptors. When the carbon dioxide level increases, breathing must be increased to blow off the excess gas. Oxygen only becomes a controlling factor when its level falls considerably below normal.

Checkpoint 18-14 What gas is the main chemical controller of respiration?

Abnormal Ventilation

In **hyperventilation** (hi-per-ven-tih-LA-shun), an increased amount of air enters the alveoli. This condition results from deep and rapid respiration that commonly occurs during anxiety attacks, or when a person is experiencing pain or other forms of stress. Hyperventilation causes an increase in the oxygen level and a decrease in the carbon dioxide level of the blood, a condition called **hypocapnia** (hi-po-KAP-ne-ah). The loss of carbon dioxide increases the blood's pH (alkalosis) by removing acidic products, as shown by the equation cited previously. The change in pH results in dizziness and tingling sensations. Breathing may stop because the respiratory control center is not stimulated. Gradually, the carbon dioxide level returns to normal, and a regular breathing pattern is resumed. In extreme cases, a person may faint, and then breathing will involuntarily return to normal. In assisting a person who is hyperventilating, one should speak calmly, reassure him or her that the situation is not dangerous, and encourage even breathing from the diaphragm.

In **hypoventilation,** an insufficient amount of air enters the alveoli. The many possible causes of this condition include respiratory obstruction, lung disease, injury to the respiratory center, depression of the respiratory center, as by drugs, and chest deformity. Hypoventilation results in an increase in the carbon dioxide concentration in the blood, leading to a decrease in the blood's pH (acidosis), again according to the equation previously mentioned.

Breathing Patterns

Normal rates of breathing vary from 12 to 20 times per minute for adults. In children, rates may vary from 20 to 40 times per minute, depending on age and size. In infants, the respiratory rate may be more than 40 times per minute. Changes in respiratory rates are important in various disorders and should be recorded carefully. To determine the respiratory rate, the healthcare worker counts the client's breathing for at least 30 seconds, usually by watching the chest rise and fall with each inhalation and exhalation. The count is then multiplied to obtain the rate in breaths per minute. It is best if the person does not realize that he or she is being observed because awareness of the measurement may cause a change in the breathing rate.

Some Terms for Altered Breathing The following is a list of terms designating various abnormalities of respiration. These are symptoms, not diseases. Note that the word ending *-pnea* refers to breathing.

- **Hyperpnea** (hi-PERP-ne-ah) refers to an abnormal increase in the depth and rate of respiration.
- **Hypopnea** (hi-POP-ne-ah) is a decrease in the rate and depth of breathing.
- **Tachypnea** (tak-IP-ne-ah) is an excessive rate of breathing that may be normal, as in exercise.
- **Apnea** (AP-ne-ah) is a temporary cessation of breathing. Short periods of apnea occur normally during deep sleep. More severe sleep apnea can result from obstruction of the respiratory passageways or, less commonly, by failure in the central respiratory center.
- **Dyspnea** (disp-NE-ah) is a subjective feeling of difficult or labored breathing.
- **Orthopnea** (or-THOP-ne-ah) refers to a difficulty in breathing that is relieved by sitting in an upright position, either against two pillows in bed or in a chair.
- **Kussmaul** (KOOS-mowl) **respiration** is deep, rapid respiration characteristic of acidosis (overly acidic body fluids) as seen in uncontrolled diabetes.
- **Cheyne-Stokes** (CHANE-stokes) **respiration** is a rhythmic variation in the depth of respiratory movements alternating with periods of apnea. It is caused by depression of the breathing centers and is seen in certain critically ill patients.

Results of Inadequate Breathing Conditions that may result from decreased respiration include the following:

- **Cyanosis** (si-ah-NO-sis) is a bluish color of the skin and mucous membranes caused by an insufficient amount of oxygen in the blood.
- **Hypoxia** (hi-POK-se-ah) means a lower than normal oxygen level in the tissues. The term anoxia (ah-NOK-se-ah) is sometimes used instead, but is not as accurate because it means a total lack of oxygen.

Box 18-2 A Closer Look

Adaptations to High Altitude: Living With Hypoxia

Our bodies work best at low altitudes where oxygen is plentiful. However, people are able to live at high altitudes where oxygen is scarce and can even survive climbing Mount Everest, the tallest peak on our planet, showing that the human body can adapt to hypoxic conditions. This adaptation process compensates for decreased atmospheric oxygen by increasing the efficiency of the respiratory and cardiovascular systems.

The body's immediate response to high altitude is to increase the rate of ventilation (hyperventilation) and raise heart rate to increase cardiac output. Hyperventilation makes more oxygen available to the cells and increases blood pH (alkalosis), which boosts hemoglobin's capacity to bind oxygen. Over time, the body adapts in additional ways. Hypoxia stimulates the kidneys to secrete erythropoietin, prompting red bone marrow to manufacture more erythrocytes and hemoglobin. Also, capillaries proliferate, increasing blood flow to the tissues. Some people are unable to adapt to high altitudes, and for them, hypoxia and alkalosis lead to potentially fatal **altitude sickness.**

Successful adaptation to high altitude illustrates the principle of homeostasis and also helps to explain how the body adjusts to hypoxia associated with disorders such as chronic obstructive pulmonary disease.

- **Hypoxemia** (hi-pok-SE-me-ah) refers to a lower than normal oxygen concentration in arterial blood.
- **Suffocation** is the cessation of respiration, often the result of a mechanical blockage of the respiratory passages.

Box 18-2 offers information on adjusting to high altitudes and other hypoxic conditions.

Disorders of the Respiratory System

Infection is a major cause of respiratory disorders. These may involve any portion of the system. Allergies and environmental factors also affect respiration, and lung cancer is a major cause of cancer deaths in both men and women.

Disorders of the Nasal Cavities and Related Structures

The paranasal sinuses are located in the skull bones in the vicinity of the nasal cavities. Infection may easily travel into these sinuses from the mouth, nose, and throat along the mucous membranes that line them. The resulting inflammation is called **sinusitis.** Chronic (long-standing) sinus infection may cause changes in the epithelial cells, resulting in tumor formation. Some of these growths have a grapelike appearance and cause obstruction of the air pathway; these tumors are called **polyps** (POL-ips).

The partition separating the two nasal cavities is called the *nasal septum.* Because of minor structural defects, the nasal septum is rarely exactly in the midline. If it is markedly to one side, it is described as a **deviated septum.** In this condition, one nasal space may be considerably smaller than the other. If an affected person has an attack of hay fever or develops a cold with accompanying swelling of the mucosa, the smaller nasal cavity may be completely closed. Sometimes, the septum is curved in such a way that both nasal cavities are occluded, forcing the person to breathe through his or her mouth. Such an occlusion may also prevent proper drainage from the sinuses and aggravate a case of sinusitis.

The most common cause of nosebleed, also called **epistaxis** (ep-e-STAK-sis) (from a Greek word meaning "to drip"), is injury to the mucous membranes in the nasal cavity. Causes of injury include infection, drying of the membranes, picking the nose, or other forms of trauma. These simple nosebleeds usually stop on their own, but some measures that help are applying pressure to the upper lip under the nose, pinching the nose together, or applying ice to the forehead. Epistaxis may signal more serious problems, such as blood clotting abnormalities, excessively high blood pressure, or tumors. Serious injuries that lead to nosebleed, or a nosebleed that will not stop, require professional medical care. Treatment may include packing the nose with gauze or other material, administering vasoconstrictors, or cauterizing the wound.

Infection

The respiratory tract mucosa is one of the most important portals of entry for disease-producing organisms. The transfer of disease organisms from the respiratory system of one person to that of another occurs most rapidly in crowded places, such as schools, theaters, and institutions. Droplets from one sneeze may be loaded with many billions of disease-producing organisms.

To some degree, the mucous membranes can protect themselves by producing larger quantities of mucus. The runny nose, an unpleasant symptom of the common cold, is the body's attempt to wash away the pathogens and protect deeper tissues from further infection. If the resistance of the mucous membrane is reduced, however, the membrane may act as a pathway for the spread of disease. The infection may travel along the membrane into the nasal sinuses, or middle ear, along the respiratory passageways, or into the lung. Each infection is named according to the part involved, such as pharyngitis (commonly called a *sore throat*), laryngitis, or bronchitis.

Among the infections transmitted through the respiratory passageways are the common cold, diphtheria, chickenpox, measles, influenza, pneumonia, and tuberculosis. Any infection that is confined to the nose and throat is called an **upper respiratory infection** (URI). Very often, an upper respiratory infection is the first evidence of infectious disease in children. Such an infection may precede the onset of a serious disease, such as rheumatic fever, which may follow a streptococcal throat infection.

The Common Cold The common cold is the most widespread of all respiratory diseases—of all communicable diseases, for that matter. More time is lost from school and work because of the common cold than any other disorder. (See Box 5-2 in Chapter 5: The Cold Facts About the Common Cold.) The causative agents are viruses that probably number more than 200 different types. Medical science has yet to establish the effectiveness of any method for preventing the common cold. Because there are so many organisms involved, the production of an effective vaccine against colds seems unlikely.

The symptoms of the common cold are familiar: first the swollen and inflamed mucosa of the nose and the throat, then the copious discharge of watery fluid from the nose, and finally the thick and ropy discharge that occurs when the cold is subsiding. The scientific name for the common cold is **acute coryza** (ko-RI-zah); the word coryza can also mean simply "a nasal discharge."

Respiratory Syncytial Virus (RSV) RSV is the most common cause of lower respiratory tract infections in infants and young children worldwide. The name comes from the fact that the virus induces fusion of cultured cells (formation of a syncytium) when grown in the laboratory. Infection may result in bronchiolitis or pneumonia, but the virus may affect the upper respiratory tract as well. Most susceptible are premature infants, those with congenital heart disease, and those who are immunodeficient. Exposure to cigarette smoke is a definite risk factor.

The virus usually enters through the eyes and nose following contact with contaminated air, nasal secretions or objects. The incubation period is 3 to 5 days, and an infected person sheds virus particles during the incubation period and up to 2 weeks thereafter. Thorough handwashing helps to reduce spread of the virus. Infection usually resolves in 5 to 7 days, although some cases require hospitalization and antiviral drug treatments.

Croup **Croup** usually affects children under 3 years of age and is associated with a number of different infections that result in upper respiratory inflammation. Constriction of the airways produces a loud, barking cough, wheezing, difficulty in breathing, and hoarseness. If croup is severe, the child may produce a harsh, squeaking noise (stridor) when breathing in through a narrowed trachea. Viral infections, such as those involving parainfluenza, adenovirus, RSV, influenza, or measles, are usually the cause. Although croup may be frightening to parents and children, recovery is complete in most cases within a week. Home treatments include humidifying room air or having the child breathe in steam. Also, cool air may shrink the respiratory tissues enough to bring relief.

Influenza **Influenza** (in-flu-EN-zah), or "flu," is an acute contagious disease characterized by an inflammatory condition of the upper respiratory tract accompanied by generalized aches and pains. It is caused by a virus and may spread to the sinuses and downward to the lungs. Inflammation of the trachea and the bronchi causes the characteristic cough of influenza, and the general infection causes an extremely weakened condition. The great danger of influenza is its tendency to develop into a particularly severe form of pneumonia. At intervals in history, there have been tremendous epidemics of influenza in which millions of people have died. Vaccines have been effective, although the protection is of short duration.

Pneumonia **Pneumonia** (nu-MO-ne-ah) is an inflammation of the lungs in which the air spaces become filled with fluid. A variety of organisms, including staphylococci, pneumococci, streptococci, *Legionella pneumophila* (as in Legionnaires disease), chlamydias, and viruses may be responsible. Many of these pathogens may be carried by a healthy person in the mucosa of the upper respiratory tract. If the person remains in good health, they may be carried for a long time with no ill effect. If the patient's resistance to infection is lowered, however, the pathogens may invade the tissues and cause disease.

Susceptibility to pneumonia is increased in patients with chronic, debilitating illness or chronic respiratory disease, in smokers, and in people with alcoholism. It is also increased in cases of exposure to toxic gases, suppression of the immune system, or viral respiratory infections.

There are two main kinds of pneumonia as determined by the extent of lung involvement and other factors:

- **Bronchopneumonia,** in which the disease process is scattered throughout the lung. The cause may be infection with a staphylococcus, gram-negative *Proteus* species, colon bacillus (not normally pathogenic), or a virus. Bronchopneumonia most often is secondary to an infection or to some agent that has lowered the patient's resistance to disease. This is the most common form of pneumonia.
- **Lobar pneumonia,** in which an entire lobe of the lung is infected at one time. The causitive organism is usually a pneumococcus, although other pathogens may also cause this disease. *Legionella* is the causative agent of a severe lobar pneumonia that occurs mostly in localized epidemics.

Most types of pneumonia are characterized by the formation of a fluid, or **exudate,** in the infected alveoli; this fluid consists chiefly of serum and pus, products of infection. Some red blood cells may be present, as indicated by red streaks in the sputum. Sometimes, so many air sacs become filled with fluid that the victim finds it hard to absorb enough oxygen to maintain life.

Pneumocystis Pneumonia (PCP) **PCP** occurs mainly in people with weakened immune systems, such as HIV-positive individuals or transplant recipients on immunosuppressant drugs. The infectious agent was originally called *P. carinii* and classified as a protozoon. It has now been reclassified as an atypical fungus and renamed *P. jiroveci*. The organism grows in the fluid that lines the alveoli of the lungs. Laboratories diagnose the disease by microscopic identification of the organism in a sputum sample, bronchoscopy specimen, or lung biopsy specimen. PCP is treated with antimicrobial drugs, although these medications may cause serious side effects in immunocompromised patients.

Tuberculosis **Tuberculosis** (tu-ber-ku-LO-sis) (**TB**) is an infectious disease caused by the bacillus *Mycobacterium tuberculosis*. Although the tubercle bacillus may invade any body tissue, it usually grows in the lung. Tuberculosis remains a leading cause of death from communicable disease, primarily because of the relatively large numbers of cases among recent immigrants, elderly people, and poor people in metropolitan areas. The spread of AIDS has been linked with a rising incidence of TB because this viral disease weakens host defenses.

The name *tuberculosis* comes from the small lesions, or tubercles, that form where the organisms grow. If unchecked, these lesions degenerate and may even liquefy to cause cavities within an organ. In early stages, the disease may lie dormant, only to flare up at a later time. The tuberculosis organism can readily spread into the lymph nodes or into the blood and be carried to other organs. The lymph nodes in the thorax, especially those surrounding the trachea and bronchi, are frequently involved. Infection of the pleura results in tuberculous pleurisy (inflammation of the pleura). In this case, a collection of fluid, known as an **effusion** (e-FU-zhun), accumulates in the pleural space.

Drugs can be used successfully in many cases of tuberculosis, although strains of the TB organism that are resistant to multiple antibiotics have appeared recently. The best results have been obtained by use of a combination of several drugs, with prompt, intensive, and uninterrupted treatment once a program is begun. Therapy is usually continued for a minimum of 6 to 18 months; therefore, close supervision by the healthcare practitioner is important. Adverse drug reactions are rather common, necessitating changes in the drug combinations. Drug treatment of patients whose infection has not progressed to active disease is particularly effective.

Hay Fever and Asthma

Hypersensitivity to plant pollens, dust, certain foods, and other allergens may lead to **hay fever** or **asthma** (AZ-mah) or both. Hay fever, known medically as *allergic rhinitis,* is characterized by a watery discharge from the eyes and nose. Hay fever often appears in a seasonal pattern due to pollen allergy. The response may be chronic if the allergen is present year round. The symptoms of asthma are caused by reversible changes, which include inflammation of airway tissues and spasm of the involuntary muscle in bronchial tubes. Spasm constricts the tubes, causing resistance to air flow. The person experiences a sense of suffocation and has labored breathing (dyspnea), often with wheezing. Treatment may include inhaled steroids to prevent inflammation and inhaled bronchodilators to open airways during acute episodes.

Patients vary considerably in their responses, and most cases of asthma involve multiple causes. Respiratory infection, noxious fumes, or drug allergy can initiate episodes, but one of the more common triggers for asthma attacks is exercise. The rapid air movement in sensitive airways causes smooth muscle spasm in the breathing passages.

A great difficulty in the treatment of hay fever or asthma is identification of the particular substance to which the patient is allergic. Allergists usually give a number of skin tests, but in most cases, the results are inconclusive. People with allergies may benefit from a series of injections to reduce their sensitivity to specific substances.

Chronic Obstructive Pulmonary Disease (COPD)

Chronic obstructive pulmonary disease (COPD) is the term used to describe several lung disorders, including **chronic bronchitis** and **emphysema** (em-fih-SE-mah). Most affected patients have symptoms and lung damage characteristic of both diseases. In chronic bronchitis, the airway linings are chronically inflamed and produce excessive secretions. Emphysema is characterized by dilation and finally destruction of the alveoli.

In COPD, respiratory function is impaired by obstruction to normal air flow, reducing exchange of oxygen and carbon dioxide. There is air trapping and over-inflation of parts of the lungs. In the early stages of these diseases, the small airways are involved, and several years may pass before symptoms become evident. Later, the affected person develops dyspnea as a result of difficulty in exhaling air through the obstructed air passages.

In certain smokers, COPD may result in serious disability and death within 10 years of the onset of symptoms. Giving up smoking may reverse progression of the disorder, especially when it is diagnosed early and other respiratory irritants also are eliminated. Sometimes, the word *emphysema* is used to mean COPD.

COPD is also called COLD (chronic obstructive lung disease).

Sudden Infant Death Syndrome (SIDS)

SIDS, also called "crib death," is the unexplained death of a seemingly healthy infant under 1 year of age. Death usually occurs during sleep, leaving no signs of its cause. Neither autopsy nor careful investigation of family history and circumstances of death provides any clues. Certain maternal conditions during pregnancy are associated with an increased risk of SIDS, although none is a sure predictor. These include cigarette smoking, age under 20, low weight gain, anemia, illegal drug use, and infections of the reproductive or urinary tracts.

Some guidelines that have reduced the incidence SIDS are:

- Place the baby supine (on its back) for sleep, unless there is some medical reason not to do so. A reminder for parents and other caregivers is the slogan "Back to sleep." A side position is not as effective, as the baby can roll over, and it should never be put to sleep prone (face down). In the prone position, the baby can rebreathe its own CO_2, building up CO_2 and diminishing blood O_2 levels. The position may also cause obstruction in the upper airways or lead to overheating by reducing loss of body heat.
- Keep the baby in a smoke-free environment. Maternal smoking during pregnancy, or smoking in the baby's environment after birth, increases the risk of SIDS.

- Use a firm, flat baby mattress, no soft foam, fur, or fiber-filled bedding.
- Avoid overheating the baby with room air, clothing or bedding, especially when the baby has a cold or other infection.

Checkpoint 18-15 What does COPD mean and what two diseases are commonly involved in COPD?

Respiratory Distress Syndrome (RDS)

RDS covers a range of inflammatory disorders that result from other medical problems or from direct injury to the lungs. **Acute respiratory distress syndrome** (ARDS), or shock lung, usually appears in adults, in contrast to a form of the syndrome that occurs in premature newborns, as described later. Some causes of ARDS are:

- Airway obstruction as from mucus, foreign bodies, emboli or tumors
- Sepsis (systemic infection)
- Aspiration (inhalation) of stomach contents
- Allergy
- Lung trauma

Inflammation and damage to the alveoli results in pulmonary edema, dyspnea (difficulty in breathing), decreased compliance, hypoxemia, and formation of fibrous scar tissue in the lungs. The incomplete expansion of a lung or portion of a lung, such as results from ARDS, is called **atelectasis** (at-e-LEK-tah-sis), or collapsed lung.

In premature newborns, atelectasis may result from insufficient production of surfactant by the immature lungs. **Respiratory distress syndrome of the newborn** is now treated by administration of surfactant that is produced in bacteria by genetic engineering. The syndrome was formerly called *hyaline membrane disease* because of the clear membrane formed from lung exudates in the alveoli.

Cancer

Tumors can arise in all portions of the respiratory tract. Two common sites are described as follows.

Lung Cancer Cancer of the lungs is the most common cause of cancer-related deaths in both men and women. The incidence rate in women continues to increase, whereas the rate in men has been decreasing recently. By far, the most important cause of lung cancer is cigarette smoking. Smokers suffer from lung cancer 10 times as often as do nonsmokers. The risk of getting lung cancer is increased in people who started smoking early in life, smoke large numbers of cigarettes daily, and inhale deeply. Smokers who are exposed to toxic chemicals or particles in the air have an even higher rate of lung cancer. Smoking has also been linked with an increase in COPD and cancers of respiratory passages.

A common form of lung cancer is **bronchogenic** (brong-ko-JEN-ik) **carcinoma**, so called because the malignancy originates in a bronchus. The tumor may grow until the bronchus is blocked, cutting off the supply of air to that lung. The lung then collapses, and the secretions trapped in the lung spaces become infected, with a resulting pneumonia or formation of a lung abscess. This type of lung cancer can spread, causing secondary growths in the lymph nodes of the chest and neck and in the brain and other parts of the body. A treatment that offers a possibility of cure before secondary growths have had time to form is complete removal of the lung. This operation is called a **pneumonectomy** (nu-mo-NEK-to-me).

Malignant tumors of the stomach, breast, and other organs may spread to the lungs as secondary growths (metastases).

Cancer of the Larynx Cancer of the larynx usually involves squamous cell carcinoma, and its incidence is definitely linked to cigarette smoking and alcohol consumption. Symptoms include sore throat, hoarseness, ear pain, and enlarged cervical lymph nodes. The cure rate is high for small tumors that have not spread when treated with radiation and (sometimes) surgery. Total or partial removal of the larynx is necessary in cases of advanced cancer that do not respond to radiation or chemotherapy. During and after laryngectomy a patient may need to have an opening, or stoma, created in the trachea with a tube (tracheostomy tube) for breathing. Patients have to care for the stoma and the "trach" (trake) tube. If the vocal cords are removed, a patient can learn to speak by using air forced out of the esophagus or by using a mechanical device to generate sound.

Disorders Involving the Pleura

Pleurisy (PLUR-ih-se), or inflammation of the pleura, usually accompanies a lung infection—particularly pneumonia or tuberculosis. This condition can be quite painful because the inflammation produces a sticky exudate that roughens the pleura of both the lung and the chest wall; when the two surfaces rub together during ventilation, the roughness causes acute irritation. The sticking together of two surfaces is called an **adhesion** (ad-HE-zhun). Infection of the pleura also causes an increase in the amount of pleural fluid. This fluid may accumulate in the pleural space in quantities large enough to compress the lung, resulting in an inability to obtain enough air.

Pneumothorax (nu-mo-THOR-aks) is an accumulation of air in the pleural space (Fig. 18-11). The lung on the affected side collapses, causing the patient to have great difficulty breathing. Pneumothorax may be caused by a wound in the chest wall or by rupture of lung air spaces. In pneumothorax caused by a penetrating wound in the chest wall, an airtight cover over the opening pre-

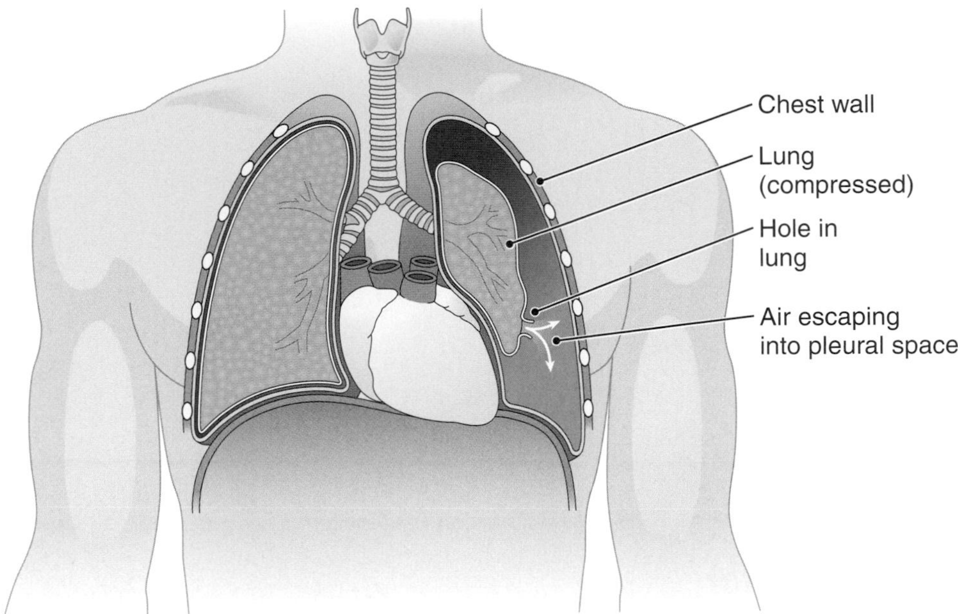

Figure 18-11 **Pneumothorax.** Injury to lung tissue allows air to leak into the pleural space and put pressure on the lung. (Reprinted with permission from Cohen BJ. Medical Terminology. 4th ed. Philadelphia: Lippincott Williams & Wilkins, 2004.)

vents further air from entering. The remaining lung can then function to provide adequate amounts of oxygen.

Blood in the pleural space, a condition called **hemothorax**, is also caused by penetrating chest wounds. In such cases, the first priority is to stop the bleeding.

The abnormal accumulation of fluid or air in the pleural space from any of the above conditions may call for procedures to promote lung expansion. In **thoracentesis** (thor-ah-sen-TE-sis) a large-bore needle is inserted between ribs into the pleural space to remove fluid (Fig. 18-12). The presence of both air and fluid in the pleural space may require insertion of a chest tube, a large tube with several openings along the internal end. The tube is securely connected to a chest drainage system. These procedures restore negative pressure in the pleural space and allow re-expansion of the lung.

Age and the Respiratory Tract

With age, the tissues of the respiratory tract lose elasticity and become more rigid. Similar rigidity in the chest wall, combined with arthritis and loss of strength in the breathing muscles, results in an overall decrease in compliance and in lung capacity. Reduction in protective mechanisms, such as phagocytosis in the lungs, leads to increased susceptibility to infection. The incidence of emphysema increases with age, hastened by cigarette smoking and by exposure to other environmental irritants. Although there is much individual variation, especially related to one's customary level of activity, these changes gradually lead to reduced capacity for exercise.

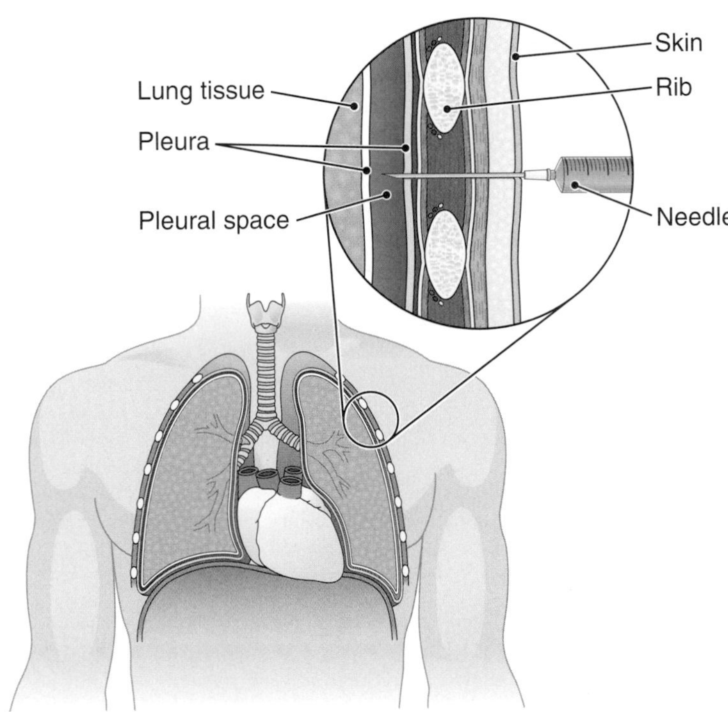

Figure 18-12 **Thoracentesis.** A needle is inserted into the pleural space to withdraw fluid. (Reprinted with permission from Cohen BJ. Medical Terminology. 4th ed. Philadelphia: Lippincott Williams & Wilkins, 2004.)

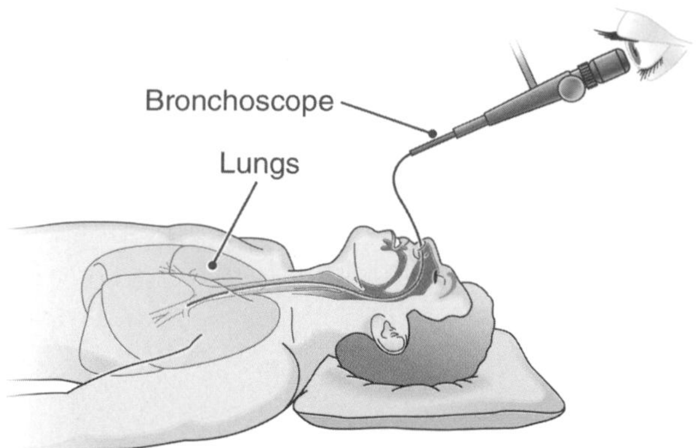

Figure 18-13 Use of a bronchoscope. (Reprinted with permission from Cohen BJ. Medical Terminology. 4th ed. Philadelphia: Lippincott Williams & Wilkins, 2004.)

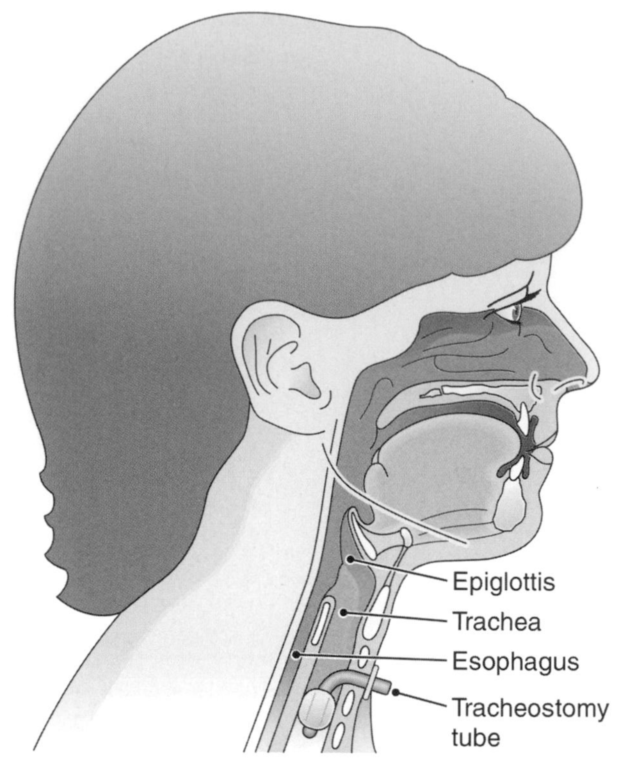

Figure 18-14 A tracheostomy tube in place. (Reprinted with permission from Cohen BJ. Medical Terminology. 4th ed. Philadelphia: Lippincott Williams & Wilkins, 2004.) *ZOOMING IN ✦ What structure is posterior to the trachea?*

Special Equipment for Respiratory Treatment

The **bronchoscope** (BRONG-ko-skope) is a rigid or flexible fiberoptic tubular instrument used for inspection of the primary bronchi and the larger bronchial tubes (Fig. 18-13). Most bronchoscopes are now attached to video recording equipment. The bronchoscope is passed into the respiratory tract by way of the nose or mouth and the pharynx. It may be used to remove foreign bodies, inspect and take tissue samples (biopsies) from tumors, or collect other specimens. Children inhale a variety of objects, such as pins, beans, pieces of nuts, and small coins, all of which a physician may remove with the aid of a bronchoscope. If such items are left in the lung, they may cause an abscess or other serious complication and may even lead to death.

Oxygen therapy is used to sustain life when a condition interferes with adequate oxygen supply to the tissues. The oxygen must first have moisture added by bubbling it through water that is at room temperature or heated. Oxygen may be delivered to the patient by mask, catheter, or nasal prongs. Because there is danger of fire when oxygen is being administered, no one in the room can smoke.

A **suction apparatus** is used for removing mucus or other substances from the respiratory tract by means of negative pressure. A container to trap secretions is located between the patient and the machine. The tube leading to the patient has an opening to control the suction. When

Box 18-3 · Health Professions

Careers in Respiratory Therapy

Respiratory therapists and respiratory therapy technicians specialize in evaluating and treating breathing disorders. Respiratory therapists evaluate the severity of their clients' conditions by taking complete histories and testing respiratory function with specialized equipment. Based on their findings, and in consultation with a physician, therapists design and implement individualized treatment plans, which may include oxygen therapy and chest physiotherapy. They also educate clients on the use of ventilators and other medical devices. Respiratory therapy technicians assist in carrying out evaluations and treatments.

To perform their duties, both types of practitioners need a thorough understanding of anatomy and physiology. Most respiratory therapists in the United States receive their training from an accredited college or university and take a national licensing exam. Respiratory therapists and technicians work in a variety of settings, such as hospitals, nursing care facilities, and private clinics. As the American population continues to age, the prevalence of respiratory ailments is expected to increase. Thus, job prospects are good. For more information about careers in respiratory therapy, contact the American Association for Respiratory Care.

suction is applied, the drainage flows from the patient's respiratory tract into the collection container.

A **tracheostomy** (tra-ke-OS-to-me) **tube** is used if the pharynx or the larynx is obstructed. It is a small metal or plastic tube that is inserted through a cut made in the trachea, and it acts as an artificial airway for ventilation (Fig. 18-14). The procedure for the insertion of such a tube is a *tracheostomy*. The word **tracheotomy** (tra-ke-OT-o-me) refers to the incision in the trachea.

Artificial respiration is used when a patient has temporarily lost the capacity to perform the normal motions of respiration. Such emergencies include cases of gas or smoke inhalation, electric shock, drowning, poisoning or paralysis of the breathing muscles. A number of different apparatuses are used for artificial respiration in a clinical setting. There are also some techniques that can be used in an emergency.

Many public agencies offer classes in the techniques of mouth-to-mouth respiration and cardiac massage to revive people experiencing respiratory or cardiac arrest. This technique is known as **cardiopulmonary resuscitation, or CPR.** These classes also include instruction in emergency airway clearance using abdominal thrusts (Heimlich maneuver), chest thrusts, or back blows to open obstructed airways.

Box 18-3 provides information on the work of respiratory therapists.

Word Anatomy

Medical terms are built from standardized word parts (prefixes, roots, and suffixes). Learning the meanings of these parts can help you remember words and interpret unfamiliar terms.

WORD PART	MEANING	EXAMPLE
The Respiratory System		
nas/o	nose	The *nasopharynx* is behind the nasal cavity.
or/o	mouth	The *oropharynx* is behind the mouth.
laryng/o	larynx	The *laryngeal* pharynx opens into the pharynx.
pleur/o	side, rib	The *pleura* covers the lung and lines the chest wall (rib cage).
The Process of Respiration		
spir/o	breathing	A *spirometer* is an instrument used to record breathing volumes.
capn/o	carbon dioxide	*Hypercapnia* is a rise in the blood level of carbon dioxide.
-pnea	breathing	*Hypopnea* is a decrease in the rate and depth of breathing.
orth/o-	straight	*Orthopnea* can be relieved by sitting in an upright position.
Disorders of the Respiratory System		
pneumon/o	lung	*Pneumonia* is inflammation of the lung.
atel/o	incomplete	*Atelectasis* is incomplete expansion of the lung.
pneum/o	air, gas	*Pneumothorax* is accumulation of air in the pleural space.
–centesis	tapping, perforation	In *thoracentesis* a needle is inserted into the pleural space to remove fluid.

Summary

I. Phases of Respiration
1. Pulmonary ventilation
2. External gas exchange
3. Internal gas exchange

II. The respiratory system
A. Nasal cavities—filter, warm, and moisten air
B. Pharynx (throat)—carries air into respiratory tract and food into digestive tract
C. Larynx (voice box)—contains vocal cords
   1. Glottis- space between the vocal cords
   2. Epiglottis—covers larynx on swallowing to help prevent food from entering
D. Trachea (windpipe)
E. Bronchi—branches of trachea that enter lungs and then subdivide
   1. Bronchioles—smallest subdivisions
F. Lungs
   1. Organs of gas exchange
   2. Lobes: three on right; two on left
   3. Alveoli
      a. Tiny air sacs where gases are exchanged
      b. Surfactant—reduces surface tension in alveoli; eases expansion of lungs
   4. Pleura—membrane that encloses the lung
      a. Visceral pleura—attached to surface of lung
      b. Parietal pleura—attached to chest wall
      c. Pleural space—between layers
   5. Mediastinum—space and organs between lungs

III. The process of respiration
A. Pulmonary ventilation
   1. Inhalation—drawing of air into lungs
      a. Compliance—ease with which lungs and thorax can be expanded
   2. Exhalation—expulsion of air from lungs
   3. Lung volumes—used to evaluate respiratory function

B. Gas exchange
  1. Gases diffuse from area of higher concentration to area of lower concentration
  2. In lungs—oxygen enters blood and carbon dioxide leaves (external exchange)
  3. In tissues—oxygen leaves blood and carbon dioxide enters (internal exchange)

C. Oxygen transport
  1. Almost totally bound to heme portion of hemoglobin in red blood cells
  2. Separates from hemoglobin when oxygen concentration is low (in tissues)
    a. Carbon monoxide replaces oxygen on hemoglobin

D. Carbon dioxide transport
  1. Most carried as bicarbonate ion
  2. Regulates pH of blood

E. Regulation of respiration
  1. Nervous control—centers in medulla and pons
  2. Chemical control
    a. Central chemoreceptors respond to CO_2, which decreases pH
    b. Peripheral chemorecptors—respond to low levels of O_2

F. Abnormal ventilation
  1. Hyperventilation—rapid, deep respiration
  2. Hypoventilation—inadequate air in alveoli

G. Breathing patterns
  1. Normal—12 to 20 times per minute in adult
  2. Types of altered breathing
    a. Hyperpnea—increase in depth and rate of breathing
    b. Tachypnea—excessive rate of breathing
    c. Apnea—temporary cessation of breathing
    d. Dyspnea—difficulty in breathing
    e. Orthopnea—difficulty relieved by upright position
    f. Kussmaul—characterizes acidosis
    g. Cheyne-Stokes—irregularity found in critically ill
  3. Possible results—cyanosis, hypoxia (anoxia), hypoxemia, suffocation

IV. Disorders of the respiratory system

A. Disorders of the nasal cavities and related structures—sinusitis, polyps, deviated septum, nosebleed (epistaxis)

B. Infection—colds, RSV, croup, influenza, pneumonia, tuberculosis

C. Hay fever and asthma—hypersensitivity (allergy)

D. COPD—involves emphysema and bronchitis

E. SIDS—sudden infant death syndrome

F. Respiratory distress syndrome (RDS)
  1. Acute (ARDS)—due to other medical problem or direct injury to lung
  2. RDS of newborn—due to lack of surfactant

G. Cancer—smoking a major causative factor

H. Disorders involving the pleural space
  1. Pleurisy—inflammation of pleura
  2. Pneumothorax—air in pleural space
  3. Hemothorax—blood in pleural space

V. Age and the respiratory tract

VI. Special equipment for respiratory treatment

1. Bronchoscope—tube used to examine air passageways and remove foreign bodies
2. Oxygen therapy
3. Suction apparatus—removes mucus and other substances
4. Tracheostomy—artificial airway
   a. Tracheotomy—incision into trachea
5. Artificial respiration—cardiopulmonary resuscitation (CPR)

Questions for Study and Review

Building Understanding

Fill in the blanks

1. The exchange of air between the atmosphere and the lungs is called ______.
2. The space between the vocal cords is the ______.
3. The ease with which the lungs and thorax can be expanded is termed ______.
4. A lower than normal level of oxygen in the tissues is called ______.
5. Inflammation of the pleura is termed ______.

Matching

Match each numbered item with the most closely related lettered item.

___ 6. A decrease in the rate and depth of breathing
___ 7. An increase in the rate and depth of breathing
___ 8. A temporary cessation of breathing
___ 9. Difficult or labored breathing
___ 10. Difficult breathing that is relieved by sitting up

a. dyspnea
b. hyperpnea
c. orthopnea
d. hypopnea
e. apnea

Multiple choice

___ 11. The bony projections in the nasal cavities that increase surface area are called
a. nares
b. septae
c. conchae
d. sinuses

___ 12. Which of the following structures produces speech?
a. pharynx
b. larynx
c. trachea
d. lungs

___ 13. The leaf-shaped cartilage that covers the larynx during swallowing is the
a. epiglottis
b. glottis
c. conchae
d. sinus

___ 14. Respiration is centrally regulated by the
a. cerebral cortex
b. diencephalon
c. brain stem
d. cerebellum

___ 15. Incomplete expansion of a lung or portion of a lung is called
a. effusion
b. adhesion
c. epistaxis
d. atelectasis

Understanding Concepts

16. Differentiate between the terms in each of the following pairs:
a. internal and external gas exchange
b. pleura and diaphragm
c. inhalation and exhalation
d. spirometer and spirogram

17. Trace the path of air from the nostrils to the lung capillaries.

18. What is the function of the cilia on cells that line the respiratory passageways?

19. Compare and contrast the transport of oxygen and carbon dioxide in the blood.

20. Define hyperventilation and hypoventilation. What is the effect of each on blood CO_2 levels and blood pH?

21. What are chemoreceptors and how do they function to regulate breathing?

22. Describe the structural and functional changes that occur in the respiratory system in chronic obstructive pulmonary disease.

23. Compare and contrast the following disease conditions:
a. Kussmaul and Cheyne-Stokes respiration
b. acute coryza and influenza
c. bronchopneumonia and lobar pneumonia
d. pneumothorax and hemothorax

Conceptual Thinking

24. Jake, a sometimes exasperating 4-year-old, threatens his mother that he will hold his breath until "he dies." Should his mother be concerned that he might succeed?

25. Why is it important that airplane interiors are pressurized? If the cabin lost pressure, what physiological adaptations to respiration might occur in the passengers?

Selected Key Terms

The following terms and other boldface terms in the chapter are defined in the Glossary

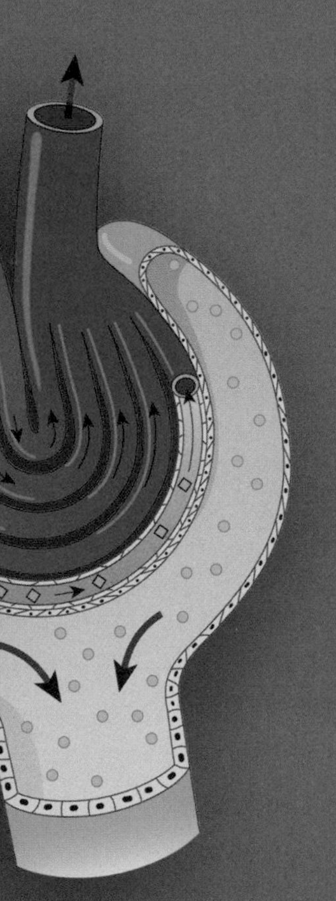

absorption
bile
chyle
chyme
defecation
deglutition
digestion
duodenum
emulsify
enzyme
esophagus
gallbladder
hydrolysis
intestine
lacteal
liver
mastication
pancreas
peristalsis
peritoneum
saliva
stomach
ulcer
villi

Learning Outcomes

After careful study of this chapter, you should be able to:

1. Name the three main functions of the digestive system
2. Describe the four layers of the digestive tract wall
3. Differentiate between the two layers of the peritoneum
4. Name and locate the different types of teeth
5. Name and describe the functions of the organs of the digestive tract
6. Name and describe the functions of the accessory organs of digestion
7. Describe how bile functions in digestion
8. Name and locate the ducts that carry bile from the liver into the digestive tract
9. Explain the role of enzymes in digestion and give examples of enzymes
10. Name the digestion products of fats, proteins, and carbohydrates
11. Define *absorption*
12. Define *villi* and state how villi function in absorption
13. Explain the use of feedback in regulating digestion and give several examples
14. List several hormones involved in regulating digestion
15. Describe common disorders of the digestive tract and the accessory organs
16. Show how word parts are used to build words related to digestion (see Word Anatomy at the end of the chapter)

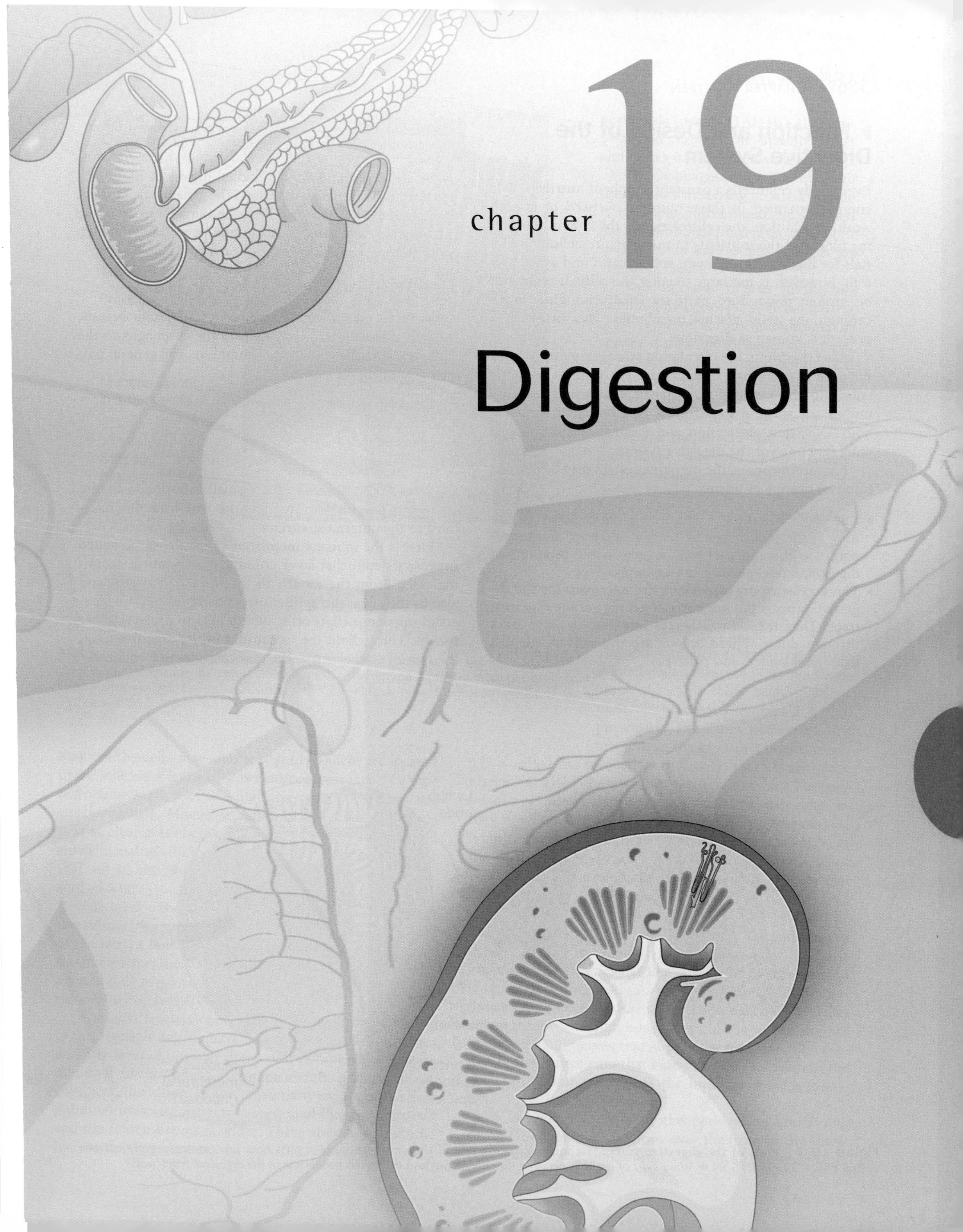

chapter 19

Digestion

c. Examples—gastrin, GIP, secretin, CCK

A. Hunger and appetite

B. Eating disorders- e.g. anorexia, bulimia

VII. Disorders of the digestive system

A. Peritonitis

B. Diseases of the mouth and teeth—caries, gingivitis, periodontitis, Vincent disease, leukoplakia

C. Disorders involving the esophagus and stomach

1. Hiatal hernia—protrusion of organ through diaphragm
2. Gastroesophageal reflux disease (GERD)
3. Nausea, vomiting (emesis)
4. Cancer
5. Ulcer—peptic ulcer in esophagus, stomach or duodenum
6. Pyloric stenosis

D. Intestinal disorders

1. Inflammatory diseases—appendicitis, Crohn disease, ulcerative colitis, irritable bowel syndrome (IBS), diverticulitis
2. Diarrhea
3. Constipation
4. Obstruction—intussuception, volvulus, ileus, hemorrhoids
5. Cancer

E. Infection of the salivary glands

1. Mumps—viral infection of parotid salivary gland

F. Cirrhosis and other diseases of the liver

1. Jaundice—yellow color due to bile pigments in blood
2. Hepatitis—viruses A to E
3. Cancer

G. Gallstones—cholelithiasis

H. Pancreatitis

VIII. Aging and the digestive system

Questions for Study and Review

Building Understanding

Fill in the blanks

1. The wave-like movement of the digestive tract wall is called ______.
2. The small intestine is connected to the posterior abdominal wall by ______.
3. The liver can store glucose in the form of ______.
4. The parotid glands secrete ______.
5. Inflammation of the gallbladder is termed ______.

Matching

Match each numbered item with the most closely related lettered item.

___ 6. Digests starch

___ 7. Begins protein digestion

___ 8. Digests fats

___ 9. Digests protein to amino acids

___ 10. Emulsify fats

a. lipase
b. amylase
c. trypsin
d. pepsin
e. bile salts

Multiple choice

___ 11. The teeth break up food into small parts by a process called
a. absorption
b. deglutition
c. ingestion
d. mastication

___ 12. Hydrochloric acid and pepsin are secreted by the
a. salivary glands
b. stomach
c. pancreas
d. liver

___ 13. The double layer of peritoneum that extends from the lower border of the stomach and hangs over the intestine is the
a. greater omentum
b. lesser omentum
c. mesentery
d. mesocolon

___ 14. The soft, fleshy V-shaped mass of tissue that hangs from the soft palate is the
a. epiglottis
b. esophageal hiatus
c. uvula
d. gingiva

___ 15. Thickened white patches on the oral mucous membranes characterizes the disorder called
a. peridontitis
b. cholelithiasis
c. pancreatitis
d. leukoplakia

Understanding Concepts

16. Differentiate between the terms in each of the following pairs:
a. digestion and absorption
b. parietal and visceral peritoneum
c. gastrin and gastric-inhibitory peptide
d. secretin and cholecystokinin

17. Name the four layers of the digestive tract. What tissue makes up each layer? What is the function of each layer?
18. Trace the path of a bolus of food through the digestive system.
19. Describe the structure and function of the liver, pancreas, and gallbladder. How are the products of these organs delivered to the digestive tract?
20. Where does absorption occur in the digestive tract, and what structures are needed for absorption? What types of nutrients are absorbed into the blood? Into the lymph?
21. Name several hormones that regulate digestion.
22. Compare and contrast the following disorders:
    a. anorexia and bulimia
    b. inflammatory bowel disease and irritable bowel syndrome
    c. intussusception and volvulus
23. What are the causes and effects of hepatitis?

Conceptual Thinking

24. Why should a person who suffers from peptic ulcers avoid the use of aspirin (acetylsalicylic acid)?
25. Cholelithiasis can cause pancreatitis. Why?

Selected Key Terms

The following terms and other boldface terms in the chapter are defined in the Glossary

anabolism
catabolism
fever
glucose
glycogen
hypothalamus
hypothermia
kilocalorie
malnutrition
metabolic rate
mineral
oxidation
pyrogen
vitamin

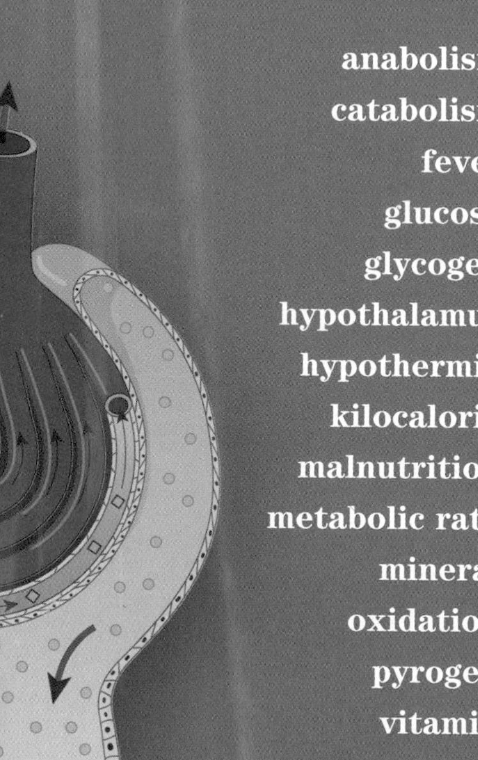

Learning Outcomes

After careful study of this chapter, you should be able to:

1. Differentiate between catabolism and anabolism
2. Differentiate between the anaerobic and aerobic phases of cellular respiration and give the end products and the relative amount of energy released by each
3. Define *metabolic rate* and name several factors that affect the metabolic rate
4. Explain the roles of glucose and glycogen in metabolism
5. Compare the energy contents of fats, proteins, and carbohydrates
6. Define *essential amino acid*
7. Explain the roles of minerals and vitamins in nutrition and give examples of each
8. List the recommended percentages of carbohydrate, fat and protein in the diet
9. Distinguish between simple and complex carbohydrates, giving examples of each
10. Compare saturated and unsaturated fats
11. List some adverse effects of alcohol consumption
12. Describe some nutritional disorders
13. Explain how heat is produced and lost in the body
14. Describe the role of the hypothalamus in regulating body temperature
15. Explain the role of fever in disease
16. Describe some adverse effects of excessive heat and cold
17. Show how word parts are used to build words related to metabolism, nutrition and body temperature (see Word Anatomy at the end of the chapter)

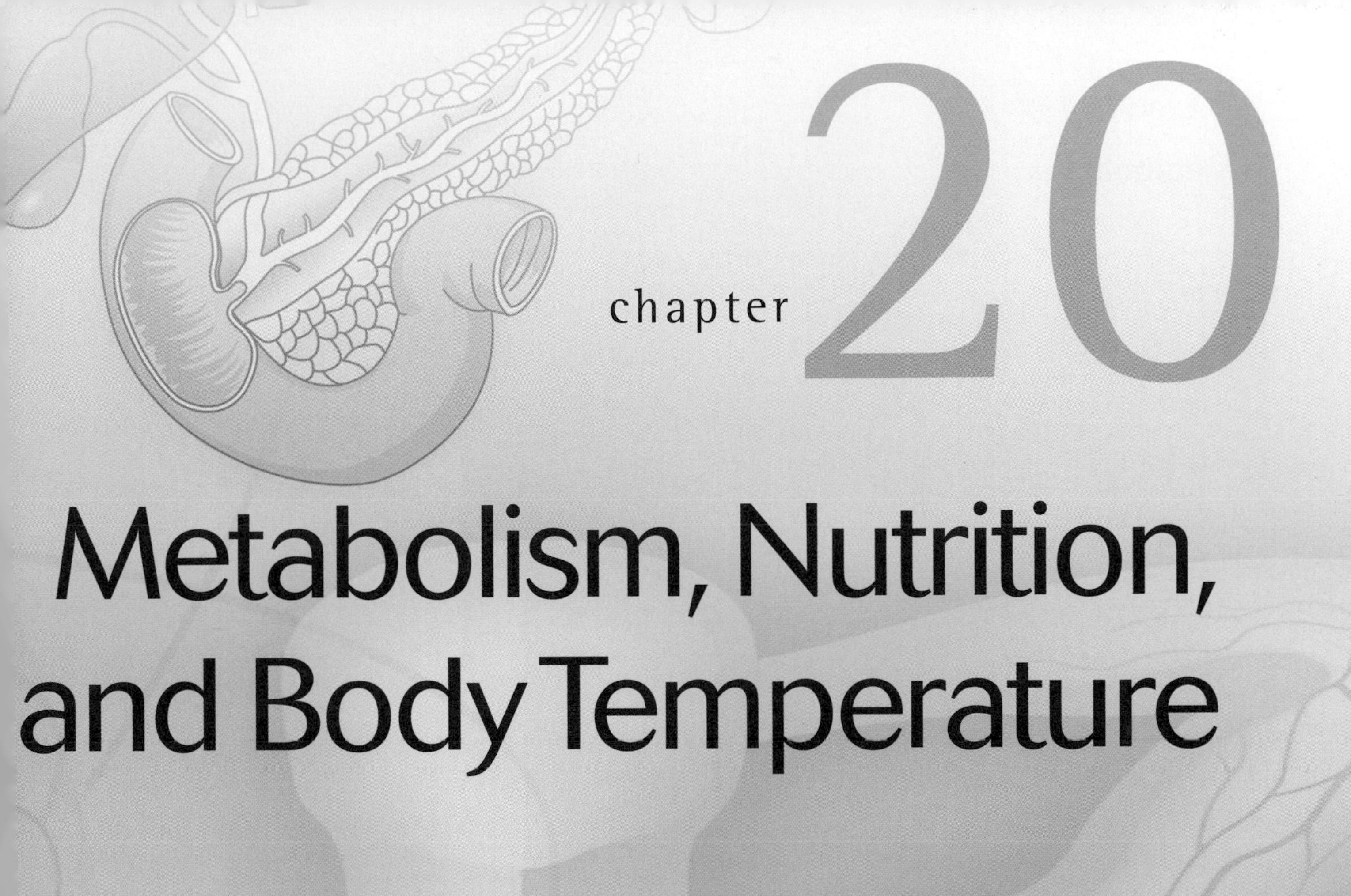

chapter 20

Metabolism, Nutrition, and Body Temperature

Metabolism

Nutrients absorbed from the digestive tract are used for all the cellular activities of the body, which together make up **metabolism**. These activities fall into two categories:

- **Catabolism**, which is the breakdown of complex compounds into simpler compounds. Catabolism includes the digestion of food into small molecules and the release of energy from these molecules within the cell.
- **Anabolism**, which is the building of simple compounds into substances needed for cellular activities and for the growth and repair of tissues.

Through the steps of catabolism and anabolism, there is a constant turnover of body materials as energy is consumed, cells function and grow, and waste products are generated.

Checkpoint 20-1 What are the two phases of metabolism?

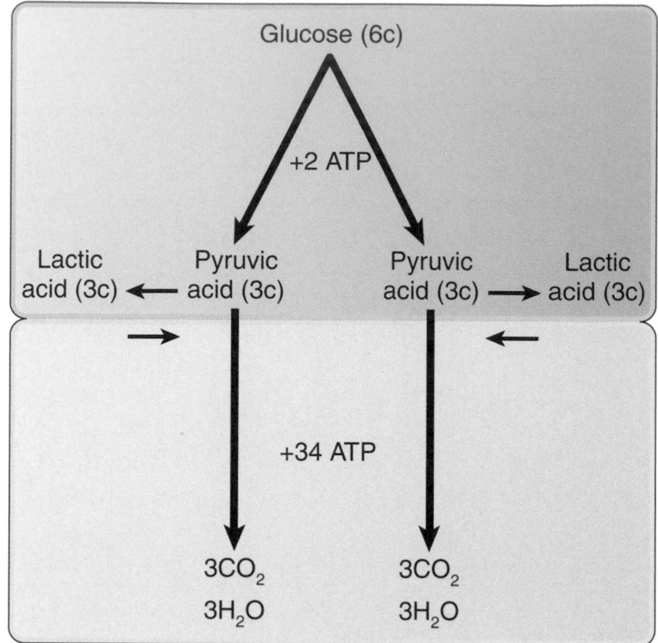

Figure 20-1 **Cellular respiration.** This diagram shows the catabolism of glucose without oxygen (anaerobic) and with oxygen (aerobic). (C = carbon atoms in one molecule of a substance.) In cellular respiration, glucose first yields two molecules of pyruvic acid, which will convert to lactic acid under anaerobic conditions, as during intense exercise. (Lactic acid must eventually be converted back to pyruvic acid.) Typically, however, pyruvic acid is broken down aerobically (using oxygen) to CO_2 and H_2O (aerobically). *ZOOMING IN ✦ What does pyruvic acid produce in cellular respiration under anaerobic conditions? Under aerobic conditions?*

Cellular Respiration

Energy is released from nutrients in a series of reactions called **cellular respiration** (see Table 20-1 and Fig. 20-1). Early studies on cellular respiration were done with **glucose** as the starting compound. Glucose is a simple sugar that is the main energy source for the body.

The Anaerobic Phase The first steps in the breakdown of glucose do not require oxygen; that is, they are **anaerobic**. This phase of catabolism, known as **glycolysis** (gli-KOL-ih-sis), occurs in the cytoplasm of the cell. It yields a small amount of energy, which is used to make ATP (adenosine triphosphate), the cells' energy compound. Each glucose molecule yields enough energy by this process to produce 2 molecules of ATP.

The anaerobic breakdown of glucose is incomplete and ends with formation of an organic product called **pyruvic** (pi-RU-vik) **acid**. This organic acid is further metabolized in the next phase of cellular respiration, which requires oxygen. In muscle cells operating briefly under anaerobic conditions, pyruvic acid is converted to lactic acid, which accumulates as the cells build up an oxygen debt (described in Chapter 8). Lactic acid induces muscle fatigue, so the body is forced to rest and recover. During the recovery phase immediately after exercise, breathing restores the oxygen needed to convert lactic acid back to pyruvic acid, which is then metabolized further. During this recovery phase, reserves stored in muscles are also replenished. These compounds are myoglobin, which stores oxygen; glycogen, which can be broken down for glucose; and creatine phosphate, which stores energy.

The Aerobic Phase To generate enough energy for survival, the body's cells must break pyruvic acid down more completely in the second phase of cellular respiration, which requires oxygen. These **aerobic** reactions occur within the mitochondria of the cell. They result in transfer of most of the energy remaining in the nutrients to ATP. On average, about 34 to 36 molecules of ATP can be formed aerobically per glucose molecule—quite an increase over anaerobic metabolism.

Table 20•1 Summary of Cellular Respiration of Glucose

PHASE	LOCATION IN CELL	END PRODUCT(S)	ENERGY YIELD/GLUCOSE
Anaerobic (glycolysis)	Cytoplasm	Pyruvic acid	2 ATP
Aerobic	Mitochondria	Carbon dioxide and water	34–36 ATP

During the aerobic steps of cellular respiration, the cells form carbon dioxide, which then must be transported to the lungs for elimination. In addition, water is formed by the combination of oxygen with the hydrogen that is removed from nutrient molecules. Because of the type of chemical reactions involved, and because oxygen is used in the final steps, cellular respiration is described as an **oxidation** of nutrients. Note that enzymes are required as catalysts in all the reactions of cellular respiration. Many of the vitamins and minerals described later in this chapter are parts of these enzymes.

Although the oxidation of food is often compared to the burning of fuel, this comparison is inaccurate. Burning fuel results in a sudden and often wasteful release of energy in the form of heat and light. In contrast, metabolic oxidation occurs in small steps, and much of the energy released is stored as ATP for later use by the cells; some of the energy is released as heat, which is used to maintain body temperature, as discussed later in this chapter.

For those who know how to read chemical equations, the net balanced equation for cellular respiration, starting with glucose, is as follows:

$$\underset{\text{glucose}}{C_6H_{12}O_6} + \underset{\text{oxygen}}{6O_2} \rightarrow \underset{\text{carbon dioxide}}{6CO_2} + \underset{\text{water}}{6H_2O}$$

Checkpoint 20-2 What name is given to the series of cellular reactions that releases energy from nutrients?

Metabolic Rate **Metabolic rate** refers to the rate at which energy is released from nutrients in the cells. It is affected by a person's size, body fat, sex, age, activity, and hormones, especially thyroid hormone (thyroxine). Metabolic rate is high in children and adolescents and decreases with age. **Basal metabolism** is the amount of energy needed to maintain life functions while the body is at rest.

The unit used to measure energy is the kilocalorie (kcal), which is the amount of heat needed to raise 1 kilogram of water 1°C. To estimate the daily calories needed taking activity level into account, see Box 20-1.

The Use of Nutrients for Energy

As noted, glucose is the main source of energy in the body. Most of the carbohydrates in the diet are converted to glucose in the course of metabolism. Reserves of glucose are stored in liver and muscle cells as **glycogen** (GLI-ko-jen), a compound built from glucose molecules. When glucose is needed for energy, glycogen is broken down to yield glucose. Glycerol and fatty acids (from fat digestion)

Box 20-1 A Closer Look

Calorie Counting: Estimating Daily Energy Needs

Basal energy requirements for a day can be estimated with a simple formula. An average woman requires 0.9 kcal/kg/hour, and a man, 1.0 kcal/kg/hour. Multiplying 0.9 by body weight in kilograms* by 24 for a woman, or 1.0 by body weight in kilograms by 24 for a man, yields the daily basal energy requirement. For example, if a woman weighed 132 pounds, the equation would be as follows:

132 pounds ÷ 2.2 pounds/kg = 60 kg

0.9 kcal/kg/hour x 60 kg = 54 kcal/hour

54 kcal/hour x 24 hours/day = 1,296 kcal/day

To estimate total energy needs for a day, a percentage based on activity level ("couch potato" to serious athlete) must also be added to the basal requirement. These percentages are shown in the table below.

The equation to calculate total energy needs for a day is:

Basal energy requirement + (basal energy requirement × activity level)

Using our previous example, and assuming light activity levels, the following equations apply:

At 40% activity:

1,296 kcal/day + (1,296 kcal/day × 40%) = 1,814.4 kcal/day

At 60% activity:

1,296 kcal/day + (1,296 kcal/day × 60%) = 2,073.6 kcal/day

Therefore, the woman in our example would require between 1,814 and 2,073 Kcal/day.

ACTIVITY LEVEL	MALE	FEMALE
Little activity ("couch potato")	25–40%	25–35%
Light activity (*e.g.*, walking to and from class, but little or no intentional exercise)	50–75%	40–60%
Moderate activity (*e.g.*, aerobics several times a week)	65–80%	50–70%
Heavy activity (serious athlete)	90–120%	80–100%

*To convert pounds to kilograms, divide weight in pounds by 2.2.

and amino acids (from protein digestion) can also be used for energy, but they enter the breakdown process at different points.

Fat in the diet yields more than twice as much energy as do protein and carbohydrate (*e.g.*, it is more "fattening"); fat yields 9 kcal of energy per gram, whereas protein and carbohydrate each yield 4 kcal per gram. Calories that are ingested in excess of need are converted to fat and stored in adipose tissue.

Before they are oxidized for energy, amino acids must have their nitrogen (amine) groups removed. This removal, called **deamination** (de-am-ih-NA-shun), occurs in the liver, where the nitrogen groups are then formed into urea by combination with carbon dioxide. The blood transports urea to the kidneys to be eliminated.

There are no specialized storage forms of proteins, as there are for carbohydrates (glycogen) and fats (adipose tissue). Therefore, when one needs more proteins than are supplied in the diet, they must be obtained from body substance, such as muscle tissue or plasma proteins. Drawing on these resources becomes dangerous when needs are extreme. Fats and carbohydrates are described as "protein sparing," because they are used for energy before proteins are and thus spare proteins for the synthesis of necessary body components.

Checkpoint 20-3 What is the main energy source for the cells?

Anabolism

Nutrient molecules are built into body materials by anabolic steps, all of which are catalyzed by enzymes.

Essential Amino Acids Eleven of the 20 amino acids needed to build proteins can be synthesized internally by metabolic reactions. These 11 amino acids are described as *nonessential* because they need not be taken in as food (Table 20-2). The remaining 9 amino acids cannot be made by the body and therefore must be taken in as part of the diet; these are the **essential amino acids**. Note that some nonessential amino acids may become essential under certain conditions, as during extreme physical stress, or in certain hereditary metabolic diseases.

Essential Fatty Acids There are also two essential fatty acids (linoleic acid and linolenic acid) that must be taken in as food. These are easily obtained through a healthful, balanced diet.

Checkpoint 20-4 What is meant when an amino acid or a fatty acid is described as essential?

Table 20•2 Amino acids

NONESSENTIAL AMINO ACIDS*		ESSENTIAL AMINO ACIDS**	
Name	Pronunciation	Name***	Pronunciation
Alanine	AL-ah-nene	Histidine	HIS-tih-dene
Arginine	AR-jih-nene	Isoleucine	i-so-LU-sene
Asparagine	ah-SPAR-ah-jene	Leucine	LU-sene
Aspartic acid	ah-SPAR-tik AH-sid	Lysine	LI-sene
Cysteine	SIS-teh-ene	Methionine	meh-THI-o-nene
Glutamic acid	glu-TAM-ik AH-sid	Phenylalanine	fen-il-AL-ah-nene
Glutamine	GLU-tah-mene	Threonine	THRE-o-nene
Glycine	GLY-sene	Tryptophan	TRIP-to-fane
Proline	PRO-lene	Valine	VA-lene
Serine	SERE-ene		
Tyrosine	TI-ro-sene		

**Nonessential amino acids can be synthesized by the body.*

***Essential amino acids cannot be synthesized by the body; they must be taken in as part of the diet.*

****If you are ever called upon to memorize the essential amino acids, the mnemonic (memory device) Pvt. T. M. Hill gives the first letter of each name.*

Minerals and Vitamins

In addition to needing fats, proteins, and carbohydrates, the body requires minerals and vitamins.

Minerals are chemical elements needed for body structure, fluid balance, and such activities as muscle contraction, nerve impulse conduction, and blood clotting. Some minerals are components of vitamins. A list of the main minerals needed in a proper diet is given in Table 20-3. Some additional minerals not listed are also required for good health. Minerals needed in extremely small amounts are referred to as **trace elements**.

Vitamins are complex organic substances needed in very small quantities. Vitamins are parts of enzymes or other substances essential for metabolism, and vitamin deficiencies lead to a variety of nutritional diseases.

The water-soluble vitamins are the B vitamins and vitamin C. These are not stored and must be taken in regularly with food. The fat-soluble vitamins are A, D, E, and K. These vitamins are kept in reserve in fatty tissue. Excess intake of the fat-soluble vitamins can lead to toxicity. A list of vitamins is given in Table 20-4.

Certain substances are valuable in the diet as **antioxidants**. They defend against the harmful effects of **free radicals**, highly reactive and unstable molecules produced from oxygen in the normal course of metabolism (and also from UV radiation, air pollution and tobacco smoke). Free radicals contribute to aging and disease. Antioxidants react with free radicals to stabilize them and minimize their harmful effects on cells. Vitamins C and E and beta carotene, an orange pigment found in plants that is converted to vitamin A, are

Table 20•3 Minerals

MINERAL	FUNCTIONS	SOURCES	RESULTS OF DEFICIENCY
Calcium (Ca)	Formation of bones and teeth, blood clotting, nerve conduction, muscle contraction	Dairy products, eggs, green vegetables, legumes (peas and beans)	Rickets, tetany, osteoporosis
Phosphorus (P)	Formation of bones and teeth; found in ATP, nucleic acids	Meat, fish, poultry, egg yolk, dairy products	Osteoporosis, abnormal metabolism
Sodium (Na)	Fluid balance; nerve impulse conduction, muscle contraction	Most foods, especially processed foods, table salt	Weakness, cramps, diarrhea, dehydration
Potassium (K)	Fluid balance, nerve and muscle activity	Fruits, meats, seafood, milk, vegetables, grains	Muscular and neurologic disorders
Chloride (Cl)	Fluid balance, hydrochloric acid in stomach	Meat, milk, eggs, processed foods, table salt	Rarely occurs
Iron (Fe)	Oxygen carrier (hemoglobin, myoglobin)	Meat, eggs, fortified cereals, legumes, dried fruit	Anemia, dry skin, indigestion
Iodine (I)	Thyroid hormones	Seafood, iodized salt	Hypothyroidism, goiter
Magnesium (Mg)	Catalyst for enzyme reactions, carbohydrate metabolism	Green vegetables, grains, nuts, legumes	Spasticity, arrhythmia, vasodilation
Manganese (Mn)	Catalyst in actions of calcium and phosphorus; facilitator of many cell processes	Many foods	Possible reproductive disorders
Copper (Cu)	Necessary for absorption and use of iron in formation of hemoglobin; part of some enzymes	Meat, water	Anemia
Chromium (Cr)	Works with insulin to regulate blood glucose levels	Meat, unrefined food, fats and oils	Inability to use glucose
Cobalt (Co)	Part of vitamin B12	Animal products	Pernicious anemia
Zinc (Zn)	Promotes carbon dioxide transport and energy metabolism; found in enzymes	Meat, fish, poultry, grains, vegetables	Alopecia (baldness); possibly related to diabetes
Fluoride (F)	Prevents tooth decay	Fluoridated water, tea, seafood	Dental caries

antioxidants. There are also many compounds found in plants (*e.g.*, soybeans and tomatoes) that are antioxidants.

Checkpoint 20-5 Both vitamins and minerals are needed in metabolism. What is the difference between vitamins and minerals?

Nutritional Guidelines

The relative amounts of carbohydrates, fats and proteins that should be in the daily diet vary somewhat with the individual. Typical recommendations for the number of calories derived each day from the three types of food are as follows:

- Carbohydrate: 55%-60%.
- Fat: 30% or less.
- Protein: 15%-20%.

It is important to realize that the type as well as the amount of each is a factor in good health. A weight loss diet should follow the same proportions as given above, but with a reduction in portion sizes.

Carbohydrates

Carbohydrates in the diet should be mainly complex, naturally occurring carbohydrates, and simple sugars should be kept to a minimum. Simple sugars are monosaccharides, such as glucose and fructose (fruit sugar), and disaccharides, such as sucrose (table sugar) and lactose (milk sugar). Simple sugars are a source of fast energy because they are metabolized rapidly. However, they boost pancreatic insulin output, and as a result, they cause blood glucose levels to rise and fall rapidly. It is healthier to maintain steady glucose levels, which normally range from approximately 85 to125 mg/dL throughout the day.

The **glycemic effect** is a measure of how rapidly a particular food raises the blood glucose level and stimulates the release of insulin. The effect is generally low for whole grains, fruit and dairy products and high for sweets and refined ("white") grains. Note, however, that the glycemic effect of a food also depends on when it is eaten during the day, and if or how it is combined with other foods.

Complex carbohydrates are polysaccharides. Examples are:

Table 20•4 Vitamins

VITAMINS	FUNCTIONS	SOURCES	RESULTS OF DEFICIENCY
A (retinol)	Required for healthy epithelial tissue and for eye pigments; involved in reproduction and immunity	Orange fruits and vegetables, liver, eggs, dairy products, dark green vegetables	Night blindness; dry, scaly skin; decreased immunity
B1 (thiamin)	Required for enzymes involved in oxidation of nutrients; nerve function	Pork, cereal, grains, meats, legumes, nuts	Beriberi, a disease of nerves
B2 (riboflavin)	In enzymes required for oxidation of nutrients	Milk, eggs, liver, green leafy vegetables, grains	Skin and tongue disorders
B3 (niacin, nicotinic acid)	Involved in oxidation of nutrients	Yeast, meat, liver, grains, legumes, nuts	Pellagra with dermatitis, diarrhea, mental disorders
B6 (pyridoxine)	Amino acid and fatty acid metabolism; formation of niacin; manufacture of red blood cells	Meat, fish, poultry, fruit, grains, legumes, vegetables	Anemia, irritability, convulsions, muscle twitching, skin disorders
Pantothenic acid	Essential for normal growth; energy metabolism	Yeast, liver, eggs, and many other foods	Sleep disturbances, digestive upset
B12 (cyanocobalamin)	Production of cells; maintenance of nerve cells; fatty acid and amino acid metabolism	Animal products	Pernicious anemia
Biotin	Involved in fat and glycogen formation, amino acid metabolism	Peanuts, liver, tomatoes, eggs, and many other foods	Lack of coordination, dermatitis, fatigue
Folate (folic acid)	Required for amino acid metabolism, DNA synthesis, maturation of red blood cells	Vegetables, liver, legumes, seeds	Anemia, digestive disorders, neural tube defects in the embryo
C (ascorbic acid)	Maintains healthy skin and mucous membranes; involved in synthesis of collagen; antioxidant	Citrus fruits, green vegetables, potatoes, orange fruits	Scurvy, poor wound healing, anemia, weak bones
D (calciferol)	Aids in absorption of calcium and phosphorus from intestinal tract	Fatty fish, liver, eggs, fortified milk	Rickets, bone deformities
E (tocopherol)	Protects cell membranes; antioxidant	Seeds, green vegetables, nuts, grains, oils,	Anemia, muscle and liver degeneration, pain
K	Synthesis of blood clotting factors, bone formation	Bacteria in digestive tract, liver, cabbage, and leafy green vegetables	Hemorrhage

- Starches, found in grains, legumes, and potatoes.
- Fibers, such as cellulose, pectins, and gums, which are the structural materials of plants.

Fiber adds bulk to the stool and promotes elimination of toxins and waste. It also slows the digestion and absorption of carbohydrates, thus regulating the release of glucose. It helps in weight control by providing a sense of fullness and limiting caloric intake. Adequate fiber in the diet lowers cholesterol and helps to prevent diabetes, colon cancer, hemorrhoids, appendicitis, and diverticulitis.

Box 20-2 • Health Maintenance

Dietary Fiber: Bulking Up

Dietary fiber is best known for its ability to improve bowel habits and ease weight loss. But fiber may also help to prevent diabetes, heart disease, and certain digestive disorders such as diverticulitis and gallstones.

Dietary fiber is an indigestible type of carbohydrate found in fruit, vegetables, and whole grains. The amount of fiber recommended for a 2,000-calorie diet is 25 grams per day, but most people in the United States tend to get only half this amount. One should eat fiber-rich foods throughout the day to meet the requirement. It is best to increase fiber in the diet gradually to avoid unpleasant symptoms, such as intestinal bloating and flatulence. If your diet lacks fiber, try adding the following foods over a period of several weeks:

- Whole grain breads, cereals, pasta, and brown rice. These add 1 to 3 more grams of fiber per serving than the "white" product.
- Legumes, which include beans, peas, and lentils. These add 4 to 12 grams of fiber per serving.
- Fruits and vegetables. Whole, raw, unpeeled versions contain the most fiber, and juices, the least. Apple juice has no fiber, whereas a whole apple has 3 grams.
- Unprocessed bran. This can be sprinkled over almost any food: cereal, soups, and casseroles. One tablespoon adds 2 grams of fiber. Be sure to take adequate fluids with bran.

Foods high in fiber, such as whole grains, fruits, and vegetables, are also rich in vitamins and minerals (see Box 20-2).

Checkpoint 20-6 What is the normal range of blood glucose?

Fats

Fats are subdivided into saturated and unsaturated forms based on their chemical structure. The fatty acids in **saturated fats** have more hydrogen atoms in their molecules and fewer double bonds between carbons atoms than do those of unsaturated fats (Fig. 20-2). Most saturated fats are from animal sources and are solid at room temperature, such as butter and lard. Also included in this group are the so-called "tropical oils": coconut oil and palm oil. **Unsaturated fats** are derived from plants. They are liquid at room temperature and are generally referred to as oils, such as corn, peanut, olive and canola oils.

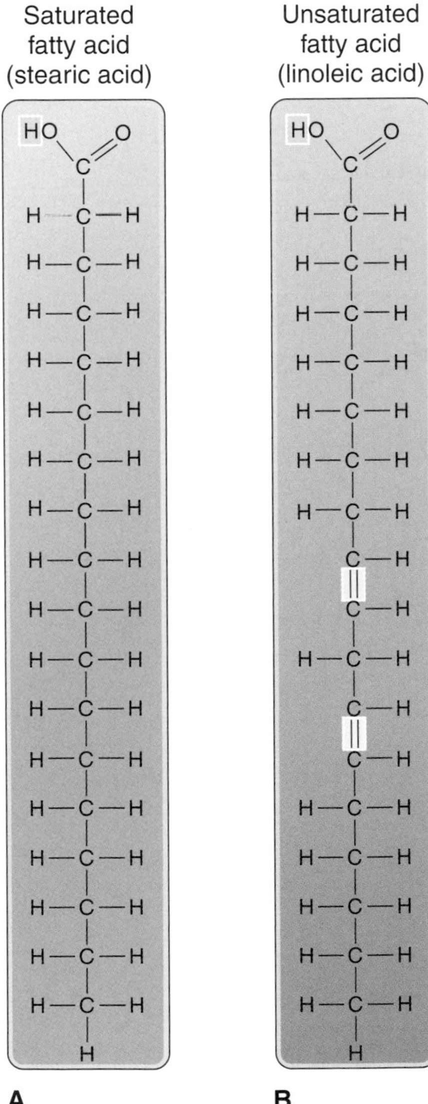

Figure 20-2 **Saturated and unsaturated fats. (A)** Saturated fatty acids contain the maximum numbers of hydrogen atoms attached to carbons and no double bonds between carbon atoms. **(B)** Unsaturated fatty acids have less than the maximum number of hydrogen atoms attached to carbons and one or more double bonds between carbon atoms (highlighted).

Saturated fats should make up less than one third of the fat in the diet (less than 10% of total calories). Diets high in saturated fats are associated with a higher than normal incidence of cancer, heart disease, and cardiovascular problems, although the relation between these factors is not fully understood.

Many commercial products contain fats that are artificially saturated to prevent rancidity and provide a more solid consistency. These are listed on food labels as partially hydrogenated (HI-dro-jen-a-ted) vegetable oils and are found in baked goods, processed peanut butter, vegetable shortening, and solid margarine. Evidence shows that components of hydrogenated fats, known as *trans-fatty acids*, may be just as harmful, if not more so, than natural saturated fats and should be avoided.

Proteins

Because proteins, unlike carbohydrates and fats, are not stored in special reserves, protein foods should be taken in on a regular basis, with attention to obtaining the essential amino acids. Most animal proteins supply all of the essential amino acids and are described as complete proteins. Most vegetables are lacking in one or more of the essential amino acids. People on strict vegetarian diets must learn to combine foods, such as legumes (*e.g.*, beans and peas) with grains (*e.g.*, rice, corn, or wheat), to obtain all the essential amino acids each day. Table 20-5 demonstrates the principles of combining two foods, legumes and grains, to supply essential amino acids that might be missing in one food or the other. Legumes are rich in isoleucine and lysine but poor in methonine and tryptophan, while grains are just the opposite. For illustration purposes, the table includes only the 4 missing essential amino acids (there are 9 total). Traditional ethnic diets reflect these healthy combinations, for example, beans with corn or rice in Mexican dishes or chickpeas and lentils with wheat in Middle Eastern fare.

Vitamin and Mineral Supplements

The need for mineral and vitamin supplements to the diet is a subject of controversy. Some researchers maintain that adequate amounts of these substances can be obtained from a varied, healthful diet. Many commercial foods, including milk, cereal and bread, are already fortified with minerals and vitamins. Others hold that pollution, depletion of the soils, and the storage, refining, and processing of foods make additional supplementation beneficial. Most agree, however, that children, elderly people, pregnant and lactating women, and teenagers, who often do not get enough of the proper foods, would profit from additional minerals and vitamins.

Table 20•5 Combining Foods for Essential Amino Acids

	ESSENTIAL AMINO ACIDS*			
	ISOLEUCINE	LYSINE	METHIONINE	TRYPTOPHAN
Legumes	x	x		
Grains			x	x
Legumes and grains combined	x	x	x	x

There are 9 essential amino acids; the table includes 4 for the purposes of illustration.

When required, supplements should be selected by a physician or nutritionist to fit an individual's particular needs. Megavitamin dosages may cause unpleasant reactions and in some cases are hazardous. Vitamins A and D have both been found to cause serious toxic effects when taken in excess.

The Food Guide Pyramid

In 1992, the USDA (United States Department of Agriculture) developed a pyramid to represent the quantities of foods in the different food groups recommended each day for good health (Fig. 20-3). This symbol is under revision, and some suggested improvements include:

- Distinguish between unrefined and refined carbohydrates.
- Distinguish between healthful unsaturated fats, which can be eaten in moderation, and less healthful saturated and processed (trans-) fats, which should be restricted.
- Accommodate vegetarians, who may avoid not only meats, but dairy products and eggs as well.

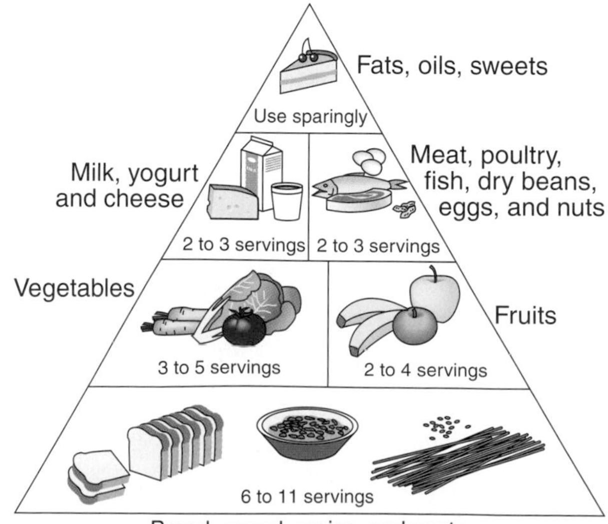

Figure 20-3 The Food Guide Pyramid. (From U.S. Department of Agriculture/U.S. Department of Health and Human Services.)

- Specify portion sizes, which are smaller than most people think.
- Include the need for water.
- Indicate possible need for vitamin supplements.

Governments in the U.S. and other countries will continue to study this topic with input from nutritionists and other scientists. The best nutrition guidelines, however, will be of no benefit unless people are educated and motivated to follow them.

Alcohol

Alcohol yields energy in the amount of 7 kcal per gram, but it is not considered a nutrient because it does not yield useful end products. In fact, alcohol interferes with metabolism and contributes to a variety of disorders.

The body can metabolize about one-half ounce of pure alcohol (ethanol) per hour. This amount translates into one glass of wine, one can of beer, or one shot of hard liquor. Consumed at a more rapid rate, alcohol enters the bloodstream and affects many cells, notably in the brain.

Alcohol is rapidly absorbed through the stomach and small intestine and is detoxified by the liver. When delivered in excess to the liver, alcohol can lead to the accumulation of fat as well as inflammation and scarring of liver tissue. It can eventually cause cirrhosis (*sih-RO-sis*), which involves irreversible changes in liver structure. Alcohol metabolism ties up enzymes needed for oxidation of nutrients and also results in byproducts that acidify body fluids. Other effects of alcoholism include obesity, malnutrition, cancer, ulcers, and fetal alcohol syndrome. Pregnant women are advised not to drink any alcohol. In addition, alcohol impairs judgment and leads to increased involvement in accidents.

Although alcohol consumption is compatible with good health and may even have a beneficial effect on the cardiovascular system, alcohol should be consumed only in moderation.

Checkpoint 20-7 What are typical recommendations for the relative amounts of carbohydrates, fats, and proteins in the diet?

Nutritional Disorders

Diet-related problems may originate from an excess or shortage of necessary nutrients. Another issue in the news today is weight control. Food allergies may also affect some people.

Food Allergies

Some people develop clear allergic (hypersensitive) symptoms if they eat certain foods. Common food allergens are wheat, nuts, milk, shellfish, and eggs, but almost any food might cause an allergic reaction in a given individual. People may also have allergic reactions to food additives, such as flavorings, colorings, or preservatives. Signs of allergic reactions usually involve the skin, respiratory tract, or gastrointestinal tract. Food allergies may provoke potentially fatal anaphylactic shock in extremely sensitive individuals.

Malnutrition

If any vital nutrient is missing from the diet, the body will suffer from malnutrition. One commonly thinks of a malnourished person as someone who does not have enough to eat, but malnutrition can also occur from eating too much of the wrong foods. Factors that contribute to malnutrition are poverty, old age, chronic illness, anorexia, poor dental health, and drug or alcohol addiction.

In poor and underdeveloped countries, many children suffer from protein and energy malnutrition (PEM). **Marasmus** (mah-RAZ-mus) is a term used for severe malnutrition in infancy (from Greek meaning "dying away").

Kwashiorkor (kwash-e-OR-kor) typically affects older children when they are weaned because another child is born (and the name means just that). A low protein level in the blood plasma interferes with fluid return to the capillaries, resulting in edema. Often excess fluid accumulates in the abdomen as ascites (ah-SI-teze) fluid, causing the stomach to bulge.

Overweight and Obesity

The causes of obesity are complex, involving social, economic, genetic, psychological and metabolic factors. It is common knowledge that overweight and obesity have increased in the past several decades in many countries. In the U.S., 35% of adults are overweight and an additional 30% are obese (see "Body Mass Index" below.) Obesity shortens the life span and is associated with cardiovascular disease, diabetes, some cancers, and other diseases. The incidence of type II diabetes, once considered to have an adult onset, has increased greatly among children. Some researchers hold that obesity has a closer correlation to chronic disease than poverty, smoking, or drinking alcohol.

Scientists are studying the nervous and hormonal controls over weight, but so far they have not found any effective and safe drugs for weight control. For most people, a varied diet eaten in moderation and regular exercise are the surest ways to avoid obesity. One-half hour of vigorous exercise at least four times a week is recommended for health and weight control.

Body Mass Index **Body mass index** (BMI) is a measurement used to evaluate body size. It is based on the ratio of weight to height (Fig. 20-4). BMI is calculated by dividing weight in kilograms by height in meters squared. (For those not accustomed to using the metric system, an alternate method is to divide weight in pounds by the square of height in inches and multiply by 703.) A healthy range for this measurement is 19-24. Overweight is defined as a BMI of 25-30, and obesity as a BMI greater than 30. However, BMI does not take into account the relative amount of muscle and fat in the body. For example, a bodybuilder might be healthy with a higher than typical BMI because muscle has a higher density than fat.

Calculation of body mass index (BMI)

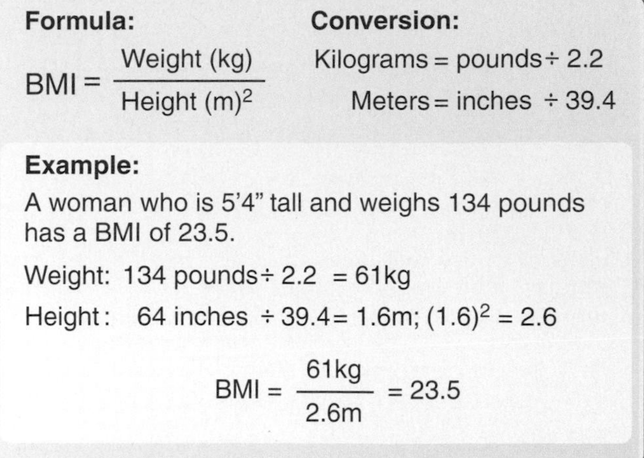

Figure 20-4 Calculation of body mass index (BMI). *ZOOMING IN ✦ What is the BMI of a male 5'10" in height who weighs 170 pounds? (Round off to one decimal place.)*

Underweight

People who are underweight have as much difficulty gaining weight as others have losing it. The problem of underweight may result from rapid growth, eating disorders, allergies, illness, or psychological factors. It is associated with low reserves of energy, reproductive disturbances, and nutritional deficiencies. A BMI of less than 18.5 is defined as underweight. To gain weight, people have to increase their intake of calories, but they should also exercise to add muscle tissue and not just fat.

Nutrition and Aging

With age, a person may find it difficult to maintain a balanced diet. Often, the elderly lose interest in buying and preparing food or are unable to do so. Because metabolism generally slows, and less food is required to meet energy needs, nutritional deficiencies may develop. Medications may interfere with appetite and with the absorption and use of specific nutrients.

It is important for older people to seek out foods that are "nutrient dense," that is, foods that have a high proportion of nutrients in comparison with the number of calories they provide. Exercise helps to boost appetite and

Box 20-3 · Health Professions

Dietitians and Nutritionists

Dietitians and nutritionists specialize in planning and supervising food programs for institutions such as hospitals, schools, and nursing care facilities. They assess their clients' nutritional needs and design individualized meal plans. Dietitians and nutritionists also work in community settings, educating the public about disease prevention through healthy eating. Increased public awareness about food and nutrition has also led to new opportunities in the food manufacturing industry. To perform their duties, dietitians and nutritionists need a thorough understanding of anatomy and physiology. Most dietitians and nutritionists in the United States receive their training from a college or university and take a licensing exam.

Job prospects for dietitians and nutritionists are good. As the American population continues to age, the need for nutritional planning in hospital and nursing care settings is expected to rise. In addition, many people now place an emphasis on healthy eating and may consult nutritionists privately. For more information about this career, contact the American Dietetic Association.

maintains muscle tissue, which is more active metabolically. Box 20-3 describes how dietitians and nutritionists can help in planning a healthful diet for people of all ages.

Body Temperature

Heat is an important byproduct of the many chemical activities constantly occurring in body tissues. At the same time, heat is always being lost through a variety of outlets. Under normal conditions, a number of regulatory devices keep body temperature constant within quite narrow limits. Maintenance of a constant temperature despite both internal and external influences is one phase of homeostasis, the tendency of all body processes to maintain a normal state despite forces that tend to alter them.

Heat Production

Heat is a byproduct of the cellular oxidations that generate energy. The amount of heat produced by a given organ varies with the kind of tissue and its activity. While at rest, muscles may produce as little as 25% of total body heat, but when muscles contract, heat production is greatly multiplied, owing to the increase in metabolic rate. Under basal conditions (at rest), the liver and other abdominal organs produce about 50% of total body heat. The brain produces only 15% of body heat at rest, and an increase in nervous tissue activity produces little increase in heat production.

Although it would seem from this description that some parts of the body would tend to become much warmer than others, the circulating blood distributes the heat fairly evenly.

Factors Affecting Heat Production The rate at which heat is produced is affected by a number of factors, including exercise, hormone production, food intake, and age. Hormones, such as thyroxine from the thyroid gland and epinephrine (adrenaline) from the adrenal medulla, increase the rate of heat production.

The intake of food is also accompanied by increased heat production. The nutrients that enter the blood after digestion are available for increased cellular metabolism. In addition, the glands and muscles of the digestive system generate heat as they set to work. These responses do not account for all the increase, however, nor do they account for the much greater increase in metabolism after a meal containing a large amount of protein. Although the reasons are not entirely clear, the intake of food definitely increases metabolism and thus adds to heat production.

Checkpoint 20-8 What are some factors that affect heat production in the body?

Heat Loss

More than 80% of heat loss occurs through the skin. The remaining 15% to 20% is dissipated by the respiratory system and with the urine and feces. Networks of blood vessels in the skin's dermis (deeper part) can bring considerable quantities of blood near the surface, so that heat can be dissipated to the outside. This release can occur in several ways.

- Heat can be transferred directly to the surrounding air by means **conduction**.
- Heat also travels from its source as heat waves or rays, a process termed **radiation**.
- If the air is moving, so that the layer of heated air next to the body is constantly being carried away and replaced with cooler air (as by an electric fan), the process is known as **convection**.
- Finally, heat may be lost by **evaporation**, the process by which liquid changes to the vapor state.

To illustrate evaporation, rub some alcohol on your skin; it evaporates rapidly, using so much heat from the skin that your arm feels cold. Perspiration does the same thing, although not as quickly. The rate of heat loss through evaporation depends on the humidity of the surrounding air. When it exceeds 60% or so, perspiration does not evaporate so readily, making one feel generally miserable unless some other means of heat loss is available, such as convection caused by a fan.

Prevention of Heat Loss Factors that play a part in heat loss through the skin include the volume of tissue compared with the amount of skin surface. A child loses heat more rapidly than does an adult. Such parts as fingers and toes are affected most by exposure to cold because they have a great amount of skin compared with total tissue volume.

If the temperature of the surrounding air is lower than that of the body, excessive heat loss is prevented by both natural and artificial means. Clothing checks heat loss by trapping "dead air" in both its material and its layers. This noncirculating air is a good insulator. An effective natural insulation against cold is the layer of fat under the skin. Even when skin temperature is low, this fatty tissue prevents the deeper tissues from losing much heat. On the average, this layer is slightly thicker in females than in males. Naturally, there are individual variations, but as a rule, the degree of insulation depends on the thickness of this subcutaneous fat layer.

Temperature Regulation

Given that body temperature remains almost constant despite wide variations in the rate of heat production or loss, there must be internal mechanisms for regulating temperature.

The Role of the Hypothalamus Many areas of the body take part in heat regulation, but the most important center is the hypothalamus, the area of the brain located just above the pituitary gland. Some of the cells in the hypothalamus control heat production in body tissues, whereas another group of cells controls heat loss. Regulation is based on the temperature of the blood circulating through the brain and also on input from temperature receptors in the skin.

If these two factors indicate that too much heat is being lost, impulses are sent quickly from the hypothalamus to the autonomic (involuntary) nervous system, which in turn causes constriction of the skin blood vessels to reduce heat loss. Other impulses are sent to the muscles to cause shivering, a rhythmic contraction of many muscles, which results in increased heat production. Furthermore, the output of epinephrine may be increased if necessary. Epinephrine increases cell metabolism for a short period, and this in turn increases heat production.

If there is danger of overheating, the hypothalamus stimulates the sweat glands to increase their activity. Impulses from the hypothalamus also cause blood vessels in the skin to dilate, so that increased blood flow to the skin will result in greater heat loss. The hypothalamus may also promote muscle relaxation to minimize heat production.

Muscles are especially important in temperature regulation because variations in the activity of these large tissue masses can readily increase or decrease heat generation. Because muscles form roughly one-third of the body, either an involuntary or an intentional increase in their activity can form enough heat to offset a considerable decrease in the temperature of the environment.

Checkpoint 20-9 What part of the brain is responsible for regulating body temperature?

Age Factors Very young and very old people are limited in their ability to regulate body temperature when exposed to environmental extremes. A newborn infant's body temperature decreases if the infant is exposed to a cool environment for a long period. Elderly people also are not able to produce enough heat to maintain body temperature in a cool environment.

With regard to overheating in these age groups, heat loss mechanisms are not fully developed in the newborn. The elderly do not lose as much heat from their skin as do younger people. Both groups should be protected from extreme temperatures.

Normal Body Temperature The normal temperature range obtained by either a mercury or an electronic thermometer may extend from 36.2°C to 37.6°C (97°F to 100°F). Body temperature varies with the time of day. Usually, it is lowest in the early morning because the muscles have been relaxed and no food has been taken in for several hours. Temperature tends to be higher in the late afternoon and evening because of physical activity and consumption of food.

Normal temperature also varies in different parts of the body. Skin temperature obtained in the axilla (armpit) is lower than mouth temperature, and mouth temperature is a degree or so lower than rectal temperature. It is believed that, if it were possible to place a thermometer inside the liver, it would register a degree or more higher than rectal temperature. The temperature within a muscle might be even higher during activity.

Although the Fahrenheit scale is used in the United States, in most parts of the world, temperature is measured with the **Celsius** (SEL-se-us) thermometer. On this scale, the ice point is at 0° and the normal boiling point of water is at 100°, the interval between these two points being divided into 100 equal units. The Celsius scale is also called the **centigrade scale** (think of 100 cents in a dollar). See Appendix 2 for a comparison of the Celsius and Fahrenheit scales and formulas for converting from one to the other.

Checkpoint 20-10 What is normal body temperature?

Fever

Fever is a condition in which the body temperature is higher than normal. An individual with a fever is described as **febrile** (FEB-ril). Usually, the presence of fever is due to an infection, but there can be many other causes, such as malignancies, brain injuries, toxic reactions, reactions to vaccines, and diseases involving the central nervous system (CNS). Sometimes, emotional upsets can bring on a fever. Whatever the cause, the effect is to reset the body's thermostat in the hypothalamus.

Curiously enough, fever usually is preceded by a chill—that is, a violent attack of shivering and a sensation of cold that blankets and heating pads seem unable to relieve. As a result of these reactions, heat is generated and stored, and when the chill subsides, the body temperature is elevated.

The old adage that a fever should be starved is completely wrong. During a fever, there is an increase in metabolism that is usually proportional to the degree of fever. The body uses available sugars and fats, and there is an increase in the use of protein. During the first week or so of a fever, there is definite evidence of protein destruction, so a high-calorie diet with plenty of protein is recommended.

When a fever ends, sometimes the drop in temperature to normal occurs very rapidly. This sudden fall in temperature is called the **crisis**, and it is usually accompanied by symptoms indicating rapid heat loss: profuse perspiration, muscular relaxation, and dilation of blood vessels in the skin. A gradual drop in temperature, in contrast, is known as **lysis**. A drug that reduces fever is described as **antipyretic** (an-ti-pi-RET-ik).

The mechanism of fever production is not completely understood, but we might think of the hypothalamus as a thermostat that is set higher during fever than normally. This change in the heat-regulating mechanism often follows the injection of a foreign protein or the entrance into the bloodstream of bacteria or their toxins. Substances that produce fever are called **pyrogens** (PI-ro-jens).

Up to a point, fever may be beneficial because it steps up phagocytosis (the process by which white blood cells destroy bacteria and other foreign material), inhibits the growth of certain organisms, and increases cellular metabolism, which may help recovery from disease.

Responses to Excessive Heat

The body's heat-regulating devices are efficient, but there is a limit to what they can accomplish. High outside temperature may overcome the body's heat loss mechanisms, in which case body temperature rises and cellular metabolism with accompanying heat production increases. When body temperature rises, the affected person is apt to suffer from a series of disorders: heat cramps are followed by heat exhaustion, which, if untreated, is followed by heat stroke.

In **heat cramps**, there is localized muscle cramping of the extremities and occasionally of the abdomen. The condition abates with rest in a cool environment and adequate fluids.

With further heat retention and more fluid loss, **heat exhaustion** occurs. Symptoms of this disorder include headache, tiredness, vomiting, and a rapid pulse. The victim feels hot, but the skin is cool due to evaporation of sweat. There may be a decrease in circulating blood volume and lowered blood pressure. Heat exhaustion is also treated by rest and fluid replacement.

Heat stroke (also called sunstroke) is a medical emergency. Heat stroke can be recognized by a body temperature of up to 41°C (105°F); hot, dry skin; and CNS symptoms, including confusion, dizziness, and loss of consciousness. The body has responded to the loss of circulating fluid by reducing blood flow to the skin and sweat glands.

It is important to lower the heatstroke victim's body temperature immediately by removing the individual's clothing, placing him or her in a cool environment, and cooling the body with cold water or ice. The patient should be treated with appropriate fluids containing necessary electrolytes, including sodium, potassium, calcium, and chloride. Supportive medical care is also needed to avoid fatal complications.

Checkpoint 20-11 What are some conditions brought on by excessive heat?

Responses to Excessive Cold

The body is no more capable of coping with prolonged exposure to cold than with prolonged exposure to heat. If, for example, the body is immersed in cold water for a time, the water (a better heat conductor than air) removes more heat from the body than can be replaced, and temperature falls. Cold air can produce the same result, particularly when clothing is inadequate. The main effects of an excessively low body temperature, termed **hypothermia** (hi-po-THER-me-ah), are uncontrolled shivering, lack of coordination, and decreased heart and respiratory rates. Speech becomes slurred, and there is overpowering sleepiness, which may lead to coma and death. Outdoor activities in cool, not necessarily cold, weather cause many unrecognized cases of hypothermia. Wind, fatigue, and depletion of water and energy stores all play a part.

When the body is cooled below a certain point, cellular metabolism slows, and heat production is inadequate to maintain a normal temperature. The person must then be warmed gradually by heat from an outside source. The best first aid measure is to remove the person's clothing and put him or her in a warmed sleeping bag with an unclothed companion until shivering stops. Administration of warm, sweetened fluids also helps.

Exposure to cold, particularly to moist cold, may result in **frostbite**, which can cause permanent local tissue damage. The areas most likely to be affected by frostbite are the face, ears, and extremities. Formation of ice crystals and reduction of blood supply to an area leads to necrosis (death) of tissue and possible gangrene. The very young, the very old, and those who suffer from disease of the circulatory system are particularly susceptible to cold injuries.

A frostbitten area should never be rubbed; rather, it should be thawed by application of warm towels or immersion in circulating lukewarm (not hot) water for 20 to 30 minutes. The affected area should be treated gently; a person with frostbitten feet should not be permitted to walk. People with cold-damaged extremities frequently have some lowering of body temperature. The whole body should be warmed at the same time that the affected part is warmed.

Hypothermia is employed in certain types of surgery. In these circumstances, drugs are used to depress the hypothalamus and reduce the body temperature to as low as 25°C (77°F) before the surgeon begins the operation. In heart surgery, the blood is cooled further 20°C (68°F) as it goes through the heart-lung machine. This method has been successful even in infants.

Checkpoint 20-12 What is the term for excessively low body temperature?

Word Anatomy

Medical terms are built from standardized word parts (prefixes, roots, and suffixes). Learning the meanings of these parts can help you remember words and interpret unfamiliar terms.

WORD PART	MEANING	EXAMPLE
Metabolism		
glyc/o	sugar, sweet	*Glycogen* yields glucose molecules when it breaks down.
-lysis	separating, dissolving	*Glycolysis* is the breakdown of glucose for energy.
Body Temperature		
pyr/o	fire, fever	An *antipyretic* drug reduces fever.
therm/o	heat	*Hypothermia* is an excessively low body temperature.

Summary

I. Metabolism—life-sustaining reactions that occur in the living cell

1. Catabolism—breakdown of complex compounds into simpler compounds
2. Anabolism—building of simple compounds into substances needed for cellular activities, growth, and repair

A. Cellular respiration—a series of reactions in which food is oxidized for energy
  1. Anaerobic phase—does not require oxygen
     a. Location—cytoplasm
     b. Yield—2 ATP per glucose
     c. End product—organic (i.e., pyruvic acid)
  2. Aerobic phase—requires oxygen
     a. Location—mitochondria
     b. Yield—34-36 ATP per glucose
     c. End products—carbon dioxide and water
  3. Metabolic rate—rate at which energy is released from food in the cells
     a. Basal metabolism—amount of energy needed to maintain life functions while at rest

B. Use of nutrients for energy
  1. Glucose—main energy source
  2. Fats—highest energy yield
  3. Proteins—can be used for energy after removal of nitrogen (deamination)

C. Anabolism
  1. Essential amino acids and fatty acids must be taken in as part of diet

D. Minerals and vitamins
  1. Minerals—elements needed for body structure and cell activities
     a. Trace elements—elements needed in extremely small amounts
  2. Vitamins—organic substances needed in small amounts
     a. Antioxidants (*e.g.*, vitamins C and E) protect against free radicals

II. Nutritional guidelines

A. Carbohydrates
  1. 55%-60% of calories
  2. Should be complex (unrefined) not simple (sugars)
     a. Glycemic effect—how quickly a food raises blood glucose and insulin
     b. Plant fiber important

B. Fats
  1. 30% or less of calories
  2. Unsaturated healthier than saturated
     a. Hydrogenated fats artificially saturated

C. Proteins
  1. 15%-20% of calories
  2. Complete—all essential amino acids
     a. Need to combine plant foods

D. Vitamin and mineral supplements

E. Food Guide Pyramid (USDA)—under revision

F. Alcohol—metabolized in liver

III. Nutritional disorders

A. Food allergies
B. Malnutrition
C. Overweight and obesity
  1. Body mass index (BMI)—weight (kg) ÷ (height [m])^2
D. Underweight

IV. Nutrition and aging

V. Body temperature

A. Heat production
  1. Most heat produced in muscles and glands
  2. Distributed by the circulation
  3. Affected by exercise, hormones, food, age
B. Heat loss
  1. Avenues—skin, urine, feces, respiratory system
  2. Mechanisms—conduction, radiation, convection, evaporation
  3. Prevention of heat loss—clothing, subcutaneous fat
C. Temperature regulation
  1. Hypothalamus—main temperature-regulating center
    a. Responds to temperature of blood in brain and temperature receptors in skin
  2. Conservation of heat
    a. Constriction of blood vessels in skin
    b. Shivering
    c. Increased release of epinephrine
  3. Release of heat
    a. Dilation of skin vessels
    b. Sweating
    c. Relaxation of muscles
  4. Age factors
  5. Normal body temperature—ranges from 36.2°C to 37.6°C; varies with time of day and location measured
D. Fever—higher than normal body temperature resulting from infection, injury, toxin, damage to CNS, etc.
  1. Pyrogen—substance that produces fever
  2. Antipyretic—drug that reduces fever
E. Response to excessive heat—heat cramps, heat exhaustion, heat stroke
F. Response to excessive cold
  1. Hypothermia—low body temperature
    a. Results—coma and death
    b. Uses—surgery
  2. Frostbite—reduction of blood supply to areas such as face, ears, toes, fingers
    a. Results—necrosis and gangrene

Questions for Study and Review

Building Understanding

Fill in the blanks

1. Building glycogen from glucose is an example of ______.
2. The amount of energy needed to maintain life functions while at rest is ______.
3. Reserves of glucose are stored in liver and muscle as ______.
4. The most important area of the brain for temperature regulation is the ______.
5. A drug that reduces fever is described as ______.

Matching

Match each numbered item with the most closely related lettered item.

___ 6. Main energy source for the body
___ 7. Chemical element required for normal body function
___ 8. Complex organic substance required for normal body function
___ 9. Energy storage molecule with only single bonds between carbon atoms
___ 10. Energy storage molecule with one or more double bonds between carbon atoms

a. saturated fat
b. vitamin
c. mineral
d. unsaturated fat
e. glucose

Multiple choice

___ 11. During amino acid catabolism, nitrogen is removed by
  a. oxidation
  b. the glycemic effect
  c. lysis
  d. deamination

___ 12. Which of the following would have the lowest glycemic effect?
  a. glucose
  b. sucrose
  c. lactose
  d. starch

___ 13. Alcohol is catabolized by the
  a. small intestine
  b. liver
  c. pancreas
  d. spleen

___ 14. Amino acids that cannot be made by metabolism are said to be
  a. essential
  b. nonessential

c. antioxidants
d. free radicals

Understanding Concepts

15. In what part of the cell does anaerobic respiration occur and what are its end products? In what part of the cell does aerobic respiration occur? What are its end products?
16. About how many kilocalories are released from a tablespoon of butter (14 grams)? a tablespoon of sugar (12 grams)? a tablespoon of egg white (15 grams)?
17. If you eat 2000 kcal a day, how many kilocalories should come from carbohydrates? from fats? from protein?
18. How is heat produced in the body? What structures produce the most heat during increased activity?
19. Emily's body temperature increased from 36.2 °C to 36.5 °C and then decreased to 36.2°C Describe the feedback mechanism regulating Emily's body temperature.
20. Define *fever*. Name some aspects of the course of fever, and list some of its beneficial and harmful effects.
21. What is hypothermia? Under what circumstances does it usually occur? List some of its effects.
22. Differentiate between the terms in the following pairs:
    a. conduction and convection
    b. radiation and evaporation
    c. marasmus and kwashiorkor
    d. lysis and crisis
    e. heat exhaustion and heat stroke

Conceptual Thinking

23. The oxidation of glucose to form ATP is often compared to the burning of fuel. Why is this analogy inaccurate?
24. Richard M, a self-described couch potato, is six feet tall and weighs 240 pounds. Calculate Richard's body mass index. Is Richard overweight or obese? List some diseases associated with obesity.

Selected Key Terms

The following terms and other boldface terms in the chapter are defined in the Glossary

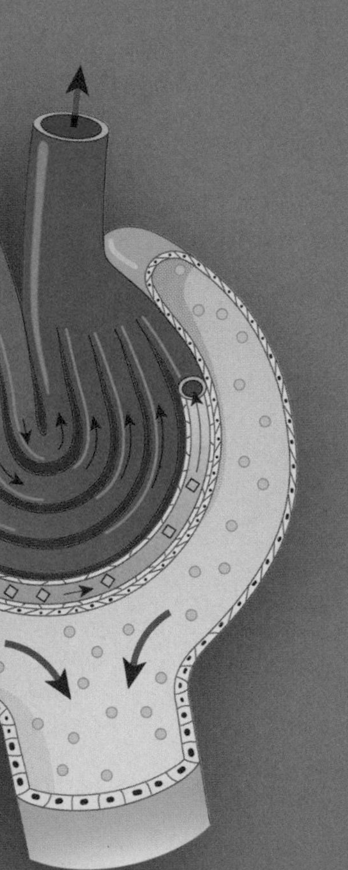

acidosis
alkalosis
ascites
buffer
dehydration
edema
effusion
electrolyte
extracellular
interstitial
intracellular
pH

Learning Outcomes

After careful study of this chapter, you should be able to:

1. Compare intracellular and extracellular fluids
2. List four types of extracellular fluids
3. Name the systems that are involved in water balance
4. Explain how thirst is regulated
5. Define *electrolytes* and describe some of their functions
6. Describe the role of hormones in electrolyte balance
7. Describe three methods for regulating the pH of body fluids
8. Compare acidosis and alkalosis, including possible causes
9. Describe three disorders involving body fluids
10. Specify some fluids used in therapy
11. Show how word parts are used to build words related to the urinary system (see Word Anatomy at the end of the chapter)

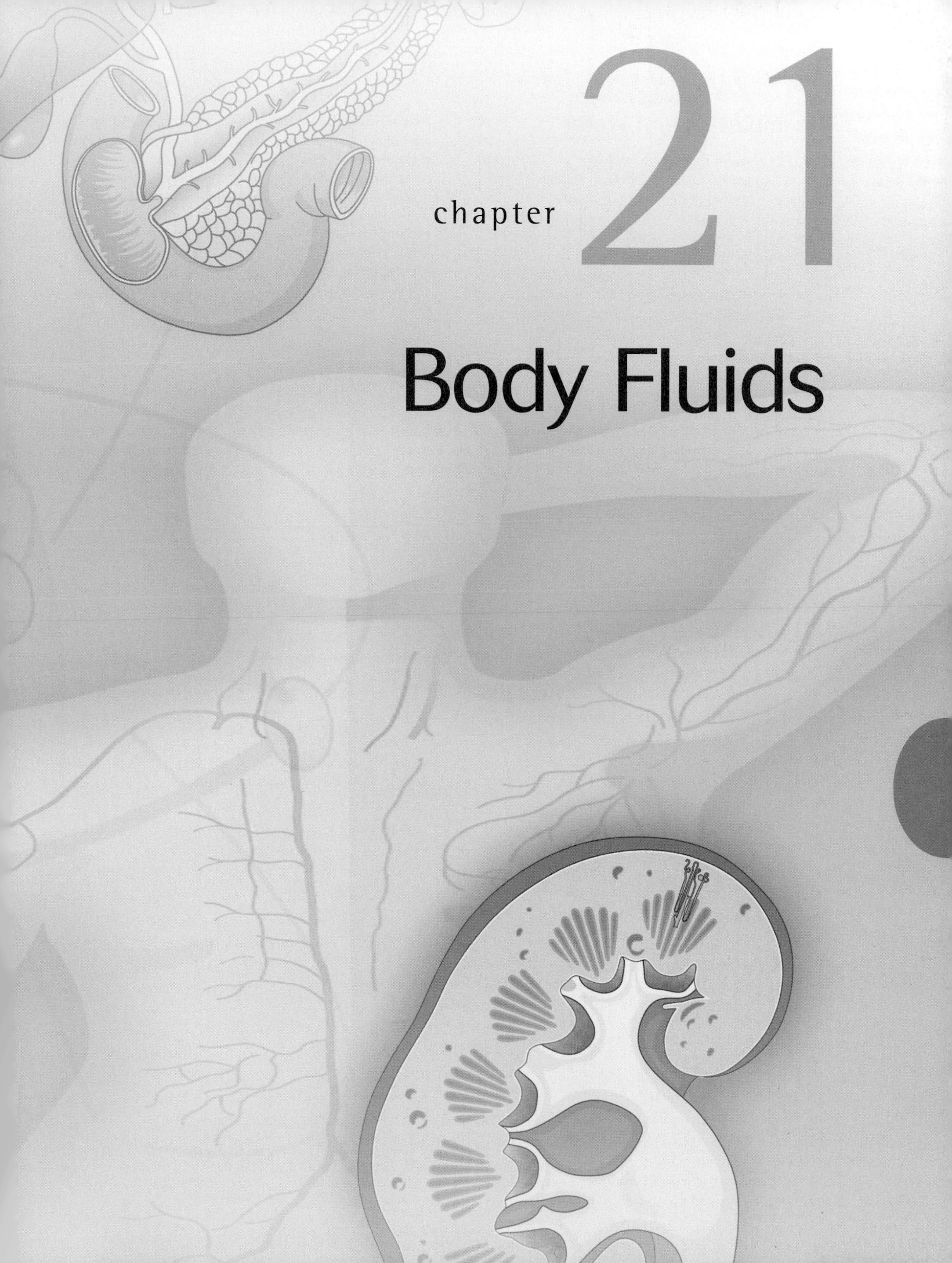

chapter 21

Body Fluids

The Importance of Water

Water is important to living cells as a solvent, a transport medium, and a participant in metabolic reactions. The normal proportion of body water varies from 50% to 70% of a person's weight. It is highest in the young and in thin, muscular individuals. In infants, water makes up 75% of the total body mass. That's why infants are in greater danger from dehydration than adults. With increase in the amount of fat, the percentage of water in the body decreases, because adipose tissue holds very little water compared with muscle tissue.

Various electrolytes (salts), nutrients, gases, waste, and special substances, such as enzymes and hormones, are dissolved or suspended in body water. The composition of body fluids is an important factor in homeostasis. Whenever the volume or chemical makeup of these fluids deviates even slightly from normal, disease results. (See Appendix 4, Table 3, for normal values.) The constancy of body fluids is maintained in the following ways:

- The thirst mechanism, which maintains the volume of water at a constant level.
- Kidney activity, which regulates the volume and composition of body fluids (see Chapter 22, The Urinary System).
- Hormones, which serve to regulate fluid volume and electrolytes.
- Regulators of pH (acidity and alkalinity), including buffers, respiration, and kidney function.

The maintenance of proper fluid balance involves many of the principles discussed in earlier chapters, such as pH and buffers, the effects of respiration on pH, tonicity of solutions, and forces influencing capillary exchange. Some of these chapters will be referenced in the following sections. Additional information follows in Chapter 22 on the urinary system.

Fluid Compartments

Although body fluids have much in common no matter where they are located, there are some important differences between fluid inside and outside cells. Accordingly, fluids are grouped into two main compartments (Fig. 21-1):

- **Intracellular fluid** (ICF) is contained within the cells. About two-thirds to three-fourths of all body fluids are in this category.
- **Extracellular fluid** (ECF) includes all body fluids outside of cells. In this group are included the following:
  - **Interstitial** (in-ter-STISH-al) **fluid,** or more simply, tissue fluid. This fluid is located in the spaces between the cells in tissues all over the body. It is estimated that tissue fluid constitutes about 15% of body weight.
  - **Blood plasma,** which constitutes about 4% of a person's body weight.
  - **Lymph,** the fluid that drains from the tissues into the lymphatic system. This is about 1% of body weight.
  - **Fluid in special compartments,** such as cerebrospinal fluid, the aqueous and vitreous humors of the eye, serous fluid, and synovial fluid. Together, these make up about 1% to 3% of total body fluids.

Fluids are not locked into one compartment. There is a constant interchange between compartments as fluids are transferred across semipermeable cell membranes by diffusion and osmosis (see Fig. 21-1). Also, fluids are lost and replaced on a daily basis.

> **Checkpoint 21-1** What are the two main compartments into which body fluids are grouped?

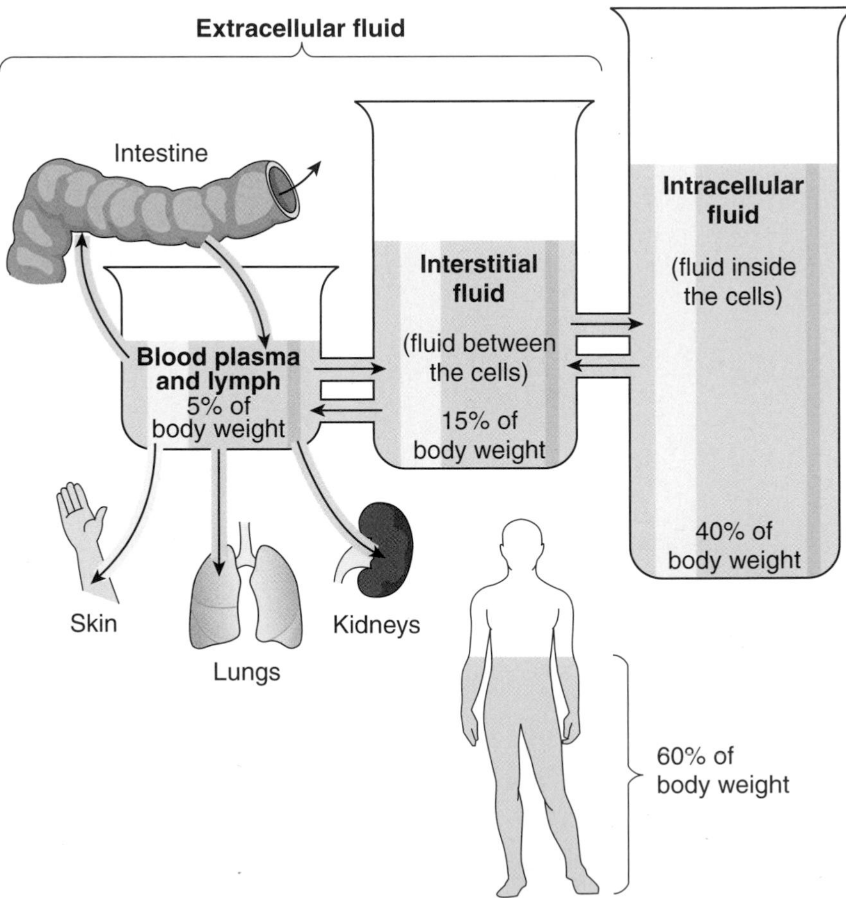

Figure 21-1 Main fluid compartments showing relative percentage by weight of body fluid. Fluid percentages vary but total about 60% of body weight. Fluids are constantly exchanged among compartments, and each day fluids are lost and replaced. *ZOOMING IN ✦ What are some avenues through which water is lost?*

Water Balance

In a person whose health is normal, the quantity of water gained in a day is approximately equal to the quantity lost (output) (Fig. 21-2). The quantity of water consumed in a day (intake) varies considerably. The average adult in a comfortable environment takes in about 2300 mL of water (about 2 1/2 quarts) daily. About two-thirds of this quantity comes from drinking water and other beverages; about one-third comes from foods—fruits, vegetables, and soups. About 200 mL of water is produced each day as a by-product of cellular respiration. This water, described as *metabolic water*, brings the total average gain to 2500 mL each day.

The same volume of water is constantly being lost from the body by the following routes:

- The **kidneys** excrete the largest quantity of water lost each day. About 1 to 1.5 liters of water are eliminated daily in the urine. (Note that beverages containing alcohol or caffeine act as diuretics and increase water loss through the kidneys.)
- The **skin.** Although sebum and keratin help prevent dehydration, water is constantly evaporating from the skin's surface. Larger amounts of water are lost from the skin as sweat when it is necessary to cool the body.
- The **lungs** expel water along with carbon dioxide.
- The **intestinal tract** eliminates water along with the feces.

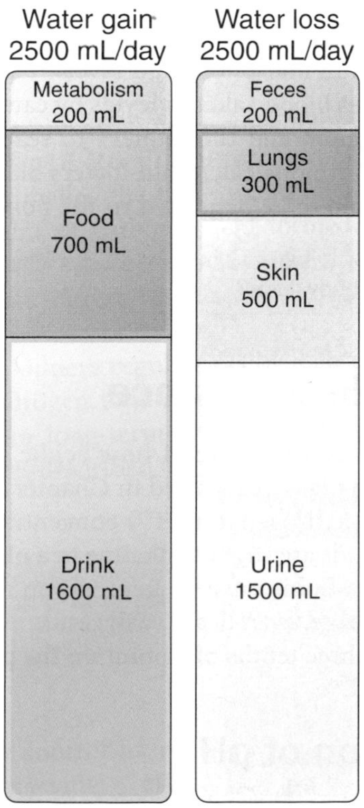

Water gain 2500 mL/day	Water loss 2500 mL/day
Metabolism 200 mL	Feces 200 mL
Food 700 mL	Lungs 300 mL
Drink 1600 mL	Skin 500 mL
	Urine 1500 mL

Figure 21-2 Daily gain and loss of water.

In many disorders, it is important for the healthcare team to know whether a patient's intake and output are equal; in such a case, a 24-hour intake–output record is kept. The intake record includes *all* the liquid the patient has taken in. This means fluids administered intravenously as well as those consumed by mouth. The healthcare worker must account for water, other beverages, and liquid foods, such as soup and ice cream. The output record includes the quantity of urine excreted in the same 24-hour period as well as an estimation of fluid losses due to fever, vomiting, diarrhea, bleeding, wound discharge, or other causes.

Checkpoint 21-2 What are three routes for water loss from the body?

Sense of Thirst

The control center for the sense of thirst is located in the brain's hypothalamus. This center plays a major role in the regulation of total fluid volume. A decrease in fluid volume or an increase in the concentration of body fluids stimulates the thirst center, causing a person to drink water or other fluids containing large amounts of water. Dryness of the mouth also causes a sensation of thirst. Excessive thirst, such as that caused by excessive urine loss in cases of diabetes, is called **polydipsia** (pol-e-DIP-se-ah).

The thirst center should stimulate enough drinking to balance fluids, but this is not always the case. During vigorous exercise, especially in hot weather, the body can dehydrate rapidly. People may not drink enough to replace needed fluids. In addition, if plain water is consumed, the dilution of body fluids may depress the thirst center. Athletes who are exercising very strenuously may need to drink beverages with some carbohydrates for energy and also some electrolytes to keep fluids in balance. (See Box 21-1, Osmoreceptors: Thinking About Thirst, for more about thirst regulation.)

Checkpoint 21-3 Where is the control center for the sense of thirst located?

Electrolytes and Their Functions

Electrolytes are important constituents of body fluids. These compounds separate into positively and negatively charged ions in solution. Positively charged ions are called *cations;* negatively charged ions are called *anions*. Electrolytes are so-named because they conduct an electrical current in solution. A few of the most important ions are reviewed next:

- Positive ions (cations):
  - **Sodium** is chiefly responsible for maintaining osmotic balance and body fluid volume. It is the main positive ion in extracellular fluids. Sodium is required for nerve

Summary

I. The importance of water

1 Functions
- a. Solvent
- b. Transport medium
- c. Participant in metabolic reactions

2. 50% to 70% of body weight
3. Contains electrolytes, nutrients, gases, wastes, hormones, and other substances
4. Important in homeostasis

II. Fluid compartments

1. Intracellular fluid—contained within the cells
2. Extracellular fluid—outside the cells
   - a. Blood plasma
   - b. Interstitial (tissue) fluid
   - c. Lymph
   - d. Fluid in special compartments

III. Water balance

1. Loss—through kidneys, skin, lungs, intestinal tract,
2. Gain—through beverages, food, metabolic water

A. Sense of thirst
1. Control center in hypothalamus
2. Responds to fluid volume and concentration of body fluids

IV. Electrolytes and their functions

1. Electrolytes release ions in solution
   - a. Positive ions (cations)—*e.g.*, sodium, potassium, calcium
   - b. Negative ions (anions)—*e.g.*, phosphate, chloride

A. Electrolyte balance
1. Kidneys—main regulators
2. Role of hormones
   - a. Aldosterone (from adrenal cortex)
     - (1) Promotes reabsorption of sodium
     - (2) Promotes excretion of potassium
   - b. ADH (from pituitary)
     - (1) Causes kidney to retain water
   - c. Parathyroid hormone (from parathyroid glands)
     - (1) Increases blood calcium level
   - d. Calcitonin (from thyroid)
     - (1) Decreases blood calcium level

V. Acid–base balance

1. Normal pH range is 7.35–7.45

A. Regulation of pH
1. Buffers—maintain constant pH
2. Respiration—release of carbon dioxide increases alkalinity; retention of carbon dioxide increases acidity
3. Kidney—regulates amount of hydrogen ion excreted

B. Abnormal pH
1. Acidosis—decrease in pH; causes: respiratory obstruction, lung disease, kidney failure, diarrhea, diabetes mellitus, starvation
2. Alkalosis—increase in pH; causes: hyperventilation, ingestion of antacids, prolonged vomiting

VI. Disorders of body fluids

1. Edema—accumulation of fluid in tissues
   - a. Causes
     - (1) Interference with fluid return to heart
     - (2) Lack of proteins in blood
     - (3) Kidney failure
     - (4) Fluid loss from capillaries
2. Water intoxication—dilution of body fluids
3. Effusion—escape of fluid into a cavity or space
4. Ascites—accumulation of fluid in abdominal cavity
5. Dehydration—deficiency of fluid

VII. Fluid therapy

1. Purpose
   - a. Correct fluid balance
   - b. Correct electrolyte balance
   - c. Provide nourishment
2. Commonly used solutions
   - a. Normal saline
   - b. 5% dextrose (glucose) in 0.45% (1/2 normal) saline
   - c. 5% dextrose in water
   - d. Ringer lactate
   - e. 25% serum albumin

Questions for Study and Review

Building Understanding

Fill in the blanks

1. Excessive thirst is termed______.
2. Loss of sodium and an excess of potassium are classic signs of ______ disease.
3. Substances in the blood that prevent sharp changes in hydrogen ion concentration are called______.
4. Effusion with accumulation of fluid within the abdominal cavity is termed ______.
5. A severe deficit in body fluid is called ______.

Matching

Match each numbered item with the most closely related lettered item.

___ 6. Essential for maintaining osmotic balance and body fluid volume; this cation is abundant in extracellular fluid

___ 7. Important in the transmission of nerve impulses and enzyme activities; this cation is abundant in intracellular fluid

___ 8. Required for bone formation, muscle contraction, and blood clotting

___ 9. Essential in bone formation and acid-base balance; this anion is found in plasma membranes, ATP and nucleic acids

___ 10. Important for gastric acid formation; this anion is abundant in extracellular fluid

a. sodium
b. potassium
c. calcium
d. phosphate
e. chloride

Multiple choice

___ 11. Body water content is greatest in
- a. infants
- b. children
- c. young adults
- d. elderly adults

___ 12. Fluid located in the spaces between the cells is called
- a. cytoplasm
- b. plasma
- c. interstitial fluid
- d. lymph

___ 13. The organ(s) responsible for water loss through evaporation is (are) the
- a. kidneys
- b. skin
- c. lungs
- d. intestinal tract

___ 14. Which of the following is responsible for long-term regulation of pH?
- a. buffer system
- b. digestive system
- c. respiratory system
- d. urinary system

___ 15. Increased blood CO_2 causes
- a. respiratory acidosis
- b. respiratory alkalosis
- c. metabolic acidosis
- d. metabolic alkalosis

Understanding Concepts

16. Compare the terms in each of the following pairs:
    - a. intracellular and extracellular fluid
    - b. aldosterone and antidiuretic hormone
    - c. calcitonin and parathyroid hormone
17. In a healthy person, what is the ratio of fluid intake to output?
18. Explain the role of the hypothalamus in water balance.
19. How do the respiratory and urinary systems regulate pH?
20. Compare and contrast the following disorders:
    - a. acidosis and alkalosis
    - b. edema and effusion
    - c. water intoxication and dehydration
21. List some causes of edema.
22. List three purposes for administering intravenous fluids.
23. Compare and contrast the following types of intravenous fluids:
    - a. normal saline and 5% dextrose saline
    - b. Ringer solution and serum albumin

Conceptual Thinking

24. Patty Grant, 55 years old, reports severe headaches and excessive thirst and urination. What is the probable cause of Patty's symptoms?
25. Why is emphysema associated with decreased urine pH?

Selected Key Terms

The following terms and other boldface terms in the chapter are defined in the Glossary

angiotensin
antidiuretic hormone (ADH)
cystitis
dialysis
erythropoietin
excretion
glomerular filtrate
glomerulonephritis
glomerulus
hemodialysis
kidney
micturition
nephron
pyelonephritis
renin
urea
ureter
urethra
urinalysis
urinary bladder
urine

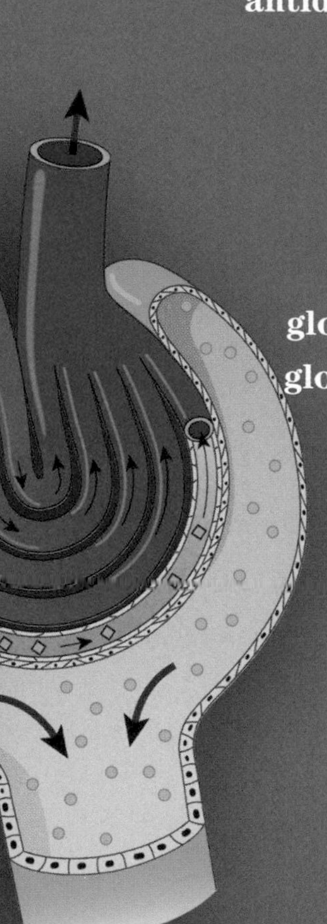

Learning Outcomes

After careful study of this chapter, you should be able to:

1. List the systems that eliminate waste and name the substances eliminated by each
2. Describe the parts of the urinary system and give the functions of each
3. Trace the path of a drop of blood as it flows through the kidney
4. Describe a nephron
5. Describe the components and functions of the juxtaglomerular (JG) apparatus
6. Name the four processes involved in urine formation and describe the action of each
7. Identify the role of ADH in urine formation
8. Describe the process of micturition
9. Name three normal and six abnormal constituents of urine
10. List the common disorders of the urinary system
11. List six signs of chronic renal failure
12. Explain the principle and the purpose of kidney dialysis
13. Show how word parts are used to build words related to the urinary system (see Word Anatomy at the end of the chapter)

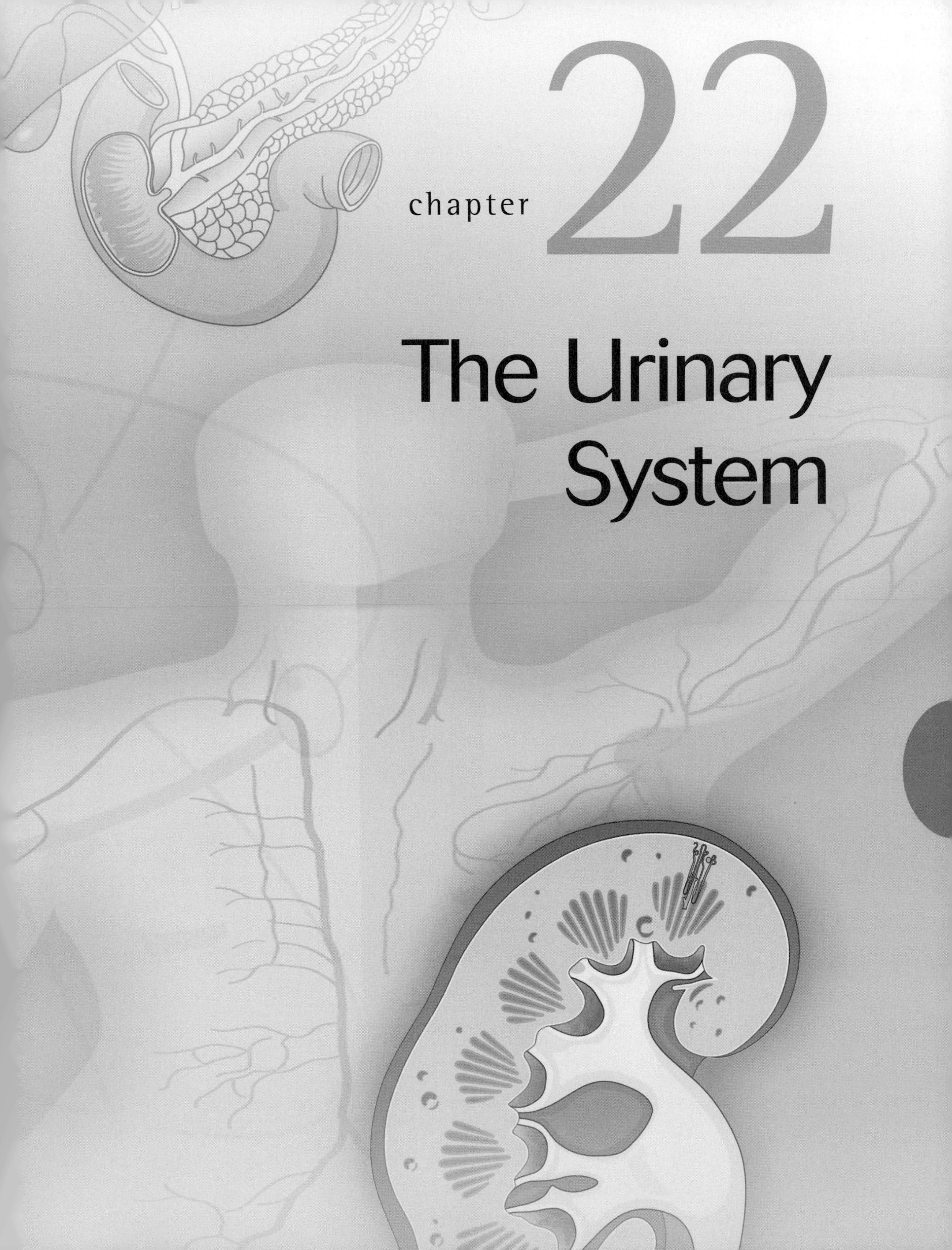

chapter 22

The Urinary System

Excretion

The urinary system is also called the *excretory system* because one of its main functions is **excretion**, removal and elimination of metabolic waste products from the blood. It has many other functions as well, including regulation of the volume, acid–base balance (pH), and electrolyte composition of body fluids.

Although the focus of this chapter is the urinary system, certain aspects of other systems are also discussed, because body systems work interdependently to maintain homeostasis (internal balance). The systems active in excretion and some of the substances they eliminate are the following:

- The **urinary system** excretes water, nitrogen-containing waste products, and salts. These are all constituents of the urine.
- The **digestive system** eliminates water, some salts, and bile in addition to digestive residue, all of which are contained in the feces. The liver is important in eliminating the products of red blood cell destruction and in breaking down certain drugs and toxins.
- The **respiratory system** eliminates carbon dioxide and water. The latter appears as vapor, as can be demonstrated by breathing on a windowpane.
- The skin, or **integumentary system**, excretes water, salts, and very small quantities of nitrogenous wastes. These all appear in perspiration, although water also evaporates continuously from the skin without our being conscious of it.

Checkpoint 22-1 The main function of the urinary system is to eliminate waste. What are some other systems that eliminate waste?

Organs of the Urinary System

The main parts of the urinary system, shown in Figure 22-1, are as follows:

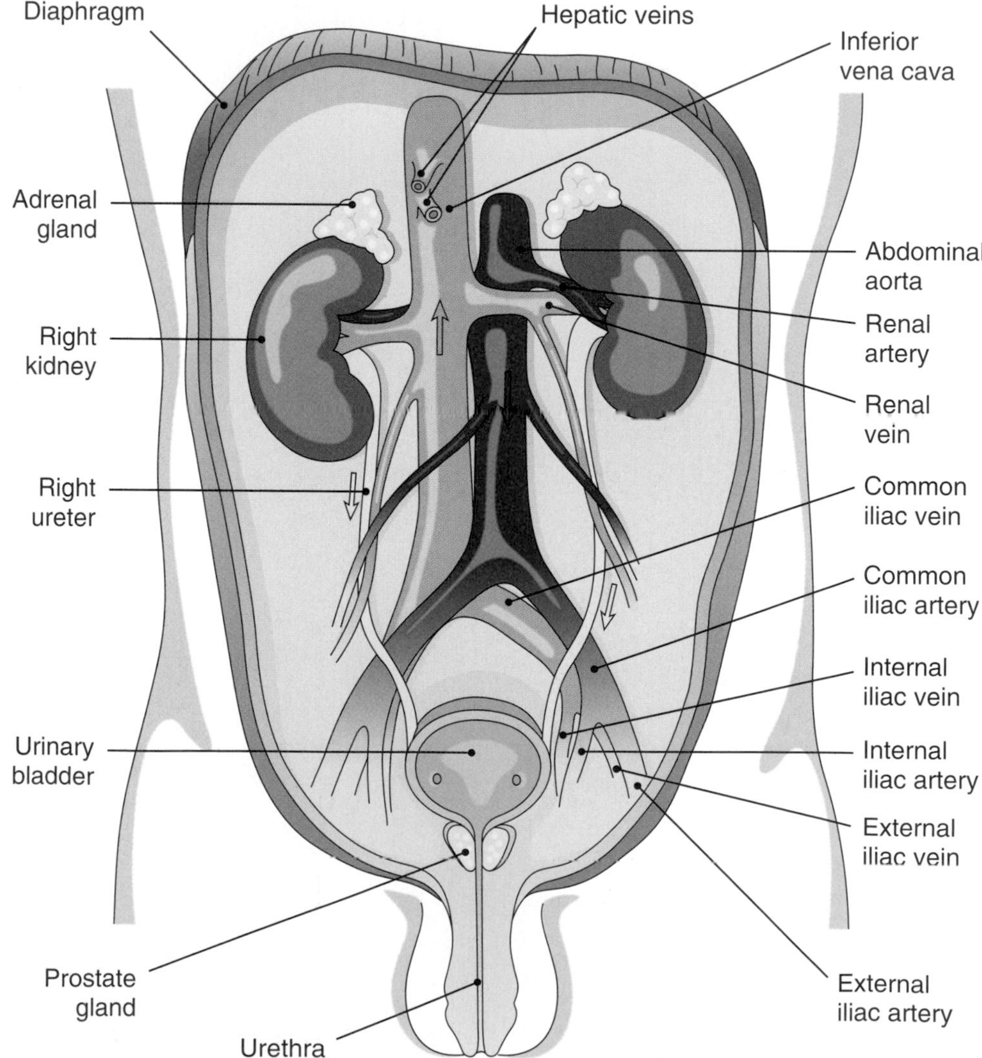

Figure 22-1 Male urinary system, showing blood vessels. *ZOOMING IN ✦ What vessel supplies blood to the kidney? What vessel drains the kidney?*

- Two **kidneys.** These organs extract wastes from the blood, balance body fluids, and form urine.
- Two **ureters** (U-re-ters). These tubes conduct urine from the kidneys to the urinary bladder.
- A single **urinary bladder**. This reservoir receives and stores the urine brought to it by the two ureters.
- A single **urethra** (u-RE-thrah). This tube conducts urine from the bladder to the outside of the body for elimination.

Checkpoint 22-2 What are the organs of the urinary system?

The Kidneys

The kidneys lie against the back muscles in the upper abdomen at about the level of the last thoracic and first three lumbar vertebrae. The right kidney is slightly lower than the left to accommodate the liver. Each kidney is firmly enclosed in a membranous **renal capsule** made of fibrous connective tissue. In addition, there is a protective layer of fat called the **adipose capsule** around the organ. An outermost layer of fascia (connective tissue) anchors the kidney to the peritoneum and abdominal wall. The kidneys, as well as the ureters, lie posterior to the peritoneum. Thus, they are not in the peritoneal cavity but rather in an area known as the **retroperitoneal** (ret-ro-per-ih-to-NE-al) **space**.

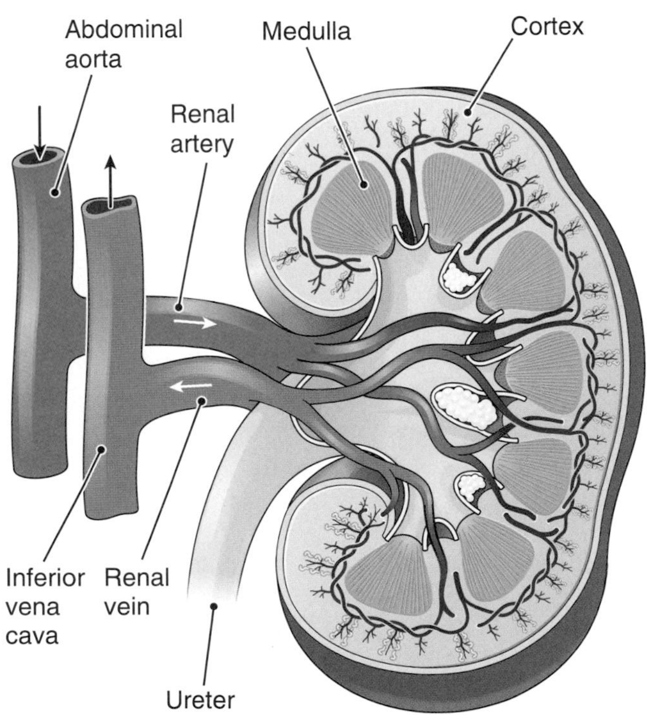

Figure 22-2 **Blood supply and circulation of the kidney.** *ZOOMING IN ✦ What vessel supplies blood to the renal artery? What vessel receives blood from the renal vein?*

Blood Supply to the Kidney

The kidney's blood supply is illustrated in Figure 22-2. Blood is brought to the kidney by a short branch of the abdominal aorta called the **renal artery**.

After entering the kidney, the renal artery subdivides into smaller and smaller branches, which eventually make contact with the functional units of the kidney, the **nephrons** (NEF-ronz). Blood leaves the kidney by vessels that finally merge to form the **renal** vein, which carries blood into the inferior vena cava for return to the heart.

Checkpoint 22-3 The kidneys are located in the retroperitoneal space. Where is this space?

Checkpoint 22-4 What vessel supplies blood to the kidney and what vessel drains blood from the kidney?

Structure of the Kidney

The kidney is a somewhat flattened organ approximately 10 cm (4 inches) long, 5 cm (2 inches) wide, and 2.5 cm (1 inch) thick (Fig. 22-3). On the medial border there is a notch called the **hilum**, where the renal artery, the renal vein, and the ureter connect with the kidney. The lateral border is convex (curved outward), giving the entire organ a bean-shaped appearance.

The kidney is divided into two regions: the renal cortex and the renal medulla (Fig. 22-3). The **renal cortex** is the kidney's outer portion. The **renal medulla** contains tubes in which urine is formed and collected. These tubes form a number of cone-shaped structures called **renal pyramids**. The tips of the pyramids point toward the **renal pelvis**, a funnel-shaped basin that forms the upper end of the ureter. Cuplike extensions of the renal pelvis surround the tips of the pyramids and collect urine; these extensions are called **calyces** (KA-lih-seze; singular, **calyx**, KA-liks). The urine that collects in the pelvis then passes down the ureters to the bladder.

Checkpoint 22-5 What are the outer and inner regions of the kidney called?

The Nephron As is the case with most organs, the most fascinating aspect of the kidney is too small to be seen with the naked eye. This basic unit, which actually does the kidney's work, is the **nephron** (Fig. 22-4). The nephron is essentially a tiny coiled tube with a bulb at one end. This bulb, known as the **glomerular** (Bowman) **capsule,** surrounds a cluster of capillaries called the **glomerulus** (glo-MER-u-lus) (pl., glomeruli [glo-MER-u-li]). Each kidney contains about 1 million nephrons; if all these coiled tubes were separated, straightened out, and laid end to end, they would span some 120 kilometers (75 miles)! Figure 22-5 is a microscopic view of kidney tissue showing several glomeruli, each surrounded by a

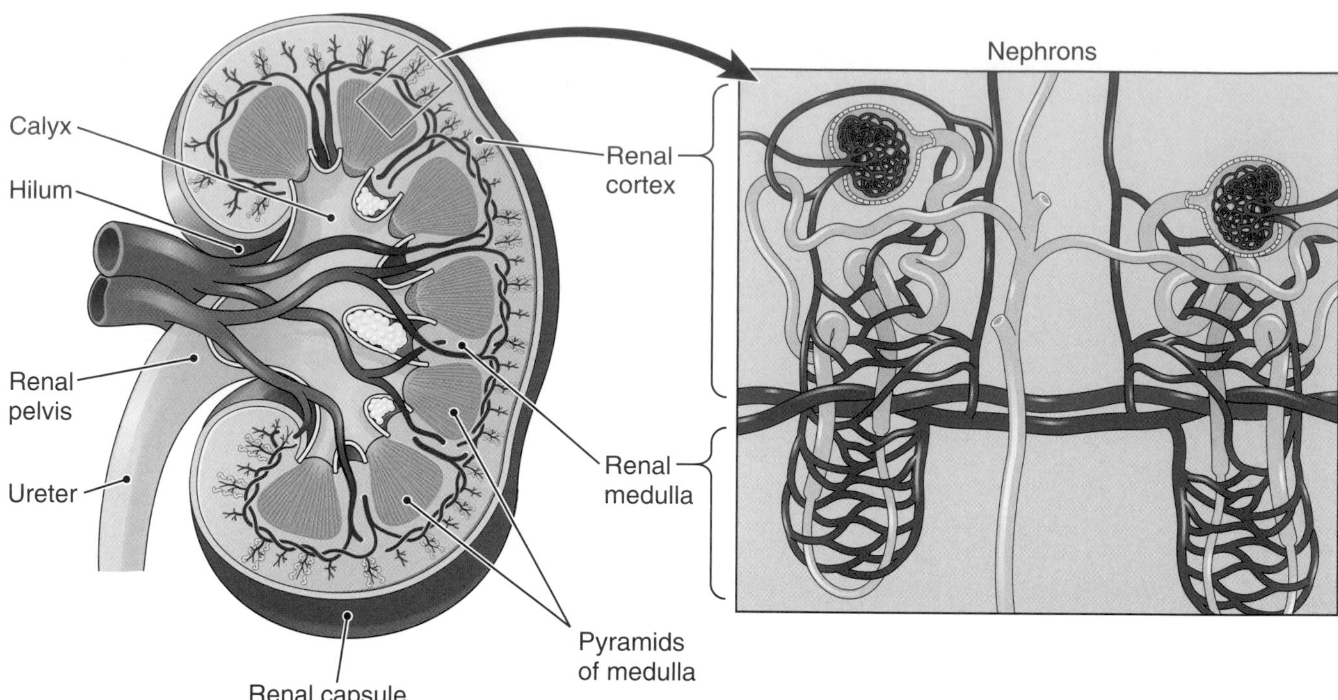

Figure 22-3 **Longitudinal section through the kidney.** Its internal structure is shown (*left*), along with an enlarged diagram of nephrons (*right*). Each kidney contains more than 1 million nephrons. *ZOOMING IN ✦ What is the outer region of the kidney called? What is the inner region of the kidney called?*

glomerular capsule. This figure also shows sections through the tubular portions of the nephrons.

A small blood vessel, the **afferent arteriole,** supplies the glomerulus with blood; another small vessel, called the **efferent arteriole,** carries blood from the glomerulus. When blood leaves the glomerulus, it does not head immediately back toward the heart. Instead, it flows into a capillary network that surrounds the nephron's tubular portion. These **peritubular capillaries,** are named for their location.

The tubular portion of the nephron consists of several parts. The coiled part leading from the glomerular capsule is called the **proximal convoluted** (KON-vo-lu-ted) **tubule** (**PCT**, or just proximal tubule). The tubule then uncoils to form a hairpin-shaped segment called the **loop of Henle**. The first part of the loop, which carries fluid toward the medulla, is the **descending limb** (see Fig. 22-4). The part that continues from the loop's turn and carries fluid away from the medulla, is the **ascending limb**. Continuing from the ascending limb, the tubule coils once again into the **distal convoluted tubule** (**DCT**, or just distal tubule), so called because it is farther along the tubule from the glomerular capsule than is the PCT. The distal end of each tubule empties into a collecting duct, which then continues through the medulla toward the renal pelvis.

The glomerulus, glomerular capsule, and the proximal and distal convoluted tubules of the nephron are within the renal cortex. The loop of Henle and collecting duct extend into the medulla (see Fig. 22-3).

Checkpoint 22-6 What is the functional unit of the kidney called?

Checkpoint 22-7 What name is given to the coil of capillaries in the glomerular (Bowman) capsule?

The Juxtaglomerular (JG) Apparatus The first portion of the DCT curves back toward the glomerulus to pass between the afferent and efferent arterioles (Fig. 22-6). At the point where the DCT makes contact with the afferent arteriole, there are specialized cells in each that together make up the **juxtaglomerular** (juks-tah-glo-MER-u-lar) (**JG**) **apparatus.** The JG apparatus helps to regulate kidney function. When blood pressure falls too low for the kidneys to function effectively, cells in the wall of the afferent arteriole secrete the enzyme **renin** (RE-nin), which raises blood pressure by a mechanism described later.

Functions of the Kidney

The kidneys are involved in the following processes:

- Excretion of unwanted substances, such as cellular metabolic waste, excess salts, and toxins. One product of amino acid metabolism is nitrogen-containing waste material, a chief form of which is **urea** (u-RE-ah). After synthesis in the liver, urea is transported in the blood to the kidneys for elimination. The kidneys have a specialized mechanism for the elimination of urea and other nitrogenous (ni-TROJ-en-us) wastes.

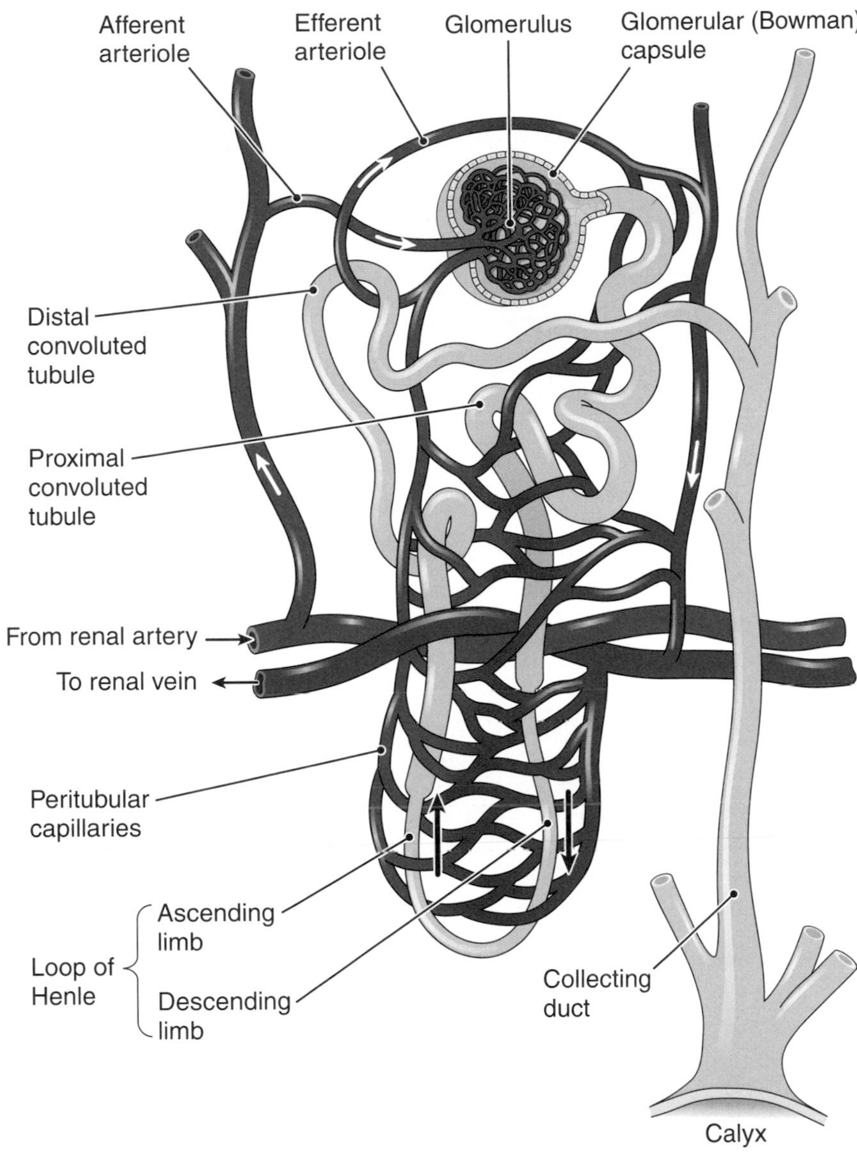

Figure 22-4 A nephron and its blood supply. The nephron regulates the proportions of water, waste, and other materials according to the body's constantly changing needs. Materials that enter the nephron can be returned to the blood through the surrounding capillaries. *ZOOMING IN ✦ Which of the two convoluted tubules is closer to the glomerular capsule? Which convoluted tubule is farther away?*

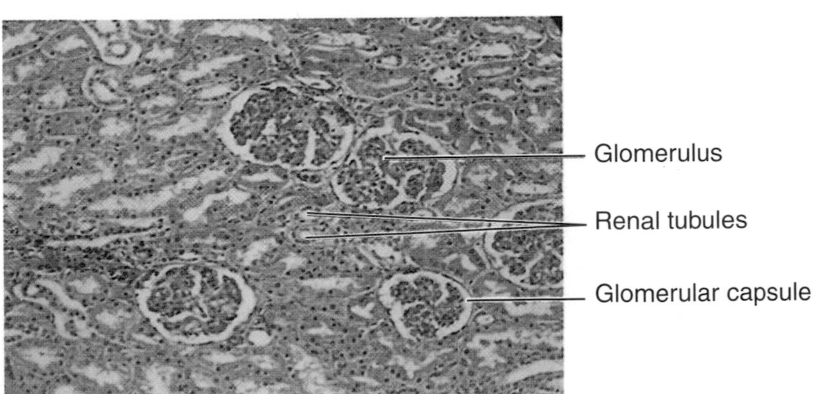

Figure 22-5 Microscopic view of the kidney. (Courtesy of Dana Morse Bittus and BJ Cohen.)

- Maintenance of water balance. Although the amount of water gained and lost in a day can vary tremendously, the kidneys can adapt to these variations, so that the volume of body water remains remarkably stable from day to day.
- Regulation of the acid–base balance of body fluids. Acids are constantly being produced by cellular metabolism. Certain foods can yield acids or bases, and people may also ingest antacids, such as bicarbonate. However, if the body is to function normally, the pH of body fluids must remain in the range of 7.35 to 7.45 (see Chapter 21).
- Regulation of blood pressure. The kidneys depend on blood pressure to filter the blood. If blood pressure falls too low for effective filtration, the cells of the JG apparatus release renin. This enzyme activates **angiotensin** (an-je-o-TEN-sin), a blood protein that causes blood vessels to constrict, thus raising blood pressure (Table 22-1). Angiotensin also stimulates the adrenal cortex to produce the hormone aldosterone, which promotes retention of sodium and water, also raising blood pressure.
- Regulation of red blood cell production. When the kidneys do not get enough oxygen, they produce the hormone **erythropoietin** (eh-rith-ro-POY-eh-tin) **(EPO)**, which stimulates red cell production in the bone marrow. EPO made by genetic engineering is now available to treat severe anemia, such as occurs in the end stage of kidney failure.

Checkpoint 22-8 What substance is produced by the JG apparatus and under what conditions is it produced?

Formation of Urine

The following explanation of urine formation describes a complex process, involving many back-and-forth exchanges between the bloodstream and the kidney tubules. As fluid filtered from the blood travels slowly through the twists and turns of the nephron, there is ample time for exchanges to take place. These

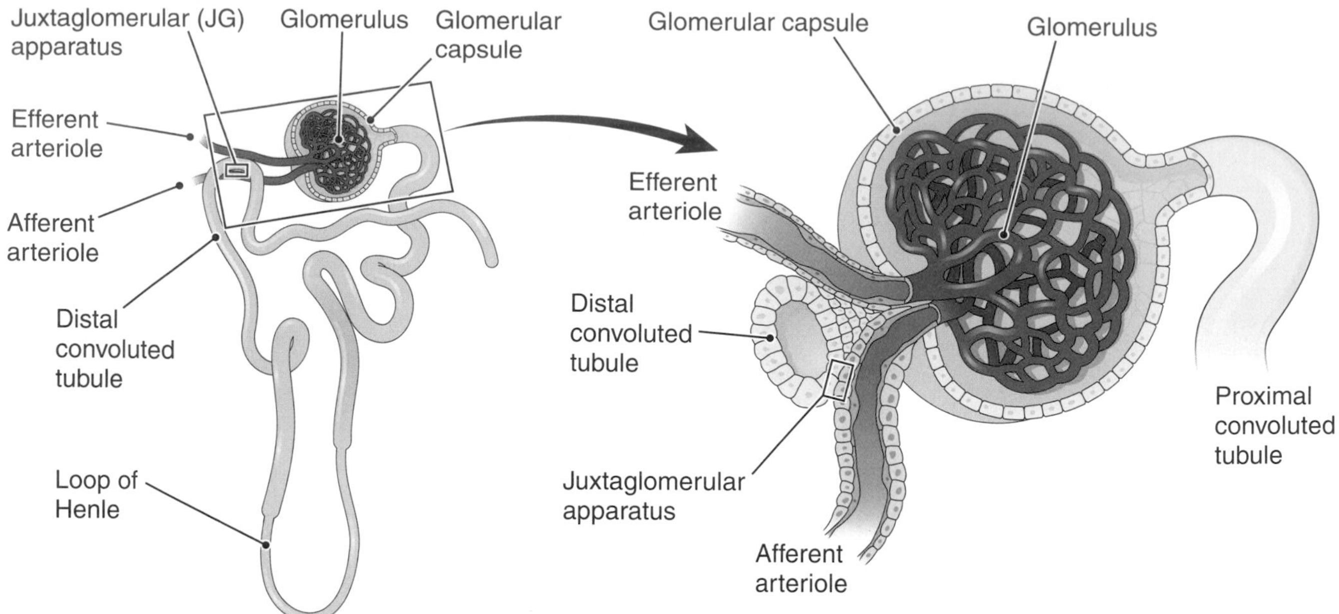

Figure 22-6 **Structure of the juxtaglomerular (JG) apparatus.** Note how the distal convoluted tubule contacts the afferent arteriole (*right*). Cells in these two structures make up the JG apparatus. *ZOOMING IN ✦ The JG apparatus is made up of cells from which two structures?*

processes together allow the kidney to "fine tune" body fluids as they adjust the composition of the urine.

Glomerular Filtration The process of urine formation begins with the glomerulus in the glomerular capsule. The walls of the glomerular capillaries are sievelike and permit the free flow of water and soluble materials through them. Like other capillary walls, however, they are impermeable (im-PER-me-abl) to blood cells and large protein molecules, and these components remain in the blood (Fig. 22-7).

Because the diameter of the afferent arteriole is slightly larger than that of the efferent arteriole (see Fig. 22-7), blood can enter the glomerulus more easily than it can leave. Thus, blood pressure in the glomerulus is about three to four times higher than it is in other capillaries. To understand this effect, think of placing your thumb over the end of a garden hose as water comes through. As you make the diameter of the opening smaller, water is forced out under higher pressure. As a result of increased fluid (hydrostatic) pressure in the glomerulus, materials are constantly being pushed out of the blood and into the nephron's glomerular capsule. As described in Chapter 3, movement of water and dissolved materials through a membrane under pressure is called *filtration*. This movement of materials under pressure from the blood into the capsule is therefore known as **glomerular filtration**.

Table 22•1 Substances that Affect Renal Function

SUBSTANCE	SOURCE	ACTION
Renin (RE-nin)	Enzyme produced by renal cells when blood pressure falls too low for effective filtration	Activates angiotensin in the blood
Angiotensin (an-je-o-TEN-sin)	Protein in the blood that is activated by renin	Causes constriction of blood vessels to raise blood pressure; also stimulates release of aldosterone from the adrenal cortex
Aldosterone (al-DOS-ter-one)	Hormone released from the adrenal cortex under effects of angiotensin	Promotes reabsorption of sodium and water in the kidney to conserve water and increase blood pressure
Antidiuretic hormone (an-te-di-u-RET-ik) (ADH)	Made in the hypothalamus and released from the posterior pituitary; released when blood becomes too concentrated	Promotes reabsorption of water from the distal convoluted tubule and collecting duct to concentrate the urine and conserve water

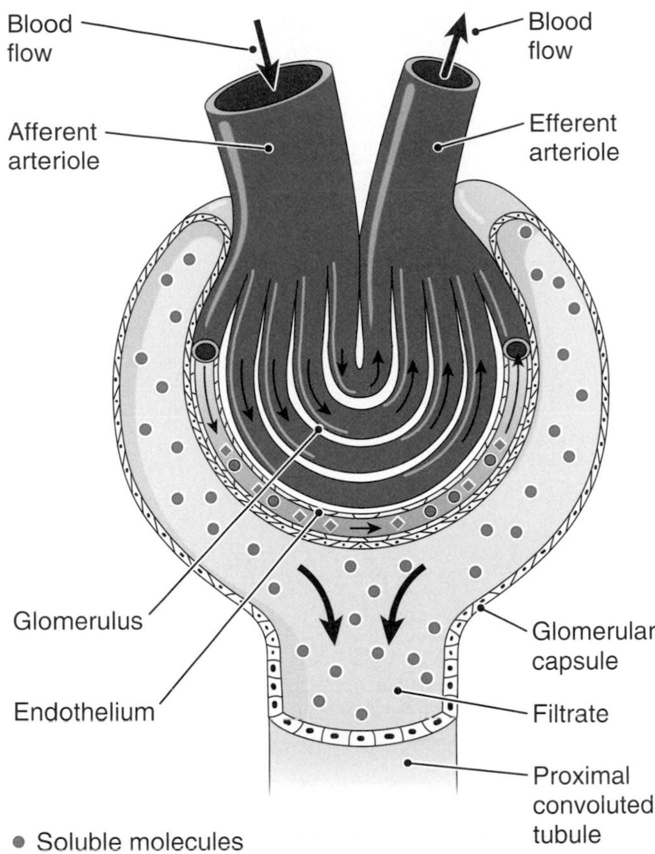

Figure 22-7 **Filtration process in the formation of urine.** Blood pressure inside the glomerulus forces water and dissolved substances into the glomerular (Bowman) capsule. Blood cells and proteins remain behind in the blood. The smaller diameter of the efferent arteriole as compared with that of the afferent arteriole maintains the hydrostatic (fluid) pressure. *ZOOMING IN ✦ Which arteriole associated with the glomerulus has the wider diameter?*

The fluid that enters the glomerular capsule, called the **glomerular filtrate**, begins its journey along the tubular system of the nephron. In addition to water and the normal soluble substances in the blood, other substances, such as vitamins and drugs, also may be filtered and become part of the glomerular filtrate.

> **Checkpoint 22-9** The first step in urine formation is glomerular filtration. What is glomerular filtration?

Tubular Reabsorption The kidneys form about 160 to 180 liters of filtrate each day. However, only 1 to 1.5 liters of urine are eliminated daily. Clearly, most of the water that enters the nephron is not excreted with the urine, but rather, is returned to the circulation. In addition to water, many other substances the body needs, such as nutrients and ions, pass into the nephron as part of the filtrate, and these also must be returned. Therefore, the process of filtration that occurs in the glomerular capsule is followed by a process of **tubular reabsorption**. As the filtrate travels through the nephron's tubular system, water and other needed substances leave the tubule and enter the surrounding tissue fluid, or interstitial fluid (IF). They move by several processes previously described in Chapter 3, including:

- Diffusion. The movement of substances from an area of higher concentration to an area of lower concentration (following the concentration gradient).
- Osmosis. Diffusion of water through a semipermeable membrane.
- Active transport. Movement of materials through the plasma membrane against the concentration gradient using energy and transporters

The substances that leave the nephron and enter the interstitial fluid then enter the peritubular capillaries and return to the circulation. In contrast, most of the urea and other nitrogenous waste materials are kept within the tubule to be eliminated with the urine. Box 22-1 presents additional information on tubular reabsorption in the nephron.

Tubular Secretion Before the filtrate leaves the body as urine, the kidney makes final adjustments in composition by the process of **tubular secretion**. In this process, some substances are actively moved from the blood into the nephron. Potassium ions are moved into the urine by this process. Importantly, the kidneys regulate the acid–base (pH) balance of body fluids by the active secretion of hydrogen ions. Some drugs, such as penicillin, also are actively secreted into the nephron for elimination.

Concentration of the Urine The amount of water that is eliminated with the urine is regulated by a complex mechanism within the nephron that is influenced by **antidiuretic hormone (ADH)**, a hormone released from the posterior pituitary gland (see Table 22-1). The process is called the **countercurrent mechanism** because it involves fluid traveling in opposite directions within the ascending and descending limbs of Henle's loop. The countercurrent mechanism is illustrated in Figure 22-8. Its essentials are as follows:

As the filtrate passes through Henle's loop, electrolytes, especially sodium, are actively pumped out by the nephron's cells, resulting in an increased concentration of the interstitial fluid. Because the ascending limb of Henle's loop is not very permeable to water, the filtrate at this point becomes increasingly dilute (see Fig. 22-8). As the filtrate then passes through the more permeable DCT and collecting duct, the concentrated fluids around the nephron draw water out to be returned to the blood. (Remember, according to the laws of osmosis, water follows salt.) In this manner, the urine becomes more concentrated as it leaves the nephron and its volume is reduced.

Box 22-1 Clinical Perspectives

Transport Maximum

The kidney works efficiently to return valuable substances to the blood after glomerular filtration. However, the carriers that are needed for active transport of these substances can become overloaded, and there is also a limit to the amount of each substance that can be reabsorbed in a given time period. The limit of this rate of reabsorption is called the **transport maximum (Tm)**, or tubular maximum, and it is measured in milligrams (mg) per minute. For example, the Tm for glucose is approximately 375 mg/minute.

If a substance is present in excess in the blood, it may exceed its transport maximum and then, because it cannot be totally reabsorbed, some will be excreted in the urine. Thus, the transport maximum determines the **renal threshold**—the plasma concentration at which a substance will begin to be excreted in the urine, which is measured in mg per deciliter (dL). For example, if the concentration of glucose in the blood exceeds its renal threshold (180 mg/dL), glucose will begin to appear in the urine, a condition called **glycosuria**. The most common cause of glycosuria is uncontrolled diabetes mellitus.

The hormone ADH makes the walls of the DCT and collecting tubule more permeable to water, so that more water will be reabsorbed and less will be excreted with the urine. The release of ADH from the posterior pituitary is regulated by a feedback system. As the blood becomes more concentrated, the hypothalamus triggers more ADH release from the posterior pituitary; as the blood becomes more dilute, less ADH is released. In the disease diabetes insipidus, there is inadequate secretion of ADH from the hypothalamus, which results in the elimination of large amounts of dilute urine accompanied by excessive thirst.

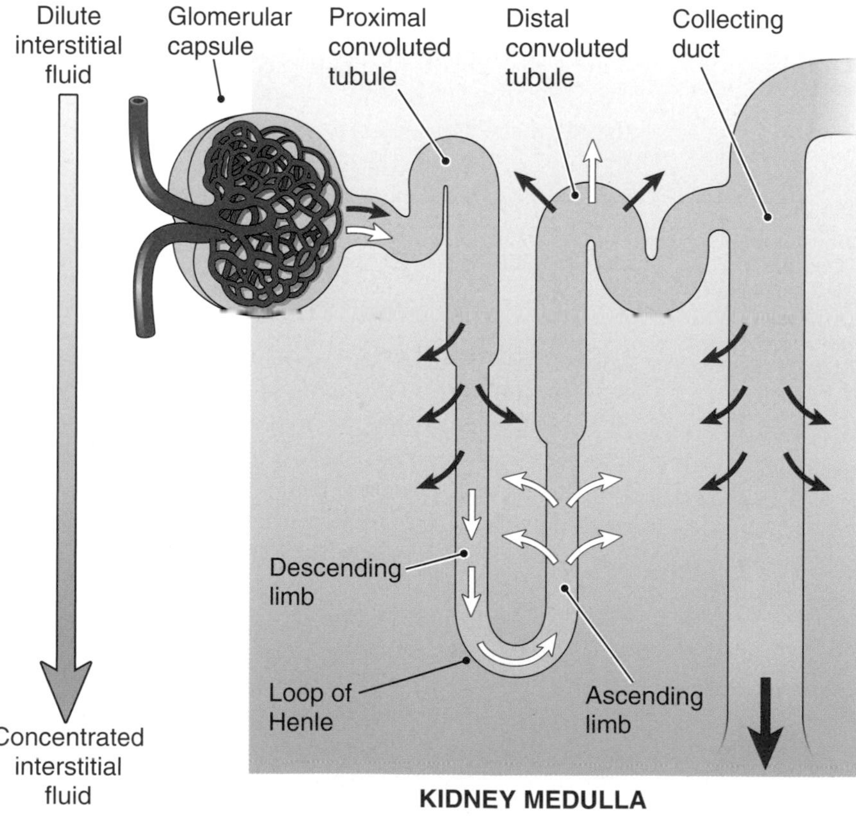

Figure 22-8 **Countercurrent mechanism for concentration of urine.** Concentration is regulated by means of intricate exchanges of water and electrolytes, mainly sodium, in the loop of Henle, distal convoluted tubule, and collecting duct. The intensity of color shows changing concentrations of the interstitial fluid and filtrate.

Summary of Urine Formation

The processes involved in urine formation are summarized below and illustrated in Figure 22-9.

1. Glomerular filtration allows diffusible materials to pass from the blood into the nephron.
2. Tubular reabsorption moves useful substances back into the blood while keeping waste products in the nephron to be eliminated in the urine.
3. Tubular secretion moves additional substances from the blood into the nephron for elimination. Movement of hydrogen ions is one means by which the pH of body fluids is balanced.
4. The countercurrent mechanism concentrates the urine and reduces the volume excreted. The pituitary hormone ADH allows more water to be reabsorbed from the nephron.

Checkpoint 22-10 What are the four processes involved in the formation of urine?

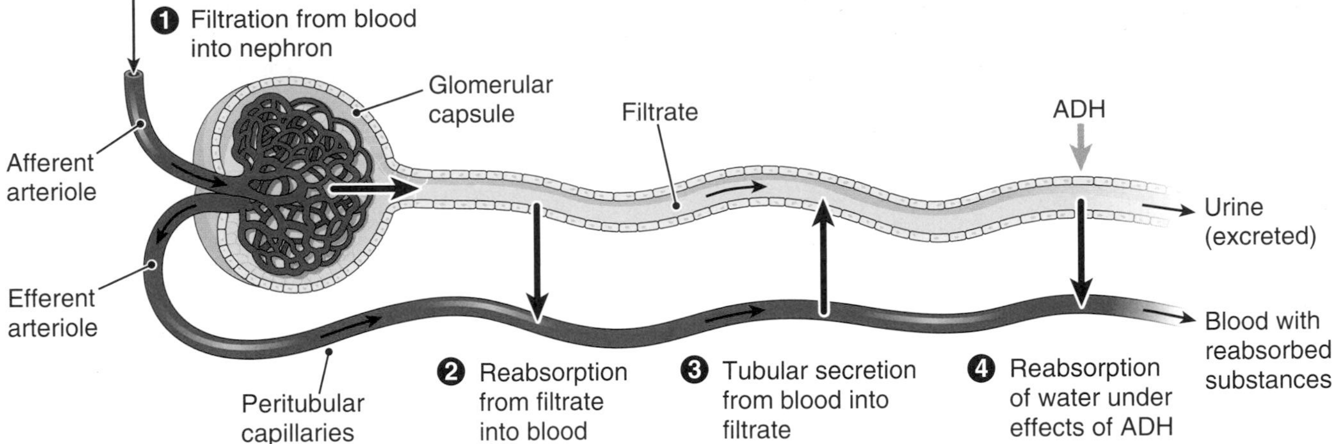

Figure 22-9 **Summary of urine formation in a nephron.**

The Ureters

Each of the two ureters is a long, slender, muscular tube that extends from the kidney down to and through the inferior portion of the urinary bladder (see Fig. 22-1). The ureters, which are located posterior to the peritoneum and, at the distal portion, below the peritoneum, are entirely extraperitoneal. Their length naturally varies with the size of the individual, and they may be anywhere from 25 cm to 32 cm (10–13 inches) long. Nearly 2.5 cm (1 inch) of the ureter's distal portion enters the bladder by passing obliquely (at an angle) through the inferior bladder wall. Because of the oblique direction the ureter takes through the wall, a full bladder compresses the ureter and prevents the backflow of urine.

The wall of the ureter includes a lining of epithelial cells, a relatively thick layer of involuntary muscle, and finally, an outer coat of fibrous connective tissue. The epithelium is the transitional type, which flattens from a cuboidal shape as the tube stretches. This same type of epithelium lines the renal pelvis, the bladder, and the proximal portion of the urethra. The ureteral muscles are capable of the same rhythmic contraction (peristalsis) that occurs in the digestive system. Urine is moved along the ureter from the kidneys to the bladder by gravity and by peristalsis at frequent intervals.

The Urinary Bladder

When it is empty, the urinary bladder (Fig. 22-10) is located below the parietal peritoneum and posterior to the pubic joint. When filled, it pushes the peritoneum upward and may extend well into the abdominal cavity proper. The urinary bladder is a temporary reservoir for urine, just as the gallbladder is a storage sac for bile.

The bladder wall has many layers. It is lined with mucous membrane containing transitional epithelium. The bladder's lining, like that of the stomach, is thrown into folds called *rugae* when the organ is empty. Beneath the mucosa is a layer of connective tissue, followed by a three-layered coat of involuntary muscle tissue that can stretch considerably. Finally, there is an incomplete coat of peritoneum that covers only the superior portion of the bladder.

When the bladder is empty, the muscular wall becomes thick, and the entire organ feels firm. As the blad-

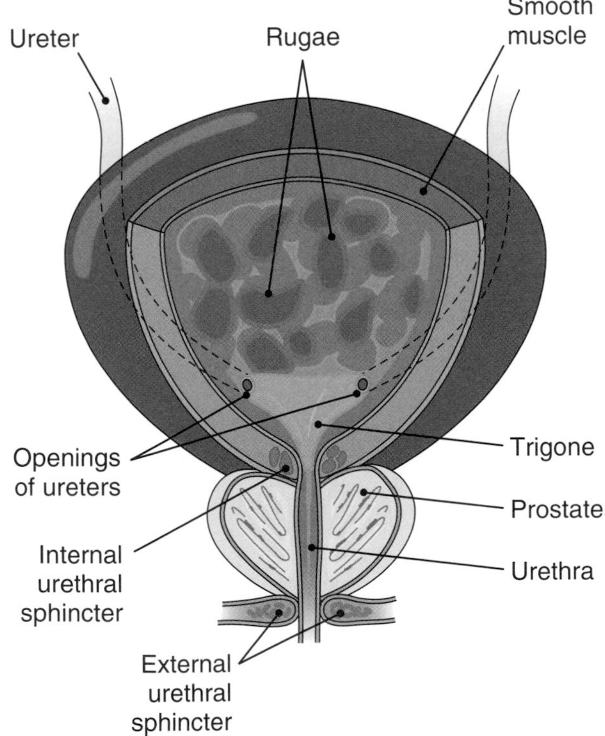

Figure 22-10 **Interior of the male urinary bladder.** The trigone is a triangular region in the floor of the bladder marked by the openings of the ureters and the urethra. *ZOOMING IN ✦ What gland does the urethra pass through in the male?*

der fills, the muscular wall becomes thinner, and the organ may increase from a length of 5 cm (2 inches) up to as much as 12.5 cm (5 inches) or even more. A moderately full bladder holds about 470 mL (1 pint) of urine.

The **trigone** (TRI-gone) is a triangular-shaped region in the floor of the bladder. It is marked by the openings of the two ureters and the urethra (see Fig. 22-10). As the bladder fills with urine, it expands upward, leaving the trigone at the base stationary. This stability prevents stretching of the ureteral openings and the possible back flow of urine into the ureters.

The Urethra

The **urethra** is the tube that extends from the bladder to the outside (see Fig. 22-1) and is the means by which the ladder is emptied. The urethra differs in men and women; in the male, it is part of both the reproductive system and the urinary system, and it is much longer than is the female urethra.

The male urethra is approximately 20 cm (8 inches) in length. Proximally, it passes through the prostate gland, where it is joined by two ducts carrying male germ cells (spermatozoa) from the testes and glandular secretions. From here, it leads to the outside through the **penis** (PE-nis), the male organ of copulation. The male urethra serves the dual purpose of conveying semen with the germ cells and draining the bladder.

The urethra in the female is a thin-walled tube about 4 cm (1.5 inches) long. It is located posterior to the pubic joint and is embedded in the muscle of the vagina's anterior wall. The external opening, called the **urinary meatus** (me-A-tus), is located just anterior to the vaginal opening between the labia minora. The female urethra drains the bladder only and is entirely separate from the reproductive system.

Urination

The process of expelling (voiding) urine from the bladder is called **urination** or **micturition** (mik-tu-RISH-un). This process is controlled both voluntarily and involuntarily with the aid of two rings of muscle (sphincters) that surround the urethra (see Fig. 22-10). Near the bladder's outlet is an involuntary **internal urethral sphincter** formed by a continuation of the smooth muscle of the bladder wall. Below this muscle is a voluntary **external urethral** sphincter formed by the muscles of the pelvic floor. By learning to control the voluntary sphincter, one can gain control over emptying of the bladder.

As the bladder fills with urine, stretch receptors in its wall send impulses to a center in the lower part of the spinal cord. Motor impulses from this center stimulate contraction of the bladder wall, forcing urine outward as both the internal and external sphincters are made to relax. In the infant, this emptying occurs automatically as a simple reflex. Early in life, a person learns to control urination from higher centers in the brain until the time is appropriate, a process known as *toilet training*. The impulse to urinate will override conscious controls if the bladder becomes too full.

The bladder can be emptied voluntarily by relaxing the muscles of the pelvic floor and increasing the pressure in the abdomen. The resulting increased pressure in the bladder triggers the spinal reflex that leads to urination.

Checkpoint 22-11 What is the name of the tube that carries urine from the kidney to the bladder?

Checkpoint 22-12 What is the name of the tube that carries urine from the bladder to the outside?

The Urine

Urine is a yellowish liquid that is approximately 95% water and 5% dissolved solids and gases. The pH of freshly collected urine averages 6.0, with a range of 4.5 to 8.0. Diet may cause considerable variation in pH.

The amount of dissolved substances in urine is indicated by its **specific gravity**. The specific gravity of pure water, used as a standard, is 1.000. Because of the dissolved materials it contains, urine has a specific gravity that normally varies from 1.002 (very dilute urine) to 1.040 (very concentrated urine). When the kidneys are diseased, they lose the ability to concentrate urine, and the specific gravity no longer varies as it does when the kidneys function normally.

Normal Constituents

Some of the dissolved substances normally found in the urine are the following:

- **Nitrogenous waste products**, including urea, uric acid, and **creatinine** (kre-AT-ih-nin).
- **Electrolytes**, including sodium chloride (as in common table salt) and different kinds of sulfates and phosphates. Electrolytes are excreted in appropriate amounts to keep their blood concentration constant.
- **Pigment**, mainly yellow pigment derived from certain bile compounds. Pigments from foods and drugs also may appear in the urine.

Abnormal Constituents

Examination of urine, called a **urinalysis** (u-rin-AL-ih-sis) (**UA**), is one of the most important parts of a medical evaluation. A routine urinalysis includes observation of color and turbidity (cloudiness) as well as measurement of pH and specific gravity. Laboratories also test for a variety of abnormal components, including:

- **Glucose** is usually an important indicator of diabetes mellitus, in which the cells do not adequately metabolize blood sugar. The excess glucose, which cannot be reabsorbed, is excreted in the urine. The presence of glucose in the urine is known as **glycosuria** (gli-ko-SU-re-ah) or glucosuria.

- **Albumin.** The presence of this protein, which is normally retained in the blood, may indicate a kidney disorder, such as glomerulonephritis. Albumin in the urine is known as **albuminuria** (al-bu-mih-NU-re-ah).
- **Blood** in the urine is usually an important indicator of urinary system disease, including nephritis. Blood in the urine is known as **hematuria** (hem-ah-TU-re-ah).
- **Ketones** (KE-tones) are produced when fats are incompletely oxidized; ketones in the urine are seen in diabetes mellitus and starvation.
- **White blood cells** (pus) are evidence of infection; they can be seen by microscopic examination of a centrifuged specimen. Pus in the urine is known as **pyuria** (pi-U-re-ah).
- **Casts** are solid materials molded within the microscopic kidney tubules. They consist of cells or proteins and, when present in large number, they usually indicate disease of the nephrons.

More extensive tests on urine may include analysis for drugs, enzymes, hormones, and other metabolites as well as cultures for microorganisms. Normal values for common urine tests are given in Appendix 4, Table 1.

Disorders of the Urinary System

The kidney is more prone to disorders than any other portion of the urinary system.

Kidney Disorders

Kidney disorders may be acute or chronic. Acute conditions usually arise suddenly, most frequently as the result of infection with inflammation of the nephrons. These diseases commonly run a course of a few weeks and are followed by complete recovery. Chronic conditions arise slowly and are often progressive, with gradual loss of kidney function.

Acute glomerulonephritis (glo-mer-u-lo-nef-RI-tis), also known as *acute poststreptococcal glomerulonephritis,* is the most common disease of the kidneys. This condition usually occurs in children about 1 to 4 weeks after a streptococcal throat infection. Antibodies formed in response to the streptococci attach to the glomerular membrane and cause injury. These damaged glomeruli allow protein, especially albumin, to filter into the glomerular capsule and ultimately to appear in the urine (albuminuria). They also allow red blood cells to filter into the urine (hematuria). Usually, the patient recovers without permanent kidney damage. In adult patients, the disease is more likely to become chronic, with a gradual decrease in the number of functioning nephrons, leading to chronic renal failure.

Pyelonephritis (pi-el-o-nef-RI-tis), an inflammation of the renal pelvis and the tissue of the kidney, may be either acute or chronic. In acute pyelonephritis, the inflammation results from a bacterial infection. Bacteria most commonly reach the kidney by ascending along the lining membrane from an infection in the distal part of the urinary tract (see Fig. 23-15 in Chapter 23). More rarely, bacteria are carried to the kidney by the blood.

Acute pyelonephritis is often seen in people with partial obstruction of urine flow with stagnation (urinary stasis). It is most likely to occur in pregnant women and in men with an enlarged prostate, because the prostate surrounds the first portion of the urethra in males. Other causes of stasis include neurogenic bladder, which is bladder dysfunction resulting from neurologic lesions, as seen in diabetes mellitus, and structural defects in the area where the ureters enter the bladder. Pyelonephritis usually responds to the administration of antibiotics, fluid replacement, rest, and fever control.

Chronic pyelonephritis, a more serious disease, is frequently seen in patients with urinary tract stasis or back flow. It may be caused by persistent or repeated bacterial infections. Progressive damage of kidney tissue is evidenced by high blood pressure, continual loss of protein in the urine, and dilute urine.

Hydronephrosis (hi-dro-nef-RO-sis) is the distention of the renal pelvis and calyces with accumulated fluid as a result of urinary tract obstruction. The most common causes of obstruction, in addition to pregnancy or an enlarged prostate, are a kidney stone that has formed in the pelvis and dropped into the ureter, a tumor that presses on a ureter, and scars due to inflammation. Prompt removal of the obstruction may result in complete recovery. If the obstruction is not removed, the kidney will be permanently damaged.

A **polycystic** (pol-e-SIS-tik) **kidney** is one in which many fluid-containing sacs develop in the active tissue and gradually destroy it by pressure. This disorder may run in families, and treatment has not proved very satisfactory, except for the use of dialysis machines or kidney transplantation.

Tumors of the kidneys usually grow rather slowly, but rapidly invading types are occasionally found. Blood in the urine and dull pain in the kidney region are warnings that should be heeded at once. Surgical removal of the kidney offers the best chance of cure because most renal cancers do not respond to chemotherapy or radiation.

Kidney Stones Kidney stones, or **calculi** (KAL-ku-li), are made of substances, such as calcium salts or uric acid, that precipitate out of the urine instead of remaining in solution. They usually form in the renal pelvis, but may also form in the bladder.

The causes of stone formation include dehydration, stasis (stagnation) of the urine, and infection of the urinary tract. The stones may vary in size from tiny grains resembling bits of gravel up to large masses that fill the renal pelvis and extend into the calyces. The latter are described as **staghorn calculi**.

There is no way of dissolving these stones because substances that could do so would also destroy kidney tissue. Sometimes, instruments can be used to crush small stones and thus allow them to be expelled with the urine, but more often, surgical removal is required. A **lithotriptor** (LITH-o-trip-tor), literally a "stone-cracker," is a device that employs external shock waves to shatter kidney stones. The procedure is called **lithotripsy** (LITH-o-trip-se).

Renal Failure **Acute renal failure** may result from a medical or surgical emergency or from toxins that damage the tubules. This condition is characterized by a sudden, serious decrease in kidney function accompanied by electrolyte and acid–base imbalances. Acute renal failure occurs as a serious complication of other severe illness and may be fatal.

Chronic renal failure results from a gradual loss of nephrons. As more and more nephrons are destroyed, the kidneys gradually lose the ability to perform their normal functions. As the disease progresses, nitrogenous waste products accumulate to high levels in the blood, causing a condition known as **uremia** (u-RE-me-ah). In many cases, there is a lesser decrease in renal function, known as **renal insufficiency**, that produces fewer symptoms.

A few of the characteristic signs and symptoms of chronic renal failure are the following:

- **Dehydration** (de-hi-DRA-shun). Excessive loss of body fluid may occur early in renal failure, when the kidneys cannot concentrate the urine and large amounts of water are eliminated.
- **Edema** (eh-DE-mah). Accumulation of fluid in the tissue spaces may occur late in chronic renal disease, when the kidneys cannot eliminate water in adequate amounts.
- **Electrolyte imbalance**, including retention of sodium and accumulation of potassium.
- **Hypertension** may occur as the result of fluid overload and the increased production of renin (see Box 22-2).
- **Anemia** occurs when the kidneys cannot produce the hormone erythropoietin to activate red blood cell production in bone marrow.
- **Uremia** (u-RE-me-ah), an excess of nitrogenous waste products in the blood. When these levels are very high, urea can be changed into ammonia in the stomach and intestine and cause ulcerations and bleeding.

Checkpoint 22-13 What is the difference between acute and chronic kidney disorders?

Renal Dialysis and Kidney Transplantation

Dialysis (di-AL-ih-sis) means "the separation of dissolved molecules based on their ability to pass through a semipermeable membrane" (Fig. 22-11 A). Molecules that can pass through the membrane move from an area of greater concentration to one of lesser concentration. In patients who have defective kidney function, the accumulation of urea and other nitrogenous waste products can be reduced by passage of the patient's blood through a dialysis machine. The principle of "molecules leaving the area of greater concentration" thus operates to remove wastes from the blood. The fluid in the dialysis machine, the dialysate, can be adjusted to regulate the flow of substances out of the blood.

There are two methods of dialysis in use: hemodialysis (blood dialysis) and peritoneal dialysis (dialysis in the

Box 22-2 A Closer Look

The Renin-Angiotensin Pathway: The Kidneys' Route to Blood Pressure Control

In addition to forming urine, the kidneys play an integral role in regulating blood pressure. When blood pressure drops, cells of the juxtaglomerular apparatus secrete the enzyme renin into the blood. Renin acts on another blood protein, **angiotensinogen**, which is manufactured by the liver. Renin converts angiotensinogen into **angiotensin I** by cleaving off some amino acids from the end of the protein. Angiotensin I is then converted into **angiotensin II** by yet another enzyme called angiotensin-converting enzyme (ACE), which is manufactured by capillary endothelium, especially in the lungs. Angiotensin II increases blood pressure in four ways:

1. It increases cardiac output and stimulates vasoconstriction.
2. It stimulates the release of aldosterone, a hormone that acts on the kidneys' distal convoluted tubules to increase sodium reabsorption, and secondarily, water reabsorption.
3. It stimulates the release of antidiuretic hormone, which acts directly on the distal convoluted tubules to increase water reabsorption.
4. It stimulates thirst centers in the hypothalamus, resulting in increased fluid consumption.

The combined effects of angiotensin II produce a dramatic increase in blood pressure. In fact, angiotensin II is estimated to be four to eight times more powerful than norepinephrine, another potent stimulator of hypertension, and thus is a good target for blood pressure-controlling drugs. One class of drugs used to treat hypertension is the **ACE inhibitors** (angiotensin-converting enzyme inhibitors), which control blood pressure by blocking the production of angiotensin II.

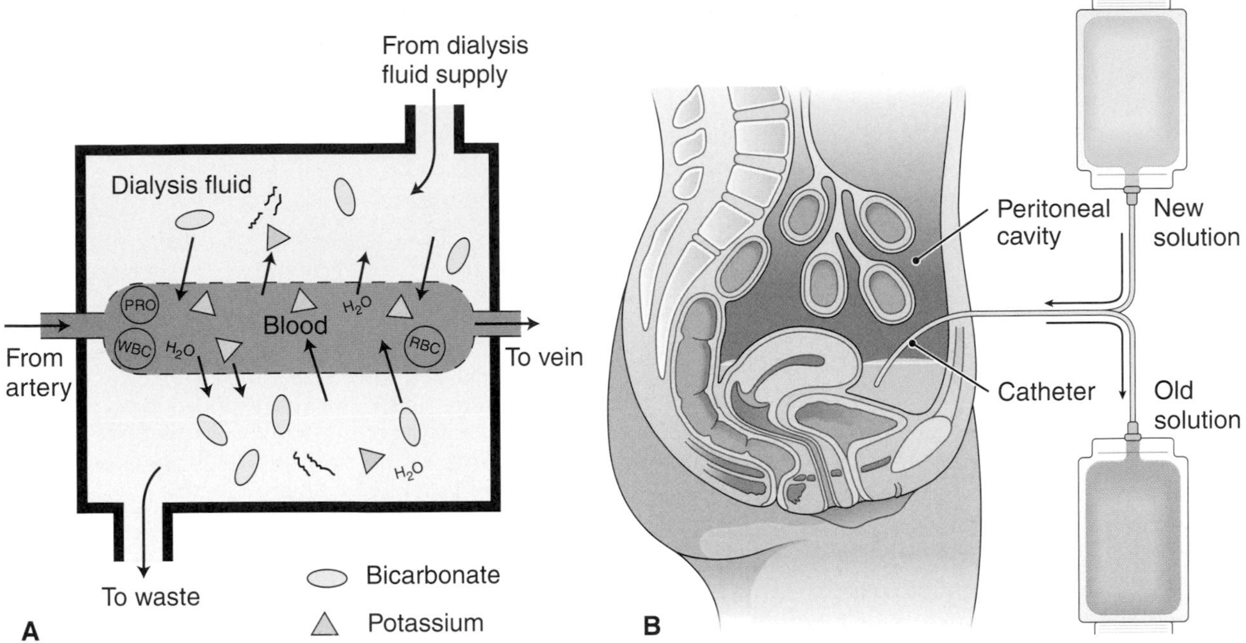

Figure 22-11 A hemodialysis system and a peritoneal dialysis system. (**A**) In hemodialysis, a cellophane membrane separates the blood compartment and dialysis fluid compartment. This membrane is porous enough to allow all of the constituents except the plasma proteins (PRO) and blood cells (WBC, RBC) to diffuse between the two compartments. (**B**) In peritoneal dialysis, a semipermeable membrane richly supplied with blood vessels lines the peritoneal cavity. With dialysate dwelling in the peritoneal cavity, waste products diffuse from the network of blood vessels into the dialysate. (A, Reprinted with permission from Porth CM. Pathophysiology. 7th ed. Philadelphia: Lippincott Williams & Wilkins, 2004; B, reprinted with permission from Cohen BJ. Medical Terminology. 4th ed. Philadelphia: Lippincott Williams & Wilkins, 2004.)

abdominal cavity). In hemodialysis, the dialysis membrane is made of cellophane or other synthetic material. In peritoneal dialysis, the surface area of the peritoneum acts as the membrane (see Fig. 22-11 B). Dialysis fluid is introduced into the peritoneal cavity and then periodically removed along with waste products. This procedure may be done at intervals through the day or during the night.

A 1973 amendment to the Social Security Act provides federal financial assistance for people who have chronic renal disease and require dialysis. Most hemodialysis is performed in freestanding clinics. Treatment time has been reduced; a typical schedule involves 2 to 3 hours, three times a week. Access to the bloodstream has been made safer and easier through surgical establishment of a permanent exchange site (shunt). Peritoneal dialysis also has been improved and simplified, enabling patients to manage treatment at home. (Box 22-3, Hemodialysis Technician, gives an overview of what to expect in a career as a hemodialysis technician.)

The final option for treatment of renal failure is kidney transplantation. Surgeons have successfully performed many of these procedures. Kidneys have so much extra functioning tissue that the loss of one kidney normally poses no problem to the donor. Records show that transplantation success is greatest when surgeons use a kidney from a living donor who is closely related to the patient. Organs from deceased donors have also proved satisfactory in many cases. The problem of tissue rejection (the rejection syndrome) is discussed in Chapter 17.

Disorders of the Ureters

Abnormalities in structure of the ureter include subdivision at the renal pelvis and constricted or abnormally narrow parts, called **strictures** (STRICK-tures). Abnormal pressure from tumors or other outside masses may cause ureteral narrowing.. Obstruction also may be caused by stones from the kidneys, or kinking of the tube because of a dropping of the kidney, a condition known as **renal ptosis** (TO-sis). In cases of **ureterocele** (u-RE-ter-o-sele), the end of the ureter bulges into the bladder (Fig. 22-12). The result is urinary obstruction that leads to distention of the ureter (hydroureter) and renal pelvis (hydronephrosis). The usual cause of ureterocele is a congenital (present at birth) narrowing of the ureteral opening.

Ureteral Stones The passage of a small stone along the ureter causes excruciating pain, called *renal colic*. Relief of this pain usually requires morphine or an equally powerful drug. The first "barber surgeons," operating without benefit of anesthesia, were permitted by their patients to cut through the skin and the muscles of the back to remove stones from the ureters. "Cutting for stone" in this way was relatively successful, despite the lack of sterile technique,

Box 22-3 · Health Professions

Hemodialysis Technician

A hemodialysis technician, also called a renal technician or a nephrology technician, specializes in the safe and effective delivery of renal dialysis therapy to patients suffering from kidney failure. Before treatment begins, the technician prepares the dialysis solutions and ensures that the dialysis machine is clean, sterile, and in proper working order. The technician measures and records the patient's weight, temperature, and vital signs, inserts a catheter into the patient's arm, and connects the dialysis machine to it. During dialysis, the technician monitors the patient for adverse reactions and guards against any equipment malfunction. After the treatment is completed, the technician again measures and records the patient's weight, temperature, and vital signs. To perform these duties, hemodialysis technicians need a thorough understanding of anatomy and physiology. Most technicians in the United States receive their training from a college or technical school, and many states require that the technician be certified.

Hemodialysis technicians work in a variety of settings such as hospitals, clinics, and patients' homes. As populations age, the incidence of kidney disease is expected to rise, as will the need for hemodialysis. For more information about this career, contact the National Association of Nephrology Technicians.

because the approach through the back avoided the peritoneal cavity and the serious risk of peritonitis.

Modern surgery employs a variety of instruments for removal of stones from the ureter, including endoscopes similar to those described in Chapter 19. The transurethral route through the urethra and urinary bladder and then into the ureter, as well as entrance through the skin and muscles of the back, may be used to remove calculi from the kidney pelvis or from the ureter.

Checkpoint 22-14 What is the scientific name for stones, as may occur in the urinary tract?

Disorders of the Bladder

A full (distended) bladder lies in an unprotected position in the lower abdomen, and a blow may rupture it, necessitating immediate surgical repair. Blood in the urine is a rather common symptom of infection or tumors, which may involve the bladder.

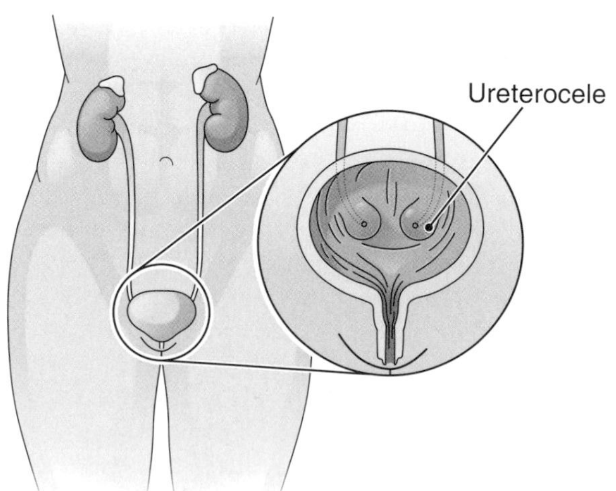

Figure 22-12 **Ureterocele.** The ureter bulges into the bladder. The resulting obstruction causes urine to back up into the ureter and renal pelvis. (Reprinted with permission from Cohen BJ. Medical Terminology. 4th ed. Philadelphia: Lippincott Williams & Wilkins, 2004.)

Cystitis Inflammation of the bladder, called **cystitis** (sis-TI-tis), is 10 times as common in women as in men. This may be due, at least in part, to the very short urethra of the female compared with that of the male. The usual path of infection is that bacteria ascend from the outside through the urethra into the bladder (see Fig. 23-15 in Chapter 23). The common contaminants are colon bacteria, such as *E. coli*, carried to the urethra from the anus. Urinary stasis and catheterization to remove urine from the bladder are other possible sources of infection. Pain, urgency to urinate, and urinary frequency are common symptoms of cystitis.

Another type of cystitis, called **interstitial cystitis,** may cause pelvic pain with discomfort before and after urination. The tissues below the mucosa are involved. The disease can be diagnosed only with the use of a **cystoscope**, a type of endoscope used to examine the bladder (Fig. 22-13). Because no bacteria are involved, antibiotics are not effective treatment and may even be harmful.

Obstruction by an enlarged prostate gland in a male or from pregnancy may lead to urinary stasis and cystitis. Reduction of a person's general resistance to infection, as in diabetes, may also lead to cystitis. The danger of cystitis is that the infection may ascend to other parts of the urinary tract.

Tumors Tumors of the bladder, which are most prevalent in men older than 50 years of age, include benign papillomas and various kinds of cancer. About 90% of bladder tumors arise from the epithelial lining. Possible causes include toxins (particularly certain aniline dyes), chronic infestations (schistosomiasis), heavy cigarette smoking, and the presence of urinary stones, which may develop and increase in size within the bladder.

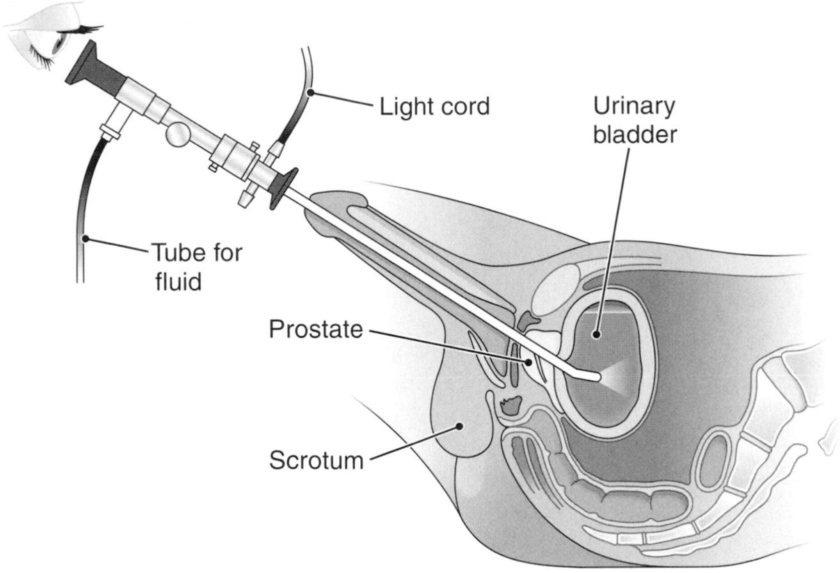

Figure 22-13 **Cystoscopy.** A lighted cystoscope is introduced through the urethra into the bladder of a male subject. Sterile fluid is used to inflate the bladder. The cystoscope is used to examine the bladder, remove specimens for biopsy, and remove tumors. (Reprinted with permission from Cohen BJ. Medical Terminology. 4th ed. Philadelphia: Lippincott Williams & Wilkins, 2004.)

Blood in the urine (hematuria) and frequent urination, in the absence of pain or fever, are early signs of a bladder tumor. A cystoscopic examination (see Fig. 22-13) and biopsy should be performed as soon as these signs are detected. Treatment includes removal of the tumor, which may be done cystoscopically, and localized chemotherapy. More serious cases may require irradiation. Removal before the tumor invades the muscle wall gives the best prognosis.

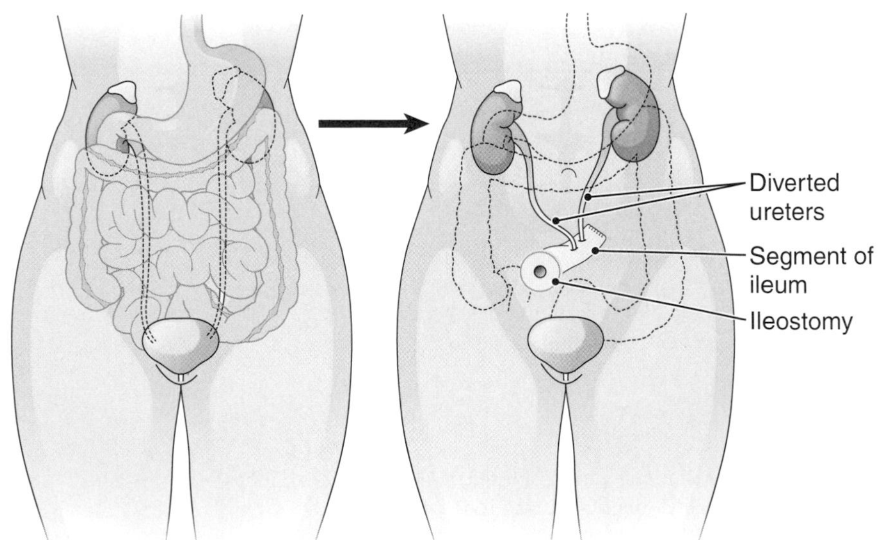

Figure 22-14 **Ileal conduit.** The ureters are vented through a segment of the ileum to open at the body surface through an ileostomy. (Reprinted with permission from Cohen BJ. Medical Terminology. 4th ed. Philadelphia: Lippincott Williams & Wilkins, 2004.)

If it is necessary to remove the bladder in a **cystectomy** (sis-TEK-to-me), the ureters must be vented elsewhere. They may be diverted to the body surface through a segment of the ileum, a procedure known as an **ileal conduit** (Fig. 22-14), or diverted to some other portion of the intestine. Alternatively, surgeons may create a bladder out of a section of the colon.

Urinary Incontinence **Urinary incontinence** (in-KON-tin-ens) refers to an involuntary loss of urine. The condition may originate with a neurologic disorder, trauma to the spinal cord, weakness of the pelvic muscles, impaired bladder function or medications. Different forms of urinary incontinence have specific names:

- Stress incontinence results from urethral incompetence that allows small amounts of urine to be released when an activity increases pressure in the abdomen. These activities include coughing, sneezing, laughing, lifting or exercising.
- Urge incontinence, also called *overactive bladder*, results from an inability to control bladder contractions once the sensation of bladder fullness is perceived.
- Overflow incontinence arises from neurologic damage or urinary obstruction that causes the bladder to overfill. Excess pressure in the bladder results in involuntary loss of urine.
- **Enuresis** (en-u-RE-sis) is involuntary urination, usually during the night (bed-wetting).

Some treatment approaches to incontinence include muscle exercises, dietary changes, biofeedback, medication, surgery or, in serious cases, self-catheterization.

Checkpoint 22-15 What is the term for inflammation of the bladder?

Disorders of the Urethra

Congenital anomalies may involve the urethra as well as other parts of the urinary tract. The opening of the urethra to the outside may be too small, or the urethra itself may be narrowed. Occasionally, an abnormal valve-like structure is found at the point where

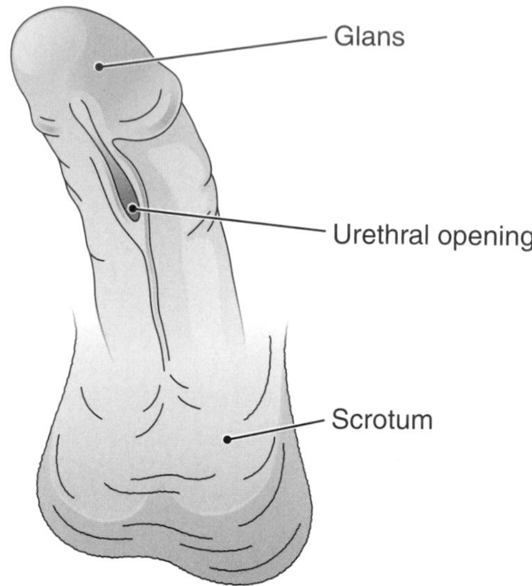

Figure 22-15 **Hypospadias.** A ventral view of the penis is shown here. (Reprinted with permission from Cohen BJ. Medical Terminology. 4th ed. Philadelphia: Lippincott Williams & Wilkins, 2004.)

the urethra enters the bladder. If it is not removed surgically, it can cause back pressure of the urine, with serious consequences. There is also a condition in the male in which the urethra opens on the undersurface of the penis instead of at the end. This is called **hypospadias** (hi-po-SPA-de-as) (Fig. 22-15).

Urethritis, which is characterized by inflammation of the mucous membrane and the glands of the urethra, is much more common in men than in women. It is often caused by infection with gonococci or chlamydias, although many other bacteria may be involved.

"Straddle" injuries to the urethra are common in men. This type of injury occurs when, for example, a man walking along a raised beam slips and lands with the beam between his legs. Such an accident may catch the urethra between the hard surfaces of the beam and the pubic arch and rupture the urethra. In accidents in which the bones of the pelvis are fractured, rupture of the urethra is fairly common.

The Effects of Aging

Even without kidney disease, aging causes the kidneys to lose some of their ability to concentrate urine. With aging, progressively more water is needed to excrete the same amount of waste. Older people find it necessary to drink more water than young people, and they eliminate larger amounts of urine (polyuria), even at night (nocturia).

Beginning at about 40 years of age, there is a decrease in the number and size of the nephrons. Often, more than half of them are lost before the age of 80 years. There may be an increase in blood urea nitrogen (BUN) without serious symptoms. Elderly people are more susceptible than young people to urinary system infections. Childbearing may cause damage to the musculature of the pelvic floor, resulting in urinary tract problems in later years.

Enlargement of the prostate, common in older men, may cause obstruction and back pressure in the ureters and kidneys. If this condition is untreated, it will cause permanent damage to the kidneys. Changes with age, including decreased bladder capacity and decreased muscle tone in the bladder and urinary sphincters, may predispose to incontinence. However, most elderly people (60% in nursing homes, and up to 85% living independently) have no incontinence.

Word Anatomy

Medical terms are built from standardized word parts (prefixes, roots, and suffixes). Learning the meanings of these parts can help you remember words and interpret unfamiliar terms.

WORD PART	MEANING	EXAMPLE
The Kidneys		
retro-	backward, behind	The *retroperitoneal* space is posterior to the peritoneal cavity.
ren/o	kidney	The *renal* artery carries blood to the kidney.
nephr/o	kidney	The *nephron* is the functional unit of the kidney.
juxta-	next to	The *juxtaglomerular* apparatus is next to the glomerulus.
The Ureters		
extra-	beyond, outside of	The ureters are *extraperitoneal*.
Disorders of the Urinary System		
pyel/o	renal pelvis	*Pyelonephritis* is inflammation of the nephrons and renal pelvis.
cyst/o	sac, bladder	A *polycystic* kidney develops many fluid-containing sacs.
dia-	through	*Dialysis* is the separation (-lysis) of molecules based on their ability to pass through a semipermeable membrane.
-cele	swelling, enlarged space	A *uterocele* is formed as the end of the ureter bulges into the bladder.
trans-	across, through	A *transurethral* route is through the urethra.
The Effects of Aging		
noct/i	night	*Nocturia* is excessive urination at night.

Summary

I. Excretion—removal and elimination of metabolic waste
1. Systems that eliminate waste
   a. Urinary—removes waste from blood
      (1) Other functions—regulates blood volume, pH, and electrolytes
   b. Digestive system—eliminates water, salts, bile with digestive residue
   c. Respiratory system—eliminates carbon dioxide, water
   d. Skin—eliminates water, salts, nitrogenous waste

II. Organs of the urinary system
   a. Kidneys (2)
   b. Ureters (2)
   c. Urinary bladder (1)
   d. Urethra (1)

III. Kidneys
1. In upper abdomen against the back
2. In retroperitoneal space (posterior to the peritoneum)

A. Blood supply to the kidney
   a. Renal artery—carries blood to kidney from aorta
   b. Renal vein—carries blood from kidney to inferior vena cava

B. Structure of the kidney
1. Cortex—outer portion
2. Medulla—inner portion
3. Pelvis
   a. Upper end of ureter
   b. Calyces—cuplike extensions that receive urine
4. Nephron
   a. Functional unit of kidney
   b. Parts
      (1) Glomerular (Bowman) capsule—around glomerulus
      (2) Proximal convoluted tubule (PCT)
      (3) Loop of Henle—descending and ascending limbs
      (4) Distal convoluted tubule (DCT)
   c. Blood supply to nephron
      (1) Afferent arteriole—enters glomerular capsule
      (2) Glomerulus—coil of capillaries in glomerular capsule
      (3) Efferent arteriole—leaves glomerular capsule
      (4) Peritubular capillaries—surround nephron
   d. Juxtaglomerular apparatus
      (1) Consists of cells in afferent arteriole and distal convoluted tubule
      (2) Releases renin to regulate blood pressure via angiotensin

C. Functions of the kidney
1. Excretion of waste, excess salts, toxins
2. Water balance
3. Acid–base balance (pH)
4. Regulation of blood pressure
5. Releases hormone erythropoietin (EPO)—stimulates red blood cell production

D. Formation of urine
1. Glomerular filtration—driven by blood pressure in glomerulus
   a. Water and soluble substances forced out of blood and into glomerular capsule
   b. Blood cells and proteins remain in blood
   c. Glomerular filtrate—material that leaves blood and enters the nephron
2. Tubular reabsorption
   a. Most of filtrate leaves nephron by diffusion, osmosis and active transport
   b. Returns to blood through peritubular capillaries
3. Tubular secretion—materials moved from blood into nephron for excretion
4. Concentration of urine
   a. Countercurrent mechanism—method for concentrating urine based on movement of ions and permeability of tubule
   b. ADH
      (1) Hormone from posterior pituitary
      (2) Promotes reabsorption of water

IV. The ureters—carry urine from the kidneys to the bladder

V. Urinary bladder
   a. Stores urine until it is eliminated
   b. Trigone—triangular region in base of bladder; remains stable as bladder fills

VI. Urethra—carries urine out of body
1. Male urethra—20 cm long; carries both urine and semen
2. Female urethra—4 cm long; opening anterior to vagina

A. Urination (micturition)
1. Both voluntary and involuntary
2. Sphincters
   a. Internal urethral sphincter—involuntary (smooth muscle)
   b. External urethral sphincter—voluntary (skeletal muscle)
3. Stretch receptors in bladder wall signal reflex emptying
4. Can be controlled through higher brain centers

VII. Urine
1. pH averages 6.0
2. Specific gravity—measures dissolved substances

A. Normal constituents—water, nitrogenous waste, electrolytes, pigments

B. Abnormal constituents—glucose, albumin, blood, ketones, white blood cells, casts

VIII. Disorders of the urinary system
A. Kidney disorders
1. Examples
   a. Acute glomerulonephritis—damages glomeruli
   b. Pyelonephritis—inflammation of kidney and renal pelvis

  c. Hydronephrosis—distention with obstructed fluids
  d. Polycystic kidney—fluid-containing sacs develop
  e. Tumors
 2. Kidney stones—calculi
 3. Renal failure
  a. Types
   1) Acute—results from medical emergency or toxins
   2) Chronic—signs include dehydration, electrolyte imbalance, edema, hypertension, anemia, uremia
 4. Renal dialysis and kidney transplantation
  a. Renal dialysis—removes unwanted substances from blood when kidneys fail
B. Disorders of the ureters
 1. Stricture (narrowing)
 2. Stones (calculi)
C. Disorders of the bladder
 1. Cystitis—inflammation; most common in females
 2. Tumors
 3. Urinary incontinence
D. Disorders of the urethra
 1. Hypospadias—urethra opens on underside of penis
 2. Urethritis—inflammation

IX. Effects of aging

 1. Polyuria—increased elimination of urine
 2. Nocturia—urination at night
 3. Incontinence
 4. Increased blood urea nitrogen (BUN)
 5. Prostate enlargement

Questions for Study and Review

Building Understanding

Fill in the blanks

1. Each kidney is located outside the abdominal cavity in a ______ space.
2. The renal artery, renal vein, and ureter connect to the kidney at the ______.
3. The part of the bladder marked by the openings of the ureters and urethra is called the ______.
4. The amount of dissolved substances in urine is indicated by its ______.
5. The presence of glucose in the urine is known as ______.

Matching

Match each numbered item with the most closely related lettered item.

___ 6. Produced by the kidney in response to low blood pressure
___ 7. Stimulates vasoconstriction
___ 8. Produced by the kidney in response to hypoxia
___ 9. Stimulates kidneys to produce concentrated urine
___ 10. Produced by the liver during protein catabolism

a. urea
b. erythropoietin
c. antidiuretic hormone
d. renin
e. angiotensin

Multiple choice

___ 11. The functional unit of the renal system is the
 a. renal capsule
 b. kidney
 c. nephron
 d. juxtaglomerular apparatus

___ 12. The loop of Henle is located in the renal
 a. cortex
 b. medulla
 c. pelvis
 d. calyx

___ 13. Fluid moves out of the glomerulus by
 a. filtration
 b. diffusion
 c. osmosis
 d. active transport

___ 14. One's ability to delay urination is due to voluntary control of the
 a. trigone
 b. internal urethral sphincter
 c. external urethral sphincter
 d. urinary meatus

___ 15. Pus in the urine is termed
 a. pyuria
 b. uremia
 c. anemia
 d. enuresis

Understanding Concepts

16. List four organ systems active in excretion. What are the products eliminated by each?
17. Compare and contrast the following terms:
 a. glomerular capsule and glomerulus
 b. afferent and efferent arteriole
 c. proximal and distal convoluted tubule
 d. ureter and urethra
18. Trace the pathway of a urea molecule from the afferent arteriole to the urinary meatus.
19. Describe the four processes involved in the formation of urine.
20. Compare the male urethra and female urethra in structure and function. Why is cystitis more common in women than in men?

21. List some of the dissolved substances normally found in the urine.
22. Differentiate between the following disorders:
    a. albuminuria and hematuria
    b. glomerulonephritis and pyelonephritis
    c. hydronephrosis and polycystic kidney
    d. renal ptosis and ureterocele
23. What is meant by the word *dialysis* and how is this principle used for patients with kidney failure? What kinds of membranes are used for hemodialysis? for peritoneal dialysis?

Conceptual Thinking

24. Christie is fourteen years old and suffers from anorexia nervosa. Her parents take her to the hospital after she reports sharp pain in the lumbar region of her back. While there, she is diagnosed with hydronephrosis. What is the relationship between her eating disorder and her renal disorder?
25. A class of antihypertensive drugs called loop diuretics prevents sodium reabsorption in the loop of Henle. How could a drug like this lower blood pressure?

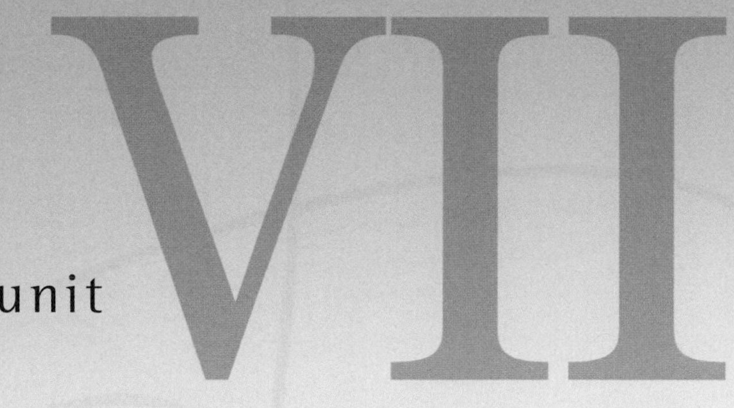

unit VII

Perpetuation of Life

The final unit includes three chapters on the structures and functions related to reproduction and heredity. The reproductive system is not necessary for the continuation of the life of the individual but rather is needed for the continuation of the human species. The reproductive cells and their genes have been studied intensively during recent years as part of the rapidly advancing science of genetics.

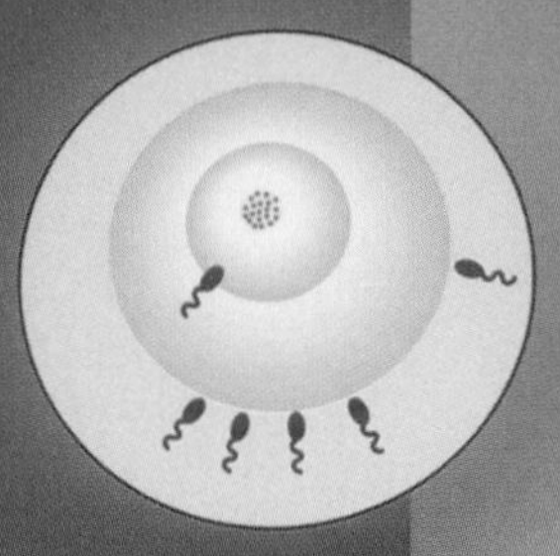

SELECTED KEY TERMS

The following terms and other boldface terms in the chapter are defined in the Glossary

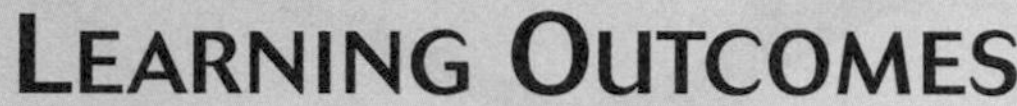

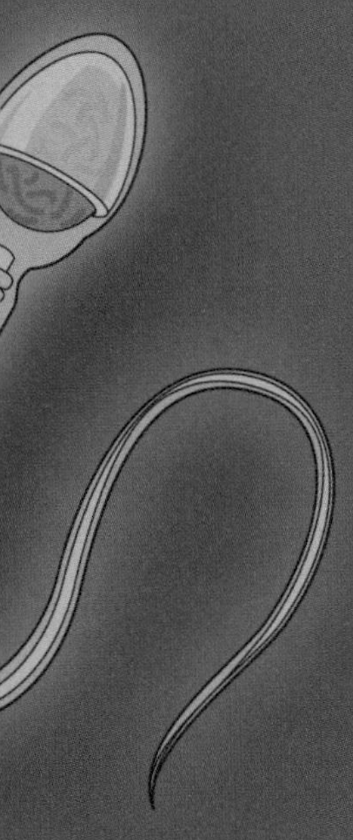

contraception
corpus luteum
endometrium
estrogen
follicle
FSH
gamete
infertility
LH
menopause
menses
menstruation
ovary
ovulation
ovum (pl., ova)
progesterone
semen
spermatozoon (pl., spermatozoa
testis (pl., testes)
testosterone
uterus

LEARNING OUTCOMES

After careful study of this chapter, you should be able to:

1. Name the male and female gonads and describe the function of each
2. State the purpose of meiosis
3. List the accessory organs of the male and female reproductive tracts and cite the function of each
4. Describe the composition and function of semen
5. Draw and label a spermatozoon
6. List in the correct order the hormones produced during the menstrual cycle and cite the source of each
7. Describe the functions of the main male and female sex hormones
8. Explain how negative feedback regulates reproductive function in both males and females
9. Describe the changes that occur during and after menopause
10. Cite the main methods of birth control in use
11. Briefly describe the major disorders of the male and female reproductive tracts
12. Show how word parts are used to build words related to the reproductive systems (see Word Anatomy at the end of the chapter)

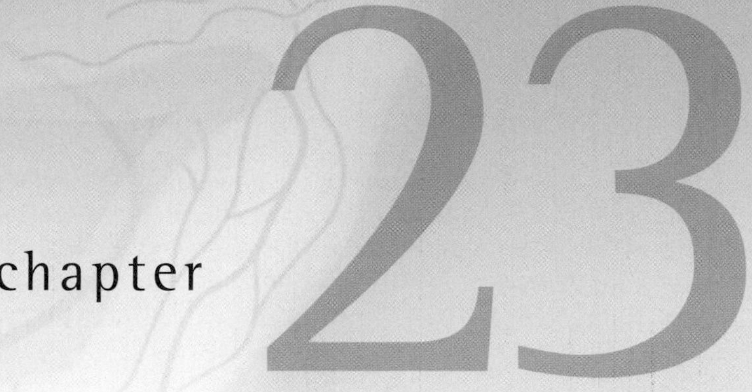

chapter 23

The Male and Female Reproductive Systems

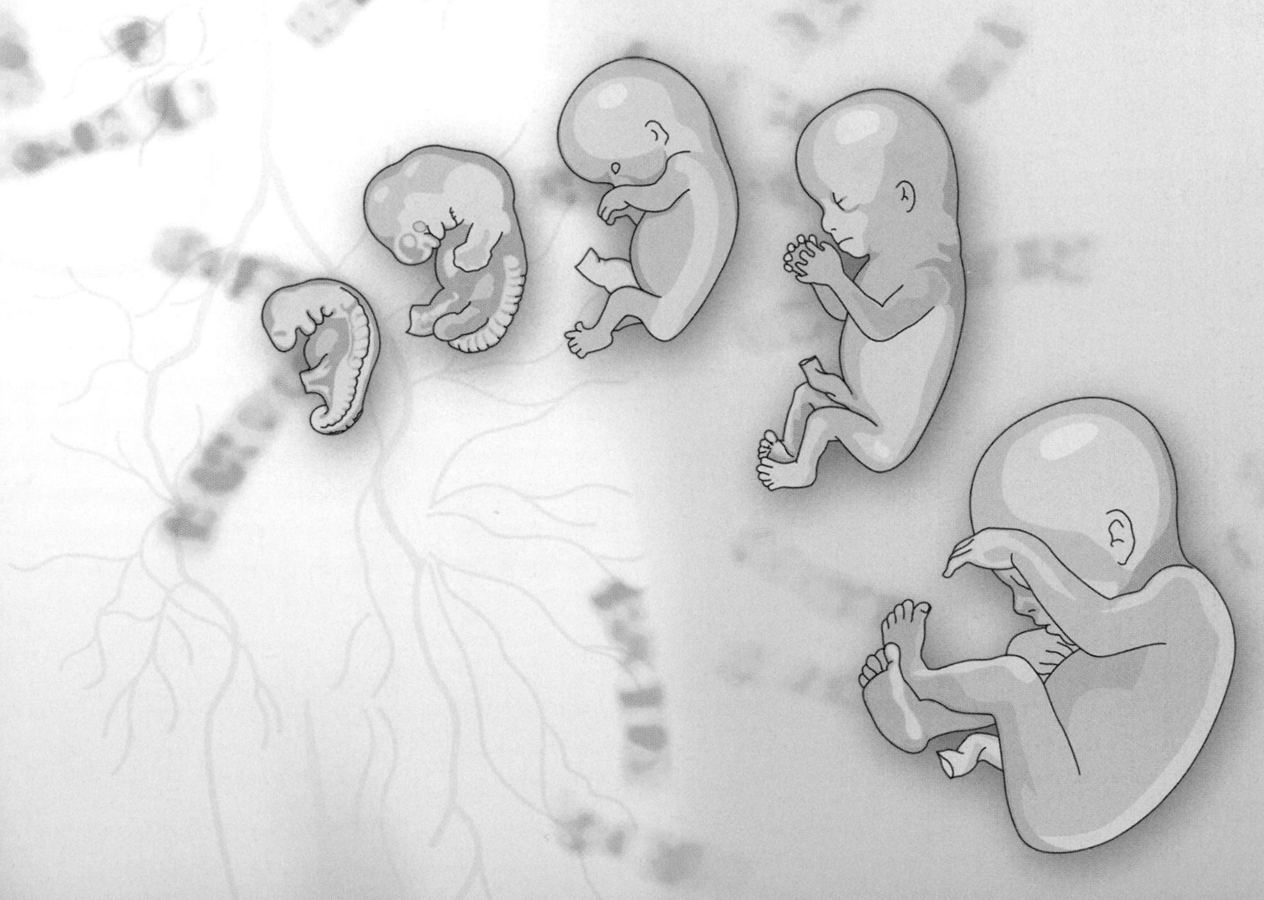

Reproduction

The chapters in this unit deal with what is certainly one of the most interesting and mysterious attributes of life: the ability to reproduce. The simplest forms of life, one-celled organisms, usually need no partner to reproduce; they simply divide by themselves. This form of reproduction is known as **asexual** (nonsexual) reproduction.

In most animals, however, reproduction is **sexual**, meaning that there are two kinds of individuals, males and females, each of which has specialized cells designed specifically for the perpetuation of the species. These specialized sex cells are known as **germ cells**, or **gametes** (GAM-etes). In the male, they are called **spermatozoa** (sper-mah-to-ZO-ah) (sing., spermatozoon), or simply sperm cells, and in the female, they are called **ova** (O-vah) (sing., ovum) or egg cells.

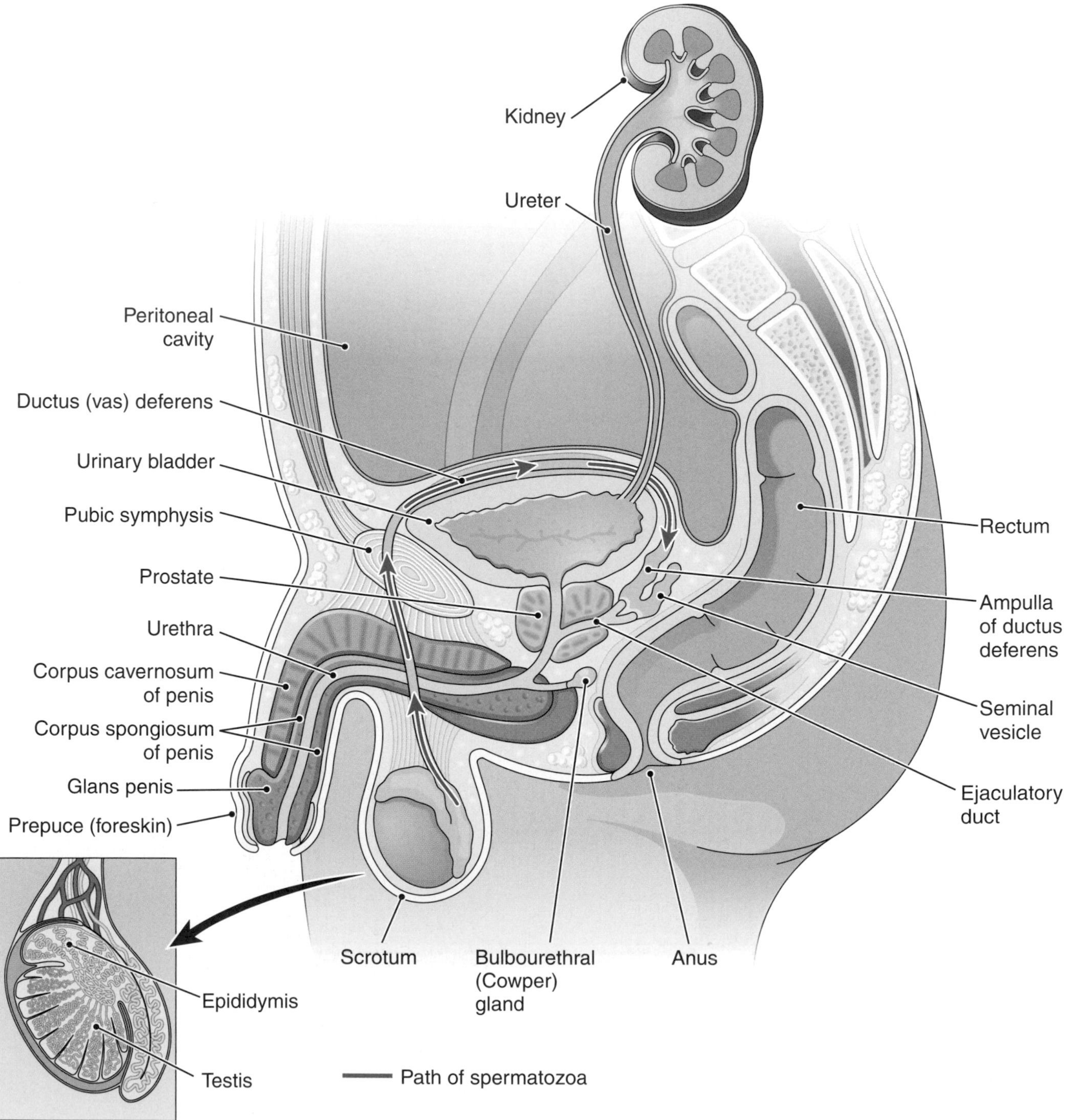

Figure 23-1 Male reproductive system. Organs of the urinary system are also shown. *ZOOMING IN ✦ What four glands empty secretions into the urethra?*

Meiosis

Gametes are characterized by having half as many chromosomes as are found in any other body cell. During their formation, they go through a special process of cell division, called **meiosis** (mi-O-sis), which halves the number of chromosomes. In humans, meiosis reduces the chromosome number in a cell from 46 to 23. The role of meiosis in reproduction is explained in more detail in Chapter 25.

Checkpoint 23-1 What is the process of cell division that halves the chromosome number in a cell to produce a gamete?

The Male Reproductive System

The male reproductive system, like that of the female, may be divided into two groups of organs: primary and accessory (see Fig. 23-1).

- The primary organs are the **gonads** (GO-nads), or sex glands; they produce the germ cells and manufacture hormones. The male gonad is the testis. (In comparison, the female gonad is the ovary, as explained below.)
- The **accessory organs** include a series of ducts that transport the germ cells as well as various exocrine glands.

The Testes

The male gonads, the **testes** (TES-teze) (sing. testis) are located outside the body proper, suspended between the thighs in a sac called the **scrotum** (SKRO-tum). The testes are oval organs measuring approximately 4.0 cm (1.5 inches) in length and approximately 2.5 cm (1 inch) in each of the other two dimensions. During embryonic life, each testis develops from tissue near the kidney.

A month or two before birth, the testis normally descends (moves downward) through the **inguinal** (ING-gwih-nal) **canal** in the abdominal wall into the scrotum. Each testis then remains suspended by a **spermatic cord** (Fig. 23-2) that extends through the inguinal canal. This cord contains blood vessels, lymphatic vessels, nerves, and the tube (ductus deferens) that transports spermatozoa away from the testis. The gland must descend completely if it is to function normally; to produce spermatozoa, the testis must be kept at the temperature of the scrotum, which is several degrees lower than that of the abdominal cavity.

Internal Structure Most of the specialized tissue of the testis consists of tiny coiled **seminiferous** (seh-mih-NIF-er-us) **tubules**. Primitive cells in the walls of these tubules develop into mature spermatozoa, aided by neighboring cells called **sustentacular** (sus-ten-TAK-u-lar) (Sertoli) **cells**. These so-called "nurse" cells nourish and protect the developing spermatozoa. They also secrete a protein that binds testosterone in the seminiferous tubules.

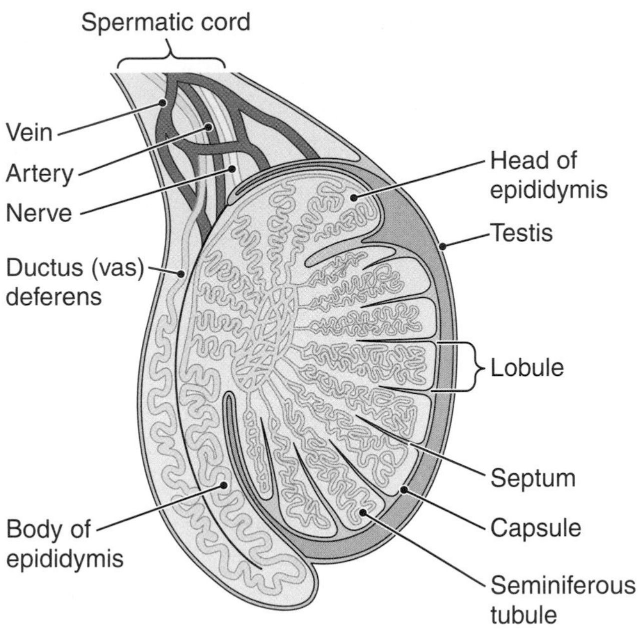

Figure 23-2 **Structure of the testis.** The epididymis and spermatic cord are also shown. *ZOOMING IN ✦ What duct receives secretions from the epididymis?*

Specialized **interstitial** (in-ter-STISH-al) **cells** that secrete the male sex hormone **testosterone** (*tes-TOS-teh-rone*) are located between the seminiferous tubules. Figure 23-3 is a microscopic view of the testis in cross-section, showing the seminiferous tubules, interstitial cells, and developing spermatozoa.

Testosterone After its secretion, testosterone is absorbed directly into the bloodstream. This hormone has three functions:

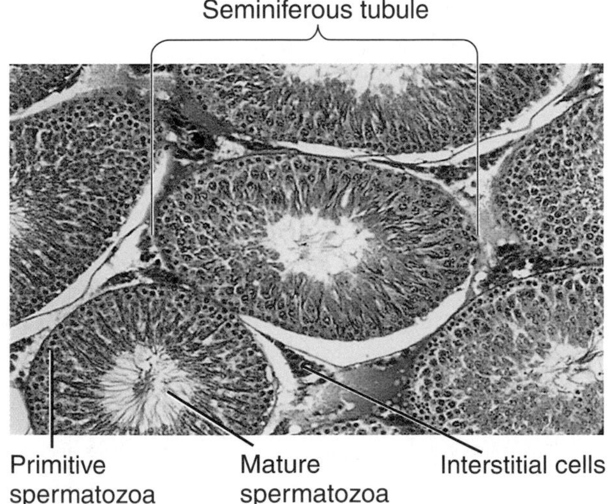

Figure 23-3 **Microscopic view of the testis.** (Courtesy of Dana Morse Bittus and BJ Cohen.)

- Development and maintenance of the reproductive structures.
- Development of spermatozoa.
- Development of **secondary sex characteristics,** traits that characterize males and females but are not directly concerned with reproduction. In males, these traits include a deeper voice, broader shoulders, narrower hips, a greater percentage of muscle tissue, and more body hair than are found in females.

The Spermatozoa Spermatozoa are tiny individual cells illustrated in Figure 23-4. They are so small that at least 200 million are contained in the average ejaculation (release of semen). After puberty, sperm cells are manufactured continuously in the seminiferous tubules of the testes.

The spermatozoon has an oval head that is largely a nucleus containing chromosomes. The **acrosome** (AK-ro-some), which covers the head like a cap, contains enzymes that help the sperm cell to penetrate the ovum.

Whiplike movements of the tail (flagellum) propel the sperm through the female reproductive system to the ovum. The cell's middle region (midpiece) contains many mitochondria that provide energy for movement.

Checkpoint 23-2 What is the male gonad? What is the main male sex hormone?

Checkpoint 23-3 What is the male sex cell (gamete) called?

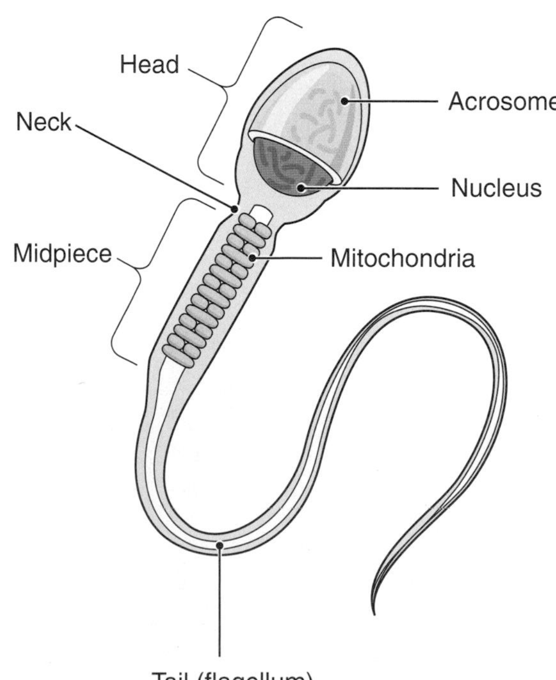

Figure 23-4 **Diagram of a human spermatozoon.** Major structural features are shown. *ZOOMING IN ✦ What organelles provide energy for sperm cell motility?*

Checkpoint 23-4 What are the main subdivisions of a spermatozoon?

Accessory Organs

The system of ducts that transports the spermatozoa begins with tubules inside the testis itself. From these tubules, the cells collect in a greatly coiled tube called the epididymis (ep-ih-DID-ih-mis), which is 6 meters (20 feet) long and is located on the surface of the testis inside the scrotal sac (see Fig. 23-2). While they are temporarily stored in the epididymis, the sperm cells mature and become motile, able to move or "swim" by themselves.

The epididymis finally extends upward as the **ductus deferens** (DEF-er-enz), also called the **vas deferens.** This tube, contained in the spermatic cord, continues through the inguinal canal into the abdominal cavity. Here, it separates from the remainder of the spermatic cord and curves behind the urinary bladder. The ductus deferens then joins with the duct of the **seminal vesicle** (VES-ih-kl) on the same side to form the **ejaculatory** (e-JAK-u-lah-to-re) **duct.** The right and left ejaculatory ducts travel through the body of the prostate gland and then empty into the urethra.

Checkpoint 23-5 What is the order in which sperm cells travel through the ducts of the male reproductive system?

Semen

Semen (*SE-men*) (meaning "seed") is the mixture of sperm cells and various secretions that is expelled from the body. It is a sticky fluid with a milky appearance. The pH is in the alkaline range of 7.2 to 7.8. The secretions in semen serve several functions:

- Nourish the spermatozoa
- Transport the spermatozoa
- Neutralize the acidity of the male urethra and the female vaginal tract
- Lubricate the reproductive tract during sexual intercourse
- Prevent infection with antibacterial enzymes and antibodies

The glands discussed next contribute secretions to the semen (see Fig. 23-1).

The Seminal Vesicles The seminal vesicles are twisted muscular tubes with many small outpouchings. They are approximately 7.5 cm (3 inches) long and are attached to the connective tissue at the posterior of the urinary bladder. The glandular lining produces a thick, yellow, alkaline secretion containing large quantities of simple sugar and other substances that provide nourishment for the sperm. The seminal fluid makes up a large part of the semen's volume.

The Prostate Gland The **prostate gland** lies immediately inferior to the urinary bladder, where it surrounds the first part of the urethra. Ducts from the prostate carry its secretions into the urethra. The thin, alkaline prostatic secretion helps neutralize the acidity of the vaginal tract and enhance the motility of the spermatozoa. The prostate gland is also supplied with muscular tissue, which, upon signals from the nervous system, contracts to aid in the expulsion of the semen from the body.

Bulbourethral Glands The **bulbourethral** (bul-bo-u-RE-thral) **glands**, also called **Cowper glands**, are a pair of pea-sized organs located in the pelvic floor just inferior to the prostate gland. They secrete mucus to lubricate the urethra and tip of the penis during sexual stimulation. The ducts of these glands extend approximately 2.5 cm (1 inch) from each side and empty into the urethra before it extends into the penis.

Other very small glands secrete mucus into the urethra as it passes through the penis.

Checkpoint 23-6 What glands, aside from the testis, contribute secretions to semen?

The Urethra and Penis

The male urethra, as discussed in Chapter 22, serves the dual purpose of conveying urine from the bladder and carrying the reproductive cells with their accompanying secretions to the outside. The ejection of semen into the receiving canal (vagina) of the female is made possible by the **erection**, or stiffening and enlargement, of the penis, through which the longest part of the urethra extends. The penis is made of spongy tissue containing many blood spaces that are relatively empty when the organ is flaccid but fill with blood and distend when the penis is erect. This tissue is subdivided into three segments, each called a **corpus** (body) (Fig. 23-5). A single, ventrally located **corpus spongiosum** contains the urethra. On either side is a larger **corpus cavernosum** (pl., corpora cavernosa). At the distal end of the penis, the corpus spongiosum enlarges to form the **glans** penis, which is covered with a loose fold of skin, the **prepuce** (PRE-puse), commonly called the *foreskin*. It is the end of the foreskin that is removed in a **circumcision** (sir-kum-SIZH-un), a surgery frequently performed on male babies for religious or cultural reasons. Experts disagree on the medical value of circumcision with regard to improved cleanliness and disease prevention.

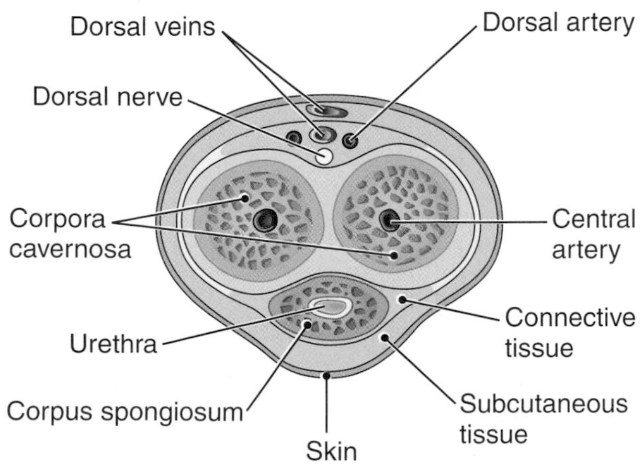

Figure 23-5 Cross-section of the penis. *ZOOMING IN ✦ What subdivision of the penis contains the urethra?*

The penis and scrotum together make up the *external genitalia* of the male.

Ejaculation **Ejaculation** (e-jak-u-LA-shun) is the forceful expulsion of semen through the urethra to the outside. The process is initiated by reflex centers in the spinal cord that stimulate smooth muscle contraction in the prostate. This is followed by contraction of skeletal muscle in the pelvic floor, which provides the force needed for expulsion. During ejaculation, the involuntary sphincter at the base of the bladder closes to prevent the release of urine.

A male typically ejaculates 2 to 5 mL of semen containing 50 to 150 million sperm cells per mL. Out of the millions of spermatozoa in an ejaculation, only one, if any, can fertilize an ovum. The remainder of the cells live from only a few hours up to a maximum of 3 days.

Hormonal Control of Male Reproduction

The activities of the testes are under the control of two hormones produced by the anterior pituitary. These hormones are named for their activity in female reproduction (described later), although they are chemically the same in both males and females.

- **Follicle-stimulating hormone (FSH)** stimulates the sustentacular (Sertoli) cells and promotes the formation of spermatozoa.
- **Luteinizing hormone (LH)** stimulates the interstitial cells between the seminiferous tubules to produce testosterone, which is also needed for sperm cell development. An older name for this hormone, which describes its action in males, is *interstitial cell–stimulating hormone* (ICSH).

Starting at puberty, the hypothalamus begins to secrete hormones that trigger the release of FSH and LH. These hormones are secreted continuously in the male.

The activity of the hypothalamus is in turn regulated by a negative feedback mechanism involving testosterone. As the blood level of testosterone increases, the hypothalamus secretes less releasing hormone; as the level of testosterone decreases, the hypothalamus secretes more releasing hormone (see Fig. 12-3 in Chapter 12).

Checkpoint 23-7 What two pituitary hormones regulate both male and female reproduction?

The Effects of Aging on Male Reproduction

A gradual decrease in the production of testosterone and spermatozoa begins as early as 20 years of age and continues throughout life. Secretions from the prostate and seminal vesicles decrease in amount and become less viscous. In a few men (less than 10%), sperm cells remain late in life, even to 80 years of age.

Disorders of the Male Reproductive System

A variety of disorders can contribute to **infertility**, a significantly lower than normal ability to reproduce. If the inability is complete, the condition is termed **sterility**. The proportion of infertility in couples that can be attributed to defects involving the male has been estimated from 40% to 50%. (See also Box 23-1 on erectile dysfunction.)

The tubules of the testes are sensitive to x-rays, infections, toxins, and malnutrition, all of which bring about degenerative changes. Such damage may cause a decrease in the numbers of spermatozoa produced, leading to a condition called **oligospermia** (ol-ih-go-SPER-me-ah). Adequate numbers of sperm are required to disperse the coating around the ovum so that one sperm can fertilize it. Absence of or an inadequate number of male sex cells is a significant cause of infertility.

A male may be intentionally sterilized by an operation called a **vasectomy** (vah-SEK-to-me). In this procedure, a portion of the ductus deferens on each side is removed, and the cut end is closed to keep spermatozoa from reaching the urethra. The tiny sperm cells are simply reabsorbed. A man who has had a vasectomy retains the ability to produce hormones and all other seminal secretions as well as the ability to perform the sex act, but no fertilization can occur.

Structural Disorders

Cryptorchidism (kript-OR-kid-izm) is a disorder characterized by failure of the testis to descend into the scrotum. Unless corrected in childhood, this condition results in sterility. Undescended testes are also particularly subject to tumor formation. Most testes that are undescended at birth descend spontaneously by 1 year of age. Surgical correction is the usual remedy in the remaining cases.

Torsion of the testis is a twisting of the spermatic cord that results from rotation of the testis (Fig. 23-6). This turning may occur during descent of the testis or later in life, most commonly between the ages of 8 to 18 years. The condition is accompanied by acute pain, swelling and shortening of the spermatic cord. It requires emergency surgery to correct the defect, and may involve removal the testis (orchiectomy). Torsion of the testis is a developmental disorder that often affects both glands, so the other testis must be examined to determine whether or not preventive surgery is needed.

Hernia (HER-ne-ah), or rupture, refers to the abnormal protrusion of an organ or organ part through the wall of the cavity in which it is normally contained (Fig. 23-7). Hernias most often occur where there is a weak

Box 23-1 Clinical Perspectives

Treating Erectile Dysfunction: When NO Means Yes

Approximately 25 million American men and their partners are affected by **erectile dysfunction** (ED), the inability to achieve an erection. Although ED is more common in men over the age of 65, it can occur at any age and can have many causes. Until recently, ED was believed to be caused by psychological factors, such as stress or depression. It is now known that many cases of ED are caused by physical factors, including cardiovascular disease, diabetes, spinal cord injury, and damage to penile nerves during prostate surgery. Antidepressant and antihypertensive medications also can produce erectile dysfunction.

Erection results from interaction between the autonomic nervous system and penile blood vessels. Sexual arousal stimulates parasympathetic nerves in the penis to release a compound called nitric oxide (NO), which activates the vascular smooth muscle enzyme guanylyl cyclase. This enzyme catalyzes production of cyclic GMP (cGMP), a potent vasodilator that increases blood flow into the penis to cause erection. Physical factors that cause ED prevent these physiologic occurrences.

Until recently, treatment options for ED, such as penile injections, vacuum pumps, and insertion of medications into the penile urethra were inadequate, inconvenient, and painful. Today, drugs that target the physiologic mechanisms that underlie erection are giving men who suffer from ED new hope. The best known of these is sildenafil (Viagra), which works by inhibiting the enzyme that breaks down cGMP, thus prolonging the effects of NO.

Although effective in about 80% of all ED cases, Viagra can cause some relatively minor side effects, including headache, nasal congestion, stomach upset, and blue-tinged vision. Viagra should never be used by men who are taking nitrate drugs to treat angina. Because nitrate drugs elevate NO levels, taking them with Viagra, a drug that prolongs the effects of NO, can cause life-threatening hypotension.

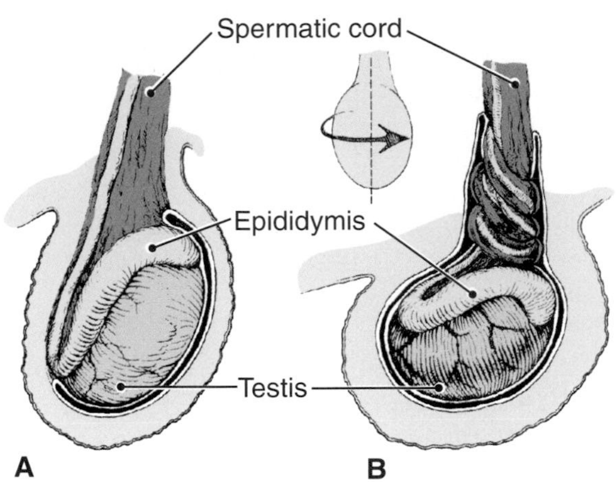

Figure 23-6 **Torsion of the testis.** (A) Normal. (B) Torsion. The testis rotates, twisting the spermatic cord. (Reprinted with permission from LifeART Pediatrics 1 [CD-ROM]. Baltimore: Lippincott Williams & Wilkins, 2000.)

area in the abdominal wall, at the inguinal canal for example. In this region, during development, the testis pushes its way through the muscles and connective tissues of the abdominal wall, carrying with it the blood vessels and other structures that form the spermatic cord.

Normally, in the adult, the inguinal area is fairly well reinforced with connective tissue, and there is no direct connection between the abdominal cavity and the scrotal sac. As in other regions where an opening permits a structure's passage through the abdominal wall, however, this area constitutes a weak place where a hernia may occur.

Phimosis (fi-MO-sis) is a tightness of the foreskin (prepuce), so that it cannot be drawn back. Phimosis may

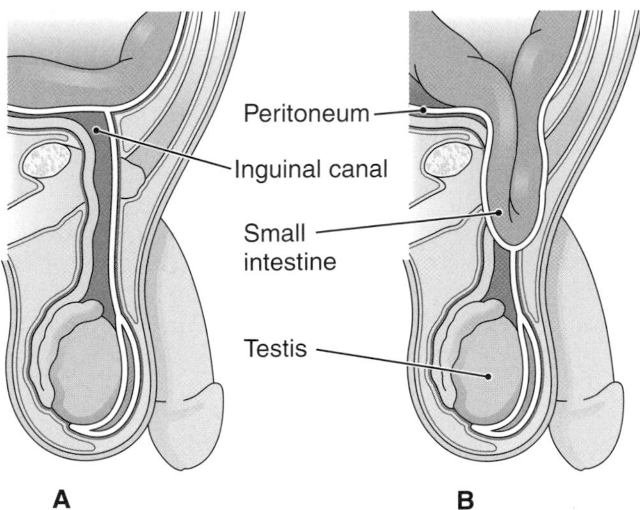

Figure 23-7 **Inguinal hernia.** (A) Normal. (B) Hernia. The intestine protrudes through a weakness in the abdominal wall at the inguinal canal. (Reprinted with permission from Cohen BJ. Medical Terminology. 4th ed. Philadelphia: Lippincott Williams & Wilkins, 2004.)

be remedied by circumcision, in which part or all of the foreskin is surgically removed.

Infections

Sexually transmitted infections (STI), formerly known as *sexually transmitted diseases* (STD) or *venereal diseases* (VD), are spread through sexual contact in both males and females. They most commonly involve chlamydial infections and gonococcal infections (gonorrhea). In males, these diseases are manifested by a discharge from the urethra, which may be accompanied by burning and pain, especially during urination. The infection may travel along the mucous membrane into the prostate gland and the epididymis; if both sides are affected and enough scar tissue is formed to destroy the tubules, sterility may result.

Another common STI is a persistent infection called **genital herpes**. Caused by a virus, this disorder is characterized by fluid-filled vesicles (blisters) on and around the genital organs.

The sexually transmitted disease **syphilis** is caused by a spirochete (*Treponema pallidum*). Because syphilis spreads quickly in the bloodstream, it is regarded as a systemic disorder (see Appendix 5, Table 1). The genital ulcers caused by syphilis increase the chances of infection with the AIDS virus. HIV itself is considered an STI because of its most common route of spread. (See Box 23-2 on lowering risks for STIs.)

Epididymitis Organisms from an STI or urinary tract infection (UTI) may travel through the ducts of the reproductive system to the epididymis. A congenital malformation in the urinary tract can predispose to **epididymitis** (ep-ih-did-ih-MI-tis), and infection may also be carried to the organ systemically by blood or lymph. Treatment includes an antibiotic along with bed rest and support of the scrotum to promote lymphatic drainage.

Prostatitis The usual cause of prostatic inflammation is bacterial infection secondary to an ascending urinary tract infection. A variety of intestinal organisms and bacteria from other sources may be involved, but *E. coli* is the most common. Treatment with antibiotics usually clears the infection, but tests to diagnose the source of infection may be needed if the condition persists. Other possible causes of **prostatitis** (pros-tah-TI-tis) are bladder-neck obstruction that forces urine into the prostate and autoimmunity.

Orchitis **Orchitis** (or-KI-tis) is inflammation of the testis, which also may follow from infection of the urinary or reproductive tract. The testes also may be involved in mumps, a viral infection of the parotid salivary gland. A mumps infection during or after puberty may result in inflammation of the testes, which could lead to sterility.

Checkpoint 23-8 What are some infectious diseases of the reproductive tract?

Box 23-2 · Health Maintenance

Sexually Transmitted Infections: Lowering Your Risks

Sexually transmitted infections (STIs) such as chlamydia, gonorrhea, genital herpes, HIV, and syphilis are some of the most common infectious diseases in the United States, affecting more than 13 million men and women each year. These diseases are associated with complications such as pelvic inflammatory disease, epididymitis, infertility, liver failure, neurological disorders, cancer, and AIDS. Women are more likely to contract STIs than are men. The same mechanisms that transport sperm cells through the female reproductive tract also move infectious organisms. The surest way to prevent STIs is to avoid sexual contact with others. If you are sexually active, the following techniques can lower your risks:

- Maintain a monogamous sexual relationship with an uninfected partner.
- Correctly and consistently use a condom. While not 100% effective, condoms greatly reduce the risk of contracting an STI.
- Avoid having sex during menstruation. Women may be more infectious as well as more susceptible to certain STIs during this time.
- Avoid contact with body fluids such as blood, semen, and vaginal fluids, all of which may harbor infectious organisms.
- Urinate and wash the genitals after sex. This may help remove infectious organisms before they cause disease.
- Have regular checkups for STIs. Most of the time STIs cause no symptoms, particularly in women.

Tumors

Tumors of the prostate may be benign or malignant. Both types cause such pressure on the urethra that urination becomes difficult. Back pressure may destroy kidney tissue and may lead to stasis of urine in the bladder with a resulting susceptibility to infection. Men with benign prostate enlargement, known as benign prostatic hyperplasia (BPH), may respond to medication to shrink the prostate. An herbal remedy that may help to slow progress of BPH is an extract of berries of the saw palmetto, a low-growing palm tree. If urinary function is threatened, however, surgery is performed to reduce the obstruction. Most commonly, surgery is performed through the urethra, in a transurethral prostatectomy (TURP). Newer methods include use of laser and ultrasound to destroy excess tissue or placement of a stent to widen the urethra.

Prostatic cancer is the most common cancer of males in the United States, especially among men older than 50 years of age. Other risk factors, in addition to age, are race, family history, and certain environmental agents. A high-fat diet may increase risk by promoting production of male sex hormones. Prostatic cancer is frequently detected as a nodule during rectal examination. Early detection has improved with annual blood tests for prostate-specific antigen (PSA). This protein increases in cases of prostate cancer, although it may increase in other prostatic disorders as well. Depending on the age of the patient and the nature of the cancer, the course of treatment may include surveillance, radiation therapy, surgery, or hormone treatments.

Testicular cancer affects young to middle-aged adults. Almost all testicular cancers arise in the germ cells, and a tumor can metastasize through the lymphatic system at an early stage of development. Early detection with regular testicular self-examination (TSE), however, improves the chances for effective treatment. The 5-year survival rate for this form of cancer is now greater than 95%. Often fertility can be preserved, although sperm banking is an option for men about to undergo treatment for testicular cancer.

The Female Reproductive System

The female gonads are the **ovaries** (O-vah-reze), where the female sex cells, or ova, are formed (Fig. 23-8). The remainder of the female reproductive tract consists of an organ (uterus) to hold and nourish a developing infant, various passageways, and the external genital organs.

Checkpoint 23-9 What is the female gonad called?

Checkpoint 23-10 What is the female gamete called?

The Ovaries

The ovary is a small, somewhat flattened oval body measuring approximately 4 cm (1.6 inches) in length, 2 cm (0.8 inch) in width, and 1 cm (0.4 inch) in depth. Like the testes, the ovaries descend, but only as far as the pelvic portion of the abdomen. Here, they are held in place by ligaments, including the broad ligament, the ovarian ligament, and others, that attach them to the uterus and the body wall.

The Ova and Ovulation

The outer layer of the ovary is made of a single layer of epithelium. Beneath this layer, the female gametes, the ova, are produced. The ovaries of a newborn female contain a large number of potential ova. Each month during the reproductive years, several ripen, but usually only one is released.

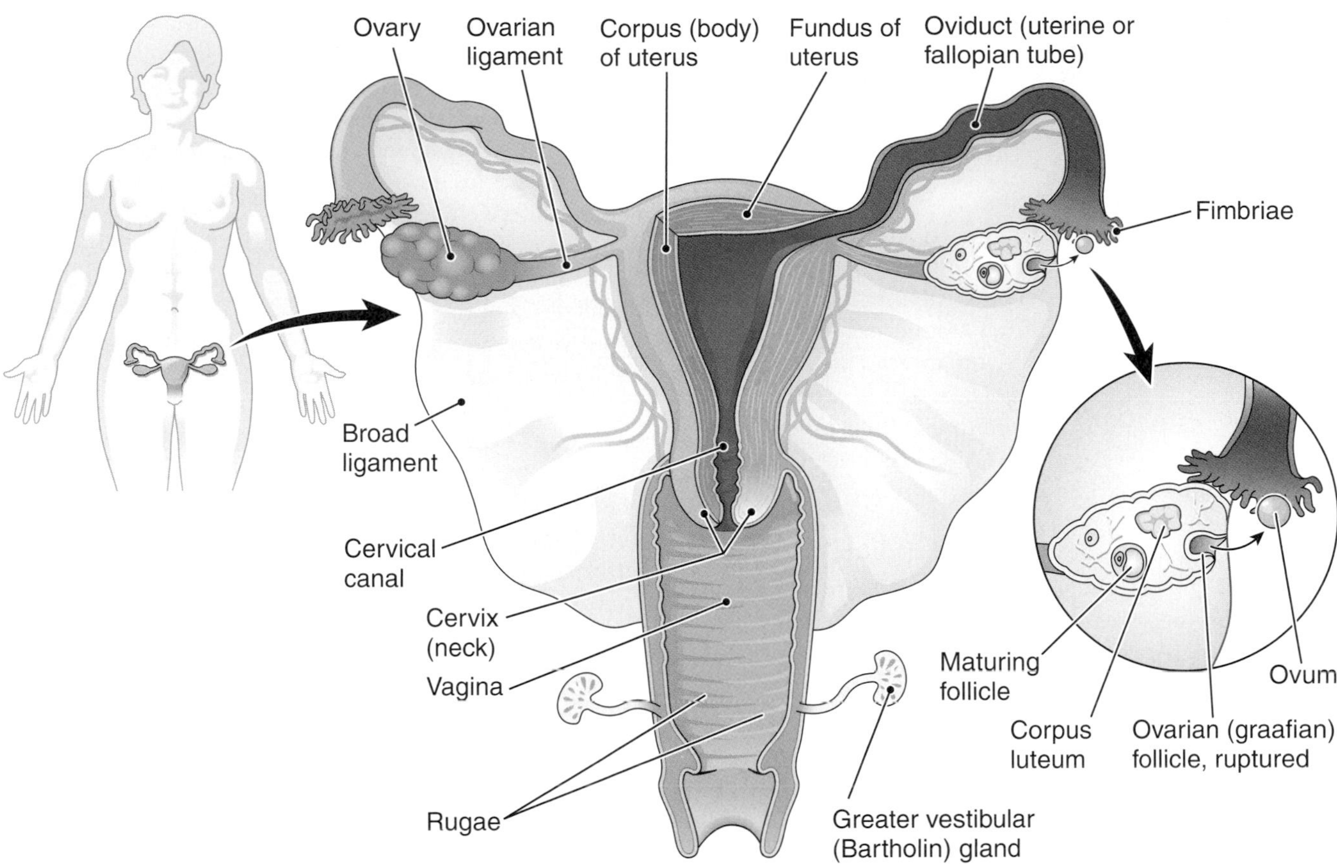

Figure 23-8 **Female reproductive system.** The enlargement (*right*) shows ovulation. *ZOOMING IN ✦ What is the deepest part of the uterus called?*

The complicated process of maturation, or "ripening," of an ovum takes place in a small fluid-filled cluster of cells called the **ovarian follicle** (o-VA-re-an FOL-ih-kl) or **graafian** (GRAF-e-an) **follicle** (Fig. 23-9). As the follicle develops, cells in its wall secrete the hormone estrogen, which stimulates growth of the uterine lining. When an ovum has ripened, the ovarian follicle may rupture and discharge the egg cell from the ovary's surface. The rupture of a follicle allowing the escape of an ovum is called **ovulation** (ov-u-LA-shun). Any developing ova that are not released simply degenerate.

After it is released, the egg cell makes its way to the nearest **oviduct** (O-vih-dukt), a tube that arches over the ovary and leads to the uterus (see Fig. 23-8).

Checkpoint 23-11 What is the structure that surrounds the egg as it ripens?

Checkpoint 23-12 What is the process of releasing an egg cell from the ovary called?

The Corpus Luteum

After the ovum has been expelled, the remaining follicle is transformed into a solid glandular mass called the **corpus luteum** (LU-te-um). This structure secretes estrogen and also progesterone, another hormone needed in the reproductive cycle. Commonly, the corpus luteum shrinks and is replaced by scar tissue. When a pregnancy occurs, however, this structure remains active. Sometimes, as a result of normal ovulation, the corpus luteum persists and forms a small ovarian cyst (fluid-filled sac). This condition usually resolves without treatment.

Checkpoint 23-13 What does the follicle become after its egg is released?

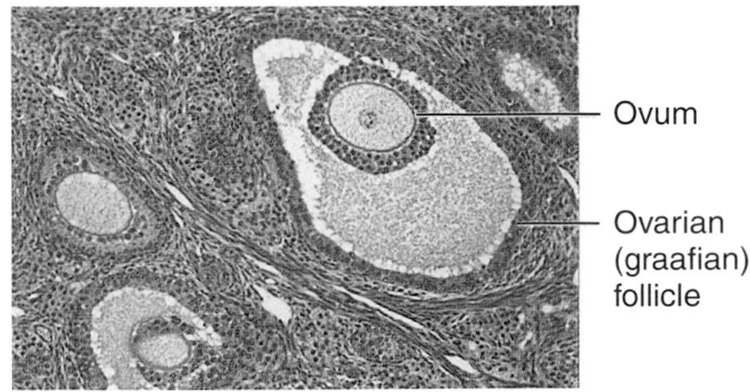

Figure 23-9 **Microscopic view of the ovary.** The photomicrograph shows egg cells (ova) developing within ovarian (graafian) follicles. (Courtesy of Dana Morse Bittus and BJ Cohen.)

Accessory Organs

The accessory organs in the female are the oviducts, the uterus, the vagina, the greater vestibular glands, and the vulva and perineum.

The Oviducts The tubes that transport the ova in the female reproductive system, the oviducts, are also known as **uterine** (U-ter-in) **tubes**, or **fallopian** (fah-LO-pe-an) **tubes.** Each is a small, muscular structure, nearly 12.5 cm (5 inches) long, extending from a point near the ovary to the uterus (womb). There is no direct connection between the ovary and this tube. The ovum is swept into the oviduct by a current in the peritoneal fluid produced by the small, fringelike extensions called **fimbriae** (FIM-bre-e) that are located at the edge of the tube's opening into the abdomen (see Fig. 23-8).

Unlike the sperm cell, the ovum cannot move by itself. Its progress through the oviduct toward the uterus depends on the sweeping action of cilia in the tube's lining and on peristalsis of the tube. It takes about 5 days for an ovum to reach the uterus from the ovary.

The Uterus The oviducts lead to the **uterus** (U-ter-us), an organ in which a fetus can develop to maturity. The uterus is a pear-shaped, muscular organ approximately 7.5 cm (3 inches) long, 5 cm (2 inches) wide, and 2.5 cm (1 inch) deep. (The organ is typically larger in women who have borne children and smaller in postmenopausal women.) The superior portion rests on the upper surface of the urinary bladder; the inferior portion is embedded in the pelvic floor between the bladder and the rectum. The wider upper region of the uterus is called the **corpus**, or *body;* the lower, narrower region is the **cervix** (SER-viks), or *neck.* The small, rounded region above the level of the tubal entrances is known as the **fundus** (FUN-dus) (see Fig. 23-8).

The broad ligaments support the uterus, extending from each side of the organ to the lateral body wall. Along with the uterus, these two portions of peritoneum form a partition dividing the female pelvis into anterior and posterior areas. The ovaries are suspended from the broad ligaments, and the oviducts lie within the upper borders. Blood vessels that supply these organs are found between the layers of the broad ligament (see Fig. 23-8).

The muscular wall of the uterus is called the **myometrium** (mi-o-ME-tre-um) (Fig. 23-10). The lining of the uterus is a specialized epithelium known as **endometrium** (en-do-ME-tre-um). This inner layer changes during the menstrual cycle, first preparing to nourish a fertilized egg, then breaking down if no fertilization occurs to be released as the menstrual flow. The cavity inside the uterus is shaped somewhat like a capital T, but it is capable of changing shape and dilating as a fetus develops.

Checkpoint 23-14 In what organ does a fetus develop?

The Vagina The cervix leads to the **vagina** (vah-JI-nah), the distal part of the birth canal, which opens to the outside of the body. The vagina is a muscular tube approximately 7.5 cm (3 inches) long. The cervix dips into the superior portion of the vagina forming a circular recess known as the **fornix** (FOR-niks). The deepest area of the fornix, located behind the cervix, is the **posterior fornix** (Fig. 23-11). This recess in the posterior vagina lies adjacent to the most infe-

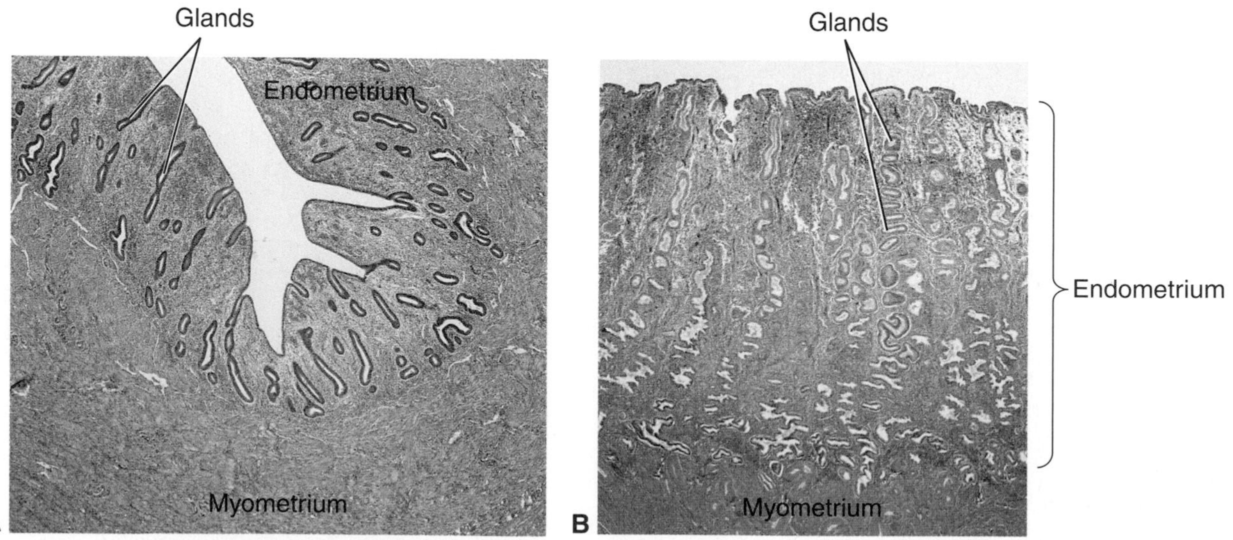

Figure 23-10 The uterus as seen under the microscope. The photomicrographs show the myometrium and endometrium and illustrate the changes that occur in the endometrium during the menstrual cycle. **(A)** Proliferative phase (first part of cycle). **(B)** Secretory phase (second part of cycle). (Reprinted with permission from Cormack DH. Essential Histology. 2nd ed. Philadelphia: Lippincott Williams & Wilkins, 2001.) *ZOOMING IN ✦ In which part of the menstrual cycle is the endometrium most highly developed?*

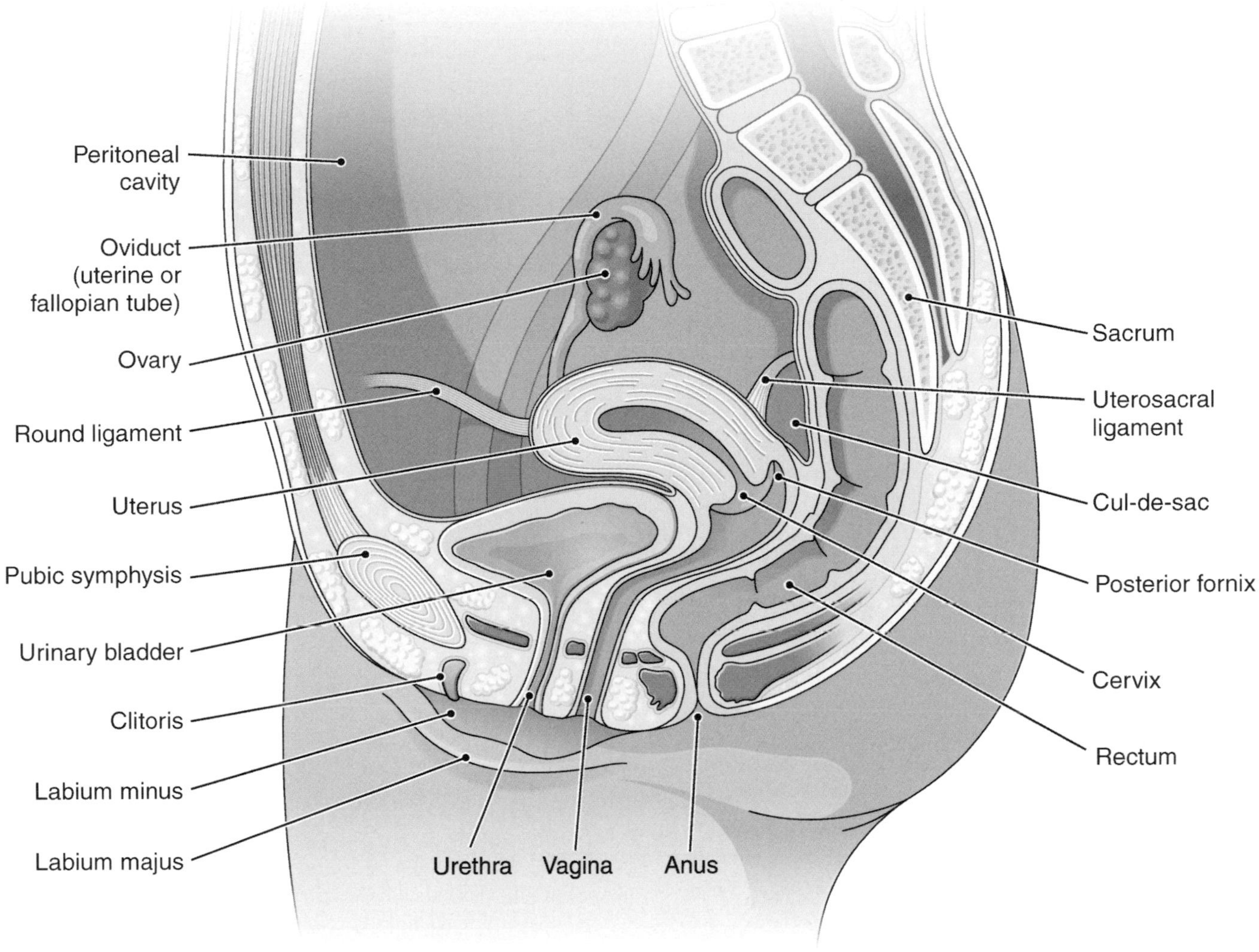

Figure 23-11 Female reproductive system (sagittal section). This view shows the relationship of the reproductive organs to each other and to other structures in the pelvic cavity. *ZOOMING IN ✦ Which has the more anterior opening, the vagina or the urethra?*

rior portion of the peritoneal cavity, a narrow passage between the uterus and the rectum named the **cul-de-sac** (from the French meaning "bottom of the sack"). This area is also known as the *rectouterine pouch* or the *pouch of Douglas*. A rather thin layer of tissue separates the posterior fornix from this region, so that abscesses or tumors in the peritoneal cavity can sometimes be detected by vaginal examination.

The lining of the vagina is a wrinkled mucous membrane similar to that found in the stomach. The folds (rugae) permit enlargement so that childbirth usually does not tear the lining. In addition to being a part of the birth canal, the vagina is the organ that receives the penis during sexual intercourse. A fold of membrane called the **hymen** (HI-men) may sometimes be found at or near the vaginal (VAJ-ih-nal) canal opening (Fig. 23-12).

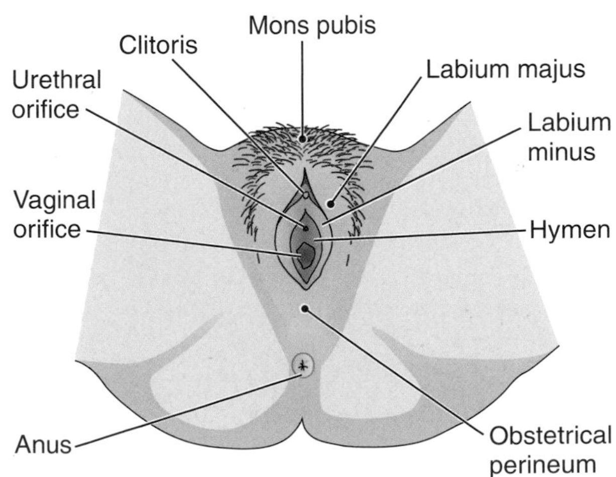

Figure 23-12 External parts of the female reproductive system. Related structures are also shown.

The Greater Vestibular Glands Just superior and lateral to the vaginal opening are the two mucus-producing

greater vestibular (ves-TIB-u-lar) (Bartholin) **glands** (see Fig. 23-8). These glands secrete into an area near the vaginal opening known as the **vestibule**. Like the Cowper glands in males, these glands provide lubrication during intercourse. If a gland becomes infected, a surgical incision may be needed to reduce swelling and promote drainage.

The Vulva and the Perineum The external parts of the female reproductive system form the **vulva** (VUL-vah), which includes two pairs of lips, or **labia** (LA-be-ah); the **clitoris** (KLIT-o-ris), which is a small organ of great sensitivity; and related structures (see Fig. 23-12). Although the entire pelvic floor in both the male and female (see Fig. 8-15 in Chapter 8) is properly called the **perineum** (per-ih-NE-um), those who care for pregnant women usually refer to the limited area between the vaginal opening and the anus as the perineum or *obstetrical perineum.*

The Menstrual Cycle

In the female, as in the male, reproductive function is controlled by pituitary hormones that are regulated by the hypothalamus. Female activity differs, however, in that it is cyclic; it shows regular patterns of increases and decreases in hormone levels. These changes are regulated by hormonal feedback. The typical length of the menstrual cycle varies between 22 and 45 days, but 28 days is taken as an average, with the first day of menstrual flow being considered the first day of the cycle (Fig. 23-13).

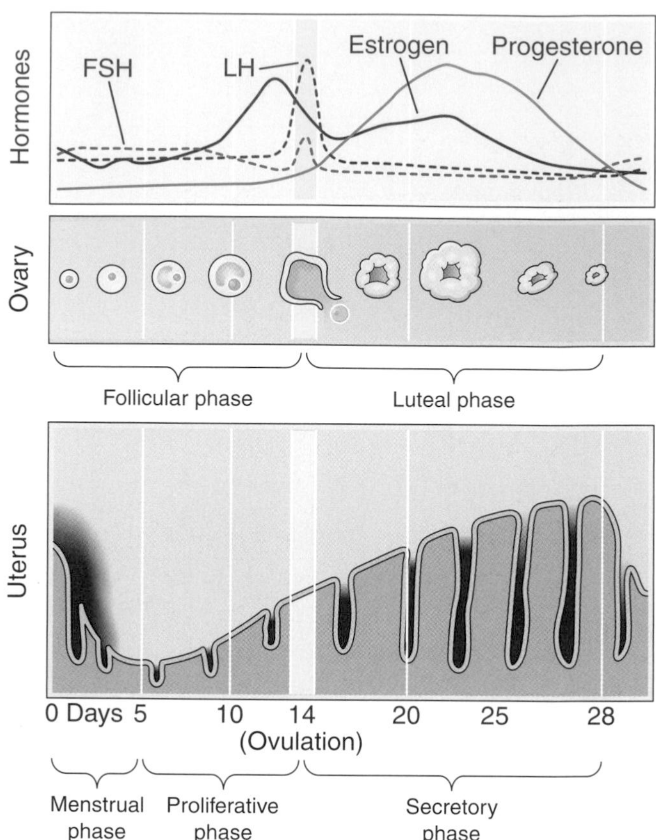

Figure 23-13 The menstrual cycle. Changes in hormones, the ovary, and the uterus are shown during a typical 28-day menstrual cycle with ovulation on day 14. (Pituitary hormones are shown with dashed lines, ovarian hormones with solid lines.) *ZOOMING IN ✦ What hormone peaks closest to ovulation?*

Beginning of the Cycle

At the start of each cycle, under the influence of pituitary FSH, several follicles, each containing an ovum, begin to develop in the ovary. Usually, only one of these follicles will ultimately release an ovum from the ovary in a single month. The follicle produces increasing amounts of **estrogen** as it matures (see Fig. 23-13). (*Estrogen* is the term used for a group of related hormones, the most active of which is estradiol.) The estrogen is carried in the bloodstream to the uterus, where it starts preparing the endometrium for a possible pregnancy. This preparation includes thickening of the endometrium and elongation of the glands that produce the uterine secretion. Estrogen in the blood also acts as a feedback messenger to inhibit the release of FSH and stimulate the release of LH from the pituitary (see Fig. 12-3 in Chapter 12). (Note that there is an unexplained rise in FSH at the time of ovulation, as shown in Fig. 23-13.)

Ovulation

In an average 28-day cycle, ovulation occurs on day 14 and is followed two weeks later by the start of the menstrual flow. However, an ovum can be released any time from day 7 to 21, thus accounting for the variation in the length of normal cycles. About 1 day before ovulation, there is an **LH surge**, a sharp rise of LH in the blood. This hormone causes ovulation and transforms the ruptured follicle into the corpus luteum, which produces some estrogen and large amounts of **progesterone**. Under the influence of these hormones, the endometrium continues to thicken, and the glands and blood vessels increase in size. The rising levels of estrogen and progesterone feed back to inhibit the release of FSH and LH from the pituitary. During this time, the ovum makes its journey to the uterus by way of the oviduct. If the ovum is not fertilized while passing through the uterine tube, it dies within 2 to 3 days and then disintegrates.

During each menstrual cycle, changes occur in both the ovary and the uterus (see Fig. 23-13). The time before ovulation is described as the follicular phase in the ovary, because it encompasses development of the ovarian follicle. The uterus during this same time is in a proliferative phase, marked by growth of the endometrium. After ovulation, the ovary is in a luteal phase, with conversion of the follicle to the corpus luteum, and the uterus is described as being in a secretory phase, based on activity of the endometrial glands.

Checkpoint 23-15 What are the two hormones produced in the ovaries?

The Menstrual Phase

If fertilization does not occur, the corpus luteum degenerates, and the levels of estrogen and progesterone decrease. Without the hormones to support growth, the endometrium degenerates. Small hemorrhages appear in this tissue, producing the bloody discharge known as **menstrual flow**, or **menses** (MEN-seze). Bits of endometrium break away and accompany the blood flow during this period of **menstruation** (men-stru-A-shun). The average duration of menstruation is 2 to 6 days.

Even before the menstrual flow ceases, the endometrium begins to repair itself through the growth of new cells. The low levels of estrogen and progesterone allow the release of FSH from the anterior pituitary. FSH causes new follicles to begin to ripen within the ovaries, and the cycle begins anew.

The activity of ovarian hormones as negative feedback messengers is the basis of hormonal methods of contraception (birth control). Estrogen and progesterone inhibit the release of FSH and LH from the pituitary, resulting in a menstrual period but no ovulation

Menopause

Menopause (MEN-o-pawz) is the period during which menstruation ceases altogether. It ordinarily occurs gradually between the ages of 45 and 55 years and is caused by a normal decline in ovarian function. The ovary becomes chiefly scar tissue and no longer produces ripe follicles or appreciable amounts of estrogen. Eventually, the uterus, oviducts, vagina, and vulva all become somewhat atrophied and the vaginal mucosa becomes thinner, dryer, and more sensitive.

Menopause is an entirely normal condition, but its onset sometimes brings about effects that are temporarily disturbing. The decrease in estrogen levels can cause nervous symptoms, such as anxiety, insomnia, and "hot flashes."

Hormone Replacement Therapy

Physicians may prescribe hormone replacement therapy (HRT) to relieve the discomforts associated with menopause. This medication is usually a combination of estrogen with a synthetic progesterone (progestin), which is included to prevent overgrowth of the endometrium and the risk of endometrial cancer. Early assumptions about the role of estrogen in preventing heart attacks have been disproved by carefully controlled studies, at least with regard to the most commonly prescribed form of HRT. The hormone therapy did lower the incidence of colorectal cancer and hip fractures, a sign of osteoporosis. Studies are continuing with estrogen alone, generally prescribed for women who have undergone a hysterectomy and do not have a uterus.

In addition to an increased risk of breast cancer, HRT also carries a risk of thrombosis and embolism, which is highest among women who smoke. All HRT risks increase with the duration of therapy. Therefore, treatment should be given for a short time and at the lowest effective dose. Women with a history or family history of breast cancer or circulatory problems should not take HRT.

Checkpoint 23-16 What is the definition of menopause?

Birth Control

Birth control is most commonly achieved by **contraception**, which is the use of artificial methods to prevent fertilization of the ovum. Birth control measures that prevent implantation of the fertilized ovum are also considered contraceptives, although technically they do not prevent conception and are more accurately called **abortifacients** (ah-bor-tih-FA-shents) (agents that cause abortion). Some of the birth control methods act by both mechanisms. Table 23-1 presents a brief description of the main contraceptive methods currently in use along with some advantages and disadvantages of each. The list is given in rough order of decreasing effectiveness. Unless specifically mentioned as doing so, a given method does *not* prevent the transmission of STIs.

The various hormonal methods of birth control basically differ in how they administer the hormones. The emergency contraceptive pill (ECP) is a synthetic progesterone (progestin) taken within 72 hours after intercourse, usually in two doses 12 hours apart. It reduces the risk of pregnancy following unprotected intercourse. This so-called "morning after pill" is intended for emergency use and not as a regular birth control method. Birth control hormones can also be implanted as capsules under the skin of the upper arm. This method is highly effective and lasts for 3–5 years, but the capsules must be implanted and removed by a health professional, and they have been difficult to remove in some cases.

The female condom is a sheath that fits into the vagina. It does protect against STIs, but is not very convenient to use. Researchers have also done trials with a male contraceptive pill, but none is on the market as yet. (See Box 23-3 on hormonal contraception for men.) Mefipristone (RU 486) is a drug taken after conception to terminate an early pregnancy. It blocks the action of progesterone, causing the uterus to shed its lining and release the fertilized egg. It must be combined with administration of prostaglandins to expel the uterine tissue. Mefipristone is not in widespread use in the United States, but it has been used in other countries.

Checkpoint 23-17 What is the definition of contraception?

Table 23•1 Main Methods of Birth Control Currently in Use

METHOD	DESCRIPTION	ADVANTAGES	DISADVANTAGES
Surgical			
Vasectomy/tubal ligation	Cutting and tying of tubes carrying gametes	Nearly 100% effective; involves no chemical or mechanical devices	Not usually reversible; rare surgical complications
Hormonal			
Birth control pills	Estrogen and progestin or progestin alone taken orally to prevent ovulation	Highly effective; requires no last-minute preparation	Alters physiology; return to fertility may be delayed. Risk of cardiovascular disease in older women who smoke or have hypertension.
Birth control shot	Injection of synthetic progesterone every 3 months to prevent ovulation	Highly effective; lasts for 3 to 4 months	Alters physiology; same possible side effects as birth control pill; also possible menstrual irregularity, amenorrhea
Birth control patch	Adhesive patch placed on body that administers estrogen and progestin through the skin; left on for 3 weeks and removed for a fourth week	Protects long-term; less chance of incorrect use; no last-minute preparation	Alters physiology; same possible side effects as birth control pill
Birth control ring	Flexible ring inserted into vagina that releases hormones internally; left in place for three weeks and removed for a fourth week	Long-lasting, highly effective; no last minute preparation	Possible infections, irritation; same possible side effects as birth control pill
Barrier			
Male condom	Sheath that fits over erect penis and prevents release of semen	Easily available; does not effect physiology; protects against sexually transmitted infection (STI)	Must be applied just before intercourse; may slip or tear
Diaphragm (with spermicide)	Rubber cap that fits over cervix and prevents entrance of sperm	Does not affect physiology; some protection against STI; no side effects	Must be inserted before intercourse and left in place for 6 hours; requires fitting by physician
Contraceptive sponge (with spermicide)	Soft, disposable foam disk containing spermicide, which is moistened with water and inserted into vagina	Protects against pregnancy for 24 hours; non-hormonal; some STI protection; available without prescription; inexpensive	85%–90% effective depending on proper use; possible skin irritation
Intrauterine device (IUD)	Metal or plastic device inserted into uterus through vagina; prevents fertilization and implantation by release of copper or birth control hormones	Highly effective for 5–10 years depending on type; reversible; no last-minute preparation	Must be introduced and removed by health professional; heavy menstrual bleeding
Other			
Spermicide	Chemicals used to kill sperm; best when used in combination with a barrier method	Available without prescription; inexpensive; does not affect physiology; some protection against STI	May cause local irritation; must be used just before intercourse
Fertility awareness	Abstinence during fertile part of cycle as determined by menstrual history, basal body temperature, or quality of cervical mucus	Does not affect physiology; accepted by certain religions	High failure rate; requires careful record keeping

Box 23-3 **Hot Topics**

Hormonal Contraception: New Options for Men

At present, sexually active men have few effective options for contraception, the most reliable being condoms or vasectomy. While condoms have the additional benefit of preventing sexually transmitted infections, their failure rate for preventing pregnancy is about 10%. With a failure rate of about 1%, vasectomies are much more reliable but are suitable only for couples who do not want children or are finished having children. A new option is on the horizon, however—male hormonal contraception.

Like female contraception, the male version of "the pill" works by suppressing the release of gonadotropin releasing hormone (GnRH) from the hypothalamus. This, in turn, blocks the pituitary's release of luteinizing hormone (LH) and follicle stimulating hormone (FSH), both of which play an important role in spermatogenesis.

Several therapies that decrease LH and FSH production in men are under investigation. One method already in clinical trials uses high levels of testosterone to negatively feed back to the hypothalamus and suppress GnRH secretion. Currently, this method requires regular testosterone injections, which makes it impractical for general use. In addition, doses of testosterone high enough to stop spermatogenesis may be associated with side effects such as acne, weight gain, mood changes, and increased risk of cardiovascular disease. More practical methods of drug delivery, such as pills, transdermal patches, and implants are being developed and may be effective at lower testosterone doses.

Another promising method uses the female hormone progesterone to block GnRH production. While this method suppresses spermatogenesis more effectively than does testosterone alone, it also suppresses normal testosterone production. Thus, the progesterone must be combined with testosterone to prevent the loss of secondary sex characteristics. Investigation is still underway to determine the best way to deliver such combination therapy.

Disorders of the Female Reproductive System

Female reproductive disorders include menstrual disturbances, various forms of tumors, and infections, any of which can contribute to infertility.

Menstrual Disorders

Absence of menstrual flow is known as **amenorrhea** (ah-men-o-RE-ah). This condition can be symptomatic of insufficient hormone secretion or congenital abnormality of the reproductive organs. Stress and other psychological factors often play a part in cessation of the menstrual flow. For example, any significant change in a woman's general state of health or change in her living habits, such as a shift in working hours, can interfere with menstruation. Very low body weight with a low percentage of body fat can lead to amenorrhea by reducing estrogen synthesis, as may occur in athletes who over-train without eating enough and in women who are starving or have eating disorders.

Dysmenorrhea (dis-men-o-RE-ah) means painful or difficult menstruation. In young women, this may be due to immaturity of the uterus. Dysmenorrhea is frequently associated with cycles in which ovulation has occurred. Often, the pain can be relieved by drugs that block prostaglandins, because some prostaglandins are known to cause painful uterine contractions.

In many cases, women have been completely relieved of menstrual cramps by their first pregnancies. Apparently, enlargement of the cervical opening remedies the condition. Artificial dilation of the cervical opening may alleviate dysmenorrhea for several months. Often, such health measures as sufficient rest, a well-balanced diet, and appropriate exercise remedy the disorder. In cases of dysmenorrhea, the application of heat over the abdomen usually relieves the pain, just as it may ease other types of muscular cramps.

Premenstrual syndrome (PMS), also called **premenstrual tension**, is a condition in which nervousness, irritability, and depression precede the menstrual period. It is thought to be caused by fluid retention in various tissues, including the brain. Sometimes, a low-salt diet and appropriate medication for 2 weeks before the menses prevent this disorder. This treatment may also avert dysmenorrhea.

Abnormal uterine bleeding includes excessive menstrual flow, too-frequent menstruation, and nonmenstrual bleeding. Any of these may cause serious anemias and deserve careful medical attention. Nonmenstrual bleeding may be an indication of a tumor, possibly cancer.

Benign and Malignant Tumors

Fibroids, which are more correctly called *myomas,* are common tumors of the uterus. Studies indicate that about 50% of women who reach the age of 50 have one or more of these growths in the uterine wall. Often, these tumors are small, and usually they remain benign and produce no symptoms. They develop between puberty and menopause and ordinarily stop growing after a woman has reached the age of 50 years. In some cases, these growths interfere with pregnancy, and in a patient younger than 40 years of age, a surgeon may simply remove the tumor and leave the uterus fairly intact. Normal pregnancies have occurred after such surgery.

Fibroids may become so large that pressure on adjacent structures causes grave disorders. In some cases, invasion of blood vessels near the uterine cavity causes serious hemorrhages. For these and other reasons, it may be necessary to remove the entire uterus or a large part of it. Surgical removal of the uterus is called a **hysterectomy** (his-ter-EK-to-me).

Breast Cancer Cancer of the breast is the most commonly occurring malignant disease in women. The risk factors in breast cancer are age past 40, family history of breast cancer, and factors that increase exposure to estrogen, such as early onset of menstruation, late menopause, late or no pregnancies, long-term HRT, and obesity (fat cells produce estrogen). Mutations in two genes (BRCA1 and BRCA2) are responsible for hereditary forms of breast cancer, which make up only about 8% of all cases. These same genetic mutations are associated with an increased risk of ovarian cancer.

The tumor is usually a painless, movable mass that is often noticed by a woman and all too frequently ignored. In recent years, however, there has been increasing emphasis on the importance of regular breast self-examination (BSE). (Most breast lumps are discovered by women themselves.) Any lump, no matter how small, should be reported to a physician immediately. The **mammogram,** a radiographic study of the breast, has improved the detection of early breast cancer. Guidelines recommend regular mammograms after the age of 40 years unless there is a history of breast cancer in the family, in which case earlier studies are recommended. Suspicious areas require further study by ultrasonography or biopsy, either a needle aspiration, removal of a core of tissue, or excision of the lump.

Breast cancer treatment consists of surgery with follow-up therapy of radiation, chemotherapy, or both. Surgical treatment by removal of the lump ("lumpectomy") or a segment of the breast is most common. Removal of the entire breast and dissection of the lymph nodes in the axilla (armpit) is called **modified radical mastectomy** (mas-TEK-to-me). The extent of tumor spread through the lymph nodes is an important factor in prognosis. In a sentinel lymph node biopsy, the first (sentinel) lymph nodes to receive lymph from the tumor are identified and tested for cancerous cells. Treatment is based on how much spread has occurred (see Box 16-2). Treatment of breast cancer is often followed by administration of drugs to block estrogen receptors in breast tissue or drugs that inhibit tumor growth factors.

Note that the incidence of the various types of cancer should not be confused with the death rates for each type. Owing to education of the public and increasingly better methods of diagnosis and treatment, some forms of cancer have a higher cure rate than others. For example, breast cancer appears much more often in women than lung cancer, but more women now die each year from lung cancer than from breast cancer.

Endometrial Cancer The most common cancer of the female reproductive tract is cancer of the endometrium (the lining of the uterus). This type of cancer usually affects women during or after menopause. It is seen most frequently in women who have been exposed to high levels of estrogen, which causes overgrowth of the endometrium. This group includes those who have received estrogen therapy unopposed by progesterone, those who have had few or no pregnancies, and the obese. Symptoms include an abnormal discharge or irregular bleeding; later there is cramping and pelvic pain. This type of cancer is diagnosed by endometrial biopsy. The usual methods of treatment include surgery and irradiation. Endometrial cancer grows slowly in its beginning stages, so early, aggressive treatment usually saves a patient's life.

Ovarian Cancer Ovarian cancer is the second most common reproductive tract cancer in the female, usually occurring in women between the ages of 40 and 65 years. It is a leading cause of cancer deaths in women. Although most ovarian cysts are not malignant, they should always be investigated for possible malignant change. Ovarian cancer is highly curable if treated before it has spread to other organs. However, these malignancies tend to progress rapidly, and they are difficult to detect because symptoms are vague, there are few recognized risk factors, and at present there is no screening test.

Cervical Cancer Cancer of the cervix is linked to infection with human papilloma virus (HPV), which causes genital warts and is spread through sexual contact. Thus, cervical cancer can be considered a sexually transmitted disease. Risk factors for the disease are related to exposure to HPV, such as early age of sexual activity and multiple sex partners. Certain strains of the virus are found in cervical carcinomas and precancerous cervical cells.

Early detection is often possible because the cancer develops slowly from atypical cervical cells. The decline in the death rate from cervical cancer is directly related to use of the **Papanicolaou** (pap-ah-nik-o-LAH-o) **test,** also known as the *Pap test* or *Pap smear.* The Pap smear is a microscopic examination of cells obtained from cervical scrapings and swabs of the cervical canal. All women should be encouraged to have this test every year. Even girls younger than 18 years of age should be tested if they are sexually active. Guidelines now recommend less frequent testing after normal results are obtained in three annual tests.

Infections

Infections that affect the male reproductive system also infect the female genital organs (Fig. 23-14), although these diseases may be less apparent in women. The most common STIs in women are chlamydial infections, gonorrhea, HIV, and genital herpes, caused by herpes simplex virus (HSV). Syphilis also occurs in women and can

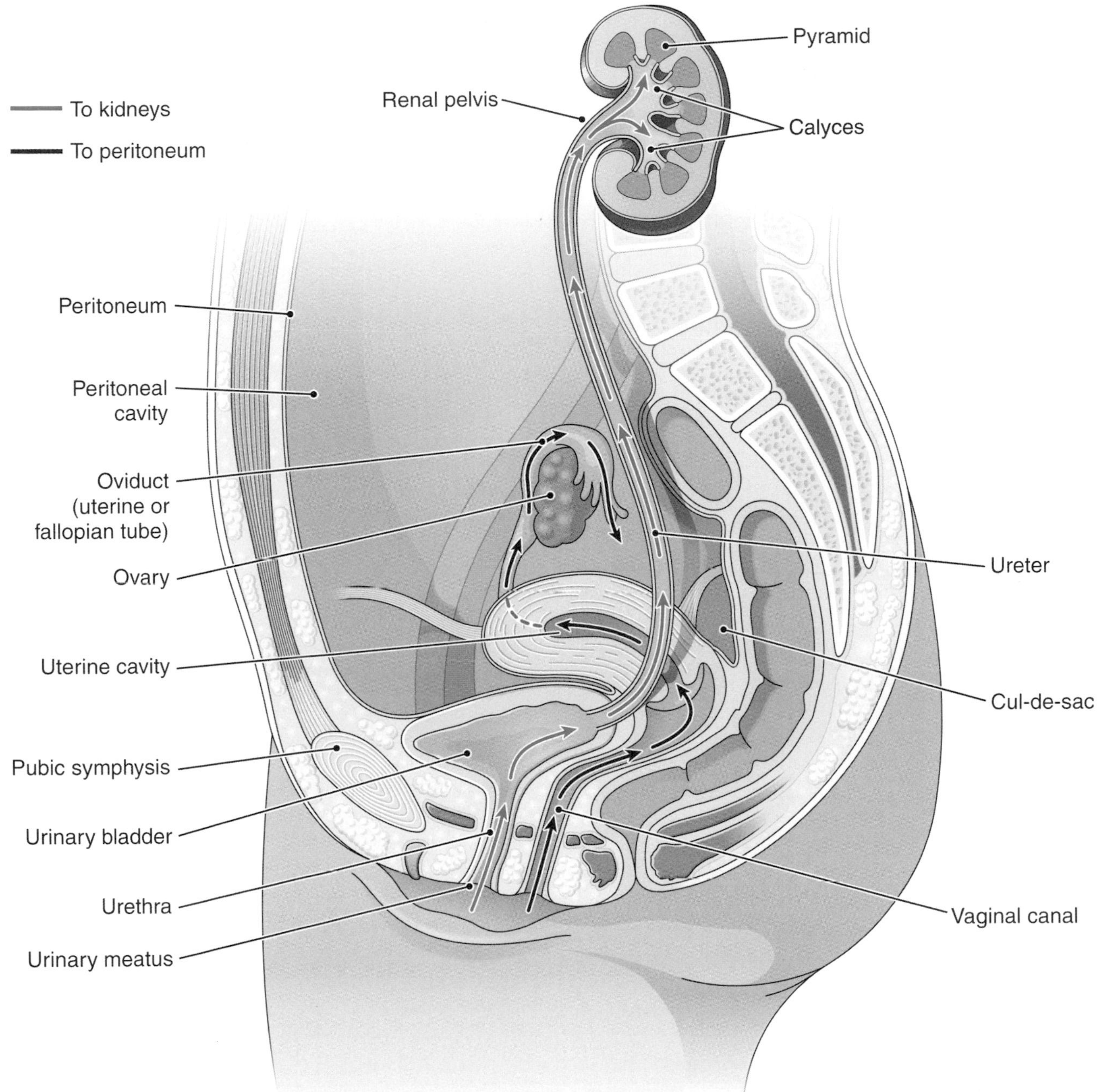

Figure 23-14 Pathway of infection. Disease organisms can travel from outside to the peritoneum and into the urinary system.

be passed through the placenta from mother to fetus, causing stillbirth or birth of an infected infant.

The incidence of **genital warts,** caused by human papillomavirus (HPV), has increased in recent years. These infections have been linked to cancer of the reproductive tract, especially as noted, cancer of the uterine cervix.

Salpingitis (sal-pin-JI-tis) means inflammation of any tube, but usually refers to disease of the uterine tubes (oviducts). Most uterine tube infections are caused by gonococci or by the bacterium *Chlamydia trachomatis,* but other bacteria may be the cause. Salpingitis may cause sterility by obstructing the tubes, thus preventing the passage of ova.

Pelvic inflammatory disease (PID) is due to extension of infections from the reproductive organs into the pelvic cavity, and it often involves the peritoneum. (See the purple arrow pathway in Fig. 23-14.) Gonococcus or chlamydia is usually the initial cause of infection, but most cases of PID involve multiple organisms.

Infertility

Infertility is much more difficult to diagnose and evaluate in the female than in the male. Whereas a microscopic examination of properly collected semen may be enough to determine the presence of abnormal or too few sperm cells in the male, no such simple study can be made in the female. Infertility in women, as in men, may be relative or absolute. Causes of female infertility include infections, endocrine disorders, psychogenic factors, and abnormalities in the structure and function of the reproductive organs themselves. In all cases of apparent infertility, the male partner should be investigated first because the procedures for determining lack of fertility in the male are much simpler and less costly than those in the female, as well as being essential for the evaluation.

Word Anatomy

Medical terms are built from standardized word parts (prefixes, roots, and suffixes). Learning the meanings of these parts can help you remember words and interpret unfamiliar terms.

WORD PART	MEANING	EXAMPLE
The Male Reproductive System		
semin/o	semen, seed	Sperm cells are produced in the *seminiferous* tubules.
test/o	testis	The hormone *testosterone* is produced in the testis.
acr/o	extreme end	The *acrosome* covers the head of a sperm cell.
fer	to carry	The ductus *deferens* carries spermatozoa away from (de-) the testis.
circum-	around	A cut is made around the glans to remove part of the foreskin in a *circumcision*.
Disorders of the Male Reproductive System		
olig/o-	few, deficiency	*Oligospermia* is a deficiency in the numbers of spermatozoa produced.
crypt/o-	hidden	*Cryptorchidism* refers to an undescended testis (orchid/o).
orchid/o, orchi/o	testis	*Orchiectomy* is removal of the testis.
The Female Reproductive System		
ov/o, ov/i	egg	An *ovum* is an egg cell.
ovar, ovari/o	ovary	The *ovarian* follicle encloses a maturing ovum.
metr/o	uterus	The *myometrium* is the muscular (my/o) layer of the uterus.
rect/o	rectum	The *rectouterine* pouch is between the uterus and rectum.
Disorders of the Female Reproductive System		
men/o	uterine bleeding; menses	*Amenorrhea* is absence of menstrual flow
hyster/o	uterus	*Hysterectomy* is surgical removal of the uterus.
mamm/o	breast, mammary gland	A *mammogram* is radiographic study of the breast.
mast/o	breast	A *mastectomy* is surgical removal of the breast.
salping/o	tube	*Salpingitis* is inflammation of a tube, such as the oviduct.

Summary

I. Reproduction

A. Meiosis—reduces chromosome number from 46 to 23
  1. Gametes (sex cells)
    a. Spermatozoa (sperm cells)—male
    b. Ova (egg cells)—female

II. Male reproductive system

  1. Primary organs—gonads
  2. Accessory organs—ducts and exocrine glands

A. Testes
  1. Scrotum—sac that holds the testes
  2. Inguinal canal—channel through which testis descends
  3. Internal structure
    a. Seminiferous tubules—tubes in which sperm cells are produced
      (1) Sustentacular (Sertoli) cells—aid in development of spermatozoa
    b. Interstitial cells (between tubules)—secrete hormones
  4. Testosterone—main male hormone
    a. Maintains reproductive structures
    b. Aids development of secondary sex characteristics
  5. Spermatozoa
    a. Head—contains chromosomes
    b. Acrosome—covers head; has enzymes to help penetration of ovum
    c. Midpiece—contains mitochondria
    d. Tail (flagellum)—propels sperm

B. Accessory organs
  1. Epididymis—stores spermatozoa until ejaculation
  2. Ductus (vas) deferens—conducts sperm cells through spermatic cord
  3. Ejaculatory duct—empties into urethra

C. Semen
  1. Functions
    a. Nourish spermatozoa
    b. Transport spermatozoa
    c. Neutralize male urethra and vaginal tract
    d. Lubricate reproductive tract during intercourse
    e. Prevent infection
  2. Seminal vesicles
  3. Prostate—around first portion of urethra
  4. Bulbourethral (Cowper) glands
D. Urethra and penis
  1. Urethra
    a. Conveys urine and semen through penis
  2. Penis
    a. Structure
      (1) Corpus spongiosum—central; contains urethra
      (2) Corpora cavernosa—lateral
      (3) Glands—distal enlargement of corpus spongiosum
      (4) Prepuce—foreskin
    b. Erection—stiffening and enlargement of penis
  3. Ejaculation—forceful expulsion of semen

III. Hormonal control of male reproduction

  1. Pituitary hormones
    a. FSH (follicle stimulating hormone)
      (1) Stimulates Sertoli cells
      (2) Promotes formation of spermatozoa
    b. LH (luteinizing hormone)
      (1) Stimulates interstitial cells to produce testosterone
      (2) Also called ICSH (interstitial cell–stimulating hormone)
A. Effects of aging on male reproduction
  1. Decline in testosterone, spermatozoa, and semen

IV. Disorders of the male reproductive system

  1. Infertility—lower than normal ability to reproduce
A. Structural disorders
  1. Cryptorchidism—failure of testis to descend
  2. Torsion of the testis—twisting of spermatic cord
  3. Inguinal hernia
  4. Phimosis—tightness of the foreskin
B. Infections
  1. Sexually transmitted infections (STI)
  2. Epididymitis—inflammation of the epididymis
  3. Prostatitis—inflammation of the prostate
  4. Orchitis—inflammation of the testis
C. Tumors
  1. Tumors of the prostate
    a. Benign prostatic hyperplasia (BPH)
  2. Cancer of the testis

V. Female reproductive system

A. Ovaries—gonads in which ova form
B. Ova and ovulation
  1. Egg ripens in graafian follicle
  2. Ovulation—release of ovum from ovary
  3. Corpus luteum
    a. Remainder of follicle in ovary
    b. Continues to function if egg fertilized
    c. Disintegrates if egg not fertilized
C. Accessory organs
  1. Oviducts (uterine tubes, fallopian tubes)
    a. Fimbriae—fringelike extensions that sweep egg into oviduct
  2. Uterus
    a. Holds developing fetus
    b. Supported by broad ligament
    c. Endometrium—lining of uterus
    d. Myometrium—muscle layer
    e. Cervix—narrow, lower part
  3. Vagina
    a. Tube connecting uterus to outside
    b. Hymen—fold of membrane over vaginal opening
    c. Greater vestibular (Bartholin) glands—secrete mucus
  4. Vulva and perineum
    a. Vulva—external genitalia
      (1) Labia—two sets of folds (majora, minora)
      (2) Clitoris—organ of great sensitivity
    b. Perineum—pelvic floor
      (1) In obstetrics—area between vagina and anus

VI. Menstrual cycle—average 28 days

A. Beginning of the cycle
  1. FSH stimulates follicle—follicular phase
  2. Follicle secretes estrogen
  3. Estrogen thickens lining of uterus—proliferative phase
B. Ovulation
  1. LH surge 1 day before
  2. Corpus luteum produces progesterone—luteal phase
  3. Progesterone continues growth of endometrium—secretory phase
  4. Ovum disintegrates if not fertilized
C. Menstrual phase (menstruation)
  1. If egg not fertilized, corpus luteum degenerates
  2. Lining of uterus breaks down releasing menses

VII. Menopause—period during which menstruation stops

A. Hormone replacement therapy (HRT)
  1. Reduces adverse symptoms of menopause
  2. Risks of HRT—cardiovascular disorders, breast cancer

VIII. Birth control

  1. Contraception—use of artificial methods to prevent fertilization or implantation of fertilized egg
  2. Methods—surgery, hormonal, barrier, IUD, spermicides, fertility awareness

IX. Disorders of the female reproductive system

A. Menstrual disorders
  1. Amenorrhea—absence of menstrual flow
  2. Dysmenorrhea—painful or difficult menstruation
  3. Premenstrual syndrome
  4. Abnormal uterine bleeding
B. Benign and malignant tumors
  1. Fibroids (myomas)—common tumors of uterus
  2. Breast cancer
    a. Mammogram—radiographic study of the breast
    b. Mastectomy—removal of breast or breast tissue

3. Endometrial cancer—cancer of uterine lining
4. Ovarian cancer
5. Cervical cancer—due to human papilloma virus (HPV) infection
    a. Pap test (smear) for cervical cancer

D. Infections
    1. Sexually transmitted infections
    2. Genital warts—caused by HPV
    3. Salpingitis—inflammation of uterine tubes
    4. Pelvic inflammatory disease (PID)

E. Infertility

Questions for Study and Review

Building Understanding

Fill in the blanks

1. Gametes go through a special process of cell division called ______.

2. Spermatozoa begin their development in tiny coiled ______.

3. An ovum matures in a small fluid-filled cluster of cells called the ______.

4. Failure of the testis to descend into the scrotum results in the disorder ______.

5. Surgical removal of the uterus is called a(n) ______.

Matching

Match each numbered item with the most closely related lettered item.

___ 6. A hormone released by the pituitary that promotes follicular development in the ovary

___ 7. A hormone released by developing follicles that promotes thickening of the endometrium

___ 8. A hormone released by the pituitary that stimulates ovulation

___ 9. A hormone released by the corpus luteum that promotes thickening of the endometrium

a. follicle stimulating hormone
b. estrogen
c. luteinizing hormone
d. progesterone

Multiple choice

___ 10. A month or two before birth, the testis travels from the abdominal cavity to the scrotum through the
a. spermatic cord
b. inguinal canal
c. seminiferous tubule
d. vas deferens

___ 11. Enzymes that help the sperm cell to penetrate the ovum are found in the
a. acrosome
b. head
c. midpiece
d. flagellum

___ 12. Inflammation of the testis is called
a. phimosis
b. epididymitis
c. prostatitis
d. orchitis

___ 13. The uterus and ovaries are supported bythe
a. uterine tubes
b. broad ligaments
c. fimbriae
d. fornix

___ 14. The area between the vaginal opening and the anus is referred to as the
a. vestibule
b. vulva
c. hymen
d. perineum

___ 15. The most common site of cancer in the female reproductive tract is the
a. endometrium
b. myometrium
c. ovaries
d. cervix

Understanding Concepts

16. Compare and contrast the following terms:
    a. asexual reproduction and sexual reproduction
    b. spermatozoa and ova
    c. sustentacular cell and interstitial cell
    d. ovarian follicle and corpus luteum
    e. myometrium and endometrium

17. Trace the pathway of sperm from the site of production to the urethra.

18. Describe the components of semen, their sites of production, and their functions.

19. List the hormones that control male reproduction and state their functions.

20. Trace the pathway of an ovum from the site of production to the site of implantation.

21. Beginning with the first day of the menstrual flow, describe the events of one complete cycle, including the role of the hormones involved.

22. Define *contraception*. Describe methods of contraception that involve (1) barriers; (2) chemicals; (3) hormones; (4) prevention of implantation.

23. Compare and contrast the following disorders:
   a. epididymitis and prostatitis
   b. benign prostatic hyperplasia and prostatic cancer
   c. amenorrhea and dysmenorrhea
   d. fibroids and endometrial cancer
   e. ovarian cancer and cervical cancer

Conceptual Thinking

24. Theoretically, it is possible for a brain-dead man to ejaculate. What anatomical and physiological feature makes this possible?

25. Nicole, a middle-aged mother of three, is considering a tubal ligation, a contraceptive procedure that involves cutting the uterine tubes. Nicole is worried that this might cause her to enter early menopause. Should she be worried?

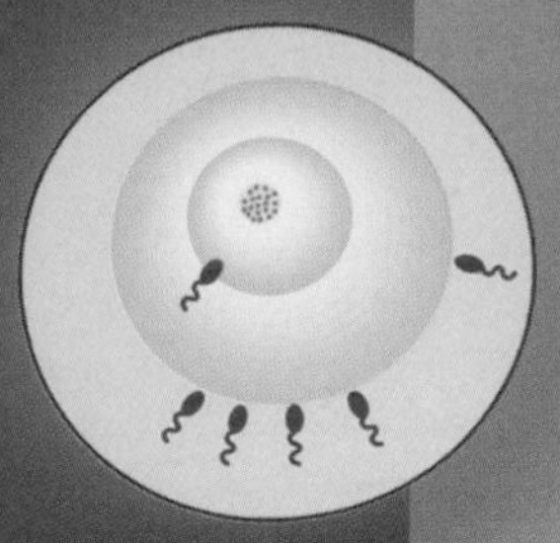

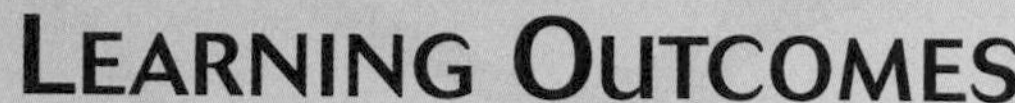

Selected Key Terms

The following terms and other boldface terms in the chapter are defined in the Glossary

abortion
amniotic sac
embryo
fertilization
fetus
gestation
human chorionic gonadotropin (hCG)
implantation
lactation
oxytocin
parturition
placenta
prolactin
umbilical cord
zygote

Learning Outcomes

After careful study of this chapter, you should be able to:

1. Describe fertilization and the early development of the fertilized egg
2. Describe the structure and function of the placenta
3. Briefly describe changes that occur in the fetus and the mother during pregnancy
4. Briefly describe the four stages of labor
5. Compare fraternal and identical twins
6. Cite the advantages of breastfeeding
7. Describe several disorders associated with pregnancy, childbirth, and lactation
8. Show how word parts are used to build words related to development and birth (see Word Anatomy at the end of the chapter)

chapter 24

Development and Birth

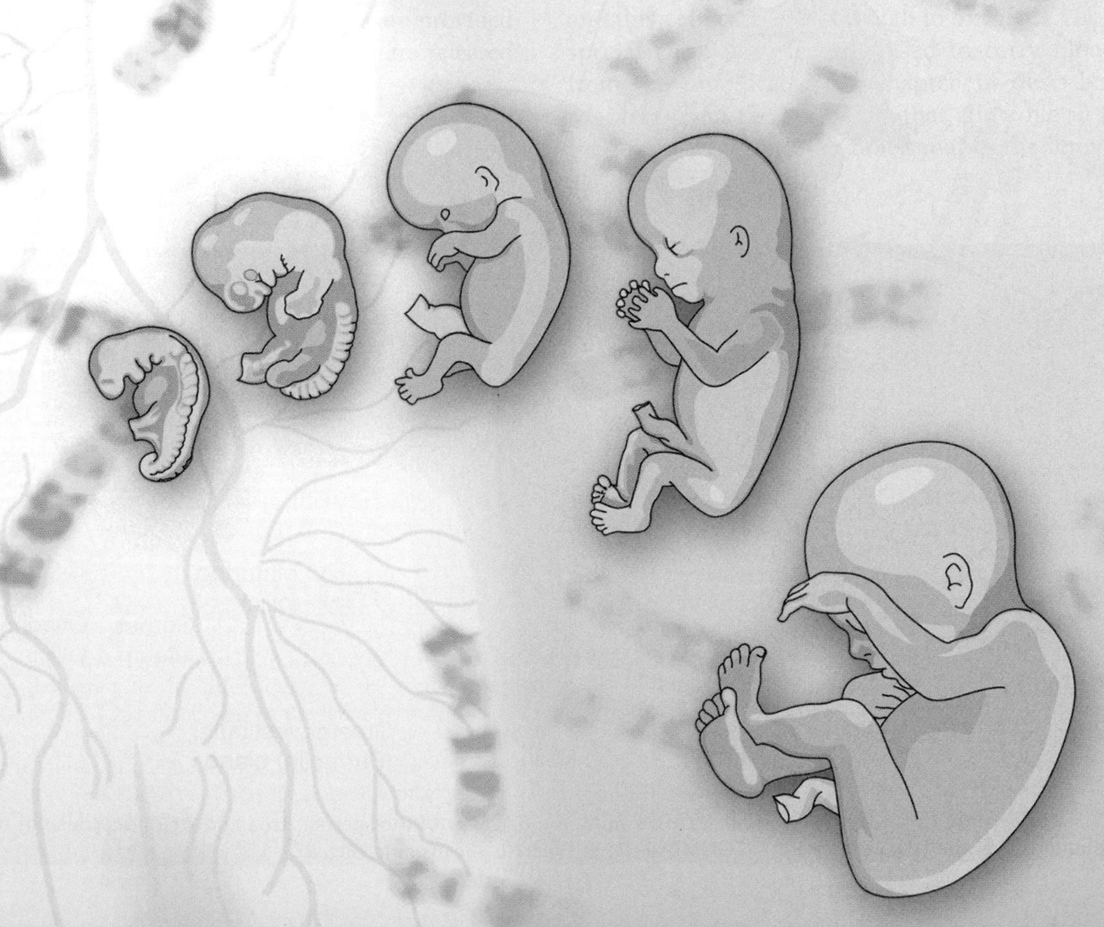

Development of the Embryo

The developing offspring is referred to as an embryo for the first 8 weeks of life (Fig. 24-3), and the study of growth during this period is called **embryology** (em-bre-OL-o-je). The beginnings of all body systems are established during this time. The heart and the brain are among the first organs to develop. A primitive nervous system begins to form in the third week. The heart and blood vessels originate during the second week, and the first heartbeat appears during week 4, at the same time that other muscles begin to develop.

By the end of the first month, the embryo is approximately 0.62 cm (0.25 inches) long, with four small swellings at the sides called **limb buds**, which will develop into the four extremities. At this time, the heart produces a prominent bulge at the anterior of the embryo.

By the end of the second month, the embryo takes on an appearance that is recognizably human. In male embryos, the primitive testes have formed and have begun to secrete testosterone, which will direct formation of the male reproductive organs as gestation continues. Figure 24-4 shows photographs of embryonic and early fetal development.

Checkpoint 24-4 All body systems originate during the early development of the embryo. At about what time in gestation does the heartbeat first appear?

The Fetus

The term *fetus* is used for the developing offspring from the beginning of the third month until birth. During this period, the organ systems continue to grow and mature. The ovaries form in the female early in this fetal period, and at this stage they contain all the primitive cells (oocytes) that can later develop into mature ova (egg cells).

For study, the entire gestation period may be divided into three equal segments or **trimesters**. The most rapid growth of the fetus occurs during the second trimester (months 4–6). By the end of the fourth month, the fetus is almost 15 cm (6 inches) long, and its external genitalia are sufficiently developed to reveal its sex. By the seventh month, the fetus is usually approximately 35 cm (14 inches) long and weighs approximately 1.1 kg (2.4 pounds). At the end of pregnancy, the normal length of the fetus is 45 to 56 cm (18–22.5 inches), and the weight varies from 2.7 to 4.5 kg (6–10 pounds).

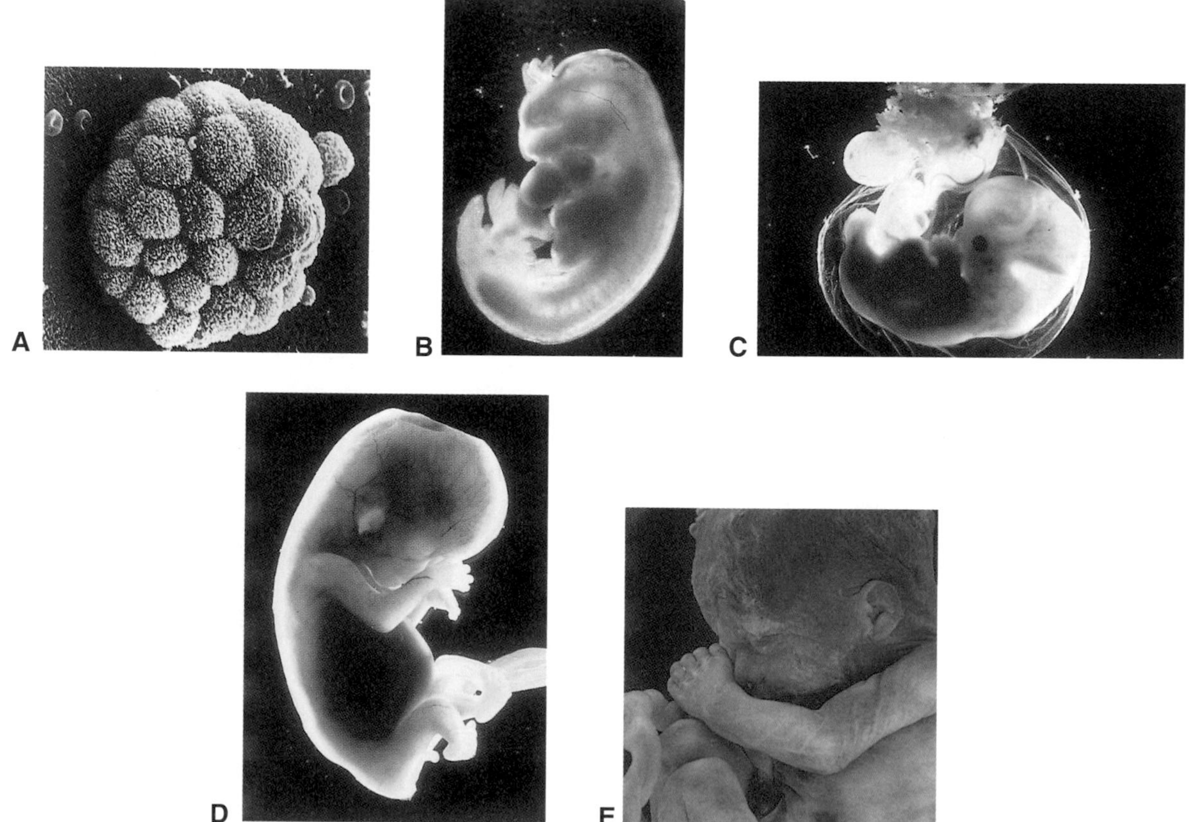

Figure 24-4 **Human embryos at different stages and early fetus.** **(A)** Implantation in uterus 7 to 8 days after conception. **(B)** Embryo at 32 days. **(C)** At 37 days. **(D)** At 41 days. **(E)** Fetus between 12 and 15 weeks. (Reprinted with permission from Pillitteri A. Maternal and Child Health Nursing. 4th ed. Philadelphia: Lippincott Williams & Wilkins, 2003.)

The **amniotic** (am-ne-OT-ik) **sac,** which is filled with a clear liquid known as **amniotic fluid,** surrounds the fetus and serves as a protective cushion for it (Fig. 24-5). The amniotic sac ruptures at birth, an event marked by the common expression that the mother's "water broke."

During development, the fetal skin is protected by a layer of cheeselike material called the **vernix caseosa** (VER-niks ka-se-O-sah) (literally, "cheesy varnish").

Checkpoint 24-5 What is the name of the fluid-filled sac that holds the fetus?

The Mother

The total period of pregnancy, from fertilization of the ovum to birth, is approximately 266 days, also given as 280 days or 40 weeks from the last menstrual period (LMP). During this time, the mother must supply all the food and oxygen for the fetus and eliminate its waste materials. To support the additional demands of the growing fetus, the mother's metabolism changes markedly, and several organ systems increase their output:

- The heart pumps more blood to supply the needs of the uterus and the fetus.
- The lungs provide more oxygen by increasing the rate and depth of respiration.
- The kidneys excrete nitrogenous wastes from both the fetus and the mother.
- The digestive system supplies additional nutrients for the growth of maternal organs (uterus and breasts) and growth of the fetus, as well as for subsequent labor and milk secretion.

Nausea and vomiting are common discomforts in early pregnancy. These most often occur upon arising or during periods of fatigue, and are more common in women who smoke cigarettes. The specific cause of these symptoms is not known, but they may be a result of the great changes in hormone levels that occur at this time. The nausea and vomiting usually last for only a few weeks to several months.

Urinary frequency and constipation are often present during the early stages of pregnancy and then usually disappear. They may reappear late in pregnancy as the head of the fetus drops from the abdominal region down into the pelvis, pressing on the rectum and the urinary bladder.

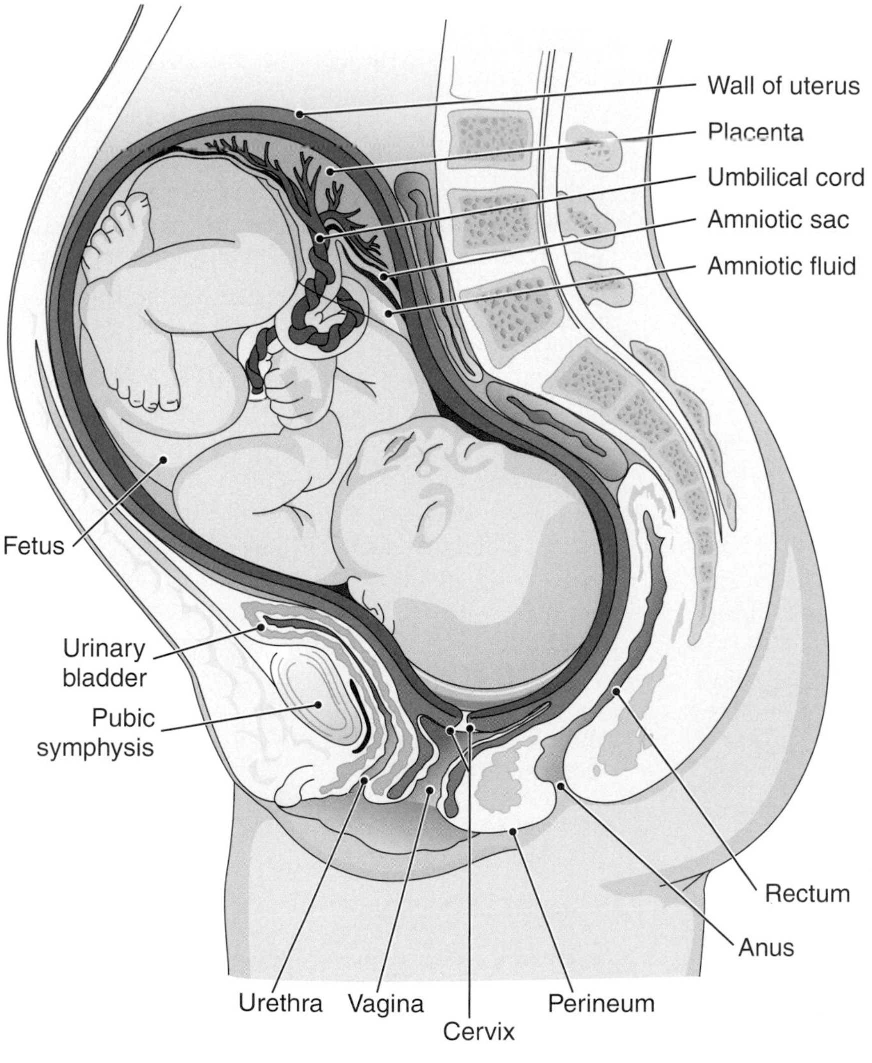

Figure 24-5 Midsagittal section of a pregnant uterus with intact fetus. *ZOOMING IN ✦ What structure connects the fetus to the placenta?*

Checkpoint 24-6 What is the approximate duration of pregnancy in days?

The Use of Ultrasound in Obstetrics

Ultrasonography (ul-trah-son-OG-rah-fe) is a safe, painless, and noninvasive method for studying soft tissue. It has proved extremely valuable for monitoring pregnancies and deliveries.

An ultrasound image, called a *sonogram,* is made by sending high-frequency sound waves into the body (Fig. 24-6). Each time a wave meets an interface between two tissues of different densities, an echo is produced. An instrument called a *transducer* converts the reflected sound waves into electrical energy, and a computer is used to generate an image on a viewing screen.

Ultrasound scans can be used in

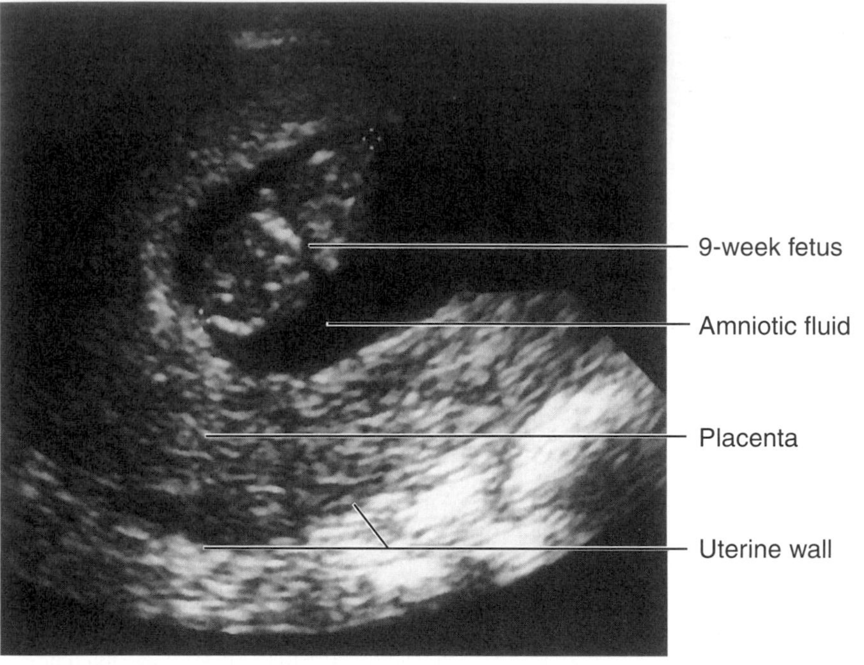

Figure 24-6 **Sonogram showing a 9-week-old fetus.** (Reprinted with permission from Erkonen WE. Radiology 101: Basics and Fundamentals of Imaging. Philadelphia: Lippincott Williams & Wilkins, 1998.)

obstetrics to diagnose pregnancy, judge fetal age, and determine the location of the placenta. The technique can also show the presence of excess amniotic fluid and fetal abnormalities.

Childbirth

The exact mechanisms that trigger the beginning of uterine contractions for childbirth are still not completely known. Some fetal and maternal factors that probably work in combination to start labor are:

- Stretching of the uterine muscle stimulates production of prostaglandin, which promotes uterine contractions.
- Pressure on the cervix from the baby stimulates release of **oxytocin** (ok-se-TO-sin) from the posterior pituitary. The uterine muscle becomes increasingly sensitive to this hormone late in pregnancy.
- Changes in the placenta that occur with time may contribute to the start of labor.
- Cortisol from the fetal adrenal cortex inhibits the mother's progesterone. Increase in the relative amount of estrogen as compared to progesterone stimulates uterine contractions.

After labor begins, stimuli from the cervix and vagina produce reflex secretion of oxytocin, which in turn increases the uterine contractions (an example of positive feedback).

The Four Stages of Labor

The process by which the fetus is expelled from the uterus is known as **labor** and **delivery**; it also may be called **parturition** (par-tu-RISH-un). It is divided into four stages:

1. The **first stage** begins with the onset of regular uterine contractions. With each contraction, the cervix becomes thinner and the opening larger. Rupture of the amniotic sac may occur at any time, with a gush of fluid from the vagina.
2. The **second stage** begins when the cervix is completely dilated and ends with the delivery of the baby. This stage involves the passage of the fetus, usually head first, through the cervical canal and the vagina to the outside.
3. The **third stage** begins after the child is born and ends with the expulsion of the **afterbirth**. The afterbirth includes the placenta, the membranes of the amniotic sac, and the umbilical cord, except for a small portion remaining attached to the baby's **umbilicus** (um-BIL-ih-kus), or navel. (Box 24-3 discusses the medical uses of cord blood.)
4. The **fourth stage** begins after expulsion of the afterbirth and constitutes a period in which bleeding is controlled. Contraction of the uterine muscle acts to close off the blood vessels leading to the placental site.

To prevent tissues of the pelvic floor from being torn during childbirth, as often happens, the obstetrician may cut the mother's perineum just before her infant is born and then repair this clean cut immediately after childbirth; such an operation is called an **episiotomy** (eh-piz-e-OT-o-me). The area between the vagina and the anus that is cut in an episiotomy is referred to as the *surgical* or *obstetrical perineum* (see Fig. 23-12 in Chapter 23).

Checkpoint 24-7 What is parturition?

Cesarean Section

A **cesarean** (se-ZAR-re-an) **section** (C section) is an incision made in the abdominal wall and uterine wall for delivery of a fetus. A cesarean section may be required for a variety of reasons, including placental abnormalities, abnormal fetal position, disproportion between the head of the fetus and the mother's pelvis that makes vaginal de-

Box 24-3 **Hot Topics**

Umbilical Cord Blood: Giving Life After Birth

Following childbirth, the umbilical cord and placenta are usually discarded. However, research suggests that blood harvested from these structures could save lives. Like bone marrow, umbilical cord blood contains stem cells capable of differentiating into all blood cell types. Cancer patients whose bone marrow is destroyed by chemotherapy often require stem cell transplants, as do those with leukemia, anemia, or certain immune disorders.

Stem cells obtained from umbilical cord blood offer some important advantages over those acquired from bone marrow. These advantages include:

- Greater ease of collection and storage. Whereas bone marrow collection is a surgical procedure, cord blood can be collected immediately after the umbilical cord is cut. The blood can then be stored frozen in a blood bank.
- No risk to the donor. Because cord blood is collected after the cord is cut, the procedure is not dangerous to the donor.
- Lower risk to the recipient. Since cord blood is immature, it does not have to match the recipient's tissues as closely as bone marrow does, so there is less chance of transplant rejection and graft-versus-host disease than with bone marrow. In addition, umbilical cord blood is less likely to contain infectious organisms than is bone marrow.
- Higher chance of finding a donor. Since umbilical cord blood need not closely match a recipient's tissues, the likelihood of finding a match between donor and recipient is higher.

Although umbilical cord blood is a promising stem cell source, only enough cells to treat a child or small adult can be harvested from a single donor. Scientists hope that improved collection techniques and advances in cell culture will increase the number of stem cells available from a single donor, enabling all patients in need to benefit from this treatment.

livery difficult or dangerous, and other problems that may arise during pregnancy and delivery.

Checkpoint 24-8 What is a cesarean section?

Multiple Births

Until recently, statistics indicated that twins occurred in about 1 of every 80 to 90 births, varying somewhat in different countries. Triplets occurred much less frequently, usually once in several thousand births, whereas quadruplets occurred very rarely. The birth of quintuplets represented a historic event unless the mother had taken fertility drugs. Now these fertility drugs, usually gonadotropins, are given more commonly, and the number of multiple births has increased significantly. Multiple fetuses tend to be born prematurely and therefore have a high death rate. However, better care of infants and newer treatments have resulted in more living multiple births than ever.

Twins originate in two different ways, and on this basis are divided into two types:

- **Fraternal twins** result from the fertilization of two different ova by two spermatozoa. Two completely different individuals, as distinct from each other as brothers and sisters of different ages, are produced. Each fetus has its own placenta and surrounding sac.
- **Identical twins** develop from a single zygote formed from a single ovum fertilized by a single spermatozoon. Sometime during the early stages of development, the embryonic cells separate into two units. Usually, there is a single placenta, although there must be a separate umbilical cord for each fetus. Identical twins are always the same sex and carry the same inherited traits.

Other multiple births may be fraternal, identical, or combinations of these. The tendency to multiple births seems to be hereditary.

Termination of Pregnancy

A pregnancy may end before its full term has been completed. The term **live birth** is used if the baby breathes or shows any evidence of life such as heartbeat, pulsation of the umbilical cord, or movement of voluntary muscles. An **immature** or **premature** infant is one born before the organ systems are mature. Infants born before the 37th week of gestation or weighing less than 2500 grams (5.5 pounds) are considered **preterm**.

Loss of the fetus is classified according to the duration of the pregnancy:

- The term **abortion** refers to loss of the embryo or fetus before the 20th week or weight of about 500 grams (1.1 pound). This loss can be either spontaneous or induced.
- **Spontaneous abortion** occurs naturally with no interference. The most common causes are related to an abnormality of the embryo or fetus. Other causes include abnormality of the mother's reproductive organs, infections, or chronic disorders, such as kidney disease or hypertension. **Miscarriage** is the lay term for spontaneous abortion.

- **Induced abortion** occurs as a result of artificial or mechanical interruption of pregnancy. A **therapeutic abortion** is an abortion performed by a physician as a treatment for a variety of reasons. More liberal access to this type of abortion has dramatically reduced the incidence of death related to illegal abortion.
- The term **fetal death** refers to loss of the fetus after the eighth week of pregnancy. **Stillbirth** refers to the delivery of an infant who is lifeless.

Immaturity is a leading cause of death in the newborn. After the 20th week of pregnancy, the fetus is considered **viable,** that is, able to live outside the uterus. A fetus expelled before the 24th week or before reaching a weight of 1000 grams (2.2 pounds) has little more than a 50% chance of survival. One born at a point closer to the full 40 weeks stands a much better chance of living. Increasing numbers of immature infants are being saved because of advances in neonatal intensive care.

Checkpoint 24-9 What does the term *viable* mean with reference to a fetus?

The Mammary Glands and Lactation

The **mammary glands,** or breasts, of the female are accessories of the reproductive system. They provide nourishment for the baby after its birth. The mammary glands are similar in construction to the sweat glands. Each gland is divided into a number of lobes composed of glandular tissue and fat, and each lobe is further subdivided. Secretions from the lobes are conveyed through **lactiferous** (lak-TIF-er-us) **ducts,** all of which converge at the papilla (nipple) (Fig. 24-7).

The mammary glands begin developing during puberty, but they do not become functional until the end of a pregnancy. Placental lactogen (hPL) helps to prepare the breasts for lactation, and the hormone **prolactin (PRL),** produced by the anterior pituitary gland, stimulates the secretory cells of the mammary glands. The first mammary gland secretion is a thin liquid called **colostrum** (ko-LOS-trum). It is nutritious but has a somewhat different composition from milk. Milk secretion begins within a few days following birth and can continue for several years as long as milk is frequently removed by the suckling baby or by pumping. Stimulation of the breast by the suckling infant causes oxytocin release from the posterior pituitary. This hormone causes the milk ducts to contract, resulting in the ejection, or *letdown,* of milk.

The digestive tract of the newborn baby is not ready for the usual adult mixed diet. Mother's milk is more desirable for the young infant than milk from other animals for several reasons, some of which are listed below:

- Infections that may be transmitted by foods exposed to the outside air are avoided by nursing.
- Both breast milk and colostrum contain maternal antibodies that help protect the baby against pathogens.
- The proportions of various nutrients and other substances in human milk are perfectly suited to the human infant. Substitutes are not exact imitations of human milk. Nutrients are present in more desirable amounts if the mother's diet is well balanced.
- The psychological and emotional benefits of nursing are of infinite value to both the mother and the infant.

Checkpoint 24-10 What is lactation?

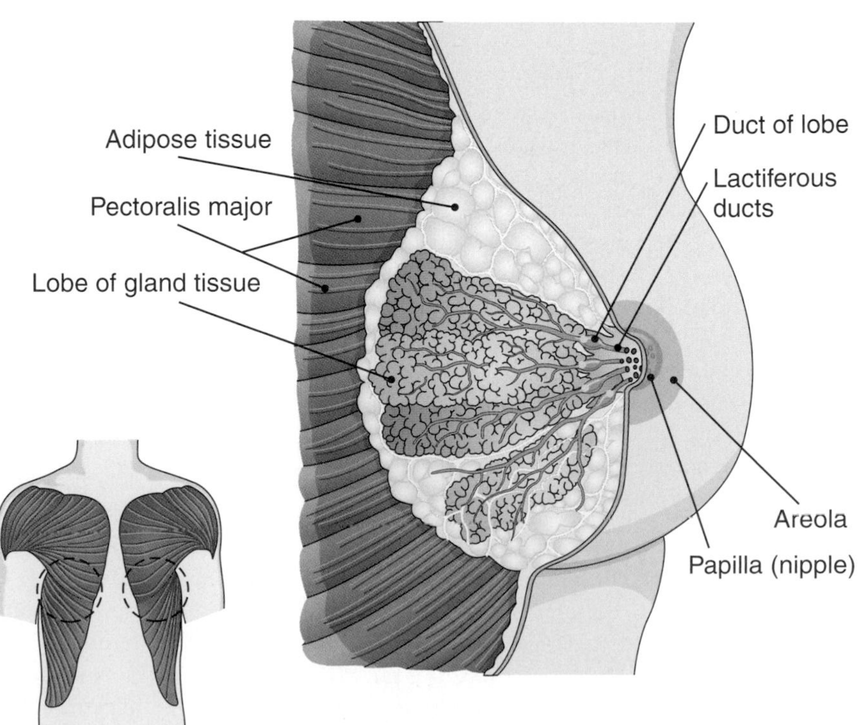

Figure 24-7 Section of the breast (mammary gland). *ZOOMING IN ✦ What muscle underlies the breast?*

Disorders of Pregnancy, Childbirth, and Lactation

A pregnancy that develops in a location outside the uterine cavity is said to be an **ectopic** (ek-TOP-ik) **pregnancy** (Fig. 24-8). The most common type is the tubal ectopic

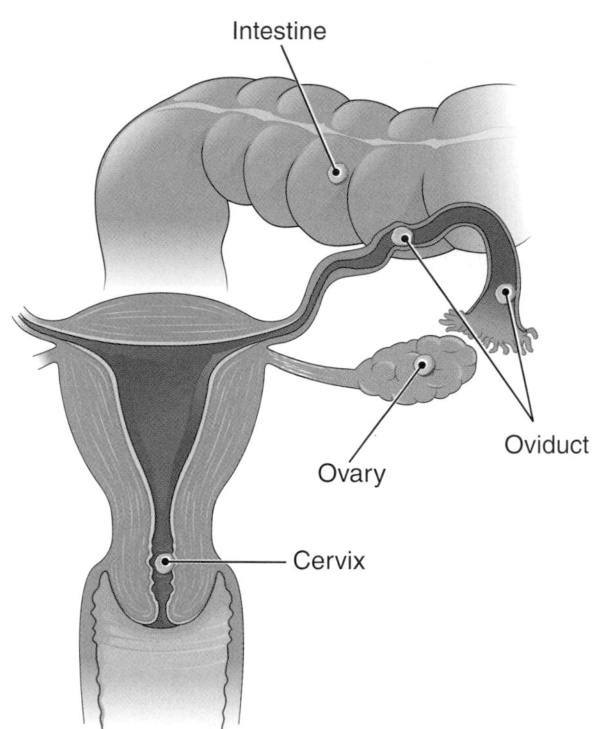

Figure 24-8 **Ectopic pregnancy sites.** The most common site is the oviduct, in which case it is a tubal ectopic pregnancy. (Reprinted with permission from Cohen BJ. Medical Terminology. 4th ed. Philadelphia: Lippincott Williams & Wilkins, 2004.)

pregnancy, in which the embryo begins to grow in the oviduct. This structure cannot expand to contain the growing embryo and may rupture. Ectopic pregnancy may threaten the mother's life if it does not receive prompt surgical treatment.

In **placenta previa** (PRE-ve-ah) the placenta, which is usually attached to the superior part of the uterus, instead becomes attached at or near the internal opening of the cervix. The normal cervical softening and dilation that occur in later pregnancy separate part of the placenta from its attachment. The result is painless bleeding and interference with the fetal oxygen supply.

Sometimes the placenta separates from the uterine wall prematurely, often after the 20th week of pregnancy, causing hemorrhage. This disorder, known as **abruptio placentae** (ab-RUP-she-o plah-SEN-te), or *placental abruption*, occurs most often in multigravidas (mul-te-GRAV-ih-dahz), meaning women who have had more than one pregnancy, older than 35 years of age. Placental abruption is a common cause of bleeding during the second half of pregnancy and may require termination of pregnancy to save the mother's life.

Pregnancy-Induced Hypertension

A serious disorder that can develop in the latter part of pregnancy is **pregnancy-induced hypertension** (PIH), also called *preeclampsia* (pre-eh-KLAMP-se-ah) or *toxemia of pregnancy*. Symptoms include hypertension, protein in the urine (proteinuria), general edema, and sudden weight gain. The cause of this disorder is a hormone imbalance that results in constriction of blood vessels. It is most often seen in women whose nutritional state is poor and who have received little or no health care during pregnancy. If PIH remains untreated, it may lead to **eclampsia** (eh-KLAMP-se-ah) with the onset of kidney failure, convulsions, and coma during pregnancy or after delivery. The result may be the death of both the mother and the infant.

Checkpoint 24-11 What is an ectopic pregnancy?

Postpartum Disorders

Childbirth-related deaths are often due to infections. **Puerperal** (pu-ER-per-al) **infections**, those related to childbirth, were once the cause of death in as many as 10% to 12% of women going through labor. Cleanliness and sterile techniques have improved the chances of avoiding such outcomes of pregnancies. Nevertheless, in the United States, puerperal infection still develops in about 6% of maternity patients. Antibiotics have dramatically improved the chances of recovery for both the mother and the child.

A **hydatidiform** (hi-dah-TID-ih-form) **mole**, or hydatid mole, is a benign overgrowth of placental tissue. The placenta dilates and resembles grapelike cysts. The growth may invade the wall of the uterus, causing it to rupture.

A very malignant tumor that is made of placental tissue is **choriocarcinoma** (ko-re-o-kar-sih-NO-mah). Although rare, this tumor spreads rapidly, and if the mother is not treated, it may be fatal within 3 to 12 months. With the use of modern chemotherapy, the outlook for cure is very good. If metastases have developed, irradiation and other forms of treatment may be necessary.

Checkpoint 24-12 What is puerperal infection?

Lactation Disturbances

Disturbances in lactation may have a variety of causes, including the following:

- Malnutrition or anemia, which may prevent lactation entirely.
- Emotional disturbances, which may affect lactation (as they may affect other glandular activities).
- Abnormalities of parts of the mammary glands or injuries to these organs, which may cause interference with their functioning.
- **Mastitis** (mas-TI-tis), or "inflammation of the breast," which is caused by infection. Antibiotic treatment usually allows for the continuation of nursing.

Word Anatomy

Medical terms are built from standardized word parts (prefixes, roots, and suffixes). Learning the meanings of these parts can help you remember words and interpret unfamiliar terms.

WORD PART	MEANING	EXAMPLE
Pregnancy		
zyg/o	joined	An ovum and spermatozoon join to form a *zygote*.
chori/o	membrane, chorion	Human *chorionic* gonadotropin is produced by the outermost cells (chorion) of the embryo and acts on the corpus luteum in the ovary.
somat/o	body	Human chorionic *somatomammotropin* controls nutrients for the body and acts on the mammary glands (mamm/o).
Childbirth		
ox/y	sharp, acute	*Oxytocin* is a hormone that stimulates labor.
toc/o	labor	See preceding example.
Disorders of Pregnancy, Childbirth, and Lactation		
ecto-	outside, external	An *ectopic* pregnancy occurs outside of the uterine cavity.

Summary

I. **Pregnancy (gestation)**—lasts about 38 weeks

A. Fertilization and the start of pregnancy
   1. Fertilization occurs in oviduct
   2. Zygote (fertilized egg)—formed by fusion of egg and sperm nuclei
      a. Divides rapidly
      b. Travels to uterus
      c. Implants in lining and becomes embryo

B. The placenta
   1. Formed by tissue around embryo and in lining of uterus
   2. Functions
      a. Nourishment
      b. Gas exchange
      c. Removal of waste
      d. Production of hormones
   3. Umbilical cord—connects fetus to placenta
   4. Placental hormones
      a. Human chorionic gonadotropin (hCG)—maintains corpus luteum for 11–12 weeks
      b. Human placental lactogen (hPL)
      c. Relaxin—relaxes birth canal

C. Development of the embryo
   1. First 8 weeks
   2. All body systems begin to develop

D. The fetus
   1. Third month to birth
   2. Amniotic sac
      a. Surrounds fetus
      b. Contains fluid to cushion and protect fetus

E. The mother
   1. Increased demands on heart, lungs, kidneys
   2. Increased nutritional needs
   3. Ultrasound used to monitor pregnancy and delivery

II. **Childbirth**— initiated by changes in uterus, placenta, fetus

A. Four stages of labor
   1. Contractions
   2. Delivery of baby
   3. Expulsion of afterbirth
   4. Contraction of uterus

B. Cesarean section
   1. Incision to remove fetus

C. Multiple births
   1. Fraternal twins formed from two different ova
   2. Identical twins develop from a single zygote
   3. Larger multiples follow either pattern or a combination
   4. Increased by fertility drugs

D. Termination of pregnancy
   1. Immature (premature) infant—born before organ system mature
   2. Preterm—born before 37th week or weighing less than 2500 grams
   3. Abortion—loss of fetus before 20th week or weighing less than 500 grams
   4. Fetal death—loss of fetus after 8 weeks of pregnancy

III. **Mammary glands and lactation**

1. Lactation—secretion of milk
   a. Colostrum—first mammary secretion
2. Hormones
   a. HPL—prepares prepares breasts for lactation
   b. Prolactin—stimulates secretory cells
   c. Oxytocin—promotes letdown (ejection) of milk
3. Advantages of breastfeeding
   a. Reduces infections
   b. Transfers antibodies

c. Provides best form of nutrition
d. Emotional satisfaction

IV. Disorders of pregnancy, childbirth, and lactation

1. Ectopic pregnancy—pregnancy outside of uterus; commonly in oviduct
2. Placenta previa—improper attachment of placenta to uterus
3. Placental abruption—separation of placenta from uterus

A. Pregnancy-induced hypertension (PIH)
1. Also called preeclampsia, toxemia of pregnancy
2. Eclampsia—results from untreated PIH

B. Postpartum disorders
1. Puerperal infection
2. Hydatidiform mole—benign overgrowth of placenta
3. Choriocarcinoma—malignant tumor of placental tissue

C. Lactation disturbances
1. Possible causes
a. Malnutrition
b. Emotional disturbances
c. Abnormalities of mammary glands
d. Mastitis—inflammation of the breast

Questions for Study and Review

Building Understanding

Fill in the blanks

1. Fetal skin is protected by a cheeselike material called______.
2. The first mammary secretion is called ______.
3. Sound waves can be used to safely monitor pregnancy with a technique called ______.
4. A pregnancy that develops in a location outside the uterine cavity is said to be a(n) ______ pregnancy.
5. Inflammation of the breast as a result of infection is named______.

Matching

Match each numbered item with the most closely related lettered item.

___ 6. A placental hormone that stimulates the ovaries to secrete progesterone and estrogen
___ 7. A placental hormone that regulates maternal blood nutrient levels
___ 8. A placental hormone that softens the cervix, which widens the birth canal
___ 9. A pituitary hormone that stimulates uterine contractions
___ 10. A pituitary hormone that stimulates maternal milk production

a. human placental lactogen
b. prolactin
c. oxytocin
d. relaxin
e. human chorionic gonadotropin

Multiple choice

___ 11. For a few days after implantation, the embryo is nourished by the
a. endometrium
b. placenta
c. yolk sac
d. umbilical cord

___ 12. By what month can the sex of the fetus be accurately determined?
a. second
b. third
c. fourth
d. fifth

___ 13. The total period of pregnancy, from fertilization to birth, is about
a. 37 weeks
b. 38 weeks
c. 39 weeks
d. 40 weeks

___ 14. With regard to identical twins, which of the following statements is incorrect?
a. they develop from a single zygote
b. they each have their own placenta
c. they are always the same sex
d. they carry the same inherited traits

___ 15. The earliest that a fetus could survive outside of the uterus is after the
a. 20th week
b. 24th week
c. 28th week
d. 30th week

Understanding Concepts

16. Distinguish among the following: zygote, embryo, and fetus.
17. Explain the role of the placenta in fetal development.
18. Is blood in the umbilical arteries relatively high or low in oxygen? In the umbilical vein?
19. Describe some of the changes that take place in the mother's body during pregnancy.
20. What is the major event of each of the four stages of parturition?
21. List several reasons why breast milk is best for baby.

22. What is a cesarean section? List several reasons why it may be required.
23. Compare and contrast the following disease-related terms:
    a. fetal death and still birth
    b. spontaneous abortion and induced abortion
    c. placenta previa and abruptio placentae
    d. pregnancy-induced hypertension and eclampsia
    e. hydatidiform mole and choriocarcinoma

Conceptual Thinking

24. Why is the risk of miscarriage highest at week 12 of pregnancy?
25. Although it is strongly suggested that a woman not drink alcohol during her entire pregnancy, why is this advice particularly important during the first trimester?

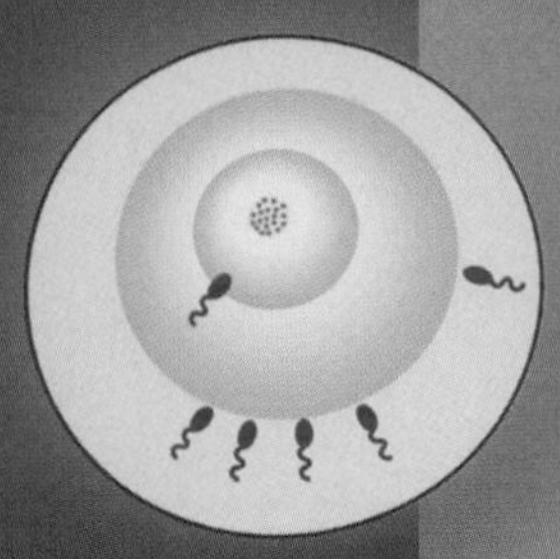

Selected Key Terms

The following terms and other boldface terms in the chapter are defined in the Glossary

allele
amniocentesis
autosome
carrier
chromosome
congenital
dominant
gene
genetic
genotype
heredity
heterozygous
homozygous
karyotype
meiosis
mutagen
mutation
pedigree
phenotype
progeny
recessive
sex-linked
trait

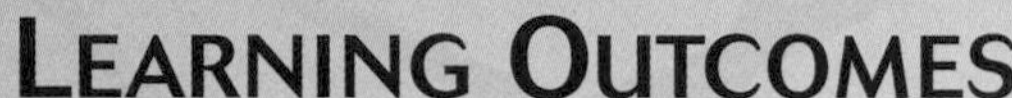

Learning Outcomes

After careful study of this chapter, you should be able to:

1. Briefly describe the mechanism of gene function
2. Explain the difference between dominant and recessive genes
3. Compare *phenotype* and *genotype* and give examples of each.
4. Describe what is meant by a *carrier* of a genetic trait
5. Define *meiosis* and explain its function in reproduction
6. Explain how sex is determined in humans
7. Describe what is meant by the term *sex-linked* and list several sex-linked traits
8. List several factors that may influence the expression of a gene
9. Define *mutation*
10. Differentiate among congenital, genetic, and hereditary disorders and give several examples of each
11. List several factors that may produce genetic disorders
12. Define *karyotype* and explain how karyotypes are used in genetic counseling
13. Briefly describe several methods used to treat genetic disorders
14. Show how word parts are used to build words related to heredity (see Word Anatomy at the end of the chapter)

chapter 25

Heredity and Hereditary Diseases

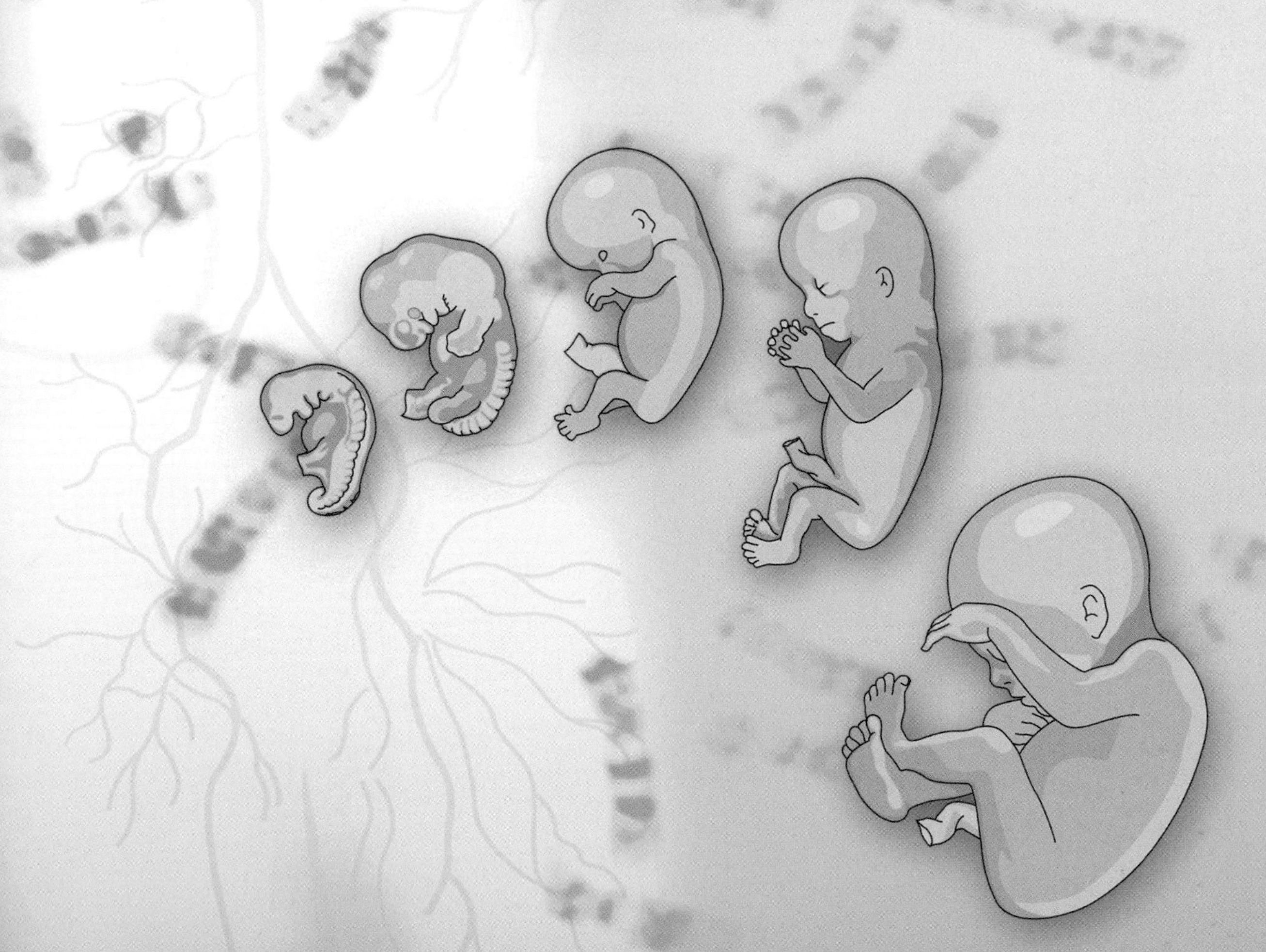

We are often struck by the resemblance of a baby to one or both of its parents, yet rarely do we stop to consider *how* various traits are transmitted from parents to offspring. This subject—heredity—has fascinated humans for thousands of years. The *Old Testament* contains numerous references to heredity (although, of course, the word was unknown in biblical times). It was not until the 19th century, however, that methodical investigation into heredity was begun. At that time, an Austrian monk, Gregor Mendel, discovered through his experiments with garden peas that there was a precise pattern in the appearance of differences among parents and their **progeny** (PROJ-eh-ne), their offspring or descendents. Mendel's most important contribution to the understanding of heredity was the demonstration that there are independent units of heredity in the cells. Later, these independent units were given the name **genes**.

Genes and Chromosomes

Genes are actually segments of DNA (deoxyribonucleic acid) contained in the threadlike chromosomes within the nucleus of each cell. Genes govern the cell by controlling the manufacture of proteins, especially enzymes, which are necessary for all the chemical reactions that occur within the cell. Other proteins regulated by genes are those used for structural materials, hormones, and growth factors.

When body cells divide by the process of mitosis, the DNA that makes up the chromosomes is duplicated and distributed to the daughter cells, so that each daughter cell gets exactly the same kind and number of chromosomes as were in the original cell. Each chromosome (aside from the Y chromosome, which determines sex) may carry thousands of genes, and each gene carries the code for a specific trait (characteristic). These traits constitute the physical, biochemical, and physiologic makeup of every cell in the body. (See Box 25-1 to learn about the Human Genome Project.)

In humans, every cell except the gametes (sex cells) contains 46 chromosomes. The chromosomes exist in pairs. One member of each pair was received at the time of fertilization from the offspring's father, and one was received from the mother. The paired chromosomes, except for the pair that determines sex, are alike in size and appearance. Thus, each body cell has one pair of sex chromosomes and 22 pairs (44 chromosomes) that are not involved in sex determination and are known as **autosomes** (AW-to-somes).

The paired autosomes carry genes for the same traits at exactly the same sites on each. The genes for each trait thus exist in pairs; each member of the gene pair that controls a given trait is known as an **allele** (al-LELE).

Checkpoint 25-1 What is a gene? What is a gene made of?

Dominant and Recessive Genes

Another of Mendel's discoveries was that genes can be either dominant or recessive. A **dominant** gene is one that expresses its effect in the cell regardless of whether its allele on the matching chromosome is the same as or different from the dominant gene. The gene need be received from only one parent to be expressed in the offspring. When the matching genes for a trait are different, the alleles are described as **heterozygous** (het-er-o-ZI-gus), or hybrid.

The effect of a **recessive** gene is not evident unless its paired allele on the matching chromosome is also recessive. Thus, a recessive trait appears only if the recessive genes for that trait are received from both parents. For ex-

Box 25-1 Hot Topics

The Human Genome Project: Reading the Book of Life

Packed tightly in nearly every one of your body cells (except the red blood cells) is a complete copy of your genome—the genetic instructions that direct all of your cellular activities. Written in the language of DNA, these instructions consist of genes parceled into 46 chromosomes that code for proteins. In 1990, a consortium of scientists from around the world set out to crack the genetic code and read the human genome, our "book of life." This monumental task, called the Human Genome Project, was completed in 2003 and succeeded in mapping the entire human genome—3 billion DNA base pairs arranged into about 30,000 genes. Now, scientists can pinpoint the exact location and chemical code of every gene in the body.

The human genome was decoded using a technique called sequencing. Samples of human DNA were fragmented into smaller pieces and then inserted into bacteria. As the bacteria multiplied, they produced more and more copies of the human DNA fragments, which the scientists extracted. The DNA copies were loaded into a sequencing machine capable of "reading" the string of DNA nucleotides that composed each fragment. Then, using computers, the scientists put all of the sequences from the fragments back together to get the entire human genome.

Now, scientists hope to use all these pages of the book of life to revolutionize the treatment of human disease. The information obtained from the Human Genome Project may lead to improved disease diagnosis, new drug treatments, and even gene therapy.

ample, the gene for brown eyes is dominant over the gene for blue eyes, which is recessive. Blue eyes appear in the offspring only if genes for blue eyes are received from both parents. When both the genes for a trait are the same, that is, both dominant or both recessive, the alleles are said to be **homozygous** (ho-mo-ZI-gus), or pure-bred. A recessive trait only appears if a person's genes are homozygous for that trait.

Any characteristic that can be observed or can be tested for is part of a person's **phenotype** (FE-no-tipe). Eye color, for example, can be seen when looking at a person. Blood type is not visible but can be determined by testing and is also a part of a person's phenotype. When someone has the recessive phenotype, his or her genetic make-up, or **genotype** (JEN-o-tipe), is obviously homozygous recessive. When a dominant phenotype appears, the person's genotype can be either homozygous dominant or heterozygous. Only genetic studies or family studies can reveal which it is.

A recessive gene is not expressed if it is present in the cell together with a dominant allele. However, the recessive gene can be passed on to offspring and may thus appear in future generations. An individual who shows no evidence of a trait but has a recessive gene for that trait is described as a **carrier** of the gene. Using genetic terminology, that person shows the dominant phenotype but has a heterozygous genotype for that trait.

Checkpoint 25-2 What is the difference between a dominant and a recessive gene?

Distribution of Chromosomes to Offspring

The reproductive cells (ova and spermatozoa) are produced by a special process of cell division called **meiosis** (mi-O-sis). This process divides the chromosome number in half, so that each reproductive cell has 23 chromosomes. Moreover, the division occurs in such a way that each cell receives one member of each chromosome pair that was present in the original cell. The separation occurs at random, meaning that either member of the original pair may be included in a given germ cell. Thus, the maternal and paternal sets of chromosomes get mixed up and redistributed at this time, leading to increased variety within the population. Children in a family resemble each other, but no two look exactly alike (unless they are identical twins), because they receive different combinations of maternal and paternal chromosomes.

Geneticists use a grid called a **Punnett square** to show all the combinations of genes that can result from a given parental cross (Fig. 25-1). In these calculations, a capital letter is used for the dominant gene and the recessive gene is represented by the lower case of the same letter. For example, if *B* is the gene for the dominant trait brown eyes, then *b* would be the recessive gene for blue eyes. In

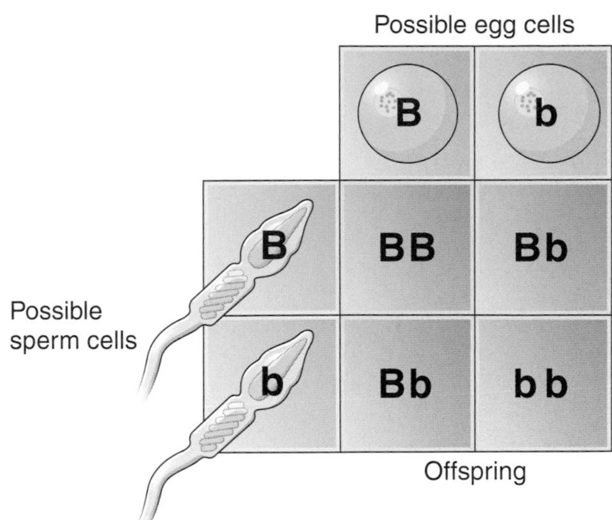

Figure 25-1 A Punnett square. Geneticists use this grid to show all the possible combinations of a given cross. *ZOOMING IN ✦ What percentage of children will show the recessive phenotype blond hair?*

the offspring, the genotype BB is homozygous dominant and the genotype Bb is heterozygous, both of which will show the dominant phenotype brown eyes. The homozygous recessive genotype bb will show the recessive phenotype blue eyes.

A Punnett square shows all the possible gene combinations of a given cross and the theoretical ratios of all the genotypes produced. Actual ratios may differ if the number of offspring is small. For example, the chances of having a male or female baby are 50-50 with each birth, but a family might have several girls before having a boy, and vice versa. The chances of seeing the theoretical ratios improve as the number of offspring increases.

Checkpoint 25-3 What is the process of cell division that forms the gametes?

Sex Determination

The two chromosomes that determine the offspring's sex, unlike the autosomes (the other 22 pairs of chromosomes), are not matched in size and appearance. The female X chromosome is larger than most other chromosomes and carries genes for other characteristics in addition to that for sex. The male Y chromosome is smaller than other chromosomes and mainly determines sex. A female has two X chromosomes in each body cell; a male has one X and one Y.

By the process of meiosis, each male sperm cell receives either an X or a Y chromosome, whereas every egg cell receives only an X chromosome (Fig. 25-2). If a sperm cell with an X chromosome fertilizes an ovum, the resulting infant will be female; if a sperm with a Y chromosome fertilizes an ovum, the resulting infant will be male (see Fig. 25-2).

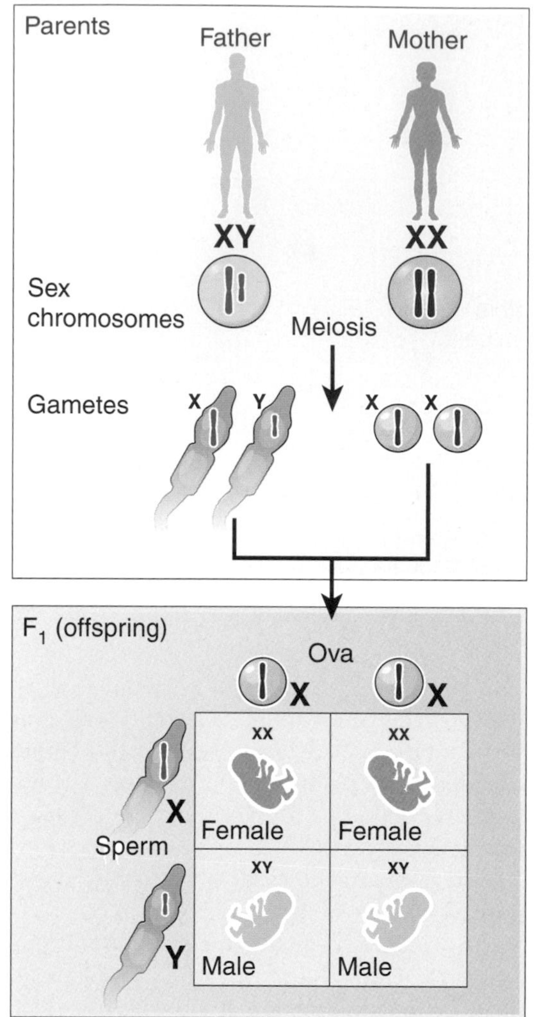

Figure 25-2 **Sex determination.** If an X chromosome from a male unites with an X chromosome from a female, the child is female (XX); if a Y chromosome from a male unites with an X chromosome from a female, the child is male (XY).

Sex-Linked Traits

Any trait that is carried on a sex chromosome is said to be **sex-linked.** Because the Y chromosome carries few traits aside from sex determination, most sex-linked traits are carried on the X chromosome and are best described as *X-linked.* Examples are hemophilia, certain forms of baldness, and red-green color blindness.

Sex-linked traits appear almost exclusively in males. The reason for this is that most of these traits are recessive, and if a recessive gene is located on the X chromosome in a male it cannot be masked by a matching dominant gene. (Remember that the Y chromosome with which the X chromosome pairs is very small and carries few genes.) Thus, a male who has only one recessive gene for a trait will exhibit that characteristic, whereas a female must have two recessive genes to show the trait. The female must inherit a recessive gene for that trait from each parent and be homozygous recessive in order for the trait to appear.

Checkpoint 25-4 What sex chromosome combination determines a female? A male?

Checkpoint 25-5 What term is used to describe a trait carried on a sex chromosome?

Hereditary Traits

Some observable hereditary traits are skin, eye, and hair color and facial features. Also influenced by genetics are less clearly defined traits, such as weight, body build, life span, and susceptibility to disease.

Some human traits, including the traits involved in many genetic diseases, are determined by a single pair of genes; most, however, are the result of two or more gene pairs acting together in what is termed **multifactorial inheritance.** This type of inheritance accounts for the wide range of variations within populations in such characteristics as coloration, height, and weight, all of which are determined by more than one pair of genes.

Gene Expression

The effect of a gene on a person's phenotype may be influenced by a variety of factors, including the individual's sex and the presence of other genes. For example, the genes for certain types of baldness and certain types of color blindness may be inherited by either males or females, but the traits appear mostly in males under the effects of male sex hormone.

Environment also plays a part in gene expression. One inherits a potential for a given size, for example, but one's actual size is additionally influenced by such factors as nutrition, development, and general state of health. The same is true of life span and susceptibility to diseases.

Genetic Mutation

As a rule, chromosomes replicate exactly during cell division. Occasionally, however, for reasons not yet totally understood, the genes or chromosomes change. This change may involve a single gene or whole chromosomes. Alternatively, it may consist of chromosomal breakage, in which there is loss or rearrangement of gene fragments. Often these changes occur during cell division (mitosis or meiosis) as chromosomes come together, re-assort and get distributed to two new cells. Such changes are termed genetic **mutations**. Mutations may occur spontaneously or may be induced by some agent, such as ionizing radiation or chemicals, described as a **mutagen** (MU-tah-jen) or mutagenic agent.

If a mutation occurs in an ovum or a sperm cell, the altered trait will be inherited by the offspring. The vast majority of harmful mutations never are expressed because the affected fetus dies and is spontaneously aborted. Most remaining mutations are so inconsequential that they have no visible effect. Beneficial mutations,

Box 25-2 Clinical Perspectives

Mitochondrial Disease: When the Powerhouses Shut Down

Mitochondria are the powerhouse organelles of cells, converting the energy in nutrients into the ATP needed for cell activities. Because they may have evolved as separate organisms early in the history of life on earth, they exist almost as special entities within the cell. They have their own DNA and multiply at their own pace, independent of the cell's pattern. When mitochondria do not function properly, disease can result.

Some mitochondrial diseases are caused by genetic mutations in mitochondrial DNA, whereas others are caused by mutations in nuclear DNA that codes for certain mitochondrial proteins. Both types of mutations disrupt ATP synthesis. Mitochondrial diseases are believed to affect several thousand children in the United States, causing serious damage to metabolically active cells in the brain, heart, liver, muscles, kidneys, and endocrine organs. The disorders are difficult to diagnose because they cause a variety of symptoms that have been confused with epilepsy, cerebral palsy, and multiple sclerosis.

If a mitochondrial defect is programmed in the nuclear DNA, it could be inherited from either parent. If, however, it is carried in the mitochondrion itself, it would be passed only from a mother to her offspring. This is because the mitochondria in the zygote come only from the ovum; sperm cells, which are much smaller, do not carry any mitochondria.

on the other hand, tend to survive and increase as a population evolves. (See Box 25-2 for information about genetic mutations and mitochondrial diseases.)

Checkpoint 25-6 What is a mutation?

Genetic Diseases

Any disorders that involve the genes may be said to be genetic, but they are not always hereditary, that is, passed from parent to offspring in the reproductive cells. Noninherited genetic disorders may begin during maturation of the sex cells or even during development of the embryo.

Advances in genetic research have made it possible to identify the causes of many hereditary disorders and to develop genetic screening methods. In people who are "at risk" for having a child with a genetic disorder, as well as fetuses and newborns with a suspected abnormality, tests can often confirm or rule out the presence of a genetic defect.

Congenital Versus Hereditary Diseases

Before we discuss hereditary diseases, we need to distinguish them from other congenital diseases. To illustrate, let us assume that two infants are born within seconds in adjoining delivery rooms of the same hospital. It is noted that one infant has a clubfoot, a condition called **talipes** (TAL-ih-pes); the second infant has a rudimentary extra finger attached to the fifth finger of each hand, a condition called **polydactyly** (pol-e-DAK-til-e). Are both conditions hereditary? Both congenital? Is either hereditary? We can answer these questions by defining the key terms, congenital and hereditary. **Congenital** means present at the time of birth; **hereditary** means genetically transmitted or transmissible. Thus, one condition may be both congenital and hereditary; another, congenital yet not hereditary.

Hereditary conditions are usually evident at birth or soon thereafter. However, certain inherited disorders, such as adult polycystic kidney disease and Huntington disease, a nervous disorder, do not manifest themselves until about midlife (40 to 50 years of age). People with these genetic defects may pass them on to their children before they are aware of them unless genetic testing reveals their presence. In the case of our earlier examples, the clubfoot is congenital, but not hereditary, having resulted from severe distortion of the developing extremities during intrauterine growth; the extra fingers are hereditary, a familial trait that appears in another relative, a grandparent perhaps, or a parent, and that is evident at the time of birth.

Causes of Congenital Disorders Although causes of congenital deformities and birth defects often are not known, in some cases, they are known and can be avoided. For example, certain infections and toxins may be transmitted from the mother's blood by way of the placenta to the fetal circulation. Some of these cause serious developmental disorders in affected babies.

German measles (rubella) is a contagious viral infection that is ordinarily a mild disease, but if maternal infection occurs during the first 3 or 4 months of pregnancy, the fetus has a 40% chance of developing defects of the eye (cataracts), ear (deafness), brain, and heart. Infection can be prevented by appropriate immunizations.

Ionizing radiation and various toxins may damage the genes, and the disorders they produce are sometimes transmissible. Environmental agents, such as mercury and some chemicals used in industry (*e.g.*, certain phenols and PCB), as well as some drugs, notably LSD, are known to disrupt genetic organization. (See Box 25-3 for information about preventing genetic damage.)

Box 25-3 · Health Maintenance

Preventing Genetic Damage

It is sometimes difficult to determine whether a genetic defect is the result of a spontaneous random mutation or is related to exposure of a germ cell to an environmental toxin. Male and female sex cells are present at birth but do not become active until the reproductive years. This leaves a long time span during which toxic exposure can occur. Most of what we know about chemicals that cause mutations has been learned from environmental accidents. For example, mercury compounds have found their way into the food chain, causing neural damage to the children of parents who consumed foods containing mercury. Lead, which is toxic when ingested, as from air or water pollution, has been implicated in sperm cell abnormalities and in reduced sperm counts. Radiation accidents have been linked to increased susceptibility to certain cancers in children born after these accidents.

Meiosis is the step most prone to genetic errors. This process can be studied in males with specimens obtained from testicular biopsy. Also, samples of sperm cells, which are produced continuously in males, can be obtained easily and studied for visible defects. Advancing age in both the mother and the father is known to increase errors in meiosis. Males between 20 and 45 years of age carry the least risk of transmitting a genetic error. For females, the least risk is between ages 15 to 35 years. Because new sperm cells are produced on a 64-day cycle, men are advised to avoid conception for a few months after exposure to x-rays, cancer chemotherapy, or other chemicals capable of causing mutations.

Intake of alcohol and cigarette smoking by a pregnant woman often cause growth retardation and low birthweight in her infant. Smaller than normal infants do not do as well as average weight babies. Some congenital brain and heart defects have been associated with a condition called **fetal alcohol syndrome**. Total abstinence from alcohol and cigarettes is strongly recommended during pregnancy.

Spina bifida (SPI-nah BIF-ih-dah) is incomplete closure of the spine, through which the spinal cord and its membranes may project (Fig. 25-3). The defect usually occurs in the lumbar region. If the meninges protrude (herniate), the defect is termed a meningocele (meh-NIN-go-sele); if both the spinal cord and meninges protrude, it is a myelomeningocele (mi-eh-lo-meh-NIN-go-sele). In the latter case, the spinal cord ends at the point of the defect, which affects function below that point. Folic acid, a B vitamin, reduces the risk of spina bifida and other CNS defects in the fetus. Women of childbearing age should eat foods high in folic acid (green leafy vegetables, fruits, and legumes) and should take folic acid supplements even before pregnancy, as the nervous system develops early. In the United States, folic acid is added to grain products, such as bread, pasta, rice and cereals.

Checkpoint 25-7 Can a disorder be congenital but not hereditary? Explain.

Examples of Genetic Diseases

The best known example of a genetic disorder that is not hereditary is the most common form of **Down syndrome,** also known as **trisomy 21** because it results from an extra chromosome number 21 in each cell. This abnormality arises during formation of a sex cell. The disorder is usually recognizable at birth by the child's distinctive facial features (Fig. 25-4). Children with Down syndrome have poor muscle tone. They have lowered immunity and are also prone to heart disease, leukemia, and Alzheimer disease. Their intellectual function is impaired. However, the amount of skill they can gain depends on the severity

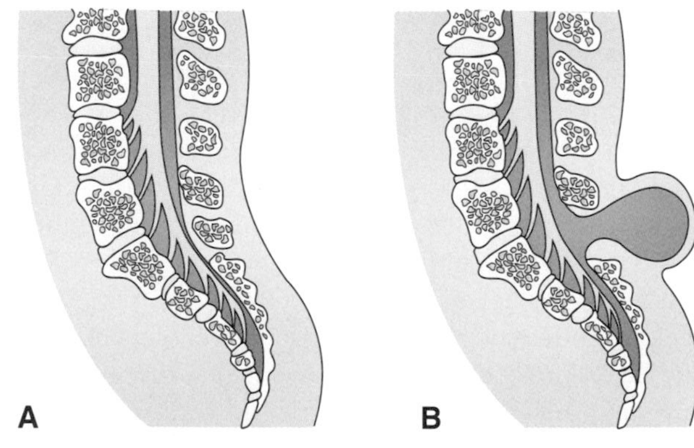

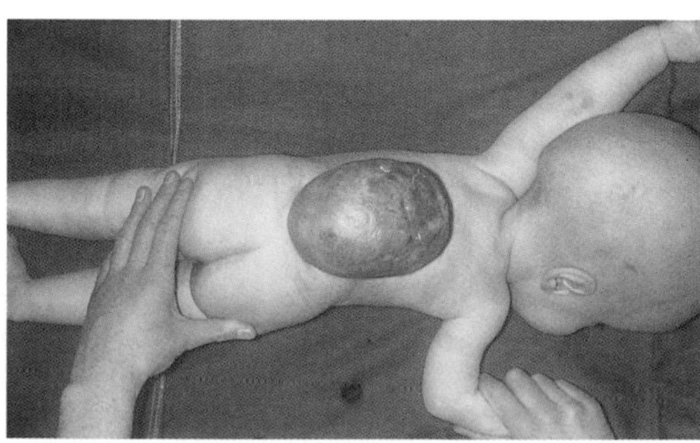

Figure 25-3 **Spina bifida, incomplete closure of the spinal cord.** (A) Normal spinal cord. (B) Spina bifida with protrusion of the meninges (meningocele). (C) Protrusion of the spinal cord and meninges (myelomeningocele). (Reprinted with permission from Pillitteri A. Maternal and Child Health Nursing. 4th ed. Philadelphia: Lippincott Williams & Wilkins, 2003.)

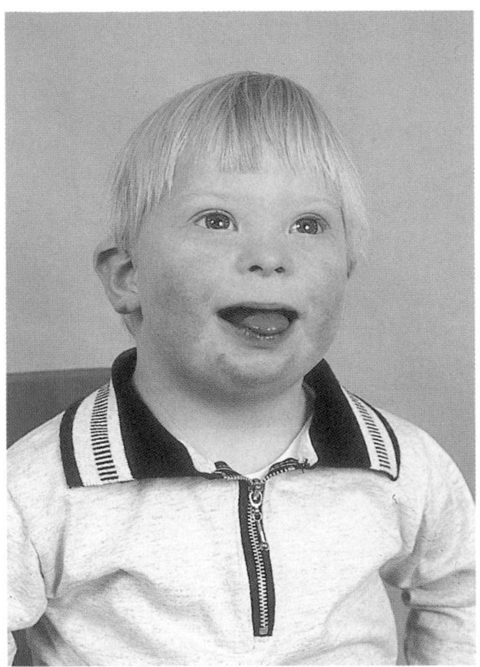

Figure 25-4 **Child with Down syndrome (trisomy 21).** The typical facial features are visible in this photo. (Reprinted with permission from Pillitteri A. Maternal and Child Health Nursing. 4th ed. Philadelphia: Lippincott Williams & Wilkins, 2003.)

of the disease and their family and school environments. Down syndrome is usually not inherited, although there is a hereditary form of the disorder. In most cases, both parents are normal, as are the child's siblings. The likelihood of having a baby with Down syndrome increases dramatically in women past the age of 35 years and may result from defects in either the male or female germ cells owing to age.

Most genetic diseases are **familial** or **hereditary**; that is, they are passed on from parent to child in the egg or sperm. In the case of a disorder carried by a dominant gene, only one parent needs to carry the abnormal gene to give rise to the disease. Any child who receives the defective gene will have the disease. Any children who do not show the disease do not have the defective gene nor are they carriers. One example is **Huntington disease**, a progressive degenerative disorder associated with rapid, involuntary muscle activity and mental deterioration. The disease does not appear until about age 40 and leads to death within 15 years. There is no cure for Huntington disease, but people with the defective gene can be identified by genetic testing. Another example is **Marfan syndrome**, a connective tissue disease. People with Marfan syndrome are tall, thin, and have heart defects.

If the disease trait is carried by a recessive gene, as is the case in most inheritable disorders, a defective gene must come from each parent. Some recessively inherited diseases are described next.

In **phenylketonuria** (fen-il-ke-to-NU-re-ah) (**PKU**), the lack of a certain enzyme prevents the proper metabolism of **phenylalanine** (fen-il-AL-ah-nin), one of the common amino acids. As a result, phenylalanine accumulates in the infant's blood and appears in the urine. If the condition remains untreated, it leads to mental retardation before the age of 2 years. Newborn infants are routinely screened for PKU.

Sickle cell disease is described in Chapter 13, where it is stated that the disease is found almost exclusively among black patients. By contrast, **cystic fibrosis** is most common in white populations; in fact, it is the most frequently inherited disease among this group. Cystic fibrosis is characterized by excessively thickened secretions in the bronchi, the intestine, and the pancreatic ducts, resulting in obstruction of these vital organs. It is associated with frequent respiratory infections, intestinal losses, particularly of fats and fat-soluble vitamins, as well as massive salt loss. Treatment includes oral administration of pancreatic enzymes and special pulmonary exercises. Cystic fibrosis was once fatal by the time of adolescence, but now, with appropriate care, life expectancies are extending into the third decade. The gene responsible for the disease has been identified, raising hope of better diagnosis, treatment, and perhaps even correction of the defective gene that causes the disorder.

In **Tay-Sachs disease**, a certain type of fat is deposited in neurons of the CNS and retina because cellular lysosomes lack an enzyme that breaks it down. The disease occurs mainly in eastern European (Ashkenazi) Jews and generally leads to death by age four. There is no cure for Tay-Sachs, but a blood test can identify genetic carriers of the disease.

Another group of heritable muscle disorders is known collectively as the **progressive muscular atrophies.** Atrophy (AT-ro-fe) means wasting due to decrease in the size of a normally developed part. The absence of normal muscle movement in the infant proceeds within a few months to extreme weakness of the respiratory muscles, until ultimately the infant is unable to breathe adequately. Most afflicted babies die within several months. The name *floppy baby syndrome,* as the disease is commonly called, provides a vivid description of its effects.

Albinism is another recessively inherited disorder that affects the cells (melanocytes) that produce the pigment melanin. The skin and hair color are strikingly white and do not darken with age. The skin is abnormally sensitive to sunlight and may appear wrinkled. People with albinism are especially susceptible to skin cancer and to some severe visual disturbances, such as myopia (nearsightedness) and abnormal sensitivity to light (photophobia).

Other inherited disorders include **osteogenesis** (os-te-o-JEN-eh-sis) **imperfecta**, or *brittle bone disease,* in which multiple fractures may occur during and shortly after fetal life, and a disorder of skin, muscles, and bones called

neurofibromatosis (nu-ro-fi-bro-mah-TO-sis). In the latter condition, multiple masses, often on stalks (pedunculated), grow along nerves all over the body.

More than 20 different cancers have been linked to specific gene mutations. These include cancers of the breast, ovary, and colon as well as some forms of leukemia. Note, however, that hereditary forms of cancer account for only about 1% of all cancers and that the development of cancer is complex, involving not only specific genes but also gene interactions and environmental factors.

Genetic components have been suggested in some other diseases as well, including certain forms of heart disease, diabetes mellitus, types of cleft lip and cleft palate, and perhaps Parkinson and Alzheimer disease.

Checkpoint 25-8 What causes phenylketonuria?

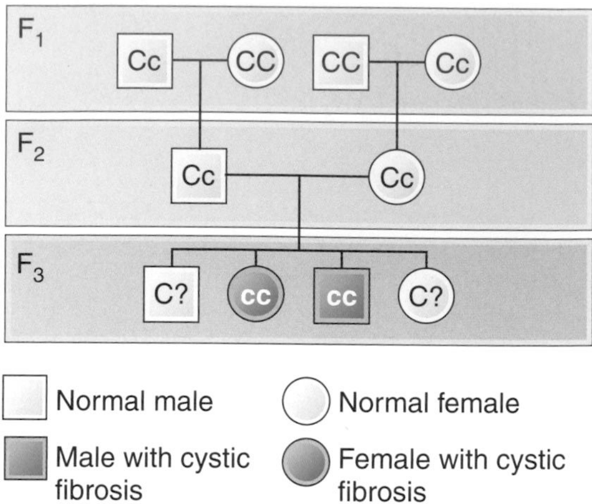

Figure 25-5 **A pedigree (family history) showing three generations (F_1-F_3).** The pedigree is a tool used in genetic studies and genetic counseling. In this example, one parent in each F_1 cross and both parents in the F_2 cross are normal but carry the recessive gene (**c**) for cystic fibrosis. For the normal children in F_3, only one gene (the dominant normal gene) is known. Note that the F_3 generation does not show strict predicted genetic ratios. Theoretically, only one in four children should be homozygous recessive (have two recessive genes). *ZOOMING IN ✦ What are the possible genotypes of the two normal children in the F_3 generation?*

Treatment and Prevention of Genetic Diseases

The number of genetic diseases is so great (more than 4000) that many pages of this book would be needed simply to list them all. Moreover, the list continues to grow as sophisticated research techniques and advances in biology make it clear that various diseases of previously unknown origin are genetic—some hereditary, others not. Can we identify which are inherited genetic disorders and which are due to environmental factors? Can we prevent the occurrence of any of them?

Genetic Counseling

It is possible to prevent genetic disorders in many cases and even to treat some of them. The most effective method of preventing genetic disease is through genetic counseling, a specialized field of health care. Genetic counseling centers use a team approach of medical, nursing, laboratory, and social service professionals to advise and care for clients. People who might consider genetic counseling include prospective parents over 35, those who have a family history of genetic disorders, and those who are considering some form of fertility treatment.

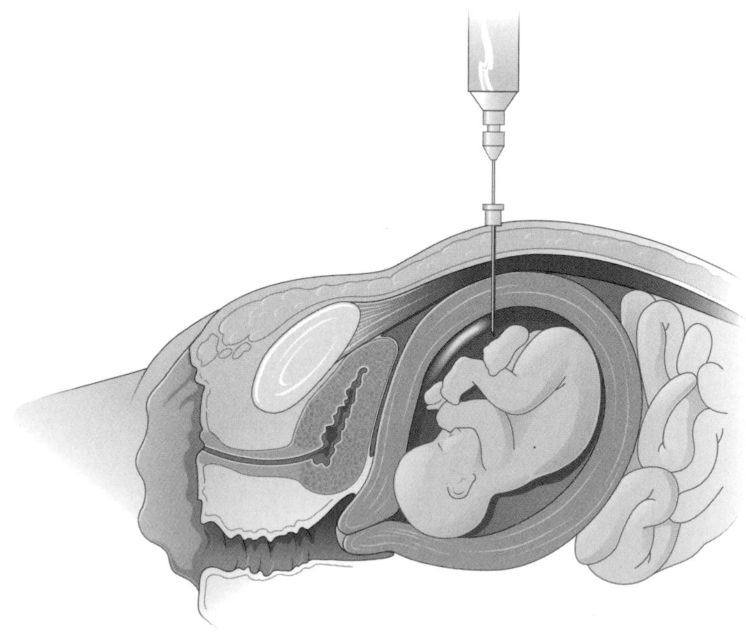

Figure 25-6 **Amniocentesis.** A sample of amniotic fluid is removed from the amniotic sac. Cells and fluid are tested for fetal abnormalities. (Reprinted with permission from Cohen BJ. Medical Terminology. 4th ed. Philadelphia: Lippincott Williams & Wilkins, 2004.)

The Family History An accurate and complete family history of both prospective parents is necessary for genetic counseling. This history should include information about relatives with respect to age, onset of a specific disease, health status, and cause of death. The families' ethnic origins may be relevant because some genetic diseases predominate in certain ethnic groups. Hospital and physician records are studied, as are photographs of family members. The ages of the prospective parents are considered as factors, as is parental or ancestral relationship (*e.g.*, marriage between first cousins). The complete, detailed family history, or tree, is called a **pedigree.** Pedigrees are used to determine the pattern of inheritance of a genetic disease within a family (Fig. 25-5). They may also indicate whether a given family member is a carrier of the disease. Note that in some cases, there is not enough family data to determine the genotype of all members with regard to a given trait. Also, small numbers of offspring may not show the strict genetic ratios expected from a given cross.

Laboratory Studies One technique that enables the geneticist to study an unborn fetus is **amniocentesis** (am-ne-o-sen-TE-sis). During this procedure, a small amount of the amniotic fluid that surrounds the fetus is withdrawn (Fig. 25-6). Fetal skin cells in the amniotic fluid are removed, grown (cultured), and separated for study. The chromosomes are examined, and the amniotic fluid is analyzed for biochemical abnormalities. With these methods, almost 200 genetic diseases can be detected before birth.

Another method for obtaining fetal cells for study involves sampling of the chorionic villi through the cervix. The chorionic villi are hairlike projections of the membrane that surrounds the embryo in early pregnancy. The method is called **chorionic villus sampling (CVS).** Samples may be taken between 8 and 10 weeks of pregnancy, and the cells obtained may be analyzed immediately. In contrast, amniocentesis cannot be done before the 14th to 16th week of pregnancy, and test results are not available for about 2 weeks.

Abnormalities in the chromosome number and some abnormalities within the chromosomes can be detected by **karyotype** (KAR-e-o-tipe) analysis. A karyotype is produced by growing cells obtained by amniocentesis or CVS in a special medium and arresting cell division at the metaphase stage. A technician uses special stains to reveal certain changes in fine structure within the chromosomes. The chromosomes, visible under the microscope, are then photographed, and the photographs are cut out and arranged in groups according to their size and form (Fig. 25-7). Errors involving abnormalities in the number or structure of the chromosomes can thereby be detected.

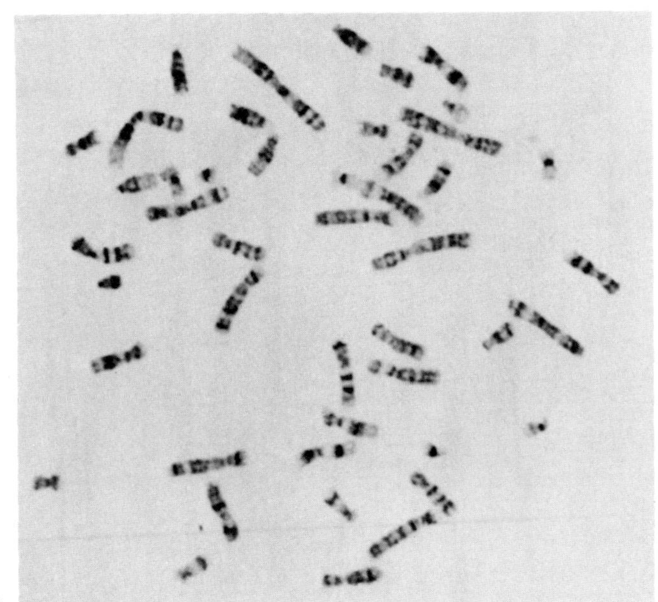

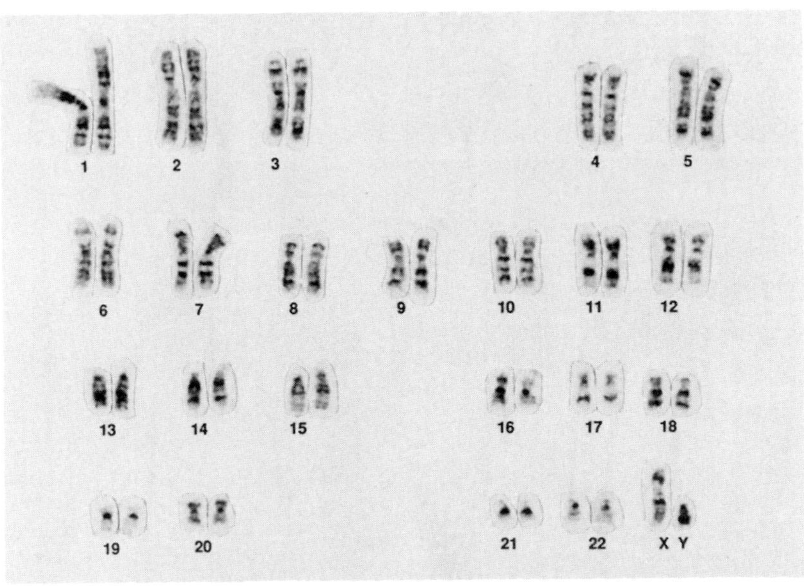

Figure 25-7 Chromosomes. (A) Metaphase spread of normal male chromosomes. The chromosomes have doubled and are ready to divide. The bands are produced by staining. (B) Karyotype. The chromosomes are arranged in matching pairs according to size and other characteristics. (Courtesy of Wenda S. Long, Thomas Jefferson University, Philadelphia.) *ZOOMING IN ✦ How many autosomes are shown in B?*

Counseling Prospective Parents Armed with all the available pertinent facts, and with knowledge of genetic inheritance patterns, the counselor is equipped to inform the prospective parents of the possibility of their having genetically abnormal offspring. The couple may then use this information to make decisions about family planning. Depending on the individuals and their situation, a couple might elect to have no children, have an adoptive family, use a donor gamete, terminate a pregnancy, or accept the risk.

Checkpoint 25-9 What is a pedigree and how is a pedigree used in genetic counseling?

Checkpoint 25-10 What is a karyotype?

Progress in Medical Treatment

The mental and physical ravages of many genetic diseases are largely preventable, provided the diseases are diagnosed and treated early in the individual's life. Some of these diseases respond well to dietary control. One such disease, called **maple syrup urine disease**, responds to very large doses of thiamin along with control of the intake of certain amino acids. The disastrous effects of Wilson disease, in which abnormal accumulations of copper in the tissue cause tremor, rigidity, uncontrollable stagger, and finally extensive liver damage, can be prevented by a combination of dietary and drug therapy.

Phenylketonuria is perhaps the best-known example of dietary management of inherited disease. If the disorder is undiagnosed and untreated, 98% of affected patients will be severely mentally retarded by 10 years of age. In contrast, if the condition is diagnosed and treated before the baby reaches the age of 6 months, and treatment is maintained until the age of 10 years, mental deficiency will be prevented, or at least minimized. A simple blood test for PKU is now done routinely in hospitals throughout the United States. Infants are usually screened immediately after birth, but they should be retested 24 to 48 hours after taking in protein.

Klinefelter (KLINE-fel-ter) **syndrome**, which occurs in about 1 in 600 males, is a common cause of underdevelopment of the gonads with resulting infertility. Victims of this disorder have abnormal sex chromosome patterns, usually an extra X chromosome. Instead of the typical male XY pattern, the cells contain an XXY combination owing to failure of the sex chromosomes to separate during cell division. Treatment of this disorder includes the use of hormones and psychotherapy.

In the future, we can anticipate greatly improved methods of screening, diagnosis, and treatment of genetic diseases. There have been reports of fetuses being treated with vitamins or hormones after prenatal diagnosis of a genetic disorder. Ahead lies the possibility of treating or correcting genetic disorders through genetic engineering—introducing genetically altered cells to produce missing factors, such as enzymes or hormones, or even correcting faulty genes in the victim's cells. Researchers have already made some attempts to supplement failed genes with healthy ones.

For the present, it is important to educate the public about the availability of screening methods for both parents and offspring. People should also be made aware of the damaging effects of radiation, drugs, and other toxic substances on the genes. Because so many congenital disorders are associated with environmental factors, public education and better health habits will probably yield greater overall benefits than genetic manipulations.

Word Anatomy

Medical terms are built from standardized word parts (prefixes, roots, and suffixes). Learning the meanings of these parts can help you remember words and interpret unfamiliar terms.

WORD PART	MEANING	EXAMPLE
Genes and Chromosomes		
chrom/o	color	*Chromosomes* color darkly with stains.
aut/o-	self	*Autosomes* are all the chromosomes aside from the two that determine sex.
heter/o	other, different	*Heterozygous* paired genes (alleles) are different from each other.
homo-	same	*Homozygous* paired genes (alleles) are the same.
phen/o	to show	Traits that can be observed or tested for make up a person's *phenotype*.
Hereditary Traits		
multi-	many	*Multifactorial* traits are determined by multiple pairs of genes.
Genetic Diseases		
dactyl/o	digit (finger or toe)	In *polydactyly* there is an extra finger on each hand.
con-	with	A *congenital* defect is present at the time of birth.
-cele	swelling	In spina bifida, the meninges can protrude through the spine as a *meningocele*.

WORD PART	MEANING	EXAMPLE
Treatment and Prevention of Genetic Diseases		
-centesis	tapping, perforation	*Amniocentesis* is a tap of the amniotic fluid.
kary/o	nucleus	A *karyotype* is an analysis of the chromosomes contained in the nucleus of a cell.

Summary

I. Genes and chromosomes

1. Genes
   a. Hereditary units
   b. Segments of DNA
   c. Control manufacture of proteins (e.g., enzymes, hormones)
2. Chromosomes
   a. Threadlike bodies in nucleus; 46 in humans
   b. Composed of genes
   c. 22 pairs autosomes (non-sex chromosomes)
   d. 1 pair sex chromosomes

A. Dominant and recessive genes
1. Dominant gene—always expressed
   a. May be heterozygous (two genes different)
   b. May be homozygous dominant (two genes the same)
2. Recessive gene—expressed only if homozygous recessive (received from both parents)
   a. Carrier—person with recessive gene that is not apparent but can be passed to offspring
   b. Phenotype—characteristic that can be seen or tested for
   c. Genotype—genetic make-up

B. Distribution of chromosomes to offspring
1. Meiosis
   a. Cell division that forms sex cells with 23 chromosomes
   b. Each cell receives one of each chromosome pair
   c. Punnett square shows results of crosses

C. Sex determination
1. X chromosome larger and carries other traits
2. Y smaller and carries mainly gene for sex determination
3. Female cells have XX; male cells have XY

D. Sex-linked traits
1. Traits carried on sex chromosome (usually X)
2. Sex-linked traits appear mostly in males
   a. Passed from mother to son on X chromosome
   b. If recessive, not masked by dominant gene on Y
   c. Examples—hemophilia, baldness, red-green color blindness

II. Hereditary traits

1. Genes determine physical, biochemical, and physiologic characteristics of every cell
2. Some traits determined by single gene pairs
3. Most determined by multifactorial inheritance
   a. Involves multiple gene pairs
   b. Produces a range of variations in a population
   c. Examples—height, weight, coloration, susceptibility to disease

A. Gene expression
1. Factors
   a. Sex
   b. Presence of other genes
   c. Environment

B. Genetic mutation
1. Change in genes or chromosomes
2. May be passed to offspring if occurs in germ cells
3. Mutagenic agents
   a. Factors causing mutation
   b. Examples—ionizing radiation, chemicals

III. Genetic diseases—disorders involving genes

A. Congenital versus hereditary diseases
1. Congenital disorders
   a. Present at birth
   b. May or may not be hereditary
2. Hereditary (familial) disorders
   a. Passed from parent to offspring in sex cells
3. Causes: infections, toxins, ionizing radiation, alcohol, smoking
   a. Examples—defects caused by rubella, fetal alcohol syndrome, spina bifida

B. Examples of genetic diseases
1. Down syndrome—results from extra chromosome 21 (trisomy 21)
2. Dominant inheritance—Huntington disease, Marfan sundrome
3. Recessive inheritance—PKU (phenylketonuria), cystic fibrosis, sickle cell anemia, Tay-Sachs disease, progressive muscular atrophies, albinism, osteogenesis imperfecta, neurofibromatosis

IV. Treatment and prevention of genetic diseases

A. Genetic counseling
1. Pedigree—family history
2. Laboratory studies
   a. Amniocentesis—withdrawal of amniotic fluid for study at 14 to 16 weeks of pregnancy
   b. Chorionic villus sampling—done at 8 to 10 weeks of pregnancy
   c. Karyotype—analysis of chromosomes
3. Counseling the prospective parents

B. Progress in medical treatment
1. Dietary control—maple syrup urine disease, Wilson disease, PKU
2. Hormone therapy—Klinefelter disease
3. Fetal therapy
4. Correction of faulty genes—experimental

Questions for Study and Review

Building Understanding

Fill in the blanks

1. The basic unit of heredity is a(n) ______.
2. Chromosomes not involved in sex determination are known as ______.
3. Any trait that is carried on a sex chromosome is said to be ______.
4. Change in a gene or chromosome is called ______.
5. Incomplete closure of the spine results in a disorder called ______.

Matching

Match each numbered item with the most closely related lettered item.

___ 6. A gene that is always expressed if present
___ 7. A gene that is not always expressed if present
___ 8. Term for paired genes for a trait that are the same
___ 9. Term for paired genes for a trait that are different

a. dominant
b. recessive
c. homozygous
d. heterozygous

Multiple choice

___ 10. The genetic code is composed of
a. deoxyribonucleic acid
b. ribonucleic acid
c. protein
d. nuclear membrane

___ 11. Genes govern the cell by controlling the manufacture of
a. carbohydrates
b. lipids
c. proteins
d. electrolytes

___ 12. Paired genes for a given trait are known as
a. chromosomes
b. ribosomes
c. nucleotides
d. alleles

___ 13. A condition characterized by extra fingers or toes is called
a. talipes
b. polydactyly
c. osteogenesis imperfecta
d. neurofibromatosis

___ 14. A complete detailed family history can be obtained by doing
a. chorionic villus sampling
b. amniocentesis
c. a karyotype
d. a pedigree

Understanding Concepts

15. How many chromosomes are there in a human body cell? In a human gamete?
16. Dana has one dominant allele for brown eyes (B) and one recessive allele for blue eyes. What is Dana's genotype? What is her phenotype?
17. Describe the process of meiosis and explain how it results in genetic variation.
18. Explain the great variation in the color of skin and hair in humans.
19. Describe how a mutagenic agent can produce genetic variation.
20. What is the difference between a congenital disease and a hereditary disease? List some congenital and hereditary diseases.
21. What is PKU and how should this disease be treated?
22. Compare and contrast amniocentesis and chorionic villus sampling. List some diseases that can be diagnosed using these techniques.
23. What is the most common inheritable disease among black people? Among white people? What are the symptoms of these two diseases?

Conceptual Thinking

24. If mitosis were used to produce gametes, what consequences would this have on the offspring's genotype, phenotype, and chromosome number?
25. Jason and Nicole are expecting their first child and are wondering what their child's eye color might be. Jason has blue eyes (a recessive trait) and Nicole has brown eyes (a dominant trait). Both of Jason's parents have blue eyes. One of Nicole's parents has brown eyes, the other has blue eyes. What are Jason's and Nicole's genotype and phenotype? What are the possible genotypes and phenotypes of their children?

Index

Page numbers in *italics* indicate figures. Page numbers followed by *t* indicate tables. Page numbers followed by *B* indicate boxed material.

U

Glossary

abdominopelvic (ab-dom-ih-no-PEL-vik) Pertaining to the abdomen and pelvis
abduction (ab-DUK-shun) Movement away from the midline
abortifacient (ah-bor-tih-FA-shent) Agent that induces an abortion
abortion (ah-BOR-shun) Loss of an embryo or fetus before the 20th week of pregnancy
abscess (AB-ses) Area of tissue breakdown; a localized space in the body containing pus and liquefied tissue
absorption (ab-SORP-shun) Transfer of digested nutrients from the digestive tract into the circulation
accommodation (ah-kom-o-DA-shun) Coordinated changes in the lens of the eye that enable one to focus on near and far objects
acetylcholine (as-e-til-KO-lene) **(ACh)** Neurotransmitter; released at synapses within the nervous system and at the neuromuscular junction
acid (AH-sid) Substance that can donate a hydrogen ion to another substance
acid-fast stain Procedure used to color cells for viewing under the microscope
acidosis (as-ih-DO-sis) Condition that results from a decrease in the pH of body fluids
acne (AK-ne) Disease of the sebaceous glands
acquired immunodeficiency syndrome (AIDS) Viral disease that attacks the immune system, specifically the T-helper lymphocytes with CD4 receptors
acromegaly (ak-ro-MEG-ah-le) Condition caused by oversecretion of growth hormone in adults; there is overgrowth of some bones and involvement of multiple body systems
acrosome (AK-ro-some) Caplike structure over the head of the sperm cell that helps the sperm to penetrate the ovum
ACTH See adrenocorticotropic hormone
actin (AK-tin) One of the two contractile proteins in muscle cells, the other being myosin
action potential Sudden change in the electrical charge on a cell membrane, which then spreads along the membrane; nerve impulse
active transport Movement of a substance into or out of a cell in an opposite direction to the way in which it would normally flow by diffusion; active transport requires energy and transporters
acupuncture (AK-u-punk-chur) Ancient Chinese method of inserting thin needles into the body at specific points to relieve pain or promote healing
acute (ah-KUTE) Referring to a severe but short-lived disease or condition
Addison disease Condition caused by hypofunction of the adrenal cortex
adduction (ad-DUK-shun) Movement toward the midline
adenosine triphosphate (ah-DEN-o-sene tri-FOS-fate) **(ATP)** Energy-storing compound found in all cells
ADH See antidiuretic hormone
adhesion (ad-HE-zhun) Holding together of two surfaces or parts; band of connective tissue between parts that are normally separate; molecular attraction between contacting bodies
adipose (AD-ih-pose) Referring to a type of connective tissue that stores fat or to fats
adrenal (ah-DRE-nal) **gland** Endocrine gland located above the kidney; suprarenal gland
adrenaline (ah-DREN-ah-lin) See Epinephrine
adrenergic (ad-ren-ER-jik) An activity or structure that responds to epinephrine (adrenaline)
adrenocorticotropic (ah-dre-no-kor-tih-ko-TRO-pik) **hormone (ACTH)** Hormone produced by the pituitary that stimulates the adrenal cortex
aerobic (air-O-bik) Requiring oxygen
afferent (AF-fer-ent) Carrying toward a given point, such as a sensory neuron that carries nerve impulses toward the central nervous system
agglutination (ah-glu-tih-NA-shun) Clumping of cells due to an antigen–antibody reaction
agranulocyte (a-GRAN-u-lo-site) Leukocyte without visible granules in the cytoplasm when stained; lymphocyte or monocyte
AIDS See acquired immunodeficiency syndrome
albinism (AL-bih-nizm) A hereditary disorder that affects melanin production
albumin (al-BU-min) Protein in blood plasma and other body fluids; helps maintain the osmotic pressure of the blood
albuminuria (al-bu-mih-NU-re-ah) Presence of albumin in the urine, usually as a result of a kidney disorder
aldosterone (al-DOS-ter-one) Hormone released by the adrenal cortex that promotes the reabsorption of sodium and water in the kidneys
alkali (AL-kah-li) Substance that can accept a hydrogen ion (H^+); substance that donates a hydroxide ion (OH^-); a base
alkalosis (al-kah-LO-sis) Condition that results from an increase in the pH of body fluids
allele (al-LELE) One member of the gene pair that controls a given trait
allergen (AL-er-jen) Substance that causes hypersensitivity; substance that induces allergy
allergy (AL-er-je) Tendency to react unfavorably to a certain substance that is normally harmless to most people; hypersensitivity
alopecia (al-o-PE-she-ah) Baldness
alveolus (al-VE-o-lus) Small sac or pouch; usually a tiny air sac in the lungs through which gases are exchanged between the outside air and the blood; tooth socket; pl., alveoli
Alzheimer (ALZ-hi-mer) **disease** Unexplained degeneration of the cerebral cortex and hippocampus with intellectual impairment, mood changes and confusion
amblyopia (am-ble-O-pe-ah) Loss of vision in a healthy eye because it cannot work properly with the other eye
amino (ah-ME-no) **acid** Building block of protein
amniocentesis (am-ne-o-sen-TE-sis) Removal of fluid and cells from the amniotic sac for prenatal diagnostic tests
amniotic (am-ne-OT-ik) Pertaining to the sac that surrounds and cushions the developing fetus or to the fluid that fills that sac
amphiarthrosis (am-fe-ar-THRO-sis) Slightly movable joint
amyotrophic (ah-mi-o-TROF-ik) **lateral sclerosis (ALS)** Disorder of the nervous system in which motor neurons are destroyed
anabolism (ah-NAB-o-lizm) Metabolic building of simple compounds into more complex substances needed by the body
anaerobic (an-air-O-bik) Not requiring oxygen
analgesic (an-al-JE-zik) Relieving pain; a pain-relieving agent that does not cause loss of consciousness
anaphase (AN-ah-faze) The third stage of mitosis in which chromosomes separate to opposite sides of the cell
anaphylaxis (an-ah-fih-LAK-sis) Severe, life-threatening allergic response
anastomosis (ah-nas-to-MO-sis) Communication between two structures, such as blood vessels
anatomy (ah-NAT-o-me) Study of body structure
anemia (ah-NE-me-ah) Abnormally low level of hemoglobin or red cells in the blood, resulting in inadequate delivery of oxygen to the tissues
androgen (AN-dro-jen) Any male sex hormone

anesthesia (an-es-THE-ze-ah) Loss of sensation, particularly of pain; drug with this effect is an anesthetic

aneurysm (AN-u-rizm) Bulging sac in the wall of a vessel

angiotensin (an-je-o-TEN-sin) Substance formed in the blood by the action of the enzyme renin from the kidneys; it increases blood pressure by causing constriction of the blood vessels and stimulating the release of aldosterone from the adrenal cortex

angina (an-JI-nah) Severe choking pain; disease or condition producing such pain. Angina pectoris is suffocating pain in the chest, usually caused by lack of oxygen supply to the heart muscle

angioplasty (AN-je-o-plas-te) Use of a balloon inserted with a catheter to open a blocked vessel

anion (AN-i-on) Negatively charged particle (ion)

anorexia (an-o-REK-se-ah) Chronic loss of appetite. Anorexia nervosa is a psychological condition in which a person may become seriously, even fatally, weakened from lack of food.

anoxia (ah-NOK-se-ah) See hypoxia

ANP See atrial natriuretic peptide

ANS See autonomic nervous system

antagonist (an-TAG-o-nist) Muscle that has an action opposite that of a given movement; substance that opposes the action of another substance

anterior (an-TE-re-or) Toward the front or belly surface; ventral

anthelmintic (ant-hel-MIN-tik) Agent that acts against worms; vermicide; vermifuge

antibiotic (an-te-bi-OT-ik) Substance produced by living cells that kills or arrests the growth of bacteria

antibody (AN-te-bod-e) **(Ab)** Substance produced in response to a specific antigen; immunoglobulin

antidiuretic (an-ti-di-u-RET-ik) **hormone (ADH)** Hormone released from the posterior pituitary gland that increases the reabsorption of water in the kidneys, thus decreasing the volume of urine excreted

antigen (AN-te-jen) **(Ag)** Foreign substance that produces an immune response

antineoplastic (an-ti-ne-o-PLAS-tik) Acting against a neoplasm (tumor)

antioxidant (an-te-OX-ih-dant) Substances in the diet that protect against harmful free radicals

antipyretic (an-ti-pi-RET-ik) Drug that reduces fever

antiseptic (an-tih-SEP-tik) Substance that prevents pathogens from multiplying but does not necessarily kill them

antiserum (an-te-SE-rum) Serum containing antibodies that may be given to provide passive immunity; immune serum

antitoxin (an-te-TOKS-in) Antibody that neutralizes a toxin

antivenin (an-te-VEN-in) Antibody that neutralizes a snake venom

anus (A-nus) Distal opening of the digestive tract

aorta (a-OR-tah) The largest artery; carries blood out of the left ventricle of the heart

apex (A-peks) The pointed region of a cone-shaped structure

aphasia (ah-FA-ze-ah) Loss or defect in language communication; loss of the ability to speak or write is expressive aphasia; loss of understanding of written or spoken language is receptive aphasia

apnea (AP-ne-ah) Temporary cessation of breathing

apocrine (AP-o-krin) Referring to a gland that releases some cellular material along with its secretions

aponeurosis (ap-o-nu-RO-sis) Broad sheet of fibrous connective tissue that attaches muscle to bone or to other muscle

appendicular (ap-en-DIK-u-lar) **skeleton** Part of the skeleton that includes the bones of the upper extremities, lower extremities, shoulder girdle, and hips

appendix (ah-PEN-diks) Fingerlike tube of lymphatic tissue attached to the first portion of the large intestine; vermiform (wormlike) appendix

aqueous (A-kwe-us) Pertaining to water; an aqueous solution is one in which water is the solvent

aqueous (A-kwe-us) **humor** Watery fluid that fills much of the eyeball anterior to the lens

arachnoid (ah-RAK-noyd) Middle layer of the meninges

areolar (ah-RE-o-lar) Referring to loose connective tissue, any small space, or to an areola, a circular area of marked color

arrector pili (ah-REK-tor PI-li) Muscle attached to a hair follicle that raises the hair

arrhythmia (ah-RITH-me-ah) Abnormal rhythm of the heartbeat; dysrhythmia

arteriole (ar-TE-re-ole) Vessel between a small artery and a capillary

arteriosclerosis (ar-te-re-o-skle-RO-sis) Hardening of the arteries

artery (AR-ter-e) Vessel that carries blood away from the heart

arthritis (arth-RI-tis) Inflammation of the joints

arthrocentesis (ar-thro-sen-TE-sis) Puncture of a joint to withdraw fluid

arthroscope (AR-thro-skope) Instrument for examining the interior of the knee and surgically repairing the knee

articular (ar-TIK-u-lar) Pertaining to a joint

ascites (ah-SI-teze) Abnormal collection of fluid in the abdominal cavity

asepsis (a-SEP-sis) Condition in which no pathogens are present; adj., aseptic

asthma (AZ-mah) Allergy-induced inflammation and constriction of the air passageways

astigmatism (ah-STIG-mah-tizm) Visual defect due to an irregularity in the curvature of the cornea or the lens

ataxia (ah-TAK-se-ah) Lack of muscular coordination; irregular muscular action

atelectasis (at-e-LEK-tah-sis) Incomplete expansion of the lung; collapsed lung

atherosclerosis (ath-er-o-skleh-RO-sis) Hardening of the arteries due to the deposit of yellowish, fatlike material in the lining of these vessels

atom (AT-om) Smallest subunit of a chemical element

atomic number The number of protons in the nucleus of an element's atoms; a number characteristic of each element

atopic dermatitis (ah-TOP-ik der-mah-TI-tis) Skin condition that may involve redness, blisters, pimples, scaling, and crusting; eczema

ATP See Adenosine triphosphate

atrial natriuretic (*na-tre-u-RET-ik*) **peptide (ANP)** Hormone produced by the atria of the heart that lowers blood pressure

atrioventricular (a-tre-o-ven-TRIK-u-lar) **(AV) node** Part of the conduction system of the heart

atrium (A-tre-um) One of the two upper chambers of the heart; adj., atrial

atrophy (AT-ro-fe) Wasting or decrease in size of a part

attenuated (ah-TEN-u-a-ted) Weakened

autoclave Instrument used to sterilize material with steam under pressure

autoimmunity (aw-to-ih-MU-nih-te) Abnormal reactivity to one's own tissues

autologous (aw-TOL-o-gus) Related to self, such as blood or tissue taken from one's own body

autonomic (aw-to-NOM-ik) **nervous system (ANS)** The part of the nervous system that controls smooth muscle, cardiac muscle, and glands; the visceral or involuntary nervous system

autosome (AW-to-some) A chromosome not involved in sex determination. There are 44 autosomes (22 pairs) in humans

AV node See Atrioventricular node

axial (AK-se-al) **skeleton** The part of the skeleton that includes the skull, spinal column, ribs, and sternum

axilla (ak-SIL-ah) Hollow beneath the arm where it joins the body; armpit

axon (AK-son) Fiber of a neuron that conducts impulses away from the cell body

bacillus (bah-SIL-us) Rod-shaped bacterium; pl., bacilli (bah-SIL-i)
bacterium (bak-TE-re-um) Type of microorganism; pl., bacteria (bak-TE-re-ah)
bacteriostasis (bak-te-re-o-STA-sis) Condition in which bacterial growth is inhibited but the organisms are not killed
band cell Immature neutrophil
basal ganglia (BA-sal GANG-le-ah) Gray masses in the lower part of the forebrain that aid in muscle coordination
base Substance that can accept a hydrogen ion (H^+); substance that donates a hydroxide ion (OH-); an alkali
basophil (BA-so-fil) Granular white blood cell that shows large, dark blue cytoplasmic granules when stained with basic stain
B cell Agranular white blood cell that gives rise to antibody-producing plasma cells in response to an antigen; B lymphocyte
Bell palsy Facial paralysis caused by damage to the facial nerve (VII), usually on one side of the face.
benign (be-NINE) Describing a tumor that does not spread; not recurrent nor becoming worse
bile Substance produced in the liver that emulsifies fats
bilirubin (BIL-ih-ru-bin) Pigment derived from the breakdown of hemoglobin and found in bile
biofeedback (bi-o-FEED-bak) A method for controling involuntary responses by means of electronic devices that monitor changes and feed information back to a person
biopsy (BI-op-se) Removal of tissue or other material from the living body for examination, usually under the microscope
blood urea nitrogen (BUN) Amount of nitrogen from urea in the blood; test to evaluate kidney function
bolus (BO-lus) A concentrated mass; the portion of food that is moved to the back of the mouth and swallowed
Bowman capsule Enlarged portion of the nephron that contains the glomerulus; glomerular capsule
bone Hard connective tissue that makes up most of the skeleton, or any structure composed of this type of tissue
bradycardia (brad-e-KAR-de-ah) Heart rate of less than 60 beats per minute
brain The central controlling area of the central nervous system (CNS)
brain stem Portion of the brain that connects the cerebrum with the spinal cord; contains the midbrain, pons, and medulla oblongata
Broca (bro-KAH) **area** Area of the cerebral cortex concerned with motor control of speech
bronchiole (BRONG-ke-ole) Microscopic branch of a bronchus
bronchoscope (BRONG-ko-skope) Endoscope for examination of the bronchi and removal of small objects from the bronchi
bronchus (BRONG-kus) Large air passageway in the lung; pl., bronchi (BRONG-ki)
buffer (BUF-er) Substance that prevents sharp changes in the pH of a solution
bulbourethral (bul-bo-u-RE-thral) **gland** Gland that secretes mucus to lubricate the urethra and tip of penis during sexual stimulation; Cowper gland
bulimia (bu-LIM-e-ah) Eating disorder also known as binge-purge syndrome
bulk transport Movement of large amounts of material through the plasma membrane of a cell
Bulla (BUL-ah) Vesicle
BUN See Blood urea nitrogen
bursa (BER-sah) Small, fluid-filled sac found in an area subject to stress around bones and joints; pl., bursae (BER-se)
bursitis (ber-SI-tis) Inflammation of a bursa

calcitonin (kal-sih-TO-nin) Hormone from the thyroid gland that lowers blood calcium levels and promotes deposit of calcium in bones; thyrocalcitonin
calcitriol (kal-sih-TRI-ol) The active form of vitamin D; dihydroxycholecalciferol (di-hi-drok-se-ko-le-kal-SIF-eh-rol)
calculus (KAL-ku-lus) Stone, such as a urinary stone; pl calculi (KAL-ku-li)
calyx (KA-liks) Cuplike extension of the renal pelvis that collects urine; pl. calyces (KA-lih-seze)
cancellous (KAN-sel-us) Referring to spongy bone tissue
cancer (KAN-ser) Tumor that spreads to other tissues; a malignant neoplasm
capillary (CAP-ih-lar-e) Microscopic vessel through which exchanges take place between the blood and the tissues
carbohydrate (kar-bo-HI-drate) Simple sugar or compound made from simple sugars linked together, such as starch or glycogen
carbon Element that is the basis of organic chemistry
carbon dioxide (di-OX-ide) **(CO2)** The gaseous waste product of cellular metabolism
carcinogen (kar-SIN-o-jen) Cancer-causing substance
carcinoma (kar-sih-NO-mah) Malignant growth of epithelial cells; a form of cancer
cardiac (KAR-de-ak) Pertaining to the heart
cardiopulmonary resuscitation (CPR) Method to restore heartbeat and breathing by mouth-to-mouth resuscitation and closed chest cardiac massage
cardiovascular system (kar-dE-o-VAS-kular) The system consisting of the heart and blood vessels that transports blood throughout the body
caries (KA-reze) Tooth decay
carotenemia (kar-o-te-NE-me-ah) Yellowish color of the skin caused by eating excessive amounts of carrots and other deeply colored vegetables
carrier Individual who has a gene that is not expressed but that can be passed to offspring
cartilage (KAR-tih-lij) Type of hard connective tissue found at the ends of bones, the tip of the nose, larynx, trachea and the embryonic skeleton
CAT See Computed tomography
catabolism (kah-TAB-o-lizm) Metabolic breakdown of substances into simpler substances; includes the digestion of food and the oxidation of nutrient molecules for energy
catalyst (KAT-ah-list) Substance that speeds the rate of a chemical reaction
cataract (KAT-ah-rakt) Opacity of the eye's lens or lens capsule
catheter (KATH-eh-ter) Tube that can be inserted into a vessel or cavity; may be used to remove fluid, such as urine or blood; v., catheterize
cation (KAT-i-on) Positively charged particle (ion)
caudal (KAWD-al) Toward or nearer to the sacral region of the spinal column
cecum (SE-kum) Small pouch at the beginning of the large intestine
cell Basic unit of life
cell membrane Outer covering of a cell; regulates what enters and leaves cell; plasma membrane
cellular respiration Series of reactions by which nutrients are oxidized for energy within the cell
central nervous system (CNS) Part of the nervous system that includes the brain and spinal cord
centrifuge (SEN-trih-fuje) An instrument that separates materials in a mixture based on density
centriole (SEN-tre-ole) Rod-shaped body near the nucleus of a cell; functions in cell division
cerebellum (ser-eh-BEL-um) Small section of the brain located under the cerebral hemispheres; functions in coordination, balance, and muscle tone
cerebral (SER-e-bral) **cortex** The very thin outer layer of gray matter on the surface of the cerebral hemispheres
cerebral palsy (PAWL-ze) Disorder caused by brain damage occurring before or during the birth process

cerebrospinal (ser-e-bro-SPI-nal) **fluid (CSF)** Fluid that circulates in and around the brain and spinal cord

cerebrovascular (ser-e-bro-VAS-ku-lar) **accident** (CVA) Condition involving obstruction of blood flow to brain tissue or bleeding into brain tissue, usually as a result of hypertension or atherosclerosis; stroke

cerebrum (SER-e-brum) Largest part of the brain; composed of two cerebral hemispheres

cerumen (seh-RU-men) Earwax; adj., ceruminous (seh-RU-min-us)

cervix (SER-vix) Constricted portion of an organ or part, such as the lower portion of the uterus; neck; adj., cervical

chemistry (KEM-is-tre) Study of the composition and properties of matter

chemoreceptor (ke-mo-re-SEP-tor) Receptor that responds to chemicals in body fluids

chemotherapy (ke-mo-THER-ah-pe) Treatment of a disease by administration of a chemical agent

Cheyne-Stokes (CHANE-stokes) **respiration** Rhythmic variation in the depth of respiratory movements alternating with periods of apnea due to depression of the breathing centers

chlamydia (klah-MID-e-ah) A type of very small bacterium that can exist only within a living cell; members of this group cause inclusion conjunctivitis, trachoma, sexually transmitted infections, and respiratory diseases

cholecystokinin (ko-le-sis-to-KI-nin) **(CCK)** Hormone from the duodenum that stimulates release of pancreatic enzymes and bile from the gallbladder

cholelithiasis (ko-le-lih-THI-ah-sis) Gallstones

cholesterol (ko-LES-ter-ol) An organic fatlike compound found in animal fat, bile, blood, myelin, liver, and other parts of the body

cholinergic (ko-lin-ER-jik) An activity or structure that responds to acetylcholine

chondrocyte (KON-dro-site) Cell that produces cartilage

chordae tendineae (KOR-de ten-DIN-e-e) Fibrous threads that stabilize the AV valve flaps in the heart

choriocarcinoma (ko-re-o-kar-sih-NO-mah) Very malignant tumor made of placental tissue

choroid (KO-royd) Pigmented middle layer of the eye

choroid plexus (KO-royd PLEKS-us) Vascular network in the ventricles of the brain that forms cerebrospinal fluid

creatinine (kre-AT-in-in) A nitrogenous waste product in the blood

chromosome (KRO-mo-some) Dark-staining, threadlike body in the nucleus of a cell; contains genes that determine hereditary traits

chronic (KRON-ik) Referring to a disease that develops slowly, persists over a long time, or is recurring

chyle (kile) Milky-appearing fluid absorbed into the lymphatic system from the small intestine. It consists of lymph and droplets of digested fat.

chyme (kime) Mixture of partially digested food, water, and digestive juices that forms in the stomach

cicatrix (SIK-ah-trix) Scar

cilia (SIL-e-ah) Hairs or hairlike processes, such as eyelashes or microscopic extensions from the surface of a cell; sing., cilium

ciliary (SIL-e-ar-e) **muscle** Eye muscle that controls the shape of the lens

circumduction (ser-kum-DUK-shun) Circular movement at a joint

circumcision (sir-kum-SIJ-un) Surgery to remove the foreskin of the penis

cirrhosis (sih-RO-sis) Chronic disease, usually of the liver, in which active cells are replaced by inactive scar tissue

cisterna chyli (sis-TER-nah KI-li) First part of the thoracic lymph duct, which is enlarged to form a temporary storage area

clitoris (KLIT-o-ris) Small organ of great sensitivity in the external genitalia of the female

CNS See Central nervous system

coagulation (ko-ag-u-LA-shun) Clotting, as of blood

coccus (KOK-us) A round bacterium; pl., cocci (KOK-si)

cochlea (KOK-le-ah) Coiled portion of the inner ear that contains the organ of hearing

colic (KOL-ik) Spasm of visceral muscle

collagen (KOL-ah-jen) Flexible white protein that gives strength and resilience to connective tissue, such as bone and cartilage

colloid (kol-OYD) Mixture in which suspended particles do not dissolve but remain distributed in the solvent because of their small size (*e.g.*, cytoplasm); colloidal suspension

colon (KO-lon) Main portion of the large intestine

colostrum (ko-LOS-trum) Secretion of the mammary glands released prior to secretion of milk

communicable (kom-MU-nih-kabl) Describing a disease that can be transmitted from one person to another

complement (KOM-ple-ment) Group of blood proteins that helps antibodies to destroy foreign cells

compliance (kom-PLI-ans) The ease with which the lungs and thorax can be expanded

compound Substance composed of two or more chemical elements

computed tomography (to-MOG-rah-fe) **(CT)** Imaging method in which multiple radiographic views taken from different angles are analyzed by computer to show a cross-section of an area; used to detect tumors and other abnormalities; also called computed axial tomography (CAT)

concha (KON-ka) Shell-like bone in the nasal cavity; pl., conchae (KON-ke)

concussion (kon-CUSH-on) Injury resulting from a violent blow or shock

condyle (KON-dile) Rounded projection, as on a bone

cone Receptor cell in the retina of the eye; used for vision in bright light

congenital (con-JEN-ih-tal) Present at birth

conjunctiva (kon-junk-TI-vah) Membrane that lines the eyelid and covers the anterior part of the sclera (white of the eye)

constipation (kon-stih-PA-shun) Infrequency of or difficulty with defecation

contraception (con-trah-SEP-shun) Prevention of an ovum's fertilization or implantation of a fertilized ovum; birth control

convergence (kon-VER-jens) The centering of both eyes on the same visual field

convulsion (kon-VUL-shun) Series of muscle spasms; seizure

cornea (KOR-ne-ah) Clear portion of the sclera that covers the anterior of the eye

coronary (KOR-on-ar-e) Referring to the heart or to the arteries supplying blood to the heart

corpus callosum (kal-O-sum) Thick bundle of myelinated nerve cell fibers, deep within the brain, that carries nerve impulses from one cerebral hemisphere to the other

corpus luteum (LU-te-um) Yellow body formed from ovarian follicle after ovulation; produces progesterone

cortex (KOR-tex) Outer layer of an organ, such as the brain, kidney, or adrenal gland

coryza (ko-RI-zah) Nasal discharge; acute coryza is the common cold

countercurrent mechanism Mechanism for concentrating urine as it flows through the distal portions of the nephron

covalent (KO-va-lent) **bond** Chemical bond formed by the sharing of electrons between atoms

CPR See Cardiopulmonary resuscitation

cranial (KRA-ne-al) Pertaining to the cranium, the part of the skull that encloses the brain; toward the head or nearer to the head.

creatine (KRE-ah-tim) **phosphate** Compound in muscle tissue that stores energy in high energy bonds

creatinine (kre-AT-ih-nin) Nitrogenous waste product eliminated in urine
crenation (kre-NA-shun) Shrinking of a cell, as when placed in a hypertonic solution
crista (KRIS-tah) Receptor for the sense of dynamic equilibrium; pl. cristae
croup (krupe) Loud barking cough associated with upper respiratory infection in children
cryoprecipitate (kri-o-pre-SIP-ih-tate) Precipitate formed when plasma is frozen and then thawed
cryptorchidism (kript-OR-kid-izm) Failure of the testis to descend into the scrotum; undescended testicle
CSF See cerebrospinal fluid
CT See computed tomography
Cushing syndrome Condition caused by overactivity of the adrenal cortex
cutaneous (ku-TA-ne-us) Referring to the skin
cuticle (KU-tih-kl) Extension of the stratum corneum that seals the space between the nail plate and the skin above the nail root
cyanosis (si-ah-NO-sis) Bluish discoloration of the skin and mucous membranes resulting from insufficient oxygen in the blood
cystic (SIS-tik) **duct** Duct that carries bile into and out of the gallbladder
cystic fibrosis (SIS-tik fi-BRO-sis) Hereditary disease involving thickened secretions and electrolyte imbalances
cystitis (sis-TI-tis) Inflammation of the urinary bladder
cytology (si-TOL-o-je) Study of cells
cytoplasm (SI-to-plazm) Substance that fills the cell, consisting of a liquid cytosol and organelles
cytosol (SI-to-sol) Liquid portion of the cytoplasm, consisting of nutrients, minerals, enzymes and other materials in water

deamination (de-am-ih-NA-shun) Removal of amino groups from proteins in metabolism
decubitus (de-KU-bih-tus) Lying down
defecation (def-eh-KA-shun) Act of eliminating undigested waste from the digestive tract
degeneration (de-jen-er-A-shun) Breakdown, as from age, injury, or disease
deglutition (deg-lu-TISH-un) Act of swallowing
dehydration (de-hi-DRA-shun) Excessive loss of body fluid
dementia (de-MEN-she-ah) Gradual and usually irreversible loss of intellectual function
denaturation (de-nah-tu-RA-shun) Change in structure of a protein, such as an enzyme, so that it can no longer function
dendrite (DEN-drite) Fiber of a neuron that conducts impulses toward the cell body
deoxyribonucleic (de-OK-se-ri-bo-nu-kle-ik) **acid (DNA)** Genetic material of the cell; makes up the chromosomes in the nucleus of the cell
depolarization (de-po-lar-ih-ZA-shun) A sudden reversal of the charge on a cell membrane.
dermal papillae (pah-PIL-le) Extensions of the dermis that project up into the epidermis; they contain blood vessels that supply the epidermis
dermatitis (der-mah-TI-tis) Inflammation of the skin
dermatome (DER-mah-tome) A region of the skin supplied by a single spinal nerve
dermatosis (der-mah-to-sis) Any skin disease
dermis (DER-mis) True skin; deeper part of the skin
dextrose (DEK-strose) Glucose, a simple sugar
diabetes insipidus (in-SIP-ih-dus) Condition due to insufficient secretion of ADH from the posterior pituitary; there is excessive loss of water
diabetes mellitus (di-ah-BE-teze mel-LI-tus) Disease of insufficient insulin in which excess glucose is found in blood and urine; characterized by abnormal metabolism of glucose, protein, and fat
diagnosis (di-ag-NO-sis) Identification of an illness
dialysis (di-AL-ih-sis) Method for separating molecules in solution based on differences in their ability to pass through a semipermeable membrane; method for removing nitrogenous waste products from the body, as by hemodialysis or peritoneal dialysis
diaphragm (DI-ah-fram) Dome-shaped muscle under the lungs that flattens during inhalation; separating membrane or structure
diaphysis (di-AF-ih-sis) Shaft of a long bone
diarrhea (di-ah-RE-ah) Abnormally frequent watery bowel movements
diarthrosis (di-ar-THRO-sis) Freely movable joint; synovial joint
diastole (di-AS-to-le) Relaxation phase of the cardiac cycle; adj., diastolic (di-as-TOL-ik)
diencephalon (di-en-SEF-ah-lon) Region of the brain between the cerebral hemispheres and the midbrain; contains the thalamus, hypothalamus, and pituitary gland
diffusion (dih-FU-zhun) Movement of molecules from a region where they are in higher concentration to a region where they are in lower concentration
digestion (di-JEST-yun) Process of breaking down food into absorbable particles
digestive system (di-JES-tiv) The system involved in taking in nutrients, converting them to a form the body can use and absorbing them into the circulation
dihydroxycholecalciferol (di-hi-drok-se-ko-le-kal-SIF-eh-rol) The active form of vitamin D
dilation (di-LA-shun) Widening of a part, such as the pupil of the eye, a blood vessel, or the uterine cervix; dilatation
disaccharide (di-SAK-ah-ride) Compound formed of two simple sugars linked together, such as sucrose and lactose
disease Illness; abnormal state in which part or all of the body does not function properly
disinfection (dis-in-FEK-shun) Killing of pathogens but not necessarily harmless microbes
dissect (dis-sekt) To cut apart or separate tissues for study
distal (DIS-tal) Farther from the origin of a structure or from a given reference point
DNA See deoxyribonucleic acid
dominant (DOM-ih-nant) Referring to a gene that is always expressed if present
dopamine (DO-pah-mene) A neurotransmitter
dorsal (DOR-sal) Toward the back; posterior
dorsiflexion (dor-sih-FLEK-shun) Bending the foot upward at the ankle
Down syndrome A congenital disorder usually due to an extra chromosome 21; trisomy 21
duct Tube or vessel
ductus deferens (DEF-er-enz) Tube that carries sperm cells from the testis to the urethra; vas deferens
duodenum (du-o-DE-num) First portion of the small intestine
dura mater (DU-rah MA-ter) Outermost layer of the meninges
dysmenorrhea (dis-men-o-RE-ah) Painful or difficult menstruation
dyspnea (disp-NE-ah) Difficult or labored breathing

eccrine (EK-rin) Referring to sweat glands that regulate body temperature and vent directly to the surface of the skin through a pore
ECG See electrocardiograph
echocardiograph (ek-o-KAR-de-o-graf) Instrument to study the heart by means of ultrasound; the record produced is an echocardiogram
eclampsia (eh-KLAMP-se-ah) Serious and sometimes fatal condition involving convulsions, liver damage, and kidney failure that can develop from pregnancy-induced hypertension
ectopic (ek-TOP-ik) Out of a normal place, as a pregnancy or heartbeat

eczema (EK-ze-mah) See atopic dermatitis
edema (eh-DE-mah) Accumulation of fluid in the tissue spaces
EEG See electroencephalograph
effector (ef-FEK-tor) Muscle or gland that responds to a stimulus; effector organ
efferent (EF-fer-ent) Carrying away from a given point, such as a motor neuron that carries nerve impulses away from the central nervous system
effusion (eh-FU-zhun) Escape of fluid into a cavity or space; the fluid itself
ejaculation (e-jak-u-LA-shun) Expulsion of semen through the urethra
EKG See electrocardiograph
electrocardiograph (e-lek-tro-KAR-de-o-graf) **(ECG, EKG)** Instrument to study the electrical activity of the heart; record made is an electrocardiogram
electroencephalograph (e-lek-tro-en-SEF-ah-lo-graf) **(EEG)** Instrument used to study electrical activity of the brain; record made is an electroencephalogram
electrolyte (e-LEK-tro-lite) Compound that separates into ions in solution; substance that conducts an electrical current in solution
electron (e-LEK-tron) Negatively charged particle located in an energy level outside the nucleus of an atom
electrophoresis (e-lek-tro-fo-RE-sis) Separation of components in a mixture by passing an electrical current through it; components separate on the basis of their charge
element (EL-eh-ment) One of the substances from which all matter is made; substance that cannot be decomposed into a simpler substance
elephantiasis (el-eh-fan-TI-ah-sis) Enlargement of the extremities due to blockage of lymph flow by small filariae (fi-LA-re-e) worms
embolism (EM-bo-lizm) The condition of having an embolus (obstruction in the circulation)
embolus (EM-bo-lus) Blood clot or other obstruction in the circulation
embryo (EM-bre-o) Developing offspring during the first 2 months of pregnancy
emesis (EM-eh-sis) Vomiting
emphysema (em-fih-SE-mah) Pulmonary disease characterized by dilation and destruction of the alveoli
emulsify (e-MUL-sih-fi) To break up fats into small particles; n., emulsification
endarterectomy (end-ar-ter-EK-to-me) Procedure to remove plaque associated with athersclerosis from the lining of a vessel
endocardium (en-do-KAR-de-um) Membrane that lines the heart chambers and covers the valves
endocrine (EN-do-krin) Referring to a gland that secretes directly into the bloodstream
endocrine system The system composed of glands that secrete hormones
endocytosis (en-do-si-TO-sis) Movement of large amounts of material into a cell (*e.g.*, phagocytosis and pinocytosis)
endolymph (EN-do-limf) Fluid that fills the membranous labyrinth of the inner ear
endomysium (en-do-MIS-e-um) Connective tissue around an individual muscle fiber
endometrium (en-do-ME-tre-um) Lining of the uterus
endoplasmic reticulum (en-do-PLAS-mik re-TIK-u-lum) **(ER)** Network of membranes in the cytoplasm of a cell; may be smooth or rough based on absence or presence of ribosomes
end-organ Modified ending on a dendrite that functions as a sensory receptor
endorphin (en-DOR-fin) Pain-relieving substance released naturally from the brain
endosteum (en-DOS-te-um) Thin membrane that lines the marrow cavity of a bone
endothelium (en-do-THE-le-um) Epithelium that lines the heart, blood vessels, and lymphatic vessels
enucleation (e-nu-kle-A-shun) Removal of the eyeball
enzyme (EN-zime) Organic catalyst; speeds the rate of a reaction but is not changed in the reaction
eosinophil (e-o-SIN-o-fil) Granular white blood cell that shows beadlike, bright pink cytoplasmic granules when stained with acid stain; acidophil
epicardium (ep-ih-KAR-de-um) Membrane that forms the outermost layer of the heart wall and is continuous with the lining of the fibrous pericardium; visceral pericardium
epicondyle (ep-ih-KON-dile) Small projection on a bone above a condyle
epidemic (ep-ih-DEM-ik) Occurrence of a disease among many people in a given region at the same time
epidermis (ep-ih-DER-mis) Outermost layer of the skin
epididymis (ep-ih-DID-ih-mis) Coiled tube on the surface of the testis in which sperm cells are stored and in which they mature
epigastric (ep-ih-GAS-trik) Pertaining to the region just inferior to the sternum (breastbone)
epiglottis (ep-e-GLOT-is) Leaf-shaped cartilage that covers the larynx during swallowing
epilepsy (EP-ih-lep-se) Chronic disorder of the nervous system involving abnormal electrical activity of the brain; characterized by seizures of varying severity
epimysium (ep-ih-MIS-e-um) Sheath of fibrous connective tissue that encloses a muscle
epinephrine (ep-ih-NEF-rin) Neurotransmitter and hormone; released from neurons of the sympathetic nervous system and from the adrenal medulla; adrenaline
epiphysis (eh-PIF-ih-sis) End of a long bone; adj epiphyseal (ep-ih-FIZ-e-al)
episiotomy (eh-piz-e-OT-o-me) Cutting of the perineum between the vaginal opening and the anus to reduce tissue tearing in childbirth
epistaxis (ep-e-STAK-sis) Nosebleed
epithelium (ep-ih-THE-le-um) One of the four main types of tissue; forms glands, covers surfaces, and lines cavities; adj., epithelial
EPO See erythropoietin
equilibrium (e-kwih-LIB-re-um) Sense of balance
ER See endoplasmic reticulum
eruption (e-RUP-shun) Raised skin lesion; rash
erythema (er-eh-THE-mah) Redness of the skin
erythrocyte (eh-RITH-ro-site) Red blood cell
erythropoietin (EPO) (eh-rith-ro-POY-eh-tin) Hormone released from the kidney that stimulates red blood cell production in the red bone marrow
esophagus (eh-SOF-ah-gus) Tube that carries food from the throat to the stomach
estrogen (ES-tro-jen) Group of female sex hormones that promotes development of the uterine lining and maintains secondary sex characteristics
etiology (e-te-OL-o-je) Study of the cause of a disease or the theory of its origin
eustachian (u-STA-shun) **tube** Tube that connects the middle ear cavity to the throat; auditory tube
eversion (e-VER-zhun) Turning outward, with reference to movement of the foot
excitability In cells, the ability to transmit an electrical current along the plasma membrane
excoriation (eks-ko-re-A-shun) Scratch into the skin
excretion (eks-KRE-shun) Removal and elimination of metabolic waste products from the blood
exfoliation (eks-fo-le-A-shun) Loss of cells from the surface of tissue, such as the skin
exhalation (eks-hah-LA-shun) Expulsion of air from the lungs; expiration
exocrine (EK-so-krin) Referring to a gland that secretes through a duct
exocytosis (eks-o-si-TO-sis) Movement of large amounts of material out of the cell using vesicles

exophthalmos (ek-sof-THAL-mos) Protrusion (bulging) of the eyes, commonly seen in Graves disease
extension (eks-TEN-shun) Motion that increases the angle at a joint
extracellular (EK-strah-sel-u-lar) Outside the cell
extremity (ek-STREM-ih-te) Limb; an arm or leg

facilitated diffusion Movement of material across the plasma membrane as it would normally flow by diffusion but using transporters to speed movement
fallopian (fah-LO-pe-an) **tube** See oviduct
fascia (FASH-e-ah) Band or sheet of fibrous connective tissue
fascicle (FAS-ih-kl) Small bundle, as of muscle cells or nerve cell fibers
fat Type of lipid composed of glycerol and fatty acids; triglyceride
febrile (FEB-ril) Pertaining to fever
fecalith (FE-kah-lith) Hardened piece of fecal material that may cause obstruction
feces (FE-seze) Waste material discharged from the large intestine; excrement; stool
feedback Return of information into a system, so that it can be used to regulate that system
fertilization (fer-til-ih-ZA-shun) Union of an ovum and a spermatozoon
fetus (FE-tus) Developing offspring from the third month of pregnancy until birth
fever (FE-ver) Abnormally high body temperature
fibrillation (fih-brih-LA-shun) Very rapid, uncoordinated beating of the heart
fibrin (FI-brin) Blood protein that forms a blood clot
fibrinogen (fi-BRIN-o-jen) Plasma protein that is converted to fibrin in blood clotting
filtration (fil-TRA-shun) Movement of material through a semipermeable membrane under mechanical force
fimbriae (FIM-bre-e) Fringelike extensions of the oviducts that sweep a released ovum into the oviduct
fissure (FISH-ure) Deep groove
flaccid (FLAK-sid) Flabby, limp, soft
flagellum (flah-JEL-lum) Long whiplike extension from a cell used for locomotion; pl., flagella
flatus (FLA-tus) Gas in the digestive tract; condition of having gas is flatulence (FLAT-u-lens)
flexion (FLEK-shun) Bending motion that decreases the angle between bones at a joint
follicle (FOL-lih-kl) Sac or cavity, such as the ovarian follicle or hair follicle
follicle-stimulating hormone (FSH) Hormone produced by the anterior pituitary that stimulates development of ova in the ovary and spermatozoa in the testes
fontanel (fon-tah-NEL) Membranous area in the infant skull where bone has not yet formed; also spelled fontanelle; "soft spot"
foramen (fo-RA-men) Opening or passageway, as into or through a bone; pl., foramina (fo-RAM-in-ah)
foramen magnum Large opening in the occipital bone of the skull through which the spinal cord passes to join the brain
formed elements Cells and cell fragments in the blood
fornix (FOR-niks) A recess or archlike structure
fossa (FOS-sah) Hollow or depression, as in a bone; pl., fossae (FOS-se)
fovea (FO-ve-ah) Small pit or cup-shaped depression in a surface; the fovea centralis near the center of the retina is the point of sharpest vision
frontal (FRONT-al) Describing a plane that divides a structure into anterior and posterior parts
FSH See follicle-stimulating hormone
fulcrum (FUL-krum) Pivot point in a lever system; joint in the skeletal system
fundus (FUN-dus) The deepest portion of an organ, such as the eye or the uterus
fungus (FUN-gus) Type of plantlike microorganism; yeast or mold; pl., fungi (FUN-ji)

gamete (GAM-ete) Reproductive cell; ovum or spermatozoon
gamma globulin (GLOB-u-lin) Protein fraction in the blood plasma that contains antibodies
ganglion (GANG-le-on) Collection of nerve cell bodies located outside the central nervous system
gangrene (GANG-grene) Death of tissue accompanied by bacterial invasion and putrefaction
gastric-inhibitory peptide (GIP) Hormone from the duodenum that inhibits release of gastric juice and stimulates release of insulin from the pancreas
gastrin (GAS-trin) Hormone released from the stomach that stimulates stomach activity
gastrointestinal (gas-tro-in-TES-tih-nal) **(GI)** Pertaining to the stomach and intestine or the digestive tract as a whole
gene Hereditary factor; portion of the DNA on a chromosome
genetic (jeh-NET-ik) Pertaining to the genes or heredity
genotype (JEN-o-tipe) Genetic make-up of an organism
gestation (jes-TA-shun) Period of development from conception to birth
GH See growth hormone
GI See gastrointestinal
gigantism (ji-GAN-tizm) Excessive growth due to oversecretion of growth hormone in childhood
gingiva (JIN-jih-vah) Tissue around the teeth; gum
glans The enlarged distal portion of the penis
glaucoma (glaw-KO-mah) Disorder involving increased fluid pressure within the eye
glial cells (GLI-al) The connective tissue cells of the nervous system; neuroglia
glioma (gli-O-mah) Tumor of neuroglial tissue
glomerular (glo-MER-u-lar) **filtrate** Fluid and dissolved materials that leave the blood and enter the kidney nephron through the glomerular (Bowman) capsule
glomerulonephritis (glo-mer-u-lo-nef-RI-tis) Kidney disease often resulting from antibodies to a streptococcal infection
glomerulus (glo-MER-u-lus) Cluster of capillaries in the glomerular (Bowman) capsule of the nephron
glottis (GLOT-is) Space between the vocal cords
glucagon (GLU-kah-gon) Hormone from the pancreatic islets that raises blood glucose level
glucocorticoid (glu-ko-KOR-tih-koyd) Steroid hormone from the adrenal cortex that raises nutrients in the blood during times of stress, *e.g.*, cortisol
glucose (GLU-kose) Simple sugar; main energy source for the cells; dextrose
glycemic (gli-SE-mik) **effect** Measure of how rapidly a food raises the blood glucose level and stimulates release of insulin
glycogen (GLI-ko-jen) Compound built from glucose molecules that is stored for energy in liver and muscles
glycolysis (gli-KOL-ih-sis) First, anaerobic phase of the metabolic breakdown of glucose for energy
glycosuria (gli-ko-SU-re-ah) Presence of glucose in the urine
goblet cell A single-celled gland that secretes mucus
goiter (GOY-ter) Enlargement of the thyroid gland
Golgi (GOL-je) **apparatus** System of membranes in the cell that formulates special substances; also called Golgi complex
gonad (GO-nad) Sex gland; ovary or testis
gonadotropin (gon-ah-do-TRO-pin) Hormone that acts on a reproductive gland (ovary or testis) *e.g.*, FSH, LH
gout Type of arthritis caused by a metabolic disturbance

Graafian (GRAF-e-an) **follicle** See ovarian follicle
gram (g) Basic unit of weight in the metric system
gram stain Procedure used to color microorganisms for viewing under the microscope
granulocyte (GRAN-u-lo-site) Leukocyte with visible granules in the cytoplasm when stained
Graves disease Common form of hyperthyroidism
gray matter Nervous tissue composed of unmyelinated fibers and cell bodies
greater vestibular (ves-TIB-u-lar) **gland** Gland that secretes mucus into the vagina; Bartholin gland
growth hormone (GH) Hormone produced by anterior pituitary that promotes growth of tissues; somatotropin
gustatory (GUS-tah-to-re) Pertaining to the sense of taste (gustation)
gyrus (JI-rus) Raised area of the cerebral cortex; pl., gyri (JI-ri)

Haversian (ha-VER-shan) **canal** Channel in the center of an osteon (haversian system), a subunit of compact bone
Haversian system See Osteon
hay fever Seasonal allergy often due to pollen
heart (hart) The organ that pumps blood through the cardiovascular system
helminth (HEL-minth) Worm
hemapheresis (hem-ah-fer-E-sis) Return of blood components to a donor following separation and removal of desired components
hematocrit (he-MAT-o-krit) **(Hct)** Volume percentage of red blood cells in whole blood; packed cell volume
hematoma (he-mah-TO-mah) Tumor or swelling filled with blood
hematuria (hem-ah-TU-re-ah) Blood in the urine
hemocytometer (he-mo-si-TOM-eh-ter) Device used to count blood cells under the microscope
hemodialysis (he-mo-di-AL-ih-sis) Removal of impurities from the blood by their passage through a semipermeable membrane in a fluid bath
hemoglobin (he-mo-GLO-bin) **(Hb)** Iron-containing protein in red blood cells that binds oxygen
hemolysis (he-MOL-ih-sis) Rupture of red blood cells; v., hemolyze (HE-mo-lize)
hemolytic (he-mo-LIT-ik) **disease of the newborn (HDN)** Condition that results from Rh incompatibility between a mother and her fetus; erythroblastosis fetalis
hemophilia (he-mo-FIL-e-ah) Hereditary bleeding disorder associated with a lack of clotting factors in the blood
hemopoiesis (he-mo-poy-E-sis) Production of blood cells; hematopoiesis
hemorrhage (HEM-eh-rij) Loss of blood
hemorrhoids (HEM-o-royds) Varicose veins in the rectum
hemostasis (he-mo-STA-sis) Stoppage of bleeding
hemothorax (he-mo-THOR-aks) Accumulation of blood in the pleural space
heparin (HEP-ah-rin) Substance that prevents blood clotting; anticoagulant
hepatitis (hep-ah-TI-tis) Inflammation of the liver
heredity (he-RED-ih-te) Transmission of characteristics from parent to offspring by means of the genes; the genetic makeup of the individual
hereditary (he-RED-ih-tar-e) Transmitted or transmissible through the genes; familial
hernia (HER-ne-ah) Protrusion of an organ or tissue through the wall of the cavity in which it is normally enclosed
heterozygous (het-er-o-ZI-gus) Having unmatched alleles for a given trait; hybrid
hilum (HI-lum) Indented region of an organ where vessels and nerves enter or leave
hippocampus (hip-o-KAM-pus) Sea horse-shaped region of the limbic system that functions in learning and formation of long-term memory
histamine (HIS-tah-mene) Substance released from tissues during an antigen–antibody reaction
histology (his-TOL-o-je) Study of tissues
HIV See human immunodeficiency virus
Hodgkin disease Chronic malignant disease of lymphoid tissue
homeostasis (ho-me-o-STA-sis) State of balance within the body; maintenance of body conditions within set limits
homozygous (ho-mo-ZI-gus) Having identical alleles for a given trait; purebred
hormone Secretion of an endocrine gland; chemical messenger that has specific regulatory effects on certain other cells
host An organism in or on which a parasite lives
human chorionic gonadotropin (ko-re-ON-ik gon-ah-do-TRO-pin) **(hCG)** Hormone produced by embryonic cells soon after implantation that maintains the corpus luteum
human immunodeficiency virus (HIV) The virus that causes AIDS
human placental lactogen (hPL) Hormone produced by the placenta that prepares the breasts for lactation and maintains nutrient levels in maternal blood
humoral (HU-mor-al) Pertaining to body fluids, such as immunity based on antibodies circulating in the blood
Huntington disease Progressive degenerative disorder carried by a dominant gene
hyaline (HI-ah-lin) Clear, glasslike; referring to a type of cartilage
hydatidiform (hi-dah-TID-ih-form) **mole** Benign overgrowth of placental tissue
hydrocephalus (hi-dro-SEF-ah-lus) Abnormal accumulation of CSF within the brain
hydrolysis (hi-DROL-ih-sis) Splitting of large molecules by the addition of water, as in digestion
hydrophilic (hi-dro-FIL-ik) Mixing with or dissolving in water, such as salts; literally "water-loving"
hydrophobic (hi-dro-FO-bik) Repelling and not dissolving in water, such as fats; literally "water-fearing"
hymen Fold of membrane near the opening of the vaginal canal
hypercapnia (hi-per-KAP-ne-ah) Increased level of carbon dioxide in the blood
hyperglycemia (hi-per-gli-SE-me-ah) Abnormal increase in the amount of glucose in the blood
hyperopia (hi-per-O-pe-ah) Farsightedness
hyperpnea (hi-PERP-ne-ah) Abnormal increase in the depth and rate of respiration
hypersensitivity (hi-per-SEN-sih-tiv-ih-te) Exaggerated reaction of the immune system to a substance that is normally harmless to most people; allergy
hypertension (hi-per-TEN-shun) High blood pressure
hypertonic (hi-per-TON-ik) Describing a solution that is more concentrated than the fluids within a cell
hypertrophy (hy-PER-tro-fe) Enlargement or overgrowth of an organ or part
hyperventilation (hi-per-ven-tih-LA-shun) Increased amount of air entering the alveoli of the lungs due to deep and rapid respiration
hypocapnia (hi-po-KAP-ne-ah) Decreased level of carbon dioxide in the blood
hypochondriac (hi-po-KON-dre-ak) Pertaining to a region just inferior to the ribs
hypogastric (hi-po-GAS-trik) Pertaining to an area inferior to the stomach or the most inferior midline region of the abdomen
hypoglycemia (hi-po-gli-SE-me-ah) Abnormal decrease in the amount of glucose in the blood
hypophysis (hi-POF-ih-sis) Pituitary gland
hypopnea (hi-POP-ne-ah) Decrease in the rate and depth of breathing
hypospadias (hi-po-SPA-de-as) Opening of the urethra on the undersurface of the penis

hypotension (hi-po-TEN-shun) Low blood pressure
hypothalamus (hi-po-THAL-ah-mus) Region of the brain that controls the pituitary and maintains homeostasis
hypothermia (hi-po-THER-me-ah) Abnormally low body temperature
hypotonic (hi-po-TON-ik) Describing a solution that is less concentrated than the fluids within a cell
hypoventilation (hi-po-ven-tih-LA-shun) Insufficient amount of air entering the alveoli
hypoxemia (hi-pok-SE-me-ah) Lower than normal concentration of oxygen in arterial blood
hypoxia (hi-POK-se-ah) Lower than normal level of oxygen in the tissues
hysterectomy (his-ter-EK-to-me) Surgical removal of the uterus

iatrogenic (i-at-ro-JEN-ik) Resulting from the adverse effects of treatment
ICSH See Luteinizing hormone
idiopathic (id-e-o-PATH-ik) Describing a disease without known cause
ileum (IL-e-um) The last portion of the small intestine
ileus (IL-e-us) Iintestinal obstruction caused by lack of peristalsis or by muscle contraction
iliac (IL-e-ak) Pertaining to the ilium, the upper portion of the hipbone
immunity (ih-MU-nih-te) Power of an individual to resist or overcome the effects of a particular disease or other harmful agent
immunization (ih-mu-nih-ZA-shun) Use of a vaccine to produce immunity; vaccination
immunodeficiency (im-u-no-de-FISH-en-se) Any failure of the immune system
immunoglobulin (im-mu-no-GLOB-u-lin) **(Ig)** See antibody
immunotherapy (im-mu-no-THER-a-pe) Stimulation of the immune system to fight disease, such as cancer
impetigo (im-peh-TI-go) Acute, contagious staphylococcal or streptococcal skin infection
implantation (im-plan-TA-shun) The embedding of the fertilized egg into the lining of the uterus
incidence (IN-sih-dense) Range of occurrence of a disease
infarct (IN-farkt) Area of tissue damaged from lack of blood supply caused by a vessel blockage
infection (in-FEK-shun) Invasion by pathogens
infectious mononucleosis (mon-o-nu-kle-O-sis) Acute viral infection associated with enlargement of the lymph nodes
inferior (in-FE-re-or) Below or lower
inferior vena cava (VE-nah KA-vah) Large vein that drains the lower part of the body and empties into the right atrium of the heart
infertility (in-fer-TIL-ih-te) Decreased ability to reproduce
inflammation (in-flah-MA-shun) Response of tissues to injury; characterized by heat, redness, swelling, and pain
influenza (in-flu-EN-zah) Acute contagious viral disease of the upper respiratory tract
infundibulum (in-fun-DIB-u-lum) Stalk that connects the pituitary gland to the hypothalamus of the brain
ingestion (in-JES-chun) The intake of food
inguinal (IN-gwih-nal) Pertaining to the groin region or the region of the inguinal canal
inhalation (in-hah-LA-shun) Drawing of air into the lungs; inspiration
insertion (in-SER-shun) Muscle attachment connected to a movable part
isthmus (IS-mus) Narrow band, such as the band that connects the two lobes of the thyroid gland
infertility Lower than normal ability to reproduce
insulin (IN-su-lin) Hormone from the pancreatic islets that lowers blood glucose level
integument (in-TEG-u-ment) Skin; adj., integumentary
integumentary system The skin and all its associated structures
intercalated (in-TER-cah-la-ted) **disk** A modified plasma membrane in cardiac tissue that allows rapid transfer of electrical impulses between cells
intercellular (in-ter-SEL-u-lar) Between cells
intercostal (in-ter-KOS-tal) Between the ribs
interferon (in-ter-FERE-on) **(IFN)** Group of substances released from virus-infected cells that prevent spread of infection to other cells; also nonspecifically boost the immune system
interleukin (in-ter-LU-kin) A substance released by a T cell or macrophage that stimulates other cells of the immune system
interneuron (in-ter-NU-ron) A nerve cell that transmits impulses within the central nervous system
interphase (IN-ter-faze) Stage in the life of a cell between one mitosis and the next when a cell is not dividing
interstitial (in-ter-STISH-al) Between; pertaining to spaces or structures in an organ between active tissues
interstitial cell–stimulating hormone (ICSH) see Luteinizing hormone
intestine (in-TES-tin) Organ of the digestive tract between the stomach and the anus, consisting of the small and large intestine
intracellular (in-trah-SEL-u-lar) Within a cell
intussusception (in-tuh-suh-SEP-shun) Slipping of a part of the intestine into a part below it
inversion (in-VER-zhun) Turning inward, with reference to movement of the foot
ion (I-on) Charged particle formed when an electrolyte goes into solution
ionic bond Chemical bond formed by the exchange of electrons between atoms
iris (I-ris) Circular colored region of the eye around the pupil
ischemia (is-KE-me-ah) Lack of blood supply to an area
islets (I-lets) Groups of cells in the pancreas that produce hormones; islets of Langerhans (LAHNG-er-hanz)
isometric (i-so-MET-rik) **contraction** Muscle contraction in which there is no change in muscle length but an increase in muscle tension, as in pushing against an immovable force
isotonic (i-so-TON-ik) Describing a solution that has the same concentration as the fluid within a cell
isotonic contraction Muscle contraction in which the tone within the muscle remains the same but the muscle shortens to produce movement
isotope (I-so-tope) Form of an element that has the same atomic number as another form of that element but a different atomic weight; isotopes differ in their numbers of neutrons

jaundice (JAWN-dis) Yellowish discoloration of the skin that is usually due to the presence of bile in the blood
jejunum (je-JU-num) Second portion of the small intestine
joint Area of junction between two or more bones; articulation
juxtaglomerular (juks-tah-glo-MER-u-lar) **(JG) apparatus** Structure in the kidney composed of cells of the afferent arteriole and distal convoluted tubule that secretes the enzyme renin when blood pressure decreases below a certain level

karyotype (KAR-e-o-tipe) Picture of the chromosomes arranged according to size and form
keloid (KE-loyd) Mass or raised area that results from excess production of scar tissue
keratin (KER-ah-tin) Protein that thickens and protects the skin; makes up hair and nails
ketoacidosis (ke-to-as-ih-DO-sis) Acidosis that results from accumulation of ketone bodies in the blood
kidney (KID-ne) Organ of excretion
kilocalorie (kil-o-KAL-o-re) A measure of the energy content of food; technically,

the amount of heat needed to raise l kg of water 1° centigrade
kinesthesia (kin-es-THE-ze-ah) Sense of body movement
Klinefelter (KLINE-fel-ter) **syndrome** Genetic disorder involving abnormal sex chromosomes, usually an extra X chromosome
Kupffer (KOOP-fer) **cells** Macrophages in the liver that help to fight infection
Kussmaul (KOOS-mowl) **respiration** Deep, rapid respiration characteristic of acidosis (overly acidic body fluids) as seen in uncontrolled diabetes.
kwashiorkor (kwash-e-OR-kor) Severe protein and energy malnutrition seen in children after weaning
kyphosis (ki-FO-sis) Exaggerated lumbar curve of the spine

labium (LA-be-um) Lip; pl labia (LA-be-ah)
labyrinth (LAB-ih-rinth) Inner ear, named for its complex shape
laceration (las-er-A-shun) Rough, jagged wound of the skin
lacrimal (LAK-rih-mal) Referring to tears or the tear glands
lactation (lak-TA-shun) Secretion of milk
lacteal (LAK-te-al) Lymphatic capillary that drains digested fats from the villi of the small intestine
lactic (LAK-tik) **acid** Organic acid that accumulates in muscle cells functioning without oxygen
laryngeal (lah-RIN-je-al) **pharynx** Lowest portion of the pharynx, opening into the larynx and esophpagus
larynx (LAR-inks) Structure between the pharynx and trachea that contains the vocal cords; voice box
laser (LA-zer) Device that produces a very intense beam of light
lateral (LAT-er-al) Farther from the midline; toward the side
lens Biconvex structure of the eye that changes in thickness to accommodate for near and far vision; crystalline lens
lesion (LE-zhun) Wound or local injury
leukemia (lu-KE-me-ah) Malignant blood disease characterized by abnormal development of white blood cells
leukocyte (LU-ko-site) White blood cell
leukocytosis (lu-ko-si-TO-sis) Increase in the number of white cells in the blood, such as during infection
leukopenia (lu-ko-PE-ne-ah) Deficiency of leukocytes in the blood
leukoplakia (lu-ko-PLA-ke-ah) Thickened white patches on the oral mucous membranes, often due to smoking
LH See luteinizing hormone
ligament (LIG-ah-ment) Band of connective tissue that connects a bone to another bone; thickened portion or fold of the peritoneum that supports an organ or attaches it to another organ
limbic (LIM- bik) **system** Area between the brain's cerebrum and diencephalon that is involved in emotional states and behavior
lipid (LIP-id) Type of organic compound, one example of which is a fat
liter (LE-ter) **(L)** Basic unit of volume in the metric system; 1000 mL; 1.06 qt.
lithotripsy (LITH-o-trip-se) Use of external shock waves to shatter stones (calculi)
loop of Henle Hairpin shaped segment of the renal tubule between the proximal and distal convoluted tubules
lordosis (lor-DO-sis) Exaggerated lumbar curve of the spine
lumbar (LUM-bar) Pertaining to the region of the spine between the thoracic vertebrae and the sacrum
lumen (LU-men) Central opening of an organ or vessel
lung Organ of respiration
lunula (LU-nu-la) The pale half-moon shaped area at the proximal end of the nail
lupus erythematosus (LU-pus er-ih-the-mah-TO-sis) Chronic inflammatory autoimmune disease that involves the skin and sometimes other organs
luteinizing (LU-te-in-i-zing) **hormone** Hormone produced by the anterior pituitary that induces ovulation and formation of the corpus luteum in females; in males, it stimulates cells in the testes to produce testosterone and may be called *interstitial cell–stimulating hormone (ICSH)*
lymph (limf) Fluid in the lymphatic system
lymphadenitis (lim-fad-en-I-tis) Inflammation of lymph nodes
lymphadenopathy (lim-fad-en-OP-ah-the) Any disorder of lymph nodes
lymphangitis (lim-fan-JI-tis) Inflammation of lymphatic vessels
lymphatic duct (lim-FAH-tic) Vessel of the lymphatic system
lymphatic system System consisting of the lymphatic vessels and lymphoid tissue; involved in immunity, digestion, and fluid balance
lymph node Mass of lymphoid tissue along the path of a lymphatic vessel that filters lymph and harbors white blood cells active in immunity
lymphadenitis (lim-fad-en-I-tis) Inflammation of lymph nodes
lymphedema (lim-feh-DE-mah) Edema due to obstruction of lymph flow
lymphocyte (LIM-fo-site) Agranular white blood cell that functions in immunity
lymphoma (lim-FO-mah) Any tumor, benign or malignant, that occurs in lymphoid tissue.
lysosome (LI-so-some) Cell organelle that contains digestive enzymes
macrophage (MAK-ro-faj) Large phagocytic cell that develops from a monocyte; presents antigen to lymphocytes in immune response
macula (MAK-u-lah) Spot; flat, discolored spot on the skin, such as a freckle or measles lesion; also called macule; Small yellow spot in the retina of the eye that contains the fovea, the point of sharpest vision; receptor for the sense of static equilibrium
magnetic resonance imaging (MRI) Method for studying tissue based on nuclear movement after exposure to radio waves in a powerful magnetic field
major histocompatibility complex (MHC) Group of genes that codes for specific proteins (antigens) on the surface of cells; these antigens are important in cross-matching for tissue transplantation; they are also important in immune reactions
malignant (mah-LIG-nant) Describing a tumor that spreads; describing a disorder that tends to become worse and cause death
malnutrition (mal-nu-TRISH-un) State resulting from lack of food, lack of an essential component of the diet, or faulty use of food in the diet
MALT Mucosal-associated lymphoid tissue; tissue in the mucous membranes that helps fight infection
mammary (MAM-er-e) **gland** Breast
mammogram (MAM-o-gram) Radiographic study of the breast
marasmus (mah-RAZ-mus) Severe malnutrition in infants
mastectomy (mas-TEK-to-me) Removal of the breast; mammectomy
mastication (mas-tih-KA-shun) Act of chewing
mastitis (mas-TI-tis) Inflammation of the breast
matrix (MA-triks) The nonliving background material in a tissue; the intercellular material
meatus (me-A-tus) Short channel or passageway, as in a bone
medial (ME-de-al) Nearer the midline of the body
mediastinum (me-de-as-TI-num) Region between the lungs and the organs and vessels it contains
medulla (meh-DUL-lah) Inner region of an organ; marrow
medullary (MED-u-lar-e) **cavity** Channel at the center of a long bone that contains bone marrow
medulla oblongata (ob-long-GAH-tah) Part of the brain stem that connects the brain to the spinal cord
megakaryocyte (meg-ah-KAR-e-o-site) Very large cell that gives rise to blood platelets

meibomian (mi-BO-me-an) **gland** Gland that produces a secretion that lubricates the eyelashes
meiosis (mi-O-sis) Process of cell division that halves the chromosome number in the formation of the reproductive cells
melanin (MEL-ah-nin) Dark pigment found in skin, hair, parts of the eye, and certain parts of the brain
melanocyte (MEL-ah-no-site) Cell that produces melanin
melanoma (mel-ah-NO-mah) Malignant tumor of melanocytes
melatonin (mel-ah-TO-nin) Hormone produced by the pineal gland
membrane Thin sheet of tissue
Mendelian (men-DE-le-en) **laws** Principles of heredity discovered by an Austrian monk named Gregor Mendel
meninges (men-IN-jeze) Three layers of fibrous membranes that cover the brain and spinal cord
menopause (MEN-o-pawz) Time during which menstruation ceases
menses (MEN-seze) Monthly flow of blood from the female reproductive tract
menstruation (men-stru-A-shun) The period of menstrual flow
mesentery (MES-en-ter-e) Membranous peritoneal ligament that attaches the small intestine to the dorsal abdominal wall
mesocolon (mes-o-KO-lon) Peritoneal ligament that attaches the colon to the dorsal abdominal wall
mesothelium (mes-o-THE-le-um) Epithelial tissue found in serous membranes
metabolic rate Rate at which energy is released from nutrients in the cells
metabolism (meh-TAB-o-lizm) All the physical and chemical processes by which an organism is maintained
metaphase (MET-ah-faze) Second stage of mitosis, during which the chromsomes line up across the equator of the cell
metarteriole (met-ar-TE-re-ole) Small vessel that connects the arterial system directly with the venous system in a blood shunt; thoroughfare channel
metastasis (meh-TAS-tah-sis) Spread of tumor cells; pl., metastases (meh-TAS-tah-seze)
meter (ME-ter) **(m)** Basic unit of length in the metric system; 1.1 yards
MHC See Major histocompatibility complex
microbiology (mi-kro-bi-OL-o-je) Study of microscopic organisms
micrometer (MI-kro-me-ter) (μm) 1/1000th of a millimeter; micron; an instrument for measuring through a microscope (pronounced mi-KROM-eh-ter)
microorganism (mi-kro-OR-gan-izm) Microscopic organism
microscope (MI-kro-skope) Magnifying instrument used to examine cells and other structures not visible with the naked eye; examples are the compound light microscope, transmission electron microscope (TEM) and scanning electron microscope (SEM)
microvilli (mi-kro-VIL-li) Small projections of the plasma membrane that increase surface area; sing., microvillus
micturition (mik-tu-RISH-un) Act of urination; voiding of the urinary bladder
midbrain Upper portion of the brainstem
mineral (MIN-er-al) Inorganic substance; in the diet, an element needed in small amounts for health
mineralocorticoid (min-er-al-o-KOR-tih-koyd) Steroid hormone from the adrenal cortex that regulates electrolyte balance, e.g. aldosterone
mitochondria (mi-to-KON-dre-ah) Cell organelles that manufacture ATP with the energy released from the oxidation of nutrients; sing., mitochondrion
mitosis (mi-TO-sis) Type of cell division that produces two daughter cells exactly like the parent cell
mitral (MI-tral) **valve** Valve between the left atrium and left ventricle of the heart; left AV valve; bicuspid valve
mixture Blend of two or more substances
molecule (MOL-eh-kule) Particle formed by chemical bonding of two or more atoms; smallest subunit of a compound
monocyte (MON-o-site) Phagocytic agranular white blood cell
monosaccharide (mon-o-SAK-ah-ride) Simple sugar; basic unit of carbohydrates
morbidity (mor-BID-ih-te) **rate** Proportion of people with a specific disease in a given population per unit of time
mortality (mor-TAL-ih-te) **rate** Percentage of a population that dies from a given disease within a period of time
motor (MO-tor) Describing structures or activities involved in transmitting impulses away from the central nervous system; efferent
motor end plate Region of a muscle cell membrane that receives nervous stimulation
motor unit Group consisting of a single neuron and all the muscle fibers it stimulates
mouth Proximal opening of the digestive tract where food is ingested, chewed, mixed with saliva and swallowed
MRI See magnetic resonance imaging
mucosa (mu-KO-sah) Lining membrane that produces mucus; mucous membrane
mucus (MU-kus) Thick protective fluid secreted by mucous membranes and glands; adj., mucous
multiple (SKLE-ro-SIS) **sclerosis** Disease that affects the myelin sheath around axons leading to neuron degeneration
murmur Abnormal heart sound
muscle (MUS-l) Tissue that contracts to produce movement; includes skeletal, smooth and cardiac types; adj., muscular
muscular (MUS-ku-lar) **system** The system of skeletal muscles that moves the skeleton, supports and protects the organs and maintains posture
mutagen (MU-tah-jen) Agent that causes mutation; adj., mutagenic (mu-tah-JEN-ik)
mutation (mu-TA-shun) Change in a gene or a chromosome
myalgia (mi-AL-je-ah) Muscular pain
mycology (mi-KOL-o-je) Study of fungi (yeasts and molds)
myelin (MI-el-in) Fatty material that covers and insulates the axons of some neurons
myocardium (mi-o-KAR-de-um) Middle layer of the heart wall; heart muscle
myoglobin (MI-o-glo-bin) Compound that stores oxygen in muscle cells
myoma (mi-O-mah) Usually benign tumor of the uterus; fibroma; fibroid
myometrium (mi-o-ME-tre-um) The muscular layer of the uterus
myopia (mi-O-pe-ah) Nearsightedness
myosin (MI-o-sin) One of the two contractile proteins in muscle cells, the other being actin
myxedema (mik-seh-DE-mah) Condition that results from hypothyroidism in adults

narcotic (nar-KOT-ik) Drug that acts on the CNS to alter perception and response to pain
nasopharynx (na-zo-FAR-inks) Upper portion of the pharynx located posterior to the nasal cavity
natural killer (NK) cell Type of lymphocyte that can nonspecifically destroy abnormal cells
naturopathy (na-chur-OP-a-the) Philosophy of helping people to heal themselves by developing healthy lifestyles
nausea (NAW-ze-ah) Unpleasant sensation due to disturbance in the upper GI tract that may precede vomiting
necrosis (neh-KRO-sis) Tissue death
negative feedback Self-regulating system in which the result of an action is the control over that action; a method for keeping body conditions within a normal range and maintaining homeostasis
neoplasm (NE-o-plazm) Abnormal growth of cells; tumor; adj., neoplastic
nephron (NEF-ron) Microscopic functional unit of the kidney
nerve Bundle of neuron fibers outside the central nervous system

nerve impulse Electrical charge that spreads along the membrane of a neuron; action potential
nervous system (NER-vus) The system that transports information in the body by means of electrical impulses
neuralgia (nu-RAL-je-ah) Pain in a nerve
neurilemma (nu-rih-LEM-mah) Thin sheath that covers certain peripheral axons; aids in axon regeneration
neuroglia (nu-ROG-le-ah) Supporting and protective cells of the central nervous system; glial cells
neuromuscular junction Point at which a nerve fiber contacts a muscle cell
neuron (NU-ron) Conducting cell of the nervous system
neurotransmitter (nu-ro-TRANS-mit-er) Chemical released from the ending of an axon that enables a nerve impulse to cross a synapse
neutron (NU-tron) Noncharged particle in the nucleus of an atom
neutrophil (NU-tro-fil) Phagocytic granular white blood cell; polymorph; poly; PMN; seg
nevus (NE-vus) Mole or birthmark
nitrogen (NI-tro-jen) Chemical element found in all proteins
node Small mass of tissue, such as a lymph node; space between cells in the myelin sheath
norepinephrine (nor-epi-ih-NEF-rin) Neurotransmitter similar to epinephrine; noradrenaline
normal saline Isotonic or physiologic salt solution
nosocomial (nos-o-KO-me-al) Acquired in a hospital, as an infection
nucleic acid (nu-KLE-ik) Complex organic substance composed of nucleotides that makes up DNA and RNA
nucleolus (nu-KLE-o-lus) Small unit within the nucleus that assembles ribosomes
nucleotide (NU-kle-o-tide) Building block of DNA and RNA
nucleus (NU-kle-us) Largest organelle in the cell, containing the DNA, which directs all cell activities; group of neurons in the central nervous system; in chemistry, the central part of an atom

obstipation (ob-stih-PA-shun) Extreme constipation
occlusion (ok-LU-zhun) Closing, as of a vessel
olfactory (ol-FAK-to-re) Pertaining to the sense of smell (olfaction)
omentum (o-MEN-tum) Portion of the peritoneum; greater omentum extends over the anterior abdomen; lesser omentum extends between the stomach and liver
oncology (on-KOL-o-je) Study of tumors
ophthalmic (of-THAL-mik) Pertaining to the eye
ophthalmoscope (of-THAL-mo-skope) Instrument for examining the posterior (fundus) of the eye
opportunistic (op-por-tu-NIS-tik) Describing an infection that takes hold because a host has been compromised (weakened) by disease
organ (OR-gan) Body part containing two or more tissues functioning together for specific purposes
organelle (or-gan-EL) Specialized subdivision within a cell
organic (or-GAN-ik) Referring to the complex compounds found in living things that contain carbon, and usually hydrogen, and oxygen
organism (OR-gan-izm) Individual plant or animal; any organized living thing
organ of Corti (KOR-te) Receptor for hearing located in the cochlea of the internal ear
origin (OR-ih-jin) Source; beginning; muscle attachment connected to a nonmoving part
oropharynx (o-ro-FAR-inks) Middle portion of the pharynx, located behind the mouth
orthopnea (or-THOP-ne-ah) Difficulty in breathing that is relieved by sitting in an upright position
osmosis (os-MO-sis) Movement of water through a semipermeable membrane
osmotic (os-MOT-ik) **pressure** Tendency of a solution to draw water into it; is directly related to the concentration of the solution
osseus (OS-e-us) Pertaining to bone tissue
ossicle (OS-ih-kl) One of three small bones of the middle ear: malleus, incus, or stapes
ossification (os-ih-fih-KA-shun) Process of bone formation
osteoblast (OS-te-o-blast) Bone-forming cell
osteoclast (OS-te-o-clast) Cell that breaks down bone
osteocyte (OS-te-o-site) Mature bone cell; maintains bone but does not produce new bone tissue
osteon (OS-te-on) Subunit of compact bone, consisting of concentric rings of bone tissue around a central channel; haversian system
osteopenia (os-te-o-PE-ne-ah) Reduction in bone density to below average levels
osteoporosis (os-te-o-po-RO-sis) Abnormal loss of bone tissue with tendency to fracture
otoliths (O-to-liths) Crystals that add weight to fluids in the inner ear and function in the sense of static equilibrium
ovarian follicle (o-VA-re-an FOL-ih-kl) Cluster of cells in which the ovum develops within the ovary; Graafian follicle
ovary (O-vah-re) Female reproductive gland
oviduct (O-vih-dukt) Tube that carries ova from the ovaries to the uterus; fallopian tube, uterine tube
ovulation (ov-u-LA-shun) Release of a mature ovum from a follicle in the ovary
ovum (O-vum) Female reproductive cell or gamete; pl., ova
oxidation (ok-sih-DA-shun) Chemical breakdown of nutrients for energy
oxygen (OK-sih-jen) **(O_2)** The gas needed to break down nutrients completely for energy within the cell
oxygen debt Amount of oxygen needed to reverse the effects produced in muscles functioning without oxygen
oxytocin (ok-se-TO-sin) Hormone from the posterior pituitary that causes uterine contraction and milk ejection ("letdown") from the breasts

pacemaker Sinoatrial (SA) node of the heart; group of cells or artificial device that sets the rate of heart contractions
palate (PAL-at) Roof of the oral cavity; anterior portion is hard palate, posterior portion is soft palate
pallor (PAL-or) Paleness of the skin
pancreas (PAN-kre-as) Large, elongated gland behind the stomach; produces digestive enzymes and hormones (*e.g.*, insulin)
pandemic (pan-DEM-ik) Disease that is prevalent throughout an entire country, continent, or the world.
Papanicolaou (pap-ah-nik-o-LAH-o) **test** Histologic test for cervical cancer; Pap test or smear
papilla (pah-PIL-ah) Small nipplelike projection or elevation
papule (PAP-ule) Firm, raised lesion of the skin
paracentesis (par-eh-sen-TE-sis) Puncture of the abdominal cavity, usually to remove a fluid accumulation, such as ascites; abdominocentesis
parasite (PAR-ah-site) Organism that lives on or within another (the host) at the other's expense
parasympathetic nervous system Craniosacral division of the autonomic nervous system; generally reverses the fight-or-flight (stress) response
parathyroid (par-ah-THI-royd) **gland** Any of four to six small glands embedded in the capsule enclosing the thyroid gland; produces parathyroid hormone, which raises the blood calcium level by causing release of calcium from bones
parietal (pah-RI-eh-tal) Pertaining to the wall of a space or cavity
Parkinson disease Progressive neurologic condition characterized by

tremors, rigidity of limbs and joints, slow movement, and impaired balance.
parturition (par-tu-RISH-un) Childbirth; labor
pathogen (PATH-o-jen) Disease-causing organism; adj., pathogenic (path-o-JEN-ik)
pathology (pah-THOL-o-je) Study of disease
pathophysiology (path-o-fiz-e-OL-o-je) Study of the physiologic basis of disease
pedigree (PED-ih-gre) Family history; used in the study of heredity; family tree
pelvic inflammatory disease (PID) Ascending infection that involves the pelvic organs; common causes are gonorrhea and chlamydia
pelvis (PEL-vis) Basinlike structure, such as the lower portion of the abdomen or the upper flared portion of the ureter (renal pelvis)
pemphigus (PEM-fih-gus) An autoimmune skin disease with blistering of the skin
penis (PE-nis) Male organ of urination and sexual intercourse
perforating canal Channel across a long bone that contains blood vessels and nerves; Volkmann canal
pericardium (per-ih-KAR-de-um) Fibrous sac lined with serous membrane that encloses the heart
perichondrium (per-ih-KON-dre-um) Layer of connective tissue that covers cartilage
perilymph (PER-e-limf) Fluid that fills the inner ear's bony labyrinth
perimysium (per-ih-MIS-e-um) Connective tissue around a fascicle of muscle tissue
perineum (per-ih-NE-um) Pelvic floor; external region between the anus and genital organs
periosteum (per-e-OS-te-um) Connective tissue membrane covering a bone
peripheral (peh-RIF-er-al) Located away from a center or central structure
peripheral nervous system (PNS) All the nerves and nervous tissue outside the central nervous system
peristalsis (per-ih-STAL-sis) Wavelike movements in the wall of an organ or duct that propel its contents forward
peritoneum (per-ih-to-NE-um) Serous membrane that lines the abdominal cavity and forms outer layer of abdominal organs; forms supporting ligaments for some organs
peritonitis (per-ih-to-NI-tis) Inflammation of the peritoneum
peroxisome (per-OK-sih-some) Cell organelle that enzymatically destroys harmful substances produced in metabolism
Peyer (PI-er) **patches** Clusters of lymphatic nodules in the mucous membranes lining the distal portion of the small intestine
pH Symbol indicating hydrogen ion (H^+) concentration; scale that measures the relative acidity and alkalinity (basicity) of a solution
phagocyte (FAG-o-site) Cell capable of engulfing large particles, such as foreign matter or cellular debris, through the plasma membrane
phagocytosis (fag-o-si-TO-sis) Engulfing of large particles through the plasma membrane
pharynx (FAR-inks) Throat; passageway between the mouth and esophagus
phenotype (FE-no-tipe) All the characteristics of an organism that can be seen or tested for
phenylketonuria (fen-il-ke-to-NU-re-ah) (**PKU**) Hereditary metabolic disorder involving inability to metabolize the amino acid phenylalanine
phimosis (fi-MO-sis) Tightness of the foreskin
phlebitis (fleh-BI-tis) Inflammation of a vein
phospholipid (fos-fo-LIP-id) Complex lipid containing phosphorus
phrenic (FREN-ik) Pertaining to the diaphragm
physiology (fiz-e-OL-o-je) Study of the function of living organisms
pia mater (PI-ah MA-ter) Innermost layer of the meninges
PID See pelvic inflammatory disease
pineal (PIN-e-al) **gland** Gland in the brain that is regulated by light; involved in sleep–wake cycles
pinna (PIN-nah) Outer projecting portion of the ear; auricle
pinocytosis (pi-no-si-TO-sis) Intake of small particles and droplets by the plasma membrane of a cell
pituitary (pih-TU-ih-tar-e) **gland** Endocrine gland located under and controlled by the hypothalamus; releases hormones that control other glands; hypophysis
placenta (plah-SEN-tah) Structure that nourishes and maintains the developing fetus during pregnancy
plaque (PLAK) A patch or flat area; fatty material that deposits in vessel linings in atherosclerosis
plasma (PLAZ-mah) Liquid portion of the blood
plasma cell Cell derived from a B cell that produces antibodies
plasma membrane Outer covering of a cell; regulates what enters and leaves cell; cell membrane
plasmapheresis (plas-mah-fer-E-sis) Separation and removal of plasma from a blood donation and return of the formed elements to the donor
platelet (PLATE-let) Cell fragment that forms a plug to stop bleeding and acts in blood clotting; thrombocyte
pleura (PLU-rah) Serous membrane that lines the chest cavity and covers the lungs
pleurisy (PLUR-ih-se) Inflammation of the pleura; pleuritis
plexus (PLEK-sus) Network of vessels or nerves
pneumonia (nu-MO-ne-ah) Inflammation of the lungs, commonly due to infection; pneumonitis
pneumothorax (nu-mo-THO-raks) Accumulation of air in the pleural space
PNS See peripheral nervous system
poliomyelitis (po-le-o-mi-eh-LI-tis) (polio) Viral disease of the nervous system that occurs most commonly in children
polycythemia (pol-e-si-THE-me-ah) Increase in the number of red cells in the blood
polydipsia (pol-e-DIP-se-ah) Excessive thirst
polyp (POL-ip) Protruding growth, often grapelike, from a mucous membrane
polysaccharide (pol-e-SAK-ah-ride) Compound formed from many simple sugars linked together, such as starch and glycogen
pons (ponz) Area of the brain between the midbrain and medulla; connects the cerebellum with the rest of the central nervous system
portal system Venous system that carries blood to a second capillary bed through which it circulates before returning to the heart
positive feedback A substance or condition that acts within a system to promote more of the same activity
positron emission tomography (to-MOG-rah-fe) (PET) Imaging method that uses a radioactive substance to show activity in an organ
posterior (pos-TE-re-or) Toward the back; dorsal
potential (po-TEN-shal) An electrical charge, as on the neuron plasma membrane
precipitation (pre-sip-ih-TA-shun) Clumping of small particles as a result of an antigen-antibody reaction; seen as a cloudiness
preeclampsia (pre-eh-KLAMP-se-ah) See pregnancy induced hypertension
pregnancy (PREG-nan-se) The period during which an embryo or fetus is developing in the body
pregnancy-induced hypertension (**PIH**) Hypertension, proteinuria and edema associated with a hormone imbalance in the latter part of pregnancy; if untreated, may lead to eclampsia; preeclampsia, toxemia of pregnancy

prepuce (PRE-puse) Loose fold of skin that covers the glans penis; foreskin
presbycusis (pres-be-KU-sis) Slowly progressive hearing loss that often accompanies aging
presbyopia (pres-be-O-pe-ah) Loss of visual accommodation that occurs with age, leading to farsightedness
prime mover Muscle that performs a given movement; agonist
prion (PRI-on) An infectious protein particle that causes progressive neurodegenerative disease
PRL see Prolactin
progeny (PROJ-eh-ne) Offspring, descendent
progesterone (pro-JES-ter-one) Hormone produced by the corpus luteum and placenta; maintains the lining of the uterus for pregnancy
prognosis (prog-NO-sis) Prediction of the probable outcome of a disease based on the condition of the patient and knowledge about the disease
prolactin (pro-LAK-tin) Hormone from the anterior pituitary that stimulates milk production in the breasts; PRL
prone Face down or palm down
prophase (PRO-faze) First stage of mitosis, during which the chromosomes become visible and the organelles disappear
prophylaxis (pro-fih-LAK-sis) Prevention of disease
proprioceptor (pro-pre-o-SEP-tor) Sensory receptor that aids in judging body position and changes in position; located in muscles, tendons, and joints
prostaglandin (pros-tah-GLAN-din) Any of a group of hormones produced by many cells; these hormones have a variety of effects
prostate (PROS-tate) **gland** Gland that surrounds the urethra below the bladder and contributes secretions to the semen
protein (PRO-tene) Organic compound made of amino acids; contains nitrogen in addition to carbon, hydrogen, and oxygen (some contain sulfur or phosphorus)
prothrombin (pro-THROM-bin) Clotting factor; converted to thrombin during blood clotting
prothrombinase (pro-THROM-bih-nase) Blood clotting factor that converts prothrombin to thrombin
proton (PRO-ton) Positively charged particle in the nucleus of an atom
protozoon (pro-to-ZO-on) Animal-like microorganism; pl., protozoa
proximal (PROK-sih-mal) Nearer to point of origin or to a reference point
pruritis (pru-RI-tis) Intense itching of the skin
psoriasis (so-RI-ah-sis) Chronic skin disease with red, flat areas covered with silvery scales
ptosis (TO-sis) Dropping down of a part
puerperal (pu-ER-per-al) Related to childbirth
pulmonary circuit Pathway that carries blood from the heart to the lungs for oxygenation and then returns the blood to the heart
pulse Wave of increased pressure in the vessels produced by contraction of the heart
pupil (PU-pil) Opening in the center of the eye through which light enters
Purkinje (pur-KIN-je) **fibers** Part of the conduction system of the heart; conduction myofibers
pus Mixture of bacteria and leukocytes formed in response to infection
pustule (PUS-tule) Vesicle filled with pus
pylorus (pi-LOR-us) Distal region of the stomach that leads to the pyloric sphincter
pyrogen (PI-ro-jen) Substance that produces fever
pyruvic (pi-RU-vik) **acid** Intermediate product in the breakdown of glucose for energy

radioactivity (ra-de-o-ak-TIV-ih-te) Emission of atomic particles from an element
radiography (ra-de-og-rah-fe) Production of an image by passage of x-rays through the body onto sensitized film; record produced is a radiograph
rash Surface skin lesion
receptor (re-SEP-tor) Specialized cell or ending of a sensory neuron that can be excited by a stimulus. A site in the cell membrane to which a special substance (*e.g.*, hormone, antibody) may attach.
recessive (re-SES-iv) Referring to a gene that is not expressed if a dominant gene for the same trait is present
reflex (RE-fleks) Simple, rapid, automatic response involving few neurons
reflex arc (ark) A pathway through the nervous system from stimulus to response; commonly involves a receptor, sensory neuron, central neuron(s), motor neuron, and effector
refraction (re-FRAK-shun) Bending of light rays as they pass from one medium to another of a different density
relaxin (re-LAKS-in) Placental hormone that softens the cervix and relaxes the pelvic joints
renin (RE-nin) Enzyme released from the kidney's juxtaglomerular apparatus that indirectly increases blood pressure by activating angiotensin
repolarization (re-po-lar-ih-ZA-shun) A sudden return to the original charge on a cell membrane following depolarizaiton.
resorption (re-SORP-shun) Loss of substance, such as that of bone or a tooth
respiration (res-pih-RA-shun) Process by which oxygen is obtained from the environment and delivered to the cells
respiratory system The system consisting of the lungs and breathing passages involved in exchange of oxygen and carbon dioxide between the outside air and the blood
reticular (reh-TIK-u-lar) **formation** Network in the limbic system that governs wakefulness and sleep
reticuloendothelial (reh-tik-u-lo-en-do-THE-le-al) **system** Protective system consisting of highly phagocytic cells in body fluids and tissues, such as the spleen, lymph nodes, bone marrow, and liver
retina (RET-ih-nah) Innermost layer of the eye; contains light-sensitive cells (rods and cones)
retroperitoneal (ret-ro-per-ih-to-NE-al) Behind the peritoneum, as are the kidneys, pancreas, and abdominal aorta
Rh factor A red cell antigen; D antigen
rheumatoid (RU-mah-toyd) **arthritis** Disease of connective tissue that affects the joints
rhodopsin (ro-DOP-sin) Light-sensitive pigment in the rods of the eye; visual purple
rib One of the slender curved bones that make up most of the thorax; costa; adj. costal
ribonucleic (RI-bo-nu-kle-ik) **acid (RNA)** Substance needed for protein manufacture in the cell
ribosome (RI-bo-some) Small body in the cell's cytoplasm that is a site of protein manufacture
rickets (RIK-ets) Softening of bone (osteomalacia) in children, usually caused by a deficiency of vitamin D
Rickettsia (rih-KET-se-ah) Extremely small oval to rod-shaped bacterium that can grow only within a living cell
RNA See ribonucleic acid
rod Receptor cell in the retina of the eye; used for vision in dim light
roentgenogram (rent-GEN-o-gram) Image produced by means of x-rays; radiograph
rotation (ro-TA-shun) Twisting or turning of a bone on its own axis
rugae (RU-je) Folds in the lining of an organ, such as the stomach or urinary bladder; sing., ruga (RU-gah)
rule of nines Method for estimating the extent of a burn based on multiples of nine

SA node See Sinoatrial node
saliva (sah-LI-vah) Secretion of the salivary glands; moistens food and contains an enzyme that digests starch
salt Compound formed by reaction between an acid and a base (e.g. NaCl, table salt)

sagittal (SAJ-ih-tal) Describing a plane that divides a structure into right and left portions
sarcoma (sar-KO-mah) Malignant tumor of connective tissue; a form of cancer
saturated fat Fat that has more hydrogen atoms and fewer double bonds between carbons than do unsaturated fats
scar Fibrous connective tissue that replaces normal tissues destroyed by injury or disease; cicatrix
Schwann cell (shvahn) Cell in the nervous system that produces the myelin sheath around peripheral axons
sclera (SKLE-rah) Outermost layer of the eye; made of tough connective tissue; "white" of the eye
scleroderma (skle-ro-DER-mah) An autoimmune disease associated with overproduction of collagen
scoliosis (sko-le-O-sis) Lateral curvature of the spine
scrotum (SKRO-tum) Sac in which testes are suspended
sebum (SE-bum) Oily secretion that lubricates the skin; adj., sebaceous (se-BA-shus)
secretin (se-KRE-tin) Hormone from the duodenum that stimulates pancreatic release of water and bicarbonate
seizure (SE-zhur) Series of muscle spasms; convulsion
selectively permeable Describing a membrane that regulates what can pass through (*e.g.*, the plasma membrane of a cell)
sella turcica (SEL-ah TUR-sih-ka) Saddlelike depression in the floor of the skull that holds the pituitary gland
semen (SE-men) Mixture of sperm cells and secretions from several glands of the male reproductive tract
semicircular canal Bony canal in the internal ear that contains receptors for the sense of dynamic equilibrium; there are three semicircular canals in each ear
semilunar (sem-e-LU-nar) Shaped like a half-moon, such as the flaps of the pulmonary and aortic valves
seminal vesicle (VES-ih-kl) Gland that contributes secretions to the semen
seminiferous (seh-mih-NIF-er-us) **tubules** Tubules in which sperm cells develop in the testis
semipermeable (sem-e-PER-me-ah-bl) Capable of being penetrated by some substances and not others
sensory (SEN-so-re) Describing cells or activities involved in transmitting impulses toward the central nervous system; afferent
sensory adaptation Gradual loss of sensation when sensory receptors are exposed to continuous stimulation
sepsis (SEP-sis) Presence of pathogenic microorganisms or their toxins in the bloodstream or other tissues; adj., septic
septicemia (sep-tih-SE-me-ah) Presence of pathogenic organisms or their toxins in the bloodstream; blood poisoning
septum (SEP-tum) Dividing wall, as between the chambers of the heart or the nasal cavities
serosa (se-RO-sah) Serous membrane; epithelial membrane that secretes a thin, watery fluid
Sertoli cells See Sustentacular cells
serum (SE-rum) Liquid portion of blood without clotting factors; thin, watery fluid; adj., serous (SE-rus)
sex-linked Referring to a gene carried on a sex chromosome, usually the X chromosome
sexually transmitted infection (STI) Communicable disease acquired through sexual relations; sexually transmitted disease (STD); venereal disease (VD)
shingles Viral infection that follows the nerve pathways; caused by the same virus that causes chicken pox; herpes zoster
shock Pertaining to the circulation: a life-threatening condition in which there is inadequate blood flow to the tissues.
sickle cell disease Hereditary disease in which abnormal hemoglobin causes red blood cells to change shape (sickle) when they release oxygen
sign Manifestation of a disease as noted by an observer
sinoatrial (si-no-A-tre-al) **(SA) node** Tissue in the upper wall of the right atrium that sets the rate of heart contractions; the heart's pacemaker
sinus (SI-nus) Cavity or channel, such as the paranasal sinuses in the skull bones
sinus rhythm A normal heart rhythm originating at the SA node
sinusoid (SI-nus-oyd) Enlarged capillary that serves as a blood channel
skeletal (SKEL-eh-tal) **system** The body system that includes the bones and joints
skeleton (SKEL-eh-ton) The complete bony framework of the body; adj., skeletal
skull Bony framework of the head
solute (SOL-ute) Substance that is dissolved in another substance (the solvent)
solution (so-LU-shun) Homogeneous mixture of one substance dissolved in another; the components in a mixture are evenly distributed and cannot be distinguished from each other
solvent (SOL-vent) Substance in which another substance (the solute) is dissolved
somatic (so-MAT-ik) **nervous system** The division of the nervous system that controls voluntary activities and stimulates skeletal muscle
somatotropin (so-mah-to-TRO-pin) Growth hormone
spasm Sudden and involuntary muscular contraction
specific gravity The weight of a substance as compared to the weight of an equal volume of pure water
spermatic (sper-MAT-ik) **cord** Cord that extends through the inguinal canal and suspends the testis; contains blood vessels nerves and ductus deferens
spermatozoon (sper-mah-to-ZO-on) Male reproductive cell or gamete; pl., spermatozoa; sperm cell
sphincter (SFINK-ter) Muscular ring that regulates the size of an opening
sphygmomanometer (sfig-mo-mah-NOM-eh-ter) Device used to measure blood pressure; blood pressure apparatus or cuff
spina bifida (SPI-nah BIF-ih-dah) Incomplete closure of the spine
spinal cord Nervous tissue contained in the spinal column; major relay area between the brain and the peripheral nervous system
spirillum (spi-RIL-um) Corkscrew or spiral-shaped bacterium; pl., spirilla
spirochete (SPI-ro-kete) Spiral-shaped microorganism that moves in a waving and twisting motion
spirometer (spi-ROM-eh-ter) Instrument for recording lung volumes; tracing is a spirogram
spleen Lymphoid organ in the upper left region of the abdomen
spore Resistant form of bacterium; reproductive cell in lower plants
squamous (SKWA-mus) Flat and irregular, as in squamous epithelium
staging A procedure for evaluating the extent of tumor spread
stain (stane) Dye that aids in viewing structures under the microscope
staphylococcus (staf-ih-lo-KOK-us) Round bacterium found in a cluster resembling a bunch of grapes; pl., staphylococci (staf-ih-lo-KOK-si)
stasis (STA-sis) Stoppage in the normal flow of fluids, such as blood, lymph, urine, or contents of the digestive tract
stem cell Cell that has the potential to develop into different types of cells
stenosis (sten-O-sis) Narrowing of a duct or canal
stent Small tube inserted into a vessel to keep it open
sterility Complete inability to reproduce
sterilization (ster-ih-li-ZA-shun) Process of killing every living microorganism on or in an object; procedure that makes an individual incapable of reproduction
steroid (STE-royd) Category of lipids that includes the hormones of the sex glands and the adrenal cortex

stethoscope (STETH-o-skope) Instrument for conveying sounds from the patient's body to the examiner's ears

STI See Sexually transmitted infection

stimulus (STIM-u-lus) Change in the external or internal environment that produces a response

stomach (STUM-ak) Organ of the digestive tract that stores food, mixes it with digestive juices and moves it into the small intestine

strabismus (strah-BIZ-mus) Deviation of the eye resulting from lack of eyeball muscle coordination

stratified In multiple layers (strata)

stratum (STRA-tum) A layer; pl. strata

stratum basale (bas-A-le) Deepest layer of the epidermis; layer that produces new epidermal cells; stratum germinativum

stratum corneum (KOR-ne-um) The thick uppermost layer of the epidermis

striations (stri-A-shuns) Stripes or bands, as seen in skeletal muscle and cardiac muscle

stricture (STRICK-ture) Narrowing of a part

stroke Damage to the brain due to lack of oxygen; usually caused by a blood clot in a vessel (thrombus) or rupture of a vessel; cerebrovascular accidnt (CVA)

subacute (sub-a-KUTE) Not as severe as an acute infection nor a long-lasting as a chronic disorder

subcutaneous (sub-ku-TA-ne-us) Under the skin

submucosa (sub-mu-KO-sah) Layer of connective tissue beneath the mucosa

substrate Substance on which an enzyme works

sudoriferous (su-do-RIF-er-us) Producing sweat; referring to the sweat glands

sulcus (SUL-kus) Shallow groove, as between convolutions of the cerebral cortex; pl., sulci (SUL-si)

superior (su-PE-re-or) Above; in a higher position

superior vena cava (VE-nah KA-vah) Large vein that drains the upper part of the body and empties into the right atrium of the heart

supine (SU-pine) Face up or palm up

surfactant (sur-FAK-tant) Substance in the alveoli that prevents their collapse by reducing surface tension of the contained fluids

suspension (sus-PEN-shun) Heterogeneous mixture that will separate unless shaken

suspensory ligaments Filaments attached to the ciliary muscle of the eye that hold the lens in place

sustentacular (sus-ten-TAK-u-lar) **cells** Cells in the seminiferous tubules that aid in development of spermatozoa; Sertoli cells

suture (SU-chur) Type of joint in which bone surfaces are closely united, as in the skull; stitch used in surgery to bring parts together or to stitch parts together in surgery

sympathetic nervous system Thoracolumbar division of the autonomic nervous system; stimulates a fight-or-flight (stress) response

symptom (SIMP-tom) Evidence of disease noted by the patient; such evidence noted by an examiner is called a sign or an objective symptom

synapse (SIN-aps) Junction between two neurons or between a neuron and an effector

synarthrosis (sin-ar-THRO-sis) Immovable joint

syndrome (SIN-drome) Group of symptoms characteristic of a disorder

synergist (SIN-er-jist) A substance or structure that enhances the work of another. A muscle that works with a prime mover to produce a given movement

synovial (sin-O-ve-al) Pertaining to a thick lubricating fluid found in joints, bursae, and tendon sheaths; pertaining to a freely movable (diarthrotic) joint

system (SIS-tem) Group of organs functioning together for the same general purposes

systemic (sis-TEM-ik) Referring to a generalized infection or condition

systemic circuit Pathway that carries blood to all tissues of the body except the lungs

systole (SIS-to-le) Contraction phase of the cardiac cycle; adj., systolic (sis-TOL-ik)

tachycardia (tak-e-KAR-de-ah) Heart rate more than 100 beats per minute

tachypnea (tak-IP-ne-ah) Excessive rate of respiration

tactile (TAK-til) Pertaining to the sense of touch

target tissue Tissue that is capable of responding to a specific hormone

Tay-Sachs disease Hereditary disease affecting fat metabolism

T cell Lymphocyte active in immunity that matures in the thymus gland; destroys foreign cells directly; T lymphocyte

tectorial (tek-TO-re-al) **membrane** Part of the hearing apparatus; generates nerve impulses as cilia move against it in response to sound waves

telophase (TEL-o-faze) Final stage of mitosis, during which new nuclei form and the cell contents usually divide

tendinitis (ten-din-I-tis) Inflammation of a tendon

tendon (TEN-don) Cord of fibrous connective tissue that attaches a muscle to a bone

teniae (TEN-e-e) **coli** Bands of smooth muscle in the wall of the large intestine

testis (TES-tis) Male reproductive gland; pl., testes (TES-teze)

testosterone (tes-TOS-ter-one) Male sex hormone produced in the testes; promotes the development of sperm cells and maintains secondary sex characteristics

tetanus (TET-an-us) Constant contraction of a muscle; infectious disease caused by a bacterium (*Clostridium tetani*); lockjaw

tetany (TET-an-e) Muscle spasms due to low blood calcium, as in parathyroid deficiency

thalamus (THAL-ah-mus) Region of the brain located in the diencephalon; chief relay center for sensory impulses traveling to the cerebral cortex

therapy (THER-ah-pe) Treatment

thoracentesis (thor-a-sen-TE-sis) Puncture of the chest for aspiration of fluid in the pleural space

thorax (THO-raks) Chest; adj., thoracic (tho-RAS-ik)

thrombocyte (THROM-bo-site) Blood platelet; cell fragment that participates in clotting

thrombocytopenia (throm-bo-si-to-PE-ne-ah) Deficiency of platelets in the blood

thrombolytic (throm-bo-LIT-ik) Dissolving blood clots

thrombosis (throm-BO-sis) Condition of having a thrombus (blood clot in a vessel)

thrombus (THROM-bus) Blood clot within a vessel

thymosin (THI-mo-sin) Hormone produced by the thymus gland

thymus (THI-mus) Endocrine gland in the upper portion of the chest; stimulates development of T cells

thyroid (THI-royd) Endocrine gland in the neck

thyroiditis (thi-royd-I-tis) Inflammation of the thyroid gland

thyroid-stimulating hormone (TSH) Hormone produced by the anterior pituitary that stimulates the thyroid gland; thyrotropin

thyroxine (thi-ROK-sin) Hormone produced by the thyroid gland; increases metabolic rate and needed for normal growth; T_4

tinea (TIN-e-ah) Common term for fungal infection of the skin

tissue Group of similar cells that performs a specialized function

tonicity (to-NIS-ih-te) The osmotic concentration or osmotic pressure of a solution. The effect that a solution will have on osmosis.

tonsil (TON-sil) Mass of lymphoid tissue in the region of the pharynx

tonus (TO-nus) Partially contracted state of muscle; also, tone

toxemia (tok-SE-me-ah) General toxic condition in which poisonous bacterial substances are absorbed into the bloodstream; presence of harmful substances in the blood as a result of abnormal metabolism
toxin (TOK-sin) Poison
toxoid (TOK-soyd) Altered toxin used to produce active immunity
trachea (TRA-ke-ah) Tube that extends from the larynx to the bronchi; windpipe
tracheostomy (tra-ke-OS-to-me) Surgical opening into the trachea for the introduction of a tube through which a person may breathe
trachoma (trah-KO-mah) Acute eye infection caused by chlamydia
tract Bundle of neuron fibers within the central nervous system
trait Characteristic
transplantation (trans-plan-TA-shun) The grafting to a recipient of an organ or tissue from an animal or other human to replace an injured or incompetent part of the body
transverse Describing a plane that divides a structure into superior and inferior parts
trauma (TRAW-mah) Injury or wound
tricuspid (tri-KUS-pid) **valve** Valve between the right atrium and right ventricle of the heart
trigeminal neuralgia (tri-JEM-ih-nal nu-RAL-je-ah) Severe spasmodic pain affecting the fifth cranial nerve; tic douloureux (tik du-lu-RU)
triglyceride (tri-GLIS-er-ide) Simple fat composed of glycerol and three fatty acids
trigone (TRI-gone) Triangulaar shaped region in the floor of the bladder that remains stable as the bladder fills
triiodothyronine (tri-i-o-do-THI-ro-nin) Thyroid hormone that functions with thyroxine to raise cellular metabolism; T_3
tropomyosin (tro-po-MI-o-sin) A protein that works with troponin to regulate contraction in skeletal muscle
troponin (tro-PO-nin) A protein that works with tropomyosin to regulate contraction in skeletal muscle
TSH See thyroid-stimulating hormone
tuberculosis (tu-ber-ku-LO-sis) (**TB**) Infectious disease, often of the lung, caused by the bacillus *Mycobacterium tuberculosis*
tumor (TU-mor) Abnormal growth or neoplasm
tympanic (tim-PAN-ik) **membrane** Membrane between the external and middle ear that transmits sound waves to the bones of the middle ear; eardrum

ulcer (UL-ser) Sore or lesion associated with death and disintegration of tissue
ultrasound (UL-trah-sound) Very high frequency sound waves
umbilical (um-BIL-ih-kal) **cord** Structure that connects the fetus with the placenta; contains vessels that carry blood between the fetus and placenta
umbilicus (um-BIL-ih-kus) Small scar on the abdomen that marks the former attachment of the umbilical cord to the fetus; navel
universal solvent Term used for water because it dissolves more substances than any other solvent
unsaturated fat Fat that has fewer hydrogen atoms and more double bonds between carbons than do saturated fats
urea (u-RE-ah) Nitrogenous waste product excreted in the urine; end product of protein metabolism
uremia (u-RE-me-ah) Accumulation of nitrogenous waste products in the blood
ureter (U-re-ter) Tube that carries urine from the kidney to the urinary bladder
urethra (u-RE-thrah) Tube that carries urine from the urinary bladder to the outside of the body
urinalysis (u-rin-AL-ih-sis) Laboratory examination of the physical and chemical properties of urine
urinary bladder Hollow organ that stores urine until it is eliminated
urinary system (U-rin-ar-e) The system involved in elimination of soluble waste, water balance and regulation of body fluids
urination (u-rin-A-shun) Voiding of urine; micturition
urine (U-rin) Liquid waste excreted by the kidneys
urticaria (ur-tih-KA-re-ah) Hives; allergic skin reaction with elevated red patches (wheals)
uterus (U-ter-us) Muscular, pear-shaped organ in the female pelvis within which the fetus develops during pregnancy
uvea (U-ve-ah) Middle coat of the eye, including the choroid, iris, and ciliary body; vascular and pigmented structures of the eye
uvula (U-vu-lah) Soft, fleshy, V-shaped mass that hangs from the soft palate

vaccination (vak-sin-A-shun) Administration of a vaccine to protect against a specific disease; immunization
vaccine (vak-SENE) Substance used to produce active immunity; usually, a suspension of attenuated or killed pathogens or some component of a pathogen given by inoculation to prevent a specific disease
vagina (vah-JI-nah) Distal part of the birth canal that opens to the outside of the body; female organ of sexual intercourse
valence (VA-lens) The combining power of an atom; the number of electrons lost or gained by atoms of an element in chemical reactions
valve Structure that prevents fluid from flowing backward, as in the heart, veins, and lymphatic vessels
varicose (VAR-ih-kose) Pertaining to an enlarged and twisted vessel, as in varicose vein
vas deferens (DEF-er-enz) Tube that carries sperm cells from the testis to the urethra; ductus deferens
vasectomy (vah-SEK-to-me) Surgical removal of part or all of the ductus (vas) deferens; usually done on both sides to produce sterility
vasoconstriction (vas-o-kon-STRIK-shun) Decrease in the diameter of a blood vessel
vasodilation (vas-o-di-LA-shun) Increase in the diameter of a blood vessel
VD Venereal disease; see sexually transmitted infection
vector (VEK-tor) An insect or other animal that transmits a disease-causing organism from one host to another
vein (vane) Vessel that carries blood toward the heart
vena cava (VE-nah KA-vah) A large vein that carries blood into the right atrium of the heart; superior vena cava or inferior vena cava
venereal (ve-NE-re-al) **disease** (**VD**) Infectious disease acquired through sexual activity; sexually transmitted infection (STI)
venous sinus (VE-nus SI-nus) Large channel that drains deoxygenated blood
ventilation (ven-tih-LA-shun) Movement of air into and out of the lungs
ventral (VEN-tral) Toward the front or belly surface; anterior
ventricle (VEN-trih-kl) Cavity or chamber; one of the two lower chambers of the heart; one of the four chambers in the brain in which cerebrospinal fluid is produced; adj., ventricular (ven-TRIK-u-lar)
venule (VEN-ule) Vessel between a capillary and a vein
vernix caseosa (VEr-niks ka-se-O-sah) Cheeselike sebaceous secretion that covers a newborn
vertebra (VER-teh-brah) A bone of the spinal column; pl., vertebrae (VER-teh-bre)
verruca (veh-RU-kah) Wart
vesicle (VES-ih-kl) Small sac or blister filled with fluid
vesicular transport Use of vesicles to move large amounts of material through the plasma membrane of a cell
vestibule (VES-tih-bule) Part of the internal ear that contains receptors for the sense of static equilibrium; any space at the entrance to a canal or organ

vibrio (VIB-re-o) Slight curved or comma-shaped bacterium; pl., vibrios

villi (VIL-li) Small fingerlike projections from the surface of a membrane; projections in the lining of the small intestine through which digested food is absorbed; sing., villus

viroid (VI-royd) Infectious agent composed of RNA with no protein. Viroids are intracellular parasites linked so far only to diseases in plants.

virulence (VIR-u-lens) Power of an organism to overcome defenses of a host

virus (VI-rus) Extremely small infectious agent that can reproduce only within a living cell

viscera (VIS-er-ah) Organs in the ventral body cavities, especially the abdominal organs; adj. visceral

viscosity (vis-KOS-ih-te) Thickness, as of the blood or other fluid

vitamin (VI-tah-min) Organic compound needed in small amounts for health

vitreous (VIT-re-us) **body** Soft, jellylike substance that fills the eyeball and holds the shape of the eye; vitreous humor

vocal cords Folds of mucous membrane in the larynx used in producing speech

Volkmann canal See perforating canal

volvulus (VOL-vu-lus) Twisting of the intestine

von Willebrand disease Hereditary blood clotting disorder in which there is a shortage of von Willebrand factor

Wernicke (VER-nih-ke) **area** Portion of the cerebral cortex concerned with speech recognition and the meaning of words

white matter Nervous tissue composed of myelinated fibers

x-ray Ray or radiation of extremely short wavelength that can penetrate opaque substances and affect photographic plates and fluorescent screens

zygote (ZI-gote) Fertilized ovum; cell formed by the union of a sperm and an egg

Glossary of Word Parts

Use of Word Parts in Medical Terminology

Medical terminology, the special language of the health occupations, is based on an understanding of a relatively few basic elements. These elements—roots, prefixes, and suffixes—form the foundation of almost all medical terms. A useful way to familiarize yourself with each term is to learn to pronounce it correctly and say it aloud several times. Soon it will become an integral part of your vocabulary.

The foundation of a word is the word root. Examples of word roots are *abdomin-*, referring to the belly region; and *aden-*, pertaining to a gland. A word root is often followed by a vowel to facilitate pronunciation, as in *abdomino-* and *adeno-*. We then refer to it as a "combining form." The hyphen appended to a combining form indicates that it is not a complete word; if the hyphen precedes the combining form, then it commonly appears as the word ending, as in *-algia*, meaning "a painful condition."

A prefix is a part of a word that precedes the word root and changes its meaning. For example, the prefix *mal-* in *malnutrition* means "abnormal." A suffix, or word ending, is a part that follows the word root and adds to or changes its meaning. The suffix *-rhea* means "profuse flow" or "discharge," as in *diarrhea*, a condition characterized by excessive discharge of liquid stools.

Many medical words are compound words; that is, they are made up of more than one root or combining form. Examples of such compound words are *erythrocyte* (red blood cell) and *hydrocele* (fluid-containing sac), and many more difficult words, such as *sternoclavicular* (indicating relations to both the sternum and the clavicle).

A general knowledge of language structure and spelling rules is also helpful in mastering medical terminology. For example, adjectives include words that end in *-al*, as in *sternal* (the noun is *sternum*), and words that end in *-ous*, as in *mucous* (the noun is *mucus*).

The following list includes some of the most commonly used word roots, combining forms, prefixes, and suffixes, as well as examples of their use. Prefixes are followed by a hyphen; suffixes are preceded by a hyphen; and word roots have no hyphen. Commonly used combining vowels are added following a slash.

Word Parts

a-, an- absent, deficient, lack of: *atrophy, anemia, anuria*
ab- away from: *abduction, aboral*
abdomin/o belly or abdominal area: *abdominocentesis, abdominoscopy*
acous, acus hearing, sound: *acoustic, presbyacusis*
acr/o- extreme end of a part, especially of the extremities: *acromegaly, acromion*
actin/o, actin/i relation to raylike structures or, more commonly, to light or roentgen (x-) rays, or some other type of radiation: *actiniform, actinodermatitis*
ad- (sometimes converted to *ac-, af-, ag-, ap-, as-, at-,*) toward, added to, near: *adrenal, accretion, agglomerated, afferent*
aden/o gland: *adenectomy, adenitis, adenocarcinoma*
aer/o air, gas: *aerobic, aerate*
-agogue inducing, leading, stimulating: *cholagogue, galactagogue*
-al pertaining to, resembling: *skeletal, surgical, ileal*
alb/i- white: *albinism, albiduria*
alge, alg/o, alges/i pain: *algetic, algophobia, analgesic*
-algia pain, painful condition: *myalgia, neuralgia*
amb/i- both, on two sides: *ambidexterity, ambivalent*
ambly- dimness, dullness: *amblyopia*
amphi on both sides, around, double: *amphiarthrosis, amphibian*
amyl/o starch: *amylase, amyloid*
an- absent, deficient, lack of: *anaerobic, anoxia, anemic*
ana- upward, back, again, excessive: *anatomy, anastomosis, anabolism*
andr/o male: *androgen, androgenous*
angi/o vessel: *angiogram, angiotensin*
ant/i- against; to prevent, suppress, or destroy: *antarthritic, antibiotic, anticoagulant*
ante- before, ahead of: *antenatal, antepartum*
anter/o- position ahead of or in front of (i.e., anterior to) another part: *anterolateral, anteroventral*
-apheresis take away, withdraw: *hemapheresis, plasmapheresis*
ap/o- separation, derivation from: *apocrine, apoptosis, apophysis*
aqu/e water: *aqueous, aquatic, aqueduct*
-ar pertaining to, resembling: *muscular, nuclear*
arthr/o joint or articulation: *arthrolysis, arthrostomy, arthritis*
-ary pertaining to, resembling: *salivary, dietary, urinary*
-ase enzyme: *lipase, protease*
-asis *see* –sis
atel/o- imperfect: *atelectasis*
ather/o gruel: *athersclerosis, atheroma*
audi/o sound, hearing: *audiogenic, audiometry, audiovisual*
aut/o- self: *autistic, autodigestion, autoimmune*

bas/o- alkaline: *basic, basophilic*
bi- two, twice: *bifurcate, bisexual*
bil/i bile: *biliary, bilirubin*
bio- life, living organism: *biopsy, antibiotic*
blast/o, -blast early stage of a cell, immature cell: *blastula, blastophore, erythroblast*
bleph, blephar/o eyelid, eyelash: *blepharism, blepharitis, blepharospasm*
brachi, brachi/o arm: *brachial, brachiocephalic, brachiotomy*
brachy- short: *brachydactylia, brachyesophagus*
brady- slow: *bradycardia*
bronch/o-, bronch/i bronchus: *bronchiectasis, bronchoscope*
bucc cheek: *buccal*

capn/o carbon dioxide: *hypocapnia, hypercapnia*
carcin/o cancer: *carcinogenic, carcinoma*
cardi/o, cardi/a heart: *carditis, cardiac, cardiologist*
cata- down: *catabolism, catalyst*
-cele swelling; enlarged space or cavity: *cystocele, meningocele, rectocele*

celi/o abdomen: *celiac, celiocentesis*
centi- relating to 100 (used in naming units of measurements): *centigrade, centimeter*
-centesis perforation, tapping: *aminocentesis, paracentesis*
cephal/o head: *cephalalgia, cephalopelvic*
cerebr/o brain: *cerobrospinal, cerebrum*
cervi neck: *cervical, cervix*
cheil/o lips; brim or edge: *cheilitis, cheilosis*
chem/o, chem/i chemistry, chemical: *chemotherapy, chemocautery, chemoreceptor*
chir/o, cheir/o hand: *cheiralgia, cheiromegaly, chiropractic*
chol/e, chol/o bile, gall: *chologogue, cholecyst, cholelith*
cholecyst/o gallbladder: *cholecystitis, cholecystokinin*
chondr/o, chondri/o cartilage: *chondric, chondrocyte, chondroma*
chori/o membrane: *chorion, choroid, choriocarcinoma*
chrom/o, chromat/o color: *chromosome, chromatin, chromophilic*
-cid, -cide to cut, kill or destroy: *bactericidal, germicide, suicide*
circum- around, surrounding: *circumorbital, circumrenal, circumduction*
-clast break: *osteoclast*
clav/o, cleid/o clavicle: *cleidomastoid, subclavian*
co- with, together: *cofactor, cohesion, coinfection*
colp/o vagina: *colpectasia, colposcope, colpotomy*
con- with: *concentric, concentrate, conduct*
contra- opposed, against: *contraindication, contralateral*
corne/o horny: *corneum, cornified, cornea*
cortic/o cortex: *cortical, corticotropic, cortisone*
cost/a, cost/o- ribs: *intercostal, costosternal*
counter- against, opposite to: *counteract, counterirritation, countertraction*
crani/o skull: *cranium, craniotomy*
cry/o- cold: *cryalgesia, cryogenic, cryotherapy*
crypt/o- hidden, concealed: *cryptic, cryptogenic, cryptorchidism*
-cusis hearing: *acusis, presbyacusis*
cut- skin: *subcutaneous*
cyan/o- blue: *cyanosis, cyanogen*
cyst/i, cyst/o sac, bladder: *cystitis, cystoscope*
cyt/o, -cyte cell: *cytology, cytoplasm, osteocyte*

dactyl/o digits (usually fingers, but sometimes toes): *dactylitis, polydactyly*
de- remove: *detoxify, dehydration*
dendr tree: *dendrite*
dent/o, dent/i tooth: *dentition, dentin, dentifrice*
derm/o, dermat/o skin: *dermatitis, dermatology, dermatosis*
di- twice, double: *dimorphism, dibasic, dihybrid*
dipl/o- double: *diplopia, diplococcus*
dia- through, between, across, apart: *diaphragm, diaphysis*
dis- apart, away from: *disarticulation, distal*
dors/i, dors/o- back (in the human, this combining form is the same as poster/o-): *dorsal, dorsiflexion, dorsonuchal*
dys- disordered, difficult, painful: *dysentery, dysphagia, dyspnea*

e- out: *enucleation, evisceration, ejection*
-ectasis expansion, dilation, stretching: *angiectasis, bronchiectasis*
ecto- outside, external: *ectoderm, ectogenous*
-ectomy surgical removal or destruction by other means: *appendectomy, thyroidectomy*
edem swelling: *edema*
-emia condition of blood: *glycemia, hyperemia*
encephal/o brain: *encephalitis, encephalogram*
end/o- in, within, innermost: *endarterial, endocardium, endothelium*
enter/o intestine: *enteritis, enterocolitis*
epi- on, upon: *epicardium, epidermis*
equi- equal: *equidistant, equivalent, equilibrium*
erg/o work: *ergonomic, energy, synergy*
eryth-, erythr/o red: *erythema, erythrocyte*
-esthesia sensation: *anesthesia, paresthesia*
eu- well, normal, good: *euphoria, eupnea*
ex/o- outside, out of, away from: *excretion, exocrine, exophthalmic*
extra- beyond, outside of, in addition to: *extracellular, extrasystole, extravasation*

fasci fibrous connective tissue layers: *fascia, fascitis, fascicle*
fer, -ferent to bear, to carry: *afferent, efferent, transfer*
fibr/o threadlike structures, fibers: *fibrillation, fibroblast, fibrositis*

gastr/o stomach: *gastritis, gastroenterostomy*
-gen an agent that produces or originates: *allergen, pathogen, fibrinogen*
-genic produced from, producing: *neurogenic, pyogenic, psychogenic*
genit/o organs of reproduction: *genitoplasty, genitourinary*
gen/o- a relationship to reproduction or sex: *genealogy, generate, genetic, genotype*
-geny manner of origin, development or production: *ontogeny, progeny*
gest/o gestation, pregnancy: *progesterone, gestagen*
glio, -glia gluey material; specifically, the support tissue of the central nervous system: *glioma, neuroglia*
gloss/o tongue: *glossitis, glossopharyngeal*
glyc/o- relating to sugar, glucose, sweet: *glycemia, glycosuria*
gnath/o related to the jaw: *prognathic, gnathoplasty*
gnos to perceive, recognize: *agnostic, prognosis, diagnosis*
gon seed, knee: *gonad, gonarthritis*
-gram record, that which is recorded: *electrocardiogram, electroencephalogram*
graph/o, -graph instrument for recording, record, writing: *electrocardiograph, electroencephalograph, micrograph*
–graphy process of recording data: *photography, radiography*
gyn/o, gyne, gynec/o female, woman: *gynecology, gynecomastia, gynoplasty*
gyr/o circle: *gyroscope, gyrus, gyration*

hema, hemo, hemat/o blood: *hematoma, hematuria, hemorrhage*
hemi- one half: *hemisphere, heminephrectomy, hemiplegia*
hepat/o liver: *hepatitis, hepatogenous*
heter/o- other, different: *heterogenous, heterosexual, heterochromia*
hist/o,histi/o tissue: *histology, histiocyte*
homeo-, homo- unchanging, the same: *hemeostasis, homosexual*
hydr/o water: *hydrolysis, hydrocephalus*
hyper- above, over, excessive: *hyperesthesia, hyperglycemia, hypertrophy*
hypo- deficient, below, beneath: *hypochondrium, hypodermic, hypogastrium*
hyster/o uterus: *hysterectomy*

-ia state of, condition of: *myopia, hypochondria, ischemia*
-iatrics, -trics medical specialty: *pediatrics, obstetrics*
iatr/o physician, medicine: *iatrogenic*
-ic pertaining to, resembling: *metric, psychiatric, geriatric*
idio- self, one's own, separate, distinct: *idiopathic, idiosyncrasy*
-ile pertaining to, resembling: *febrile, virile*
im-, in- in, into, lacking: *implantation, infiltration, inanimate*
infra- below, inferior: *infraspinous, infracortical*
insul/o pancreatic islet, island: *insulin, insulation, insuloma*
inter- between: *intercostal, interstitial*
intra- within a part or structure: *intracranial, intracellular, intraocular*
isch suppression: *ischemia*
-ism state of: *alcoholism, hyperthyroidism*
iso- same, equal: *isotonic, isometric*
–ist one who specializes in a field of study: *cardiologist, gastroenterologist*
-itis inflammation: *dermatitis, keratitis, neuritis*

juxta- next to: *juxtaglomerular, juxtaposition*

kary/o nucleus: *karyotype, karyoplasm*
kerat/o cornea of the eye, certain horny tissues: *keratin, keratitis, keratoplasty*
kine movement: *kinetic, kinesiology, kinesthesia*

lacri- tear: *lacrimal*
lact/o milk: *lactation, lactogenic*
laryng/o larynx: *laryngeal, laryngectomy, laryngitis*
later/o- side: *lateral*
-lemma sheath: *neurilemma, sarcolemma*
leuk/o- (also written as *leuc-, leuco-*) white, colorless: *leukocyte, leukoplakia*
lip/o lipid, fat: *lipase, lipoma*
lig- bind: *ligament, ligature*
lingu/o tongue: *lingual, linguodental*
lith/o stone (calculus): *lithiasis, lithotripsy*
-logy study of: *physiology, gynecology*
lute/o yellow: *macula lutea, corpus luteum*
lymph/o lymph, lymphatic system, lymphocyte: *lymphoid, lymphedema*
lyso-, -lysis, -lytic: loosening, dissolving, separating: *hemolysis, paralysis, lysosome*

macr/o- large, abnormal length: *macrophage, macroblast*. See also **-mega, mega/o-**
mal- bad, diseased, disordered, abnormal: *malnutrition, malocclusion, malunion*
malac/o, -malacia softening: *malacoma, osteomalacia*
mamm/o breast, mammary gland: *mammogram, mammoplasty, mammal*
man/o pressure: *manometer, sphygmomanometer*
mast/o breast: *mastectomy, mastitis*
meg/a-, megal/o, -megaly unusually or excessively large: *megacolon, megaloblast, splenomegaly, megakaryocyte*
melan/o dark, black: *melanin, melanocyte, melanoma*
men/o physiologic uterine bleeding, menses: *menstrual, menorrhagia, menopause*
mening/o membranes covering the brain and spinal cord: *meningitis, meningocele*
mes/a, mes/o- middle, midline: *mesencephalon, mesoderm*
meta- change, beyond, after, over, near: *metabolism, metacarpal, metaplasia*
-meter, metr/o measure: *hemocytometer, sphygmomanometer, spirometer, isometric*
metr/o uterus: *endometrium, metroptosis, metrorrhagia*
micro- very small: *microscope, microbiology, microsurgery, micrometer*
mon/o- single, one: *monocyte, mononucleosis*
morph/o shape, form: *morphogenesis, morphology*
multi- many: *multiple, multifactorial, multipara*
my/o muscle: *myenteron, myocardium, myometrium*
myc/o, mycet fungus: *mycid, mycete, mycology, mycosis, mycelium*
myel/o marrow (often used in reference to the spinal cord): *myeloid, myeloblast, osteomyelitis, poliomyelitis*
myring/o tympanic membrane: *myringotomy, myringitis*
myx/o mucus: *myxoma, myxovirus*

narc/o stupor: *narcosis, narcolepsy, narcotic*
nas/o nose: *nasopharynx, paranasal*
natri sodium: *hyponatremia, natriuretic*
necr/o death, corpse: *necrosis*
neo- new: *neoplasm, neonatal*
neph, nephr/o kidney: *nephrectomy, nephron*
neur/o, neur/i nerve, nervous tissue: *neuron, neuralgia, neuroma*
neutr/o neutral: *neutrophil, neutropenia*
noct/i night: *noctambulation, nocturia, noctiphobia*

ocul/o eye: *oculist, oculomotor, oculomycosis*
odont/o tooth, teeth: *odontalgia, orthodontics*
-odynia pain, tenderness: *myodynia, neurodynia*
-oid like, resembling: *lymphoid, myeloid*
olig/o- few, a deficiency: *oligospermia, oliguria*
-oma tumor, swelling: *hematoma, sarcoma*
-one ending for steroid hormone: *testosterone, progesterone*
onych/o nails: *paronychia, onychoma*
oo, ovum, egg: *oocyte, oogenesis*, (do not confuse with **oophor-**)
oophor/o ovary: *oophorectomy, oophoritis, oophorocystectomy*. See also **ovar-**
ophthalm/o eye: *ophthalmia, ophthalmologist, ophthalmoscope*
-opia disorder of the eye or vision: *heterotropia, myopia, hyperopia*
or/o mouth: *oropharynx, oral*
orchi/o, orchid/o testis: *orchitis, cryptorchidism*
orth/o- straight, normal: *orthopedics, orthopnea, orthosis*
-ory pertaining to, resembling: *respiratory, circulatory*
oscill/o to swing to and fro: *oscilloscope*
osmo- osmosis: *osmoreceptor; osmotic*
oss/i, osse/o, oste/o bone, bone tissue: *osseous, ossicle, osteocyte, osteomyelitis*
ot/o ear: *otalgia, otitis, otomycosis*
-ous pertaining to, resembling: *fibrous, venous, androgynous*
ov/o egg, ovum: *oviduct, ovulation*
ovar, ovari/o ovary: *ovariectomy*. See also **oophor**
ox-, -oxia pertaining to oxygen: *hypoxemia, hypoxia, anoxia*
oxy sharp, acute: *oxygen, oxytocia*

pan- all: *pandemic, panacea*
papill/o nipple: *papilloma, papillary*
para- near, beyond, apart from, beside: *paramedical, parametrium, parathyroid, parasagittal*
pariet/o wall: *parietal*
path/o, -pathy disease, abnormal condition: *pathogen, pathology, neuropathy*
ped/o, pedia child, foot: *pedophobia, pediatrician, pedialgia*
-penia lack of: *leukopenia, thrombocytopenia*
per- through, excessively: *percutaneous, perfusion*
peri- around: *pericardium, perichondrium*
-pexy fixation: *nephropexy, proctopexy*
phag/o to eat, to ingest: *phagocyte, phagosone*
-phagia, -phagy eating, swallowing: *aphagia, dysphagia*
-phasia speech, ability to talk: *aphasia, dysphasia*
phen/o to show: *phenotype*
-phil, -philic to like, have an affinity for: *eosinophilia, hemophilia, hydrophilic*
phleb/o vein: *phlebitis, phlebotomy*
-phobia fear, dread, abnormal aversion: *phobic, acrophobia, hydrophobia*
phot/o light: *photoreceptor, photophobia*
phren/o diaphragm: *phrenic, phrenicotomy*
physi/o natural, physical: *physiology, physician*
pil/e, pil/i, pil/o hair, resembling hair: *pileous, piliation, pilonidal*
pin/o to drink: *pinocytosis*
-plasty molding, surgical formation: *cystoplasty, gastroplasty, kineplasty*
-plegia stroke, paralysis: *paraplegia, hemiplegia*
pleur/o side, rib, pleura: *pleurisy, pleurotomy*
-pnea air, breathing: *dyspnea, eupnea*
pneum/o, pneumat/o air, gas, respiration: *pneumothorax, pneumograph, pneumatocele*
pneumon/o lung: *pneumonia, pneumonectomy*
pod/o foot: *podiatry, pododynia*
-poiesis making, forming: *erythropoiesis, hematopoiesis*
polio- gray: *polioencephalitis, poliomyelitis*
poly- many: *polyarthritis, polycystic, polycythemia*
post- behind, after, following: *postnatal, postocular, postpartum*
pre- before, ahead of: *precancerous, preclinical, prenatal*
presby- old age: *presbycusis, presbyopia*
pro- before, in front of, in favor of: *prodromal, prosencephalon, prolapse, prothrombin*
proct/o rectum: *proctitis, proctocele, proctologist*
propri/o own: *proprioception*
pseud/o false: *pseudoarthrosis, pseudostratified, pseudopod*
psych/o mind: *psychosomatic, psychotherapy*
-ptosis downward displacement, falling, prolapse: *blepharoptosis, enteroptosis, nephroptosis*
pulm/o, pulmon/o lung: *pulmonic, pulmonology*
py/o pus: *pyuria, pyogenic, pyorrhea*

pyel/o renal pelvis: *pyelitis, pyelogram, pyelonephrosis*
pyr/o fire, fever: *pyrogen, antipyretic, pyromania*

quadr/i- four: *quadriceps, quadriplegic*

rachi/o spine: *rachicentesis, rachischisis*
radio- emission of rays or radiation: *radioactive, radiography, radiology*
re- again, back: *reabsorption, reaction, regenerate*
rect/o rectum: *rectal, rectouterine*
ren/o kidney: *renal, renopathy*
reticul/o network: *reticulum, reticular*
retro- backward, located behind: *retrocecal, retroperitoneal*
rhin/o nose: *rhinitis, rhinoplasty*
-rhage, -rhagia* bursting forth, excessive flow: *hemorrhage, menorrhagia*
-rhaphy* suturing or sewing up a gap or defect in a part: *herniorrhaphy, gastrorrhaphy, cystorrhaphy*
-rhea* flow, discharge: *diarrhea, gonorrhea, seborrhea*

sacchar/o sugar: *monosaccharide, polysaccharide*
salping/o tube: *salpingitis, salpingoscopy*
sarc/o flesh: *sarcolemma, sarcoplasm, sarcomere*
scler/o hard, hardness; *scleroderma, sclerosis*
scoli/o- twisted, crooked: *scoliosis, scoliosometer*
-scope instrument used to look into or examine a part: *bronchoscope, endoscope, arthroscope*
semi- partial, half: *semipermeable, semicoma*
semin/o semen, seed: *seminiferous, seminal*
sep, septic poison, rot, decay: *sepsis, septicemia*

*When a suffix beginning with *rh* is added to a word root, the *r* is doubled.

sin/o sinus: *sinusitis, sinusoid, sinoatrial*
-sis condition or process, usually abnormal: *dermatosis, osteoporosis*
soma-, somat/o, -some body: *somatic, somatotype, somatotropin*
son/o sound: *sonogram, sonography*
sphygm/o pulse: *sphygmomanometer*
spir/o breathing: *spirometer, inspiration, expiration*
splanchn/o- internal organs: *splanchnic, splanchnoptosis*
splen/o spleen: *splenectomy, splenic*
staphyl/o grapelike cluster: *staphylococcus*
stat, -stasis stand, stoppage, remain at rest: *hemostasis, static, homeostasis*
sten/o- contracted, narrowed: *stenosis*
sthen/o, -sthenia, -sthenic strength: *asthenic, calisthenics, neurasthenia*
steth/o chest: *stethoscope*
stoma, stomat/o mouth: *stomatitis*
-stomy surgical creation of an opening into a hollow organ or an opening between two organs: *colostomy, tracheostomy, gastroenterostomy*
strept/o chain: *streptcoccus, streptobacillus*
sub- under, below, near, almost: *subclavian, subcutaneous, subluxation*
super- over, above, excessive: *superego, supernatant, superficial*
supra- above, over, superior: *supranasal, suprarenal*
sym-, syn- with, together: *symphysis, synapse*
syring/o fistula, tube, cavity: *syringectomy, syringomyelia*

tach/o-, tachy- rapid: *tachycardia, tachypnea*
tars/o eyelid, foot: *tarsitis, tarsoplasty, tarsoptosis*
-taxia, -taxis order, arrangement: *ataxia, chemotaxis, thermotaxis*
tel/o end: *telophase, telomere*
tens- stretch, pull: *extension, tensor*
test/o testis: *testosterone, testicular*
tetr/a four: *tetralogy, tetraplegia*
therm/o-, -thermy heat: *thermalgesia, thermocautery, diathermy, thermometer*
thromb/o blood clot: *thrombosis, thrombocyte*
toc/o labor: *eutocia, dystocia, oxytocin*
tom/o, -tomy incision of, cutting: *anatomy, phlebotomy, laparotomy*
ton/o tone, tension: *tonicity, tonic*
tox, toxic/o poison: *toxin, cytotoxic, toxemia, toxicology*
trache/o trachea, windpipe: *tracheal, tracheitis, tracheotomy*
trans- across, through, beyond: *transorbital, transpiration, transplant, transport*
tri- three: *triad, triceps*
trich/o hair: *trichiasis, trichosis, trichology*
troph/o, -trophic, -trophy nutrition, nurture: *atrophic, hypertrophy*
trop/o, -tropin, -tropic turning toward, acting on, influencing, changing: *thyrotropin, adrenocorticotropic, gonadotropic*
tympan/o drum: *tympanic, tympanum*

ultra- beyond or excessive: *ultrasound, ultraviolent, ultrastructure*
uni- one: *unilateral, uniovular, unicellular*
-uria urine: *glycosuria, hematuria, pyuria*
ur/o urine, urinary tract: *urology, urogenital*

vas/o vessel, duct: *vascular, vasectomy, vasodilation*
viscer/o internal organs, viscera: *visceral, visceroptosis*
vitre/o glasslike: *vitreous*

xer/o dryness: *xeroderma, xerophthalmia, xerosis*

-y condition of: *tetany, atony, dysentery*

zyg/o joined: zygote, heterozygous, monozygotic

Appendices

Appendix 1 Metric Measurements

UNIT	ABBREVIATION	METRIC EQUIVALENT	U.S. EQUIVALENT
Units of length			
Kilometer	km	1000 meters	0.62 miles; 1.6 km/mile
Meter*	m	100 cm; 1000 mm	39.4 inches; 1.1 yards
Centimeter	cm	1/100 m; 0.01 m	0.39 inches; 2.5 cm/inch
Millimeter	mm	1/1000 m; 0.001 m	0.039 inches; 25 mm/inch
Micrometer	μm	1/1000 mm; 0.001 mm	
Units of Weight			
Kilogram	kg	1000 g	2.2 lb
Gram*	g	1000 mg	0.035 oz.; 28.5 g/oz
Milligram	mg	1/1000 g; 0.001 g	
Microgram	μg	1/1000 mg; 0.001 mg	
Units of volume			
Liter*	L	1000 mL	1.06 qt
Deciliter	dL	1/10 L; 0.1 L	
Milliliter	mL	1/1000 L; 0.001 L	0.034 oz.; 29.4 mL/oz
Microliter	μL	1/1000 mL; 0.001 mL	

**Basic unit.*

Appendix 2 Celsius–Fahrenheit Temperature Conversion Scale

CELSIUS TO FAHRENHEIT

Use the following formula to convert Celsius readings to Fahrenheit readings:

°F= 9/5°C + 32

For example, if the Celsius reading is 37°

°F= (9/5 × 37) + 32

=6.6 + 32

=98.6°F (normal body temperature)

FAHRENHEIT TO CELSIUS

Use the following formula to convert Fahrenheit readings to Celsius readings:

°C= 5/9 (°F - 32)

For example, if the Fahrenheit reading is 68°:

°C =5/9 (68 - 32)

=5/9 × 36

=20°C (a nice spring day)

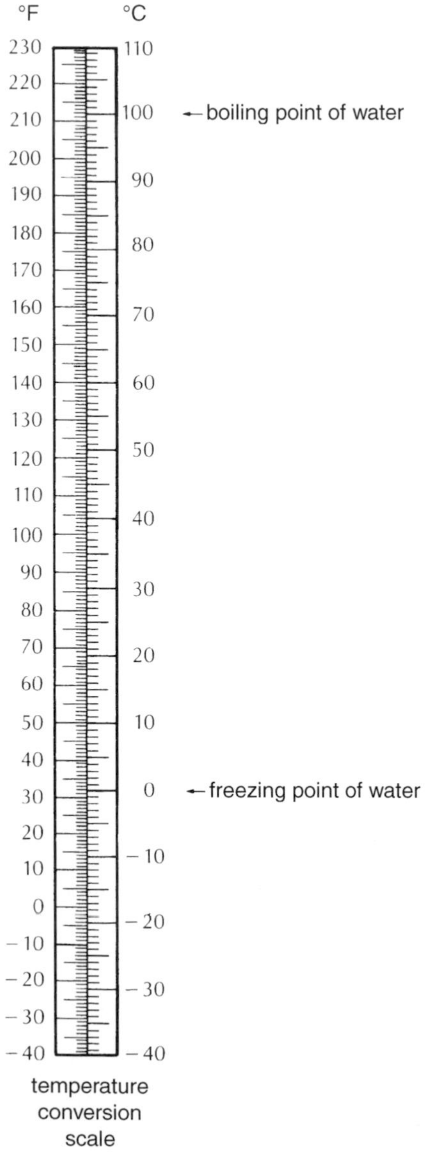

temperature conversion scale

Appendix 3 Periodic Table of Elements

The periodic table lists the chemical elements according to their atomic numbers. The boxes in the table have information about the elements, as shown by the example at the top of the chart. The upper number in each box is the atomic number, which represents the number of protons in the nucleus of the atom. Under the name of the element is its chemical symbol, an abbreviation of its modern or Latin name. The Latin names of four common elements are shown below the chart. The bottom number in each box gives the atomic weight (mass) of that element's atoms compared with the weight of carbon atoms. Atomic weight is the sum of the weights of the protons and neutrons in the nucleus.

All the elements in a column share similar chemical properties based on the number of electrons in their outermost energy levels. Those in column VIII are non-reactive (inert) and are referred to as the *noble gases*. The 26 elements found in the body are color coded according to quantity (see totals above the chart). Carbon, hydrogen, oxygen and nitrogen make up 96% of body weight. The first three of these are present in all carbohydrates, lipids, proteins and nucleic acids. Nitrogen is an additional component of all proteins. Nine other elements make up almost all the rest of body weight. The remaining 13 elements are present in very small amounts and are referred to as *trace elements*. Although needed in very small quantities, they are essential for good health, as they are parts of enzymes and other compounds used in metabolism.

PERIODIC TABLE OF THE ELEMENTS

- 96% of body weight
- 3.9% of body weight
- 0.1% of body weight

Notation:

6	Atomic number
Carbon	Name
C	Symbol
12.01	Atomic weight

I	II											III	IV	V	VI	VII	VIII
1 Hydrogen **H** 1.01																	2 Helium **He** 4.00
3 Lithium **Li** 6.94	4 Beryllium **Be** 9.01											5 Boron **B** 10.81	6 Carbon **C** 12.01	7 Nitrogen **N** 14.01	8 Oxygen **O** 16.00	9 Fluorine **F** 19.00	10 Neon **Ne** 20.18
11 Sodium **Na** 22.99	12 Magnesium **Mg** 24.31											13 Aluminum **Al** 26.98	14 Silicon **Si** 28.09	15 Phosphorus **P** 30.97	16 Sulfur **S** 32.07	17 Chlorine **Cl** 35.45	18 Argon **Ar** 39.95
19 Potassium **K** 39.10	20 Calcium **Ca** 40.08	21 Scandium **Sc** 44.96	22 Titanium **Ti** 47.88	23 Vanadium **V** 50.94	24 Chromium **Cr** 52.00	25 Manganese **Mn** 54.94	26 Iron **Fe** 55.85	27 Cobalt **Co** 58.93	28 Nickel **Ni** 58.69	29 Copper **Cu** 63.55	30 Zinc **Zn** 65.39	31 Gallium **Ga** 69.72	32 Germanium **Ge** 72.59	33 Arsenic **As** 74.92	34 Selenium **Se** 78.96	35 Bromine **Br** 79.90	36 Krypton **Kr** 83.80
37 Rubidium **Rb** 85.47	38 Strontium **Sr** 87.62	39 Yttrium **Y** 88.91	40 Zirconium **Zr** 91.22	41 Niobium **Nb** 92.91	42 Molybdenum **Mo** 95.94	43 Technetium **Tc** (98)	44 Ruthenium **Ru** 101.1	45 Rhodium **Rh** 102.9	46 Palladium **Pd** 106.4	47 Silver **Ag** 107.9	48 Cadmium **Cd** 112.4	49 Indium **In** 114.8	50 Tin **Sn** 118.7	51 Antimony **Sb** 121.8	52 Tellurium **Te** 127.6	53 Iodine **I** 126.9	54 Xenon **Xe** 131.3
55 Cesium **Cs** 132.91	56 Barium **Ba** 137.34		72 Hafnium **Hf** 178.5	73 Tantalum **Ta** 180.9	74 Tungsten **W** 183.9	75 Rhenium **Re** 186.2	76 Osmium **Os** 190.2	77 Iridium **Ir** 192.2	78 Platinum **Pt** 195.1	79 Gold **Au** 196.9	80 Mercury **Hg** 200.6	81 Thallium **Tl** 204.4	82 Lead **Pb** 207.2	83 Bismuth **Bi** 209.0	84 Polonium **Po** (210)	85 Astatine **At** (210)	86 Radon **Rn** (222)
87 Francium **Fr** (223)	88 Radium **Ra** (226)		104 Rutherfordium **Rf** (257)	105 Dubnium **Db** (260)	106 Seaborgium **Sg** (263)	107 Bohrium **Bh** (262)	108 Hassium **Hs** (265)	109 Meitnerium **Mt** (267)	110 Darmstadtium **Ds** (271)	111 Unnamed (272)	112 Unnamed (277)						

57-71 Lanthanides	57 Lanthanum **La** 138.9	58 Cerium **Ce** 140.1	59 Praseodymium **Pr** 140.9	60 Neodymium **Nd** 144.2	61 Promethium **Pm** (145)	62 Samarium **Sm** (150.4)	63 Europium **Eu** 152.0	64 Gadolinium **Gd** 157.3	65 Terbium **Tb** 158.9	66 Dysprosium **Dy** 162.5	67 Holmium **Ho** 164.9	68 Erbium **Er** 167.3	69 Thulium **Tm** 168.9	70 Ytterbium **Yb** 173.0	71 Lutetium **Lu** 175.0
89-103 Actinides	89 Actinium **Ac** (227)	90 Thorium **Th** 232.0	91 Protactinium **Pa** (231)	92 Uranium **U** (238)	93 Neptunium **Np** (237)	94 Plutonium **Pu** (244)	95 Americium **Am** (243)	96 Curium **Cm** (247)	97 Berkelium **Bk** (247)	98 Californium **Cf** (251)	99 Einsteinium **Es** (254)	100 Fermium **Fm** (257)	101 Mendelevium **Md** (256)	102 Nobelium **No** (259)	103 Lawrencium **Lr** (257)

Name	Latin name	Symbol
Copper	*cuprium*	Cu
Iron	*ferrum*	Fe
Potassium	*kalium*	K
Sodium	*natrium*	Na

Appendix 4•1 Routine Urinalysis

TEST	NORMAL VALUE	CLINICAL SIGNIFICANCE
General characteristics and measurements		
Color	Pale yellow to amber	Color change can be due to concentration or dilution, drugs, metabolic or inflammatory disorders
Odor	Slightly aromatic	Foul odor typical of urinary tract infection, fruity odor in uncontrolled diabetes mellitus
Appearance (clarity)	Clear to slightly hazy	Cloudy urine occurs with infection or after refrigeration; may indicate presence of bacteria, cells, mucus, or crystals
Specific gravity	1.003–1.030 (first morning catch; routine is random)	Decreased in diabetes insipidus, acute renal failure, water intoxication; increased in liver disorders, heart failure, dehydration
pH	4.5–8.0	Acid urine accompanies acidosis, fever, high protein diet; alkaline urine in urinary tract infection, metabolic alkalosis, vegetarian diet
Chemical determinations		
Glucose	Negative	Glucose present in uncontrolled diabetes mellitus, steroid excess
Ketones	Negative	Present in diabetes mellitus and in starvation
Protein	Negative	Present in kidney disorders, such as glomerulonephritis, acute kidney failure
Bilirubin	Negative	Breakdown product of hemoglobin; present in liver disease or in bile blockage
Urobilinogen	0.2–1.0 Ehrlich units /dL	Breakdown product of bilirubin; increased in hemolytic anemias and in liver disease; remains negative in bile obstruction
Blood (occult)	Negative	Detects small amounts of blood cells, hemoglobin, or myoglobin; present in severe trauma, metabolic disorders, bladder infections
Nitrite	Negative	Product of bacterial breakdown of urine; positive result suggests urinary tract infection and needs to be followed up with a culture of the urine
Microscopic		
Red blood cells	0–3 per high-power field	Increased because of bleeding within the urinary tract from trauma, tumors, inflammation, or damage within the kidney
White blood cells	0–4 per high-power field	Increased by kidney or bladder infection
Renal epithelial cells	Occasional	Increased number indicates damage to kidney tubules
Casts	None	Hyaline casts normal; large number of abnormal casts indicates inflammation or a systemic disorder
Crystals	Present	Most are normal; may be acid or alkaline
Bacteria	Few	Increased in urinary tract infection or contamination from infected genitalia
Others		Any yeasts, parasites, mucus, spermatozoa, or other microscopic findings would be reported here

Appendix 4•2 Complete Blood Count (CBC)

TEST	NORMAL VALUE*	CLINICAL SIGNIFICANCE
Red blood cell (RBC) count	Men: 4.2–5.4 million/μL Women: 3.6–5.0 million/μL	Decreased in anemia; increased in dehydration, polycythemia
Hemoglobin (Hb)	Men: 13.5–17.5 g/dL Women: 12–16 g/dL	Decreased in anemia, hemorrhage, and hemolytic reactions; increased in dehydration, heart and lung disease
Hematocrit (Hct) or packed cell volume(PCV)	Men: 40%–50% Women: 37%–47%	Decreased in anemia; increased in polycythemia, dehydration
Red blood cell (RBC) indices (examples)		These values, calculated from the RBC count, Hb, and Hct, give information valuable in the diagnosis and classification of anemia
Mean corpuscular volume (MCV)	87–103 μL/red cell	Measures the average size or volume of each RBC: small size (microcytic) in iron-deficiency anemia; large size (macrocytic) typical of pernicious anemia
Mean corpuscular hemoglobin (MCH)	26–34 pg/red cell	Measures the weight of hemoglobin per RBC; useful in differentiating types of anemia in a severely anemic patient
Mean corpuscular hemoglobin concentration (MCHC)	31–37 g/dL	Defines the volume of hemoglobin per RBC; used to determine the color or concentration of hemoglobin per RBC
White blood cell (WBC) count	5,000–10,000μL	Increased in leukemia and in response to infection, inflammation, and dehydration; decreased in bone marrow suppression
Platelets	150,000–350,000/μL	Increased in many malignant disorders; decreased in disseminated intravascular coagulation (DIC) or toxic drug effects; spontaneous bleeding may occur at platelet counts below 20,000 μL
Differential (Peripheral blood smear)		A stained slide of the blood is needed to perform the differential. The percentages of the different WBCs are estimated, and the slide is microscopically checked for abnormal characteristics in WBCs, RBCs, and platelets.
WBCs		
Segmented neutrophils (SEGs, POLYs)	40%–74%	Increased in bacterial infections; low numbers leave person very susceptible to infection
Immature neutrophils (BANDs)	0%–3%	Increased when neutrophil count increases
Lymphocytes (LYMPHs)	20%–40%	Increased in viral infections; low numbers leave person dangerously susceptible to infection
Monocytes (MONOs)	2%–6%	Increased in specific infections
Eosinophils (EOs)	1%–4%	Increased in allergic disorders
Basophils (BASOs)	0.5%–1%	Increased in allergic disorders

**Values vary depending on instrumentation and type of test.*

Appendix 4•3 Blood Chemistry Tests

TEST	NORMAL VALUE	CLINICAL SIGNIFICANCE
Basic panel: An overview of electrolytes, waste product management, and metabolism		
Blood urea nitrogen (BUN)	7–18 mg/dL	Increased in renal disease and dehydration; decreased in liver damage and malnutrition
Carbon dioxide (CO_2) (includes bicarbonate)	23–30 mmol/L	Useful to evaluate acid-base balance by measuring total carbon dioxide in the blood: Elevated in vomiting and pulmonary disease; decreased in diabetic acidosis, acute renal failure, and hyperventilation
Chloride (Cl)	98–106 mEq/L	Increased in dehydration, hyperventilation, and congestive heart failure; decreased in vomiting, diarrhea, and fever
Creatinine	0.6–1.2 mg/dL	Produced at a constant rate and excreted by the kidney; increased in kidney disease
Glucose	Fasting: 70–110 mg/dL Random: 85–125 mg/dL	Increased in diabetes and severe illness; decreased in insulin overdose or hypoglycemia
Potassium (K)	3.5–5 mEq/L	Increased in renal failure, extensive cell damage, and acidosis; decreased in vomiting, diarrhea, and excess administration of diuretics or IV fluids
Sodium (Na)	101–111 mEq/L or 135–148 mEq/L (depending on test)	Increased in dehydration and diabetes insipidus; decreased in overload of IV fluids, burns, diarrhea, or vomiting
Additional blood chemistry tests		
Alanine aminotransferase (ALT)	10–40 U/L	Used to diagnose and monitor treatment of liver disease and to monitor the effects of drugs on the liver; increased in myocardial infarction
Albumin	3.8–5.0 g/dL	Albumin holds water in blood; decreased in liver disease and kidney disease
Albumin-globulin ratio (A/G ratio)	Greater than 1	Low A/G ratio signifies a tendency for edema because globulin is less effective than albumin at holding water in the blood
Alkaline phosphatase (ALP)	20–70 U/L (varies by method)	Enzyme of bone metabolism; increased in liver disease and metastatic bone disease
Amylase	21–160 U/L	Used to diagnose and monitor treatment of acute pancreatitis and to detect inflammation of the salivary glands
Aspartate aminotransferase (AST)	0–41 U/L (varies)	Enzyme present in tissues with high metabolic activity; increased in myocardial infarction and liver disease
Bilirubin, total	0.2–1.0 mg/dL	Breakdown product of hemoglobin from red blood cells; increased when excessive red blood cells are being destroyed or in liver disease
Calcium (Ca)	8.8–10.0 mg/dL	Increased in excess parathyroid hormone production and in cancer; decreased in alkalosis, elevated phosphate in renal failure, and excess IV fluids
Cholesterol	120–220 mg/dL desirable range	Screening test used to evaluate risk of heart disease; levels of 200 mg/dL or above indicate increased risk of heart disease and warrant further investigation
Creatine phosphokinase (CPK or CK)	Men: 38–174 U/L Women: 96–140 U/L	Elevated enzyme level indicates myocardial infarction or damage to skeletal muscle. When elevated, specific fractions (isoenzymes) are tested for
Gamma-glutamyl transferase (GGT)	Men: 6–26 U/L Women: 4–18 U/L	Used to diagnose liver disease and to test for chronic alcoholism
Globulins	2.3–3.5 g/dL	Proteins active in immunity; help albumin keep water in blood
Iron, serum (Fe)	Men: 75–175 μg/dL Women: 65–165 μ/dL	Decreased in iron deficiency and anemia; increased in hemolytic conditions
High-density lipoproteins (HDLs)	Men: 30–70 mg/dL Women: 30–85 mg/dL	Used to evaluate the risk of heart disease
Lactic dehydrogenase (LDH or LD)	95–200 U/L (Normal ranges vary greatly)	Enzyme released in many kinds of tissue damage, including myocardial infarction, pulmonary infarction, and liver disease
Lipase	4–24 U/L (varies with test)	Enzyme used to diagnose pancreatitis

(*Continued*)

Appendix 4·3 Blood Chemistry Tests (continued)

TEST	NORMAL VALUE	CLINICAL SIGNIFICANCE
Low-density lipoproteins (LDLs)	80–140 mg/dL	Used to evaluate the risk of heart disease
Magnesium (Mg)	1.3–2.1 mEq/L	Vital in neuromuscular function; decreased levels may occur in malnutrition, alcoholism, pancreatitis, diarrhea
Phosphorus (P) (inorganic)	2.7–4.5 mg/dL	Evaluated in response to calcium; main store is in bone: elevated in kidney disease; decreased in excess parathyroid hormone
Protein, total	6–8 g/dL	Increased in dehydration, multiple myeloma; decreased in kidney disease, liver disease, poor nutrition, severe burns, excessive bleeding
Serum glutamic oxalacetic transaminase (SGOT)		See Aspartate aminotransferase (AST)
Serum glutamic pyruvic transaminase (SGPT)		See Alanine aminotransferase (ALT)
Thyroxin (T_4)	5–12.5 μg/dL (varies)	Screening test of thyroid function; increased in hyperthyroidism; decreased in myxedema and hypothyroidism
Thyroid-stimulating hormone (TSH)	0.5–6 mlU/L	Produced by pituitary to promote thyroid gland function; elevated when thyroid gland is not functioning
Triiodothyronine (T_3)	120–195 mg/dL	Elevated in specific types of hyperthyroidism
Triglycerides	Men: 40–160 mg/dL Women: 35–135 mg/dL	An indication of ability to metabolize fats; increased triglycerides and cholesterol indicate high risk of atherosclerosis
Uric acid	Men: 3.5–7.2 mg/dL Women: 2.6–6.0 mg/dL	Produced by breakdown of ingested purines in food and nucleic acids; elevated in kidney disease, gout, and leukemia

Appendix 5•1 Bacterial Diseases

ORGANISM	DISEASE AND DESCRIPTION
Cocci	
Neisseria gonorrhoeae (gonococcus)	Gonorrhea. Acute inflammation of mucous membranes of the reproductive and urinary tracts (with possible spread to the peritoneum in the female). Systemic infection may cause gonococcal arthritis and endocarditis. Organism also causes ophthalmia neonatorum, an eye inflammation of the newborn.
Neisseria meningitidis (meningococcus)	Epidemic meningitis. Inflammation of the membranes covering brain and spinal cord. A vaccine is available for use in high-risk populations.
Staphylococcus aureus and other staphylococci	Boils, carbuncles, impetigo, osteomyelitis, staphylococcal pneumonia, cystitis, pyelonephritis, empyema, septicemia, toxic shock, and food poisoning. Strains resistant to antibiotics are a cause of infections originating in hospitals, such as wound infections.
Streptococcus pneumoniae	Pneumonia; inflammation of the alveoli, bronchioles, and bronchi; middle ear infections; meningitis. May be prevented by use of polyvalent pneumococcal vaccine.
Streptococcus pyogenes, Streptococcus hemolyticus, and other streptococci	Septicemia, septic sore throat, scarlet fever, puerperal sepsis, erysipelas, streptococcal pneumonia, rheumatic fever, subacute bacterial endocarditis, acute glomerulonephritis.
Bacilli	
Bordetella pertussis	Pertussis (whooping cough). Severe infection of the trachea and bronchi. The "whoop" is caused by the effort to recover breath after coughing. All children should be immunized against pertussis.
Brucella abortus (and others)	Brucellosis, or undulant fever. Disease of animals such as cattle and goats transmitted to humans through unpasteurized dairy products or undercooked meat. Acute phase of fever and weight loss; chronic disease with abscess formation and depression.
Clostridium botulinum	Botulism. Very severe poisoning caused by eating food in which the organism has been allowed to grow and excrete its toxin. Causes muscle paralysis and may result in death from asphyxiation. Infant botulism results from ingestion of spores. It causes respiratory problems and flaccid paralysis, which usually respond to treatment.
Clostridium perfringens	Gas gangrene. Acute wound infection. Organisms cause death of tissues accompanied by the generation of gas within them.
Clostridium tetani	Tetanus. Acute, often fatal poisoning caused by introduction of the organism into deep wounds. Characterized by severe muscular spasms. Also called *lockjaw*.
Corynebacterium diphtheriae	Diphtheria. Acute inflammation of the throat with the formation of a leathery membranelike growth (pseudomembrane) that can obstruct air passages and cause death by asphyxiation. Toxin produced by this organism can damage heart, nerves, kidneys, and other organs. Disease preventable by appropriate vaccination.
Escherichia coli, Proteus *spp.,* and other colon bacilli	Normal inhabitants of the colon, and usually harmless there. Cause of local and systemic infections, food poisoning, diarrhea (especially in children), septicemia, and septic shock. *E. coli* is a common hospital-acquired infection.
Francisella tularensis	Tularemia, or deer fly fever. Transmitted by contact with an infected animal or a tick or fly bite. Symptoms are fever, ulceration of the skin, and enlarged lymph nodes.
Haemophilus influenzae type b (Hib)	Severe infections in children under 3 years of age. Causes meningitis, also epiglottitis, septicemia, pneumonia, pericarditis, and septic arthritis. Preschool vaccinations are routine.
Helicobacter pylori	Acute inflammation of the stomach (gastritis), ulcers of the stomach's pyloric area and the duodenum.
Legionella pneumophila	Legionnaires disease (pneumonia). Seen in localized epidemics; may be transmitted by air conditioning towers and by contaminated soil at excavation sites. Not spread person to person. Characterized by high fever, vomiting, diarrhea, cough, and bradycardia. Mild form of the disease called *Pontiac fever*.
Mycobacterium leprae (Hansen bacillus)	Leprosy. Chronic illness in which hard swellings occur under the skin, particularly of the face, causing a distorted appearance. In one form of leprosy, the nerves are affected, resulting in loss of sensation in the extremities.
Mycobacterium tuberculosis (tubercle bacillus)	Tuberculosis. Infectious disease in which the organism causes primary lesions called *tubercles*. These break down into cheeselike masses of tissue, a process known as *caseation*. Any body organ can be infected, but in adults, the usual site is the lungs. Still one of the most widespread diseases in the world, tuberculosis is treated with chemotherapy; strains of the bacillus have developed resistance to drugs.
Pseudomonas aeruginosa	Common organism is a frequent cause of wound and urinary infections in debilitated hospitalized patients. Often found in solutions that have been standing for long periods.

(*Continued*)

Appendix 5•1 Bacterial Diseases (continued)

ORGANISM	DISEASE AND DESCRIPTION
Salmonella typhi (and others)	Salmonellosis occurs as enterocolitis, bacteremia, localized infection, or typhoid. Depending on type, presenting symptoms may be fever, diarrhea, or abscesses; complications include intestinal perforation and endocarditis. Carried in water, milk, meat, and other food.
Shigella dysenteriae (and others)	A serious bacillary dysentery. Acute intestinal infection with diarrhea (sometimes bloody); may cause dehydration with electrolyte imbalance or septicemia. Transmitted through fecal-oral route or other poor sanitation.
Yersinia pestis	Plague, the "black death" of the Middle Ages. Transmitted by fleas from infected rodents to humans. Symptoms of the most common form are swollen, infected lymph nodes, or *buboes*. Another form may cause pneumonia. All forms may lead to a rapidly fatal septicemia.
Curved rods	
Vibrio	
Vibrio cholerae	Cholera. Acute infection of the intestine characterized by prolonged vomiting and diarrhea, leading to severe dehydration, electrolyte imbalance, and in some cases, death.
Spirochetes	
Borrelia burgdorferi	Lyme disease, transmitted by the extremely small deer tick. Usually starts with a bulls-eye rash followed by flulike symptoms, at which time antibiotics are effective. May progress to neurologic problems and joint inflammation.
Borrelia recurrentis (and others)	Relapsing fever. Generalized infection in which attacks of fever alternate with periods of apparent recovery. Organisms spread by lice, ticks, and other insects.
Treponema pallidum	Syphillis. Infectious disease transmitted mainly by sexual intercourse. Untreated syphilis is seen in the following three stages: primary—formation of primary lesion (chancre); secondary—skin eruptions and infectious patches on mucous membranes; tertiary—development of generalized lesions (gummas) and destruction of tissues resulting in aneurysm, heart disease, and degenerative changes in brain, spinal cord, ganglia, and meninges. Also a cause of intrauterine fetal death or stillbirth.
Treponema vincentii	Vincent disease (trench mouth). Infection of the mouth and throat accompanied by formation of a pseudomembrane, with ulceration.
Other bacteria (*Note:* The following organisms are smaller than other bacteria and vary in shape. Like viruses, they grow within cells, but they differ from viruses in that they are affected by antibiotics.)	
Chlamydia oculogenitalis	Inclusion conjunctivitis, acute eye infection. Carried in genital organs, transmitted during birth or through water in inadequately chlorinated swimming pools.
Chlamydia psittaci	Psittacosis, also called *ornithosis*. Disease transmitted by various birds, including parrots, ducks, geese, and turkeys. Primary symptoms are chills, headache, and fever, more severe in older people. The duration may be from 2 to 3 weeks, often with a long convalescence. Antibiotic drugs are effective remedies.
Chlamydia trachomatis	A sexually transmitted infection causing pelvic inflammatory disease and other infections of the reproductive tract. Also causes inclusion conjunctivitis, an acute eye infection, and trachoma, a chronic infection that is a common cause of blindness in underdeveloped areas of the world. Infection of the conjunctiva and cornea characterized by redness, pain, and lacrimation. Antibiotic therapy is effective if begun before there is scarring. The same organism causes lymphogranuloma venereum (LGV), a sexually transmitted infection characterized by swelling of inguinal lymph nodes and accompanied by signs of general infection.
Coxiella burnetti	Q fever. Infection transmitted from cattle, sheep, and goats to humans by contaminated dust and also carried by arthropods. Symptoms are fever, headache, chills, and pneumonitis. This disorder is almost never fatal.
Rickettsia prowazekii	Epidemic typhus. Transmitted to humans by lice; associated with poor hygiene and war. Main symptoms are headache, hypotension, delirium, and a red rash. Frequently fatal in older people.
Rickettsia rickettsii	Rocky Mountain spotted fever. Tick-borne disease occurring throughout the United States. Symptoms are fever, muscle aches, and a rash that may progress to gangrene over bony prominences. The disease is rarely fatal.
Rickettsia typhi	Endemic or murine typhus. A milder disease transmitted to humans from rats by fleas. Symptoms are fever, rash, headache, and cough. The disease is rarely fatal.

Appendix 5•2 Viral Diseases

ORGANISM	DISEASE AND DESCRIPTION
Common cold viruses	Common cold (coryza), viral infection of the upper respiratory tract. A wide variety of organisms may be involved. May lead to complications, such as pneumonia and influenza.
Cytomegalovirus (CMV)	Common mild infection of the salivary glands. In an immunosuppressed person may cause infection of the retina, lung, and liver, ulceration of GI tract, and inflammation of the brain. Causes severe fetal or neonatal damage.
Encephalitis viruses	Encephalitis, which usually refers to any brain inflammation accompanied by degenerative tissue changes. Encephalitis has many causes besides viruses. Viral forms of encephalitis include Western and Eastern epidemic, equine, St. Louis, Japanese B, and others. Some are known to be transmitted from birds and other animals to humans by insects, principally mosquitoes.
Epstein-Barr virus (EBV)	Mononucleosis, a highly infectious disease spread by saliva. Common among teenagers and young adults. There is fever, sore throat, marked fatigue, and enlargement of the spleen and lymph nodes. Infects B lymphocytes (mononuclear leukocytes) causing them to multiply. Virus remains latent for life after infection. EBV also causes Burkitt lymphoma, a malignant B lymphocyte tumor common in parts of Africa.
Hantavirus	Pulmonary syndrome with high mortality rate. Spread by inhalation of rodent droppings.
Hepatitis viruses	Liver inflammation. Varieties A through E are recognized.
Hepatitis A virus (HAV)	Transmitted by fecal contamination. Does not become chronic or produce carrier state. Infection provides lifelong immunity. Vaccine is available.
Hepatitis B virus (HBV)	Transmitted by direct exchange of blood and body fluids. Can cause rapidly fatal disease or develop into chronic disease and carrier state. Risk of progress to liver cancer. Vaccine is available.
Hepatitis C virus (HCV)	Spread through blood exchange (usually transfusions before 1992 when screening began) or shared needles. May become chronic and lead to cirrhosis, liver failure, liver cancer. Antiviral drugs may limit infection.
Hepatitis D virus (HDV)	Spread by blood exchange and occurs as coinfection with hepatitis B. Responsible for half of rapidly fatal liver failure cases and also a high rate of chronic disease that progresses to death.
Hepatitis E virus (HEV)	Transmitted by fecal contamination and occurs in epidemics in Middle East and Asia. Resembles hepatitis A. Can be fatal in pregnant women.
Herpes simplex virus type 1	Cold sores or fever blisters that appear around the mouth and nose of people with colds or other illnesses accompanied by fever.
Herpes simplex virus type 2	Genital herpes. Acute inflammatory disease of the genitalia, often recurring. A very common sexually transmitted infection.
Human immunodeficiency virus (HIV)	Acquired immunodeficiency syndrome (AIDS). Fatal disease that infects T cells of the immune system. Diagnosed by antibody tests, decline in specific (CD4) cells, and presenting disease, including *Candida albicans* infection, *Pneumocystis jirovici* pneumonia (PCP), Kaposi sarcoma, persistent swelling of lymph nodes (lymphadenopathy), chronic diarrhea, and wasting. Spread by contact with contaminated body fluids and by transplacental route.
Human papillomavirus (HPV)	Genital warts (condylomata acuminata). Sexually transmitted warts of the genital and perianal area in men and women. Associated with cervical dysplasia and cancer.
Influenza virus	An epidemic viral infection, marked by chills, fever, muscular pains, and prostration. The most serious complication is bronchopneumonia caused by *Haemophilus influenzae* (a bacillus) or streptococci.
Mumps virus	Epidemic parotitis. Acute inflammation with swelling of the parotid salivary glands. Mumps can have many complications, such as orchitis (inflammation of the testes) in young men and meningitis in young children.
Pneumonia viruses	Lung infections caused by a number of different viruses, such as the influenza and parainfluenza viruses, adenoviruses, and varicella viruses.
Poliovirus	Poliomyelitis (polio). Acute viral infection that may attack the anterior horns of the spinal cord, resulting in paralysis of certain voluntary muscles. Most countries have eliminated polio through vaccination programs.
Rhabdovirus	Rabies. An acute, fatal disease transmitted to humans through the saliva of an infected animal. Rabies is characterized by violent muscular spasms induced by the slightest sensations. Because the swallowing of water causes spasms of the throat, the disease is also call *hydrophobia* ("fear of water"). The final stage of paralysis ends in death. Rabies vaccines are available for humans and animals.
Rotavirus	Attacks lining of small intestine causing severe diarrhea in children.

(*Continued*)

Appendix 5•2 Viral Diseases (continued)

ORGANISM	DISEASE AND DESCRIPTION
Rubella virus	Rubella or German measles. A less severe form of measles, but especially dangerous during the first 3 months of pregnancy because the disease organism can cause heart defects, deafness, mental deficiency, and other permanent damage in the fetus.
Rubeola virus	Measles. An acute respiratory inflammation followed by fever and a generalized skin rash. Patients are prone to the development of dangerous complications, such as bronchopneumonia and other secondary infections caused by staphylococci and streptococci.
SARS virus	Highly infectious respiratory disease called severe acute respiratory syndrome (SARS). Emerged in China early in 2003 and spread to other countries before it was isolated and identified as a viral infection. Believed to have spread from small mammals to humans.
Varicella zoster	Chickenpox (varicella). A usually mild infection, almost completely confined to children, characterized by blisterlike skin eruptions. Vaccine now available. Shingles (herpes zoster). A very painful eruption of skin blisters that follows the course of certain peripheral nerves. These blisters eventually dry up and form scabs that resemble shingles.

Appendix 5•3 Prion Diseases

(*Note:* Prions are infectious agents that contain protein but no nucleic acid. They cause slow, spongy degeneration of brain tissue, known as spongiform encephalitis, in humans and animals.)

AGENT	DISEASE
Chronic wasting disease agent	Chronic wasting disease in deer and elk.
Creuzfeldt-Jakob agent	Cruetzfeldt-Jacob disease (CJD), a spongiform encephalopathy in humans.
Kuru agent	Kuru spongiform encephalopathy in humans.
Mad cow agent	Mad cow spongiform encephalopathy, or bovine spongiform encephalopathy (BSE) in cows and humans.
Scrapie agent	Scrapie spongiform encephalopathy in sheep.

Appendix 5•4 Fungal Diseases

DISEASE/ORGANISM	DESCRIPTION
Actinomycosis	"Lumpy jaw" in cattle and humans. The organisms cause the formation of large tissue masses, which are often accompanied by abscesses. The lungs and liver may be involved.
Blastomycosis (*Blastomyces dermatitidis*)	A general term for any infection caused by a yeastlike organism. There may be skin tumors and lesions in the lungs, bones, liver, spleen, and kidneys.
Candidiasis (*Candida albicans*)	An infection that can involve the skin and mucous membranes. May cause diaper rash, infection of the nail beds, and infection of the mucous membranes of the mouth (thrush), throat, and vagina.
Coccidioidomycosis (*Coccidioides immitis*)	A systemic fungal disease also called *San Joaquin Valley fever*. Because it often attacks the lungs, it may be mistaken for tuberculosis.
Histoplasmosis (*Histoplasma capsulatum*)	A variety of disorders, ranging from mild respiratory symptoms or enlargement of liver, spleen, and lymph nodes to cavities in the lungs with symptoms similar to those of tuberculosis.
Pneumocystis jiroveci (formerly *carinii*)	Pneumonia (PCP). Opportunistic infection in people with a depressed immune system. Invades lungs and causes a foamy exudate to collect in alveoli.
Ringworm Tinea capitis Tinea corporis Tinea pedis	Common fungal infections of the skin, many of which cause blisters and scaling with discoloration of the affected areas. All are caused by similar organisms from a group of fungi called *dermatophytes*. They are easily transmitted by person to person contact or by contaminated articles.

Appendix 5•5 Protozoal Diseases

ORGANISM	DISEASE AND DESCRIPTION
Amebae	
Entamoeba histolytica	Amebic dysentery. Severe ulceration of the wall of the large intestine caused by amebae. Acute diarrhea may be an important symptom. This organism also may cause liver abscesses.
Ciliates	
Balantidium coli	Gastrointestinal disturbances and ulcers of the colon.
Flagellates	
Giardia lamblia	Gastrointestinal disturbances.
Leishmania donovani (and others)	Kala-azar. In this disease, there is enlargement of the liver and spleen as well as skin lesions.
Trichomonas vaginalis	Inflammation and discharge from the vagina. In males, it involves the urethra and causes painful urination.
Trypanosoma	African sleeping sickness. Disease begins with a high fever, followed by invasion of the brain and spinal cord by the organisms. Usually, the disease ends with continued drowsiness, coma, and death.
Sporozoa (apicomplexans)	
Cryptosporidium	Cramps and diarrhea that can be long term and severe in people with a weakened immune system, such as those with AIDS. Spread in water and by personal contact in close quarters.
Plasmodium; varieties include *vivax, falciparum, malariae*	Malaria. Characterized by recurrent attacks of chills followed by high fever. Severe attacks of malaria can be fatal because of kidney failure, cerebral disorders, and other complications.
Toxoplasma gondii	Toxoplasmosis. Common infectious disease transmitted by cats and raw meat. Mild forms cause fever and enlargement of lymph nodes. May cause fatal encephalitis in immunosuppressed patients. Infection of a pregnant woman is a cause of fetal stillbirth or congenital damage.

Appendix 6 Answers to Chapter Checkpoint and Zooming In Questions

CHAPTER 1

Answers to Checkpoint Questions

1-1 Study of body structure is anatomy; study of body function is physiology.
1-2 The breakdown phase of metabolism is catabolism; the building phase of metabolism is anabolism.
1-3 Negative feedback systems are primarily used to maintain homeostasis.
1-4 The three planes in which the body can be cut are sagittal, frontal (coronal), and transverse (horizontal). The midsagittal plane divides the body into two equal halves.
1-5 The posterior cavity is the dorsal cavity; the anterior cavity is the ventral cavity.
1-6 The three central regions of the abdomen are the epigastric, umbilical, and hypogastric regions; the three left and right lateral regions of the abdomen are the hypochondriac, lumbar, and iliac (inguinal) regions.
1-7 The basic unit of length in the metric system is the meter; of weight, the gram; of volume, the liter.

Answers to Zooming In Questions

1-7 The small figure is standing in the anatomical position.
1-8 The transverse (horizontal) plane divides the body into superior and inferior parts. The frontal (coronal) plane divides the body into anterior and posterior parts.
1-11 The ventral cavity contains the diaphragm.

CHAPTER 2

Answers to Checkpoint Questions

2-1 Atoms are subunits of elements.
2-2 Three types of particles found in atoms are protons, neutrons, and electrons.
2-3 Molecules are units composed of two or more atoms. They are the subunits of compounds.
2-4 Water is the most abundant compound in the body.
2-5 In a solution, the components dissolve and remain evenly distributed (the mixture is homogeneous); in a suspension, the particles settle out unless the mixture is shaken (the mixture is heterogeneous).
2-6 When an electrolyte goes into solution, it separates into charged particles called ions (cations and anions).
2-7 A covalent bond is formed by the sharing of electrons.
2-8 A value of 7.0 is neutral on the pH scale. An acid measures lower than 7.0; a base measures higher than 7.0.
2-9 A buffer is a substance that maintains a steady pH of a solution.
2-10 Isotopes that break down to give off radiation are termed radioactive.
2-11 Organic compounds are found in living things.
2-12 The element carbon is the basis of organic chemistry.
2-13 The three main categories of organic compounds are carbohydrates, lipids, and proteins.
2-14 A catalyst is a compound that speeds up the rate of a chemical reaction.

Answers to Zooming In Questions

2-1 The number of protons is equal to the number of electrons. There are eight protons and eight electrons.
2-2 Two hydrogen atoms bond with an oxygen atom to form water.
2-4 Two electrons are needed to complete the energy level of each hydrogen atom.
2-5 The amount of hydroxide ion (OH^-) in a solution decreases when the amount of hydrogen ion (H^+) increases.
2-7 Monosaccharides are the building blocks of disaccharides and polysaccharides.
2-8 There are three carbon atoms in glycerol.
2-9 The amino group of an amino acid contains nitrogen.
2-10 The shape of the enzyme after the reaction is the same as it was before the reaction.

CHAPTER 3

Answers to Checkpoint Questions

3-1 The cell shows organization, metabolism, responsiveness, homeostasis, growth, and reproduction.
3-2 Three types of microscopes are the compound light microscope, transmission electron microscope (TEM), and scanning electron microscope (SEM).
3-3 The main substance of the plasma membrane is a bilayer of phospholipids. Three types of materials found within the membrane are cholesterol, proteins, and carbohydrates (glycoproteins and glycolipids).
3-4 The cell organelles are specialized structures that perform different tasks.
3-5 The nucleus is called the control center of the cell because it contains the chromosomes, hereditary units that control all cellular activities.
3-6 The two types of organelles used for movement are the cilia, which are small and hairlike, and the flagellum, which is long and whiplike.
3-7 Nucleotides are the building blocks of nucleic acids.
3-8 DNA codes for proteins in the cell.
3-9 The three types of RNA are messenger RNA (mRNA), ribosomal RNA (rRNA) and transfer RNA (tRNA).
3-10 Before mitosis can occur, the DNA must double (duplicate). The doubling occurs during interphase.
3-11 The four stages of mitosis are prophase, metaphase, anaphase, and telophase.
3-12 Diffusion, osmosis, filtration, and facilitated diffusion do not require cellular energy; active transport, endocytosis (phagocytosis and pinocytosis), and exocytosis require cellular energy.

17-4 Inborn immunity is inherited in a person's genetic material; acquired immunity develops during an individual's lifetime.
17-5 An antigen is any foreign substance, usually a protein, that induces an immune response.
17-6 Four types of T cells are cytotoxic, helper, regulatory, and memory.
17-7 An antibody is a substance produced in response to an antigen.
17-8 Plasma cells, derived from B cells, produce antibodies.
17-9 Complement is a group of proteins in the blood that sometimes is required for the destruction of foreign cells.
17-10 The active form of naturally acquired immunity comes from contact with a disease organism; the passive form comes from the passage of antibodies from a mother to her fetus through the placenta or breast milk.
17-11 Bacterial diseases for which there are vaccines include smallpox, whooping cough (pertussis), diphtheria, tetanus, Haemophilus influenzae type b (Hib), and pneumococcus.
17-12 Viral diseases for which there are vaccines include poliomyelitis, measles (rubeola), mumps, rubella (German measles), hepatitis A and B, chicken pox (varicella), influenza, and rabies.
17-13 An immune serum is an antiserum prepared in an animal; immune sera can be used in emergencies to provide passive immunization.
17-14 Disorders of the immune system include allergy, autoimmunity, and immune deficiency diseases.
17-15 The tendency of every organism to destroy foreign substances is the greatest obstacle to transplantation of tissues from one individual to another.

Answers to Zooming In Questions

17-2 Digestive enzymes are contained in the lysosome that joins the phagocytic vesicle.
17-3 Plasma cells and memory cells develop from activated B cells.

CHAPTER 18

Answers to Checkpoint Questions

18-1 The three phases of respiration are pulmonary ventilation, external exchange of gases, and internal exchange of gases.
18-2 As air passes over the nasal mucosa, it is filtered, warmed, and moistened.
18-3 The scientific name for the throat is pharynx, for the voice box is larynx, and for the windpipe is trachea.
18-4 The three regions of the pharynx are the nasopharynx, oropharynx, and laryngeal pharynx.
18-5 The cells that line the respiratory passageways have cilia to filter impurities and to move fluids.
18-6 Gas exchange in the lungs occurs in the alveoli.
18-7 The pleura is the membrane that encloses the lung.
18-8 The two phases of breathing are inhalation, which is active, and exhalation, which is passive.
18-9 Diffusion is the movement of molecules from an area in which they are in higher concentration to an area where they are in lower concentration.
18-10 Hemoglobin is the substance in red blood cells that carries almost all of the oxygen in the blood.
18-11 The main form in which carbon dioxide is carried in the blood is as bicarbonate ion.
18-12 The medulla of the brain stem sets the basic pattern of respiration.
18-13 The phrenic nerve is the motor nerve that controls the diaphragm.
18-14 Carbon dioxide is the main chemical controller of respiration.
18-15 COPD is chronic obstructive pulmonary disease. Chronic bronchitis and emphysema are commonly involved in COPD.

Answers to Zooming In Questions

18-2 The heart is located in the medial depression of the left lung.
18-4 The epiglottis is named for its position above the glottis.
18-7 The external and internal intercostals are the muscles between the ribs.
18-8 Gas pressure decreases as the volume of its container increases.
18-9 Residual volume can not be measured with a spirometer.
18-14 The esophagus is posterior to the trachea.

CHAPTER 19

Answers to Checkpoint Questions

19-1 Food must be broken down by digestion into particles small enough to pass through the plasma membrane.
19-2 The digestive tract has a wall composed of a mucous membrane (mucosa), a submucosa, smooth muscle, and a serous membrane (serosa).
19-3 The peritoneum is the large serous membrane that lines the abdominopelvic cavity and covers the organs it contains.
19-4 There are 20 baby teeth, which are also called deciduous teeth.
19-5 Proteins are digested in the stomach.
19-6 The three divisions of the small intestine are the duodenum, jejunum, and ileum.
19-7 Most digestion takes place in the small intestine under the effects of digestive juices from the small intestine and the accessory organs. Most absorption of digested food and water also occurs in the small intestine.
19-8 The divisions of the large intestine are the cecum, ascending colon, transverse colon, descending colon, sigmoid colon, and rectum.
19-9 The large intestine reabsorbs some water and stores, forms, and eliminates the stool. It also houses bacteria that provide some vitamins.

19-10 The salivary glands are the parotid, submandibular (submaxillary), and sublingual.
19-11 The gallbladder stores bile.
19-12 Bile emulsifies fats.
19-13 The pancreas produces the most complete digestive secretions.
19-14 Absorption is the movement of digested nutrients into the circulation.
19-15 The two types of control over the digestive process are nervous control and hormonal control.
19-16 Hunger is the desire for food that can be satisfied by the ingestion of a filling meal. Appetite is a desire for food that is unrelated to a need for food.
19-17 Caries, gingivitis, and periodontitis are common diseases of the mouth and teeth.
19-18 Crohn disease and ulcerative colitis are inflammatory bowel diseases.
19-19 Hepatitis is inflammation of the liver.

Answers to Zooming In Questions

19-1 Smooth muscle (circular and longitudinal) is between the submucosa and the serous membrane in the digestive tract wall.
19-3 The mesentery is the part of the peritoneum around the small intestine.
19-4 The salivary glands are the accessory organs that secrete into the mouth.
19-7 The oblique muscle layer is an additional muscle layer in the stomach as compared to the rest of the digestive tract.
19-8 The ileum of the small intestine joins the cecum.
19-10 The accessory organs shown secrete into the duodenum.

CHAPTER 20

Answers to Checkpoint Questions

20-1 The two phases of metabolism are catabolism, the breakdown phase of metabolism, and anabolism, the building phase of metabolism.
20-2 Cellular respiration is the series of reactions that releases energy from nutrients in the cell.
20-3 Glucose is the main energy source for the cells.
20-4 An essential amino acid or fatty acid cannot be made metabolically and must be taken in as part of the diet.
20-5 Minerals are chemical elements, and vitamins are complex organic substances.
20-6 The normal range of blood glucose is 85 to 125 mg/dL
20-7 Typical recommendations are 55% to 60% carbohydrate; 30% or less fat; 15% to 20% protein.
20-8 Some factors that affect heat production are exercise, hormone production, food intake, and age.
20-9 The hypothalamus of the brain is responsible for regulating body temperature.
20-10 Normal body temperature is 36.2°C to 37.68C (97°F to 100°F).
20-11 Heat cramps, heat exhaustion, and heat stroke are brought on by excessive heat.
20-12 Hypothermia is excessively low body temperature.

Answers to Zooming In Questions

20-1 Pyruvic acid produces lactic acid under anaerobic conditions; it produces CO_2 and H_20 under aerobic conditions.
20-4 The BMI is 24 (77 ÷ 3.2 = 24).

CHAPTER 21

Answers to Checkpoint Questions

21-1 Body fluids are grouped into intracelluar fluid and extracellular fluid.
21-2 Water is lost from the body through the kidneys, the skin, the lungs, and the intestinal tract.
21-3 The control center for the sense of thirst is located in the hypothalamus of the brain.
21-4 Sodium is the main cation in extracellular fluid. Potassium is the main cation in intracellular fluid.
21-5 Chloride is the main anion in extracellular fluid.
21-6 Some electrolytes are lost through the feces and sweat. The kidneys have the main job of balancing electrolytes. Several hormones, such as aldosterone, parathyroid hormone, and calcitonin, are also involved.
21-7 The acid–base balance of body fluids is maintained by buffer systems, respiration, and kidney function.
21-8 Abnormally low pH of body fluids results in acidosis; abnormally high pH of body fluids results in alkalosis.
21-9 Edema is the accumulation of excessive fluid in the intercellular spaces.

Answers to Zooming In Questions

21-1 Water is lost through the skin, lungs, kidneys, and intestine.

CHAPTER 22

Answers to Checkpoint Questions

22-1 Systems other than the urinary system that eliminate waste include the digestive, respiratory, and integumentary systems.
22-2 The urinary system consists of two kidneys, two ureters, the bladder, and the urethra.
22-3 The retroperitoneal space is posterior to the peritoneum.

22-4 The renal artery supplies blood to the kidney, and the renal vein drains blood from the kidney.
22-5 The outer region of the kidney is the renal cortex; the inner region is the renal medulla.
22-6 The nephron is the functional unit of the kidney.
22-7 The glomerulus is the coil of capillaries in the glomerular (Bowman) capsule.
22-8 The JG apparatus produces renin when blood pressure falls too low for the kidneys to function effectively.
22-9 Glomerular filtration is the movement of materials under pressure from the blood into the glomerular capsule of the nephron.
22-10 The four processes involved in the formation of urine are glomerular filtration, tubular reabsorption, tubular secretion, and the countercurrent mechanism for concentrating the urine.
22-11 The ureter carries urine from the kidney to the bladder.
22-12 The urethra carries urine from the bladder to the outside.
22-13 Acute kidney disorders arise suddenly, usually as a result of infection. Chronic conditions arise slowly and are often progressive, with gradual loss of kidney functions.
22-14 The scientific name for stones is calculi.
22-15 Inflammation of the bladder is cystitis.

Answers to Zooming In Questions

22-1 The renal artery supplies blood to the kidney. The renal vein drains blood from the kidney.
22-2 The aorta supplies blood to the renal artery. The inferior vena cava receives blood from the renal vein.
22-3 The outer region of the kidney is the renal cortex. The inner region of the kidney is the renal medulla.
22-4 The proximal convoluted tubule is closer to the glomerular capsule. The distal convoluted tubule is farther away from the glomerular capsule.
22-6 The juxtaglomerular apparatus is made up of cells from the afferent arteriole and the distal convoluted tubule.
22-7 The afferent arteriole has a wider diameter than the efferent arteriole.
22-10 The urethra passes through the prostate gland in the male.

CHAPTER 23

Answers to Checkpoint Questions

23-1 Meiosis is the process of cell division that halves the chromosome number in a cell to produce a gamete.
23-2 The testis is the male gonad. Testosterone is the main male sex hormone.
23-3 The spermatozoon, or sperm cell, is the male sex cell (gamete).
23-4 The main subdivisions of the sperm cell are the head, midpiece, and tail (flagellum).
23-5 Sperm cells leave the seminiferous tubules within the testis and then travel through the epididymis, ductus (vas) deferens, ejaculatory duct, and urethra.
23-6 Glands that contribute secretions to the semen, aside from the testes, are the seminal vesicles, prostate, and bulbourethral glands.
23-7 Follicle-stimulating hormone (FSH) and luteinizing hormone (LH), also called ICSH, are the pituitary hormones that regulate male and female reproduction.
23-8 Infectious diseases of the reproductive tract include chlamydial and gonococcal infections, genital herpes, syphilis, E. coli infections, mumps.
23-9 The ovary is the female gonad.
23-10 The ovum (egg cell) is the female gamete.
23-11 The ovarian (graafian) follicle surrounds the egg as it ripens.
23-12 Ovulation is the process of releasing an egg cell from the ovary.
23-13 The follicle becomes the corpus luteum after ovulation
23-14 The fetus develops in the uterus.
23-15 The two hormones produced in the ovaries are estrogen and progesterone.
23-16 Menopause is the period during which menstruation ceases.
23-17 Contraception is the use of artificial methods to prevent fertilization of the ovum or implantation of the fertilized ovum.

Answers to Zooming In Questions

23-1 The four glands that empty secretions into the urethra are the testes, seminal vesicles, prostate, and bulbourethral glands.
23-2 The ductus (vas) deferens receives secretions from the epididymis.
23-4 Mitochondria are the organelles that provide energy for sperm cell motility.
23-5 The corpus spongiosum of the penis contains the urethra.
23-8 The fundus of the uterus is the deepest part.
23-10 The endometrium is most highly developed in the second part of the menstrual cycle.
23-11 The opening of the urethra is anterior to the opening of the vagina.
23-13 LH shows the greatest increase at the time of ovulation.

CHAPTER 24

Answers to Checkpoint Questions

24-1 A zygote is formed by the union of an ovum and a spermatozoon.
24-2 The placenta nourishes the developing fetus.
24-3 The umbilical cord carries blood between the fetus and the placenta.
24-4 The heartbeat first appears during the fourth week of embryonic development.
24-5 The amniotic sac is the fluid-filled sac that holds the fetus.
24-6 The approximate length of pregnancy in days is 266.
24-7 Parturition is the process of labor and delivery.

24-8 A cesarean section is an incision made in the abdominal wall and the wall of the uterus for delivery of a fetus.
24-9 The term viable with reference to a fetus means able to live outside the uterus.
24-10 Lactation is the secretion of milk from the mammary glands.
24-11 An ectopic pregnancy is one that develops in a location outside the uterine cavity.
24-12 Puerperal infection is an infection that is related to childbirth.

Answers to Zooming In Questions

24-1 The ovum is fertilized in the oviduct (fallopian, uterine) tube.
24-2 The purple color signifies a mixture of oxygenated and unoxygenated blood.
24-5 The umbilical cord connects the fetus to the placenta.
24-7 The pectoralis major underlies the breast.

CHAPTER 25

Answers to Checkpoint Questions

25-1 A gene is an independent unit of heredity. Each is a segment of DNA contained in a chromosome.
25-2 A dominant gene is always expressed, regardless of the gene on the matching chromosome. A recessive gene is only expressed if the gene on the matching chromosome is also recessive.
25-3 Meiosis is the process of cell division that forms the gametes.
25-4 The sex chromosome combination that determines a female is XX; a male is XY.
25-5 A trait carried on a sex chromosome is described as sex-linked.
25-6 A mutation is a change in the genetic material (a gene or chromosome) of a cell.
25-7 A congenital disease is present at birth. A hereditary disease is genetically transmitted or transmissible. A disorder may occur during development and be present at birth but not be inherited through the genes.
25-8 Phenylketonuria is caused by a hereditary lack of an enzyme needed for the metabolism of phenylalanine.
25-9 A pedigree is a complete, detailed family history. It is used to determine the inheritance pattern of a genetic disease within a family.
25-10 A karyotype is a picture of the chromosomes cut out and arranged in groups according to size and form.

Answers to Zooming In Questions

25-1 25% of children will show the recessive phenotype blond hair. 50% of children will be heterozygous.
25-5 The possible genotypes of the two normal children in the F3 generation are CC or Cc.
25-7 There are 44 autosomes shown in B.